D1387285

PDxMD
Rheumatology

PD~x~MD

An Imprint of Elsevier Science

Philadelphia ■ St Louis ■ London ■ Sydney ■ New York ■ Toronto

PDxMD Medical Conditions Series is dedicated to health and healing professionals everywhere. We are privileged to be in your service and hope our efforts help you in your quest for better quality-of-life and optimized outcomes for all your patients.

PDxMD
An imprint of Elsevier Science

Publisher: Steven Merahn, MD
Project Managers: Caroline Barnett, Lucy Hamilton, Zak Knowles
Programmer: Narinder Chandi
Production: Aoibhe O'Shea – GMS UK, Alan Palfreyman – PTU
Designer: Jayne Jones
Layout: The Designers Collective Limited

Printed in China by RDC Group

PDxMD
Elsevier Science
The Curtis Center
625 Walnut Street,
Philadelphia, PA 19106

The
Publisher's
policy is to use
**paper manufactured
from sustainable forests**

ISBN 1-932141-09-X

Contents

Contents

Contents

Introduction

What is PDxMD?

PDxMD is a new, evidence-based primary care clinical information system designed to support your judgment with practical clinical information. The content is continuously updated by expert contributors with the latest on evaluation, diagnosis, management, outcomes and prevention – all designed for use at the point and time of care.

First and foremost, PDxMD is an electronic resource. This book gives you access to just a fraction of the content available on-line. At www.pdxmd.com, you will find:

- Over 1400 differential diagnoses for you to search for information according to your patient's chief complaint via a unique signs and symptoms matrix
- Information on more than 450 medical conditions and more than 750 drugs and other therapies, organised in condition-specific 'MediFiles'
- Patient information sheets on 300 topics for you to customize and hand to your patient during consultation

About This Book

The PDxMD Medical Conditions Series is a print version of the comprehensive approach offered on line. Concise information on medical conditions is systematically organized in a consistent MediFile format, our electronic equivalent of chapters.

Each MediFile covers summary information and background on each condition, and comprehensive information on diagnosis, treatment, outcomes, and prevention, and other resources, especially written and designed for use in practice. Each MediFile is organized identically to allow you to find information consistently and reliably for every condition. See the MediFile 'Road Map' inside the back cover for more information.

Ranging from epidemiology to risk assessment and reduction, from diagnostic evaluation and testing to therapeutic options, prognosis and outcomes - you'll find the information that you need is easier to locate with this methodical approach.

How to Use This Book

Find the MediFile for any specific medical condition in the Contents list. Familiarize yourself with the MediFile Road Map (see inside back cover) to rapidly find the precise information you require.

Information on drugs and tests are found within the MediFiles for the specific conditions. For an overview, see the 'Summary of options' sections under DIAGNOSIS and under TREATMENT in the relevant MediFile. Details of tests, drugs and other therapies then follow.

PDxMD believes that physician clinical judgment is central to appropriate diagnostic and therapeutic decision-making. The information is designed to support professional judgment and, accounting for individual patient differences, does not provide direct answers or force specific practices or policies.

Introduction

How is PDxMD created?

PDxMD is created through Collaborative Authoring. This process allows medical information to be reviewed and synthesized from multiple sources – including but not limited to peer-reviewed articles, evidence databases, guidelines and position papers – and by multiple individuals. The information is organized around and integrated into a template that matches the needs of primary care physicians in practice.

Professional medical writers begin the process of reviewing and synthesizing information for PDxMD, working from core evidence databases and other expert resources and with the guidance of Editorial Advisory Board (EAB) members. This first draft is sent to a physician 'clinical reviewer', who works with the writer to make sure the information is accurate and properly organized. A second review by the physician clinical reviewer ensures that appropriate changes are in place.

After these first two levels of clinical review, the files are reviewed and edited by the relevant specialist member of the Editorial Advisory Board. A primary care member of the EAB, who has final sign-off authority, then conducts the final review and edit. Editorial checks are conducted between all review stages and, after primary care sign-off, a pharmacist double checks the drug recommendations prior to a final editorial review.

There are a minimum of three and as many as five physicians involved in each MediFile, and additional clinical reviewers and/or EAB members are added when appropriate (e.g., alternative/complementary medicine experts, or conditions requiring multi-disciplinary approaches). The contributor team for each MediFile is listed in the Resources section.

A complete list of Editorial Faculty and staff of PDxMD is provided below. All Editorial Faculty, and specifically the Editorial Advisory Board members, participate in PDxMD as individuals and not as representatives of, or on behalf of, their affiliated institutions or associations and any indication of their affiliation with a specific institution or association should not be taken as an endorsement of PDxMD or any participation of their institution or association with PDxMD.

Continuous Product Improvement

PDxMD is committed to continuous quality improvement and welcomes any comments, suggestions and feedback from the professional community. Please send any ideas or considerations regarding this volume or any other volume in the PDxMD series via e-mail to feedback.pdxmd@elsevier.com or to PDxMD, Elsevier Science, The Curtis Center, 625 Walnut Street, Philadelphia, PA 19106.

Introduction

Evidence-Based Medicine Policies

PDxMD is committed to providing available and up-to-date evidence for the diagnostic and therapeutic recommendations provided in our knowledge base. All MediFiles begin with a core set of evidence-based references from recognized sources. These are supplemented with extensive searches of the literature and reviews of reference books, peer-reviewed journals, association guidelines and position papers, among others.

Criteria for Evidence-Based Medicine
Evidence Sources

PDxMD has taken the best evidence currently available from the following:

Published Critically Evaluated Evidence

- Cochrane Systematic Reviews – respected throughout the world as one of the most rigorous searches of medical journals with highly structured systematic reviews and use of meta-analysis to produce reliable evidence
- Clinical Evidence – produced jointly by the British Medical Journal Publishing Group and the American College of Physicians–American Society of Internal Medicine. Clinical Evidence provides a concise account of the current state of knowledge on the treatment and prevention of many clinical conditions based on the search and appraisal of the available literature
- The National Guideline Clearinghouse – a comprehensive database of evidence-based clinical practice guidelines and related documents produced by the Agency for Healthcare Research and Quality in partnership with the American Medical Association and the American Association of Health Plans

Evidence Published in Peer-Reviewed Journals

- Association Guidelines and Position Papers

Where evidence exists that has not yet been critically reviewed by one of the sources listed above, for example randomized controlled trials and clinical cohort studies, the evidence is summarized briefly, categorized, and fully referenced.

Clinical Experience

While recognizing the importance of these evidence-based resources, PDxMD also highlights the importance of experience in clinical practice. Therefore, our Editorial Advisory Board also provide advice from their own clinical experience, within Clinical Pearl sections of the MediFiles and elsewhere. Contributing expert physicians are identified in the Resources section of every MediFile.

Introduction

Evaluation of Evidence

PDxMD evaluates all cited evidence according to the AAFP Recommended Basic Model for Evaluating and Categorizing the Clinical Content of CME, based on the model used by the University of Michigan:

Level M   Evidence from either:
Meta-analysis or
Multiple randomized controlled trials

Level P   Evidence from either:
A well-designed prospective clinical trial or
Several prospective clinical cohort studies with consistent findings (without randomization)

Level S   Evidence from studies other than clinical trials, such as:
Epidemiological studies
Physiological studies

References

The information provided by PDxMD is concise and action-oriented. As a result, our editorial policy is to cite only essential reference sources. References and evidence summaries are provided in four areas:

1.   In the Diagnostic Decision section under Diagnosis
2.   In the Guidelines and Evidence sections under Treatment
3.   In the Outcomes section under Evidence
4.   In the Key Reference Section under Resources

Where on-line references to the Cochrane Abstracts, BMJ Clinical Evidence and National Guideline Clearinghouse are cited in the text, the internet addresses of the home pages are given. The internet addresses of individual reports are not given.

When references are to association guidelines and position papers, the internet address of the association home page is generally provided. When possible, the internet address of the specific report is provided.

Editorial Faculty and Staff

Executive Committee

Fred F Ferri, MD, FACP
Editorial Board & Medical Chair, Executive
Committee Family Medicine
Clinical Professor
Brown University of Medicine, Chief
Division of Internal Medicine
Fatima Hospital, St Joseph's Health Services
Providence, RI

George T Danakas, MD, FACOG
Editorial Board & Executive Committee
Obstetrics, Gynecology
Clinical Assistant Professor
SUNY at Buffalo
Williamsville, NY

David G Fairchild, MD, MPH
Editorial Board & Executive Committee
Primary Care, Signs & Symptoms
Brigham and Women's Hospital
Boston, MA

Russell C Jones, MD, MPH
Editorial Board & Executive Committee
Family Medicine
Dartmouth Medical School
New London, NH

Kathleen M O'Hanlon, MD
Editorial Board & Executive Committee
Primary Care
Professor, Marshall University School of
Medicine
Department of Family & Community Health
Huntington, WV

John L Pfenninger, MD, FAAFP
Editorial Board & Executive Committee
Primary Care, Procedures
President and Director
The National Procedures Institute
Director, The Medical Procedures Center, PC
Clinical Professor of Family Medicine
Michigan State University
Midland, MI

Joseph E Scherger, MD, MPH
Editorial Board & Executive Committee
Primary Care, Site Search
Dean, College of Medicine
Florida State University
Tallahassee, FL

Myron Yanoff, MD
Editorial Board & Executive Committee
Ophthalmology, Otolaryngology
Professor & Chair, Department of Ophthalmology
MCP Hahnemann University
Philadelphia, PA

Editorial Board

Philip J Aliotta, MD, MHA, FACS
Editorial Board, Urology
Attending Urologist and Clinical Research
Director Center for Urologic Research of
Western New York
Main Urology Associates, PC
Williamsville, NY

Gordon H Baustian, MD
Editorial Board, Family Medicine
Director of Medical Education and Residency
Cedar Rapids Medical Education Foundation
Cedar Rapids, IA

Editorial Faculty and Staff

Editorial Faculty and Staff

Editorial Faculty and Staff

Editorial Faculty and Staff

Geraldine N Urse, DO
Family Medicine
Professor of Family Medicine
Ohio University College of Osteopathic Medicine
OH

Writers

Solomon Almond, MB ChB, MRCP, DTM&H
Lory E Baraz, MD
Elly C Blake
Patricia L Carroll, RN, CEN, RRT
Rosalyn S Carson-DeWitt, MD
Simon R Cartwright, MBBS, DRCOG, MRCGP
Tony W B Crockett, BMBS, DRCOG, MRCGP
Laini Dubach
Neil D Fisher, BSc PhD
Tony C Fisher, MD
Ewan M Gerard, MB ChB, MSc, MRCGP

Sian W Gerard, BSc, BM
Muhayman N Jamil, MB ChB, FRCS
David P Kernick, MD, MB ChB, BSc
Fiona McCrimmon, MBBS MRCGP
Tim J F Mitchell, DRCOG, MRCGP
Andy R Oppenheimer
Mary E Selby, MB ChB, DRCOG, MRCGP
Janet Stephenson, PhD, BSc
Alison Whitehouse
Robert Whittle, MB BS (NSW)
Jeffrey R Wohlgethan, MD

Staff

Management Team
Fiona Foley, Steven Merahn, MD, Daniel Pollock, Zak Knowles, Howard Croft, Tanya Thomas, Lucy Hamilton, Julie Volck, Bill Bruggemeyer, Andrea Ford

Editorial Team
Anne Dyson, Sadaf Hashmi, Debbie Goring, Louise Morrison, Ellen Haigh, Robert Whittle, Claire Champion, Caroline Barnett, Laurie Smith, Li Wan, Paul Mayhew, Carmen Jones, Fi Ward

Technical Team
Martin Miller, Narinder Chandi, Roy Patterson, Aaron McGrath, John Wylie, Sarah Craze, Cameron Sangster

We would also like to acknowledge the extraordinary contributions of the following individuals to the conceptualization and realization of PDxMD over the initial years of its growth and development:

Tim Hailstone, Jonathan Black, Alison Whitehouse, Jayne Harris, Angela Baggi, Sharon Bambaji, Sam Bedser, Layla van den Bergh, Stuart Boffey, Siobhan Egan, Helen Elder, Mark Mitchenall, Chris Moodie, Tony Pollard, Simon Seljeflot, Liz Southey, Tim Stentiford, Matthew Whyte

ANKYLOSING SPONDYLITIS

SUMMARY INFORMATION

DESCRIPTION

- Low back pain, with prominent morning stiffness, sometimes nocturnal
- Often insidious in onset
- Loss of chest expansion
- Associated with peripheral arthritis, enthesitis, and extra-articular manifestations, such as iritis
- Most frequently found in young men under 40 years of age

URGENT ACTION

- Refer to rheumatologist
- Arrange for the patient to see a physical therapist
- Prescribe a nonsteroidal anti-inflammatory drug (NSAID)

KEY! DON'T MISS!

- The onset of low back pain is sometimes incorrectly attributed to athletic injuries in younger patients
- Difficulty in breathing may accompany spinal symptoms
- Sudden onset of extreme pain and tenderness in the spinal area of these patients indicates potential bony fracture. The lower neck (cervical spine) is the most common area for such fractures

ICD9 CODE
720.0 Chronic ankylosing spondylitis

SYNONYMS
- AS
- Marie-Strümpell disease

CARDINAL FEATURES
- Back pain, associated with stiffness and restriction after inactivity, often nocturnal
- Loss of chest expansion
- Progressive fixed spinal deformity, which may develop in the neck area (cervical spine) and in the lower back (thoracolumbar spine). In either case, developing rigidity of the ankylosing spondylitis spine is amenable to physical therapy intervention. A fixed 'ankylosis' makes it difficult for the patient to stand and look forward
- Progressive, ascending spinal stiffening and spinal ligament calcification, with characteristic radiological findings
- Chronic and progressive inflammation of the axial skeleton and sacroiliac joints – the earliest abnormalities (pseudo-widening from subchondral erosions, sclerosis or later narrowing) occur in the sacroiliac joints; prominent syndesmophytes and diffuse paraspinal ligamentous calcification develop in a minority of patients over an average period of 10 years
- Hips and shoulders may be involved
- Most patients are male and the disease begins in the second or third decade
- Usually milder, and therefore less frequently diagnosed, in women
- Extraskeletal disorders are present in one-third of patients – they include cardiac (aortic insufficiency, conduction abnormalities), enthesitis, pulmonary (apical fibrosis, restrictive lung disease), and ocular involvement (painful inflammation e.g. iritis/uveitis)
- AS can also affect areas where ribs attach to the upper spine, further limiting lung capacity. Late ankylosing spondylitis can cause inflammation and scarring of the lungs, causing coughing and shortness of breath, especially infections
- Mild or moderate attacks of active spondylitis alternate with periods of almost or totally inactive inflammation
- Strong link with antigen HLA-B27
- AS can begin atypically in peripheral joints in children and women, and rarely, with acute iritis (anterior uveitis)
- Prone to spinal fractures with even minimal trauma

Childhood ankylosing spondylitis:
- Ankylosing spondylitis may develop in children and resembles pauciarticular juvenile rheumatoid arthritis
- Usually in boys over 8 years of age with a family history of AS
- Asymmetric peripheral arthritis of lower extremities

CAUSES
Common causes
Cause is unknown, but enteric infection with coliform organisms is suspected to be important by creating an autoimmune reaction. Chronic tissue inflammation may therefore result from continued activation of the immune system.

Contributory or predisposing factors
- The majority (90%) of patients with ankylosing spondylitis are born with the HLA-B27 gene

- However, some additional factors, perhaps environmental, are necessary for the disease to appear or become expressed, because the majority of people carrying HLA-B27 never suffer from AS

EPIDEMIOLOGY
Incidence and prevalence
PREVALENCE

Ankylosing spondylitis afflicts an estimated 1.29 per 1000 people in the US.

Demographics
AGE

Most commonly begins between 16 and 40 years of age.

GENDER

Ankylosing spondylitis is three times more frequent in men than in women.

RACE

- Increased prevalence of HLA-B27 tissue antigen in Caucasians or HLA-B7 in African-Americans supports a genetic predisposition
- The prevalence of AS varies by ethnic group and is most common in Native Americans

GENETICS

- The majority (90%) of patients with ankylosing spondylitis are born with the HLA-B27 gene
- AS is 10–20 times more common in first-degree relatives of ankylosing spondylitis patients than in the general population
- 50% of their offspring will carry HLA-B27
- The child of an HLA-B27-positive parent has a 33% chance of developing ankylosing spondylitis
- Although environmental factors may contribute, the risk of ankylosing spondylitis in people with HLA-B27 is about 20%
- In some cases, the disease occurs in these predisposed people after exposure to bowel or urinary tract infections

SOCIOECONOMIC STATUS

This may be a factor in poor areas where back pain and resulting deformity may be endured without sufferers seeking help.

DIAGNOSIS

DIFFERENTIAL DIAGNOSIS
Herniated intervertebral disk
A very common and painful acute spinal injury, often misdiagnosed.

FEATURES
- Back pain, often intense, either sharp in lumbar or cervical region or sharp pain or chronic ache radiating down one limb (sciatica) worsened on sitting down and often with acute onset, which the patient may relate to a specific event
- Pain on movement, particularly bending or turning or sitting
- Pain may be relieved by lying down flat
- In severe cases patient is unable to straighten up and has to remain bent forward to accommodate protruding herniated disk material blocking spinal joint
- In ankylosing spondylitis flexed or bent-over posture often eases whereas in protruded intervertebral disk bending can be extremely painful. Stiffness far less prominent in herniated disk
- May be urinary incontinence or loss of reflexes in severe cases
- Limited to the spine (though there may be radiation of pain and associated neurological signs relating to the affected nerve root) and usually has no systemic manifestations (e.g. fatigue, anorexia, weight loss, gastrointestinal disturbance)
- Laboratory tests, including the erythrocyte sedimentation rate (ESR), are normal. Herniated disk may be confirmed using MRI, CT, or myelography
- Disease of a single sacroiliac joint may indicate infection or be a manifestation of an alternative seronegative arthritis (psoriatic arthritis or Reiter's syndrome)

Diffuse idiopathic skeletal hyperostosis (DISH) syndrome
FEATURES
- Occurs primarily in men older than 50 years
- May resemble ankylosing spondylitis clinically and on X-ray
- Patients are likely to present with spinal back pain. There may also be stiffness and insidious loss of range of movement
- Unlike ankylosing spondylitis, the sacroiliac and spinal apophyseal joints are not eroded, stiffness is not accentuated in the morning, the ESR is normal, and there is no link to HLA-B27
- X-ray findings include large ligamentous ossifications bridging several vertebrae and usually affecting the cervical and lower thoracic spine

Spondyloarthropathies associated with reactive arthritis
FEATURES
Causes signs and symptoms as for ankylosing spondylitis:
- Back pain, especially at night, improved by exercise but NOT improved by rest
- Morning stiffness
- Loss of lumbar motion
- Weight loss
- Fatigue
- Anorexia
- Low-grade fever
- Conjunctivitis
- Psoriasis
- Inflammatory bowel disease (colitis)
- Urethritis

SIGNS & SYMPTOMS
Signs
- Bilateral sacroiliac tenderness
- A dramatic loss of flexibility in the lumbar spine is an early sign
- Loss of chest expansion of less than 2.5cm (normal >5cm) from diffuse costovertebral involvement
- Loss of the usual spinal curvature
- Diminished chest expansion
- Weight loss (also a symptom)
- Recurrent, acute iritis (anterior uveitis) presents as a painful red eye and requires ophthalmologic assessment
- Neurologic signs, resulting from compression radiculitis or sciatica
- Anemia
- Aortic insufficiency, angina, pericarditis, and ECG conduction abnormalities are uncommon
- Rare pulmonary finding is upper lobe fibrosis, occasionally with cavitation that may be mistaken for tuberculosis and can be complicated by infection with aspergillus

Symptoms
- Back pain, especially at night, improved by exercise but NOT improved by rest
- The pain usually disturbs sleep and is associated with morning stiffness and loss of flexibility after immobility, particularly in the lower spine
- Onset is gradual and is often accompanied by constitutional disturbances
- At the disease progresses, pain is often felt in the mid-lumbar, thoracic, and cervical regions resulting in a significant reduction in the range of motion of the entire spine
- In the late stages of the disease, there may be reduction in spinal pain as the axial skeleton becomes 'ankylosed' or fixed
- Symptoms improve with exercise
- Chest pain
- Shortness of breath
- Weight loss
- Fatigue
- Anorexia
- Low-grade fever
- Onset is atypically in peripheral joints, especially in children and women, and rarely with acute iritis (anterior uveitis)
- A flexed or bent-over posture eases back pain and paraspinal muscle spasm; thus, some degree of kyphosis is common in untreated patients but leads to longer term functional impairment

ASSOCIATED DISORDERS
Ankylosing spondylitis is one of the seronegative (i.e. rheumatoid factor-negative) spondyloarthropathies (the others are Reiter's syndrome, psoriasis, reactive arthritis, ulcerative colitis, and Crohn's disease).

KEY! DON'T MISS!
- The onset of low back pain is sometimes incorrectly attributed to athletic injuries in younger patients
- Difficulty in breathing may accompany spinal symptoms
- Sudden onset of extreme pain and tenderness in the spinal area of these patients indicates potential bony fracture. The lower neck (cervical spine) is the most common area for such fractures

CONSIDER CONSULT
Refer to a rheumatologist in all cases to confirm diagnosis and to set up tests correctly.

INVESTIGATION OF THE PATIENT
Direct questions to patient

Q Do you have pain? Where is the pain? Ankylosing spondylitis typically causes lower back pain

Q How long have you had it? Ankylosing spondylitis comes on gradually

Q Have you had a fall recently? To ascertain if an acute injury

Q When is your back pain and stiffness worst? Ankylosing spondylitis pain and stiffness are usually most severe after rest – in the morning, and sometimes at night

Q Is your back painful all the time? Malignancy causes pain which is constant and will often wake the patient at night

Q Does your chest hurt and are you finding it hard to breathe? To check for classic symptom of ankylosing spondylitis – loss of chest expansion

Q Do you have severe twinges or a nagging ache down one leg or through the buttock? Both AS and herniated intervertebral disc may present as sciatica

Q Have you had back pain before? The patient may have suffered back pain over a long period, or have had previous injuries

Q Is the pain better when you lie down, or worse? May help to differentiate between AS and other disorders, and protruded intervertebral disk

Q Does the pain lessen slightly with movement and exercise? To ascertain if ankylosing spondylitis or osteoarthritis, or an injury that would disable the patient

Q Have you seen a specialist before for back pain? To ascertain if patient has sought specialist advice in the past

Q Was it diagnosed? If so, what did the physician/specialist tell you? To trace possible history of other spinal disorders or if patient has seen another practitioner who failed to diagnose the problem

Q Do you have sore eyes or ever had painful red eyes? To check for uveitis

Q Do you have shoulder, hip, or buttock pain and/or stiffness?

Q Have you got or had diarrhea or had blood in your stools? To check for ulcerative colitis or enteric infection

Q Have you had discharge from your penis recently or confirmed chlamydial infection? Both psoriatic arthritis and Reiter's syndrome can mimic ankylosing spondylitis

Contributory or predisposing factors

Q Has the patient suffered from an enteric or urinary tract infection in the past? These may predispose to ankylosing spondylitis

Family history

Q Is there a family history of similar problems or diagnosed ankylosing spondylitis? Often one parent has ankylosing spondylitis

Examination

- Gently palpate the sacroiliac joints to check for tenderness
- Ask the patient to stand up as straight as possible to check for deformity of posture
- Ask the patient to bend forward and backward (may be impossible); then laterally from the waist to check for global restriction of movement in the lumbar spine (i.e. forward flexion, extension, and lateral flexion)
- Assess lower limbs for neurologic signs resulting from compression radiculitis
- Examine for diminished chest expansion, which is a frequent finding in ankylosing spondylitis and may cause deformity
- Cardiac examination for signs of aortic insufficiency and pericarditis
- Examine the eyes for signs of inflammation – eye complications may require referral to an ophthalmologist
- Check for fever and signs of weight loss, both of which can occur in ankylosing spondylitis

▦ Check for psoriasis, which may be associated with ankylosing spondylitis

Summary of investigative tests

▦ X-rays are required to reveal bilateral sacroiliitis. In addition films of the lumbar spine may show characteristic changes of ankylosing spondylitis

▦ A CT scan may detect early changes in the sacroiliac joints

▦ ESR and C-reactive protein are elevated in most patients with ankylosing spondylitis

▦ Tests for IgM rheumatoid factor

▦ Bone scintigraphy is a very nonspecific investigation and carries a high radiation dose but may be helpful in cases where the differential diagnosis includes disseminated malignancy

▦ HLA-B27 antigen test is positive in more than 90% of patients with AS – but the test should not be used indiscriminately in patients with low back pain because the majority of patients with a positive HLA-B27 never suffer AS. Testing for HLA-B27 is both expensive and unnecessary in the great majority of cases, as diagnosis can be made on the clinical findings and X-rays. A negative HLA-B27 test may sometimes be useful in helping to exclude ankylosing spondylitis

DIAGNOSTIC DECISION

▦ Diagnosis should be confirmed by sacroiliac joint X-ray

▦ Limited lumbar motion

▦ Limited chest expansion

▦ Nocturnal pain and early-morning stiffness with above two symptoms could provide provisional diagnosis

The New York Diagnostic Criteria for ankylosing spondylitis [1]) give the following:

▦ Limitation of motion of the lumbar spine in all three planes: anterior flexion, lateral flexion, and extension

▦ History of the presence of pain at the dorsolumbar junction or in the lumbar spine

▦ Limitation of chest expansion to 1 inch (2.5cm) or less, measured at the level of the fourth intercostal space

Definite ankylosing spondylitis:

▦ Grade 3–4 sacroiliitis with at least one clinical criterion, or

▦ Grade 3–4 unilateral, or

▦ Grade 2 bilateral sacroiliitis, with clinical criterion 1, or

▦ Criterion 2 and 3

Probable ankylosing spondylitis:

▦ Grade 3–4 sacroiliitis without any clinical criteria

▦ Radiologically, the early diagnosis may be easier to see in the lower costovertebral joints or upper lumbar facet joints which frequently show early involvement with joint margins that are ill-defined in comparison to the normal appearance

▦ The ESR and other acute-phase reactants (e.g. C-reactive protein levels) are mildly elevated in most patients with active AS

(Grade 1 – suspicious change of the sacroiliac joints
Grade 2 – minimal change consistent with sacroilitis
Grade 3 – unequivocal change in the sacroiliac joint
Grade 4 – severe sacroiliitis with marked ankylosis)

CLINICAL PEARLS

- A young man with back pain (unassociated with trauma) and morning stiffness should be considered to have inflammatory spinal disease until proven otherwise
- Peripheral joint synovitis in a male patient with low back pain suggests an alternative seronegative arthritis because most AS is confined to the spine in men
- X-rays of the sacroiliac joints are unreliable until skeletal maturity at the age of 21 – this may be a practical concern in patients with early-onset disease

THE TESTS
Body fluids
ERYTHROCYTE SEDIMENTATION RATE
Description
Venous blood sample.

Advantages/Disadvantages
ADVANTAGES:
- Simple and universally available test
- May help to upport diagnosis if X-rays are normal

DISADVANTAGE:
A raised ESR can occur in may other conditions

Normal
- Males: 1-15mm/h
- Females: 0–20mm/h

Abnormal
- Males: >15mm/h
- Females: >20mm/h
- Keep in mind the possibility of a false-positive result

Cause of abnormal result
Increased fibrinogen levels in response to inflammation.

Drugs, disorders and other factors that may alter results
- Corticosteroid therapy
- Many inflammatory and autoimmune conditions cause a raised ESR

C-REACTIVE PROTEIN
Description
Venous blood sample.

Advantages/Disadvantages
ADVANTAGES:
- Usually elevated in ankylosing spondylitis and so may help to support diagnosis
- More sensitive to disease fluctuation than ESR

Normal
6.8–820mcg/dL.

Abnormal
Values outside the normal range.

Cause of abnormal result
Inflammatory reactions of any etiology cause an increase in C-reactive protein levels.

IGM RHEUMATOID FACTOR
Description
Venous blood sample.

Advantages/Disadvantages
ADVANTAGES:
- Reasonably readily available test
- May help to confirm or refute the diagnosis – test is NEGATIVE in ankylosing spondylitis

Normal
Negative.

Abnormal
Present in a titer of 1 in 20 or more.

Cause of abnormal result
Many rheumatic diseases (e.g. rheumatoid arthritis, Sjögren's syndrome, systemic lupus erythematosus) as well as some infections (infective endocarditis) and malignancies cause an elevated rheumatoid factor.

Imaging
X-RAYS
Advantages/Disadvantages
ADVANTAGES:
- X-rays show characteristic changes in ankylosing spondylitis
- Quick, inexpensive and in the right clinical setting confirm the diagnosis
- AP view of the pelvis required
- A lumbar-spinal X-ray is equivalent to around 12 months of background radiation and not necessary where bilateral sacroiliitis is present but can add useful supportive information if there are typical inflammatory changes suggestive of enthesopathy

DISADVANTAGE:
- Difficulties in interpreting X-ray of the sacroiliac joints exist in elderly individuals, in which degenerative changes of the sacroiliac joints are common, and in young patients (under 21 years) where skeletal immaturity of the sacroiliac joints makes interpretation difficult

Normal
X-ray may show no changes in early stage of AS.

Abnormal
- As the disease progresses, changes become visible on the X-rays first of the sacroiliac joints and later the thoracolumbar and cervical spine
- Erosions and sclerosis noted on both sides of sacroiliac joints
- Squaring of the vertebrae (Romanus lesion)
- Development of syndesmophytes – bony bridges between the vertebrae due to ossification of the outer layer of the annulus fibrosis of the disk and the deep layers of the longitudinal ligaments
- Syndesmophytes ascending the spine in a symmetric fashion to produce 'bamboo spine' in very late and aggressive disease

Cause of abnormal result
Inflammatory changes and later calcification around the insertion of soft tissue to bone.

CT SCAN
Advantages/Disadvantages
ADVANTAGES:
- CT scan may detect early changes of the sacroiliac joints in cases where X-ray findings are equivocal
- It may also reveal a herniated intervertebral disc and other spinal disorders

DISADVANTAGE:
- It is noninvasive but carries significant radiation dose

Abnormal
- Inflammatory changes in sacroiliac joints
- Squaring of vertebrae, syndesmophytes
- Ossification of annulus fibrosis

Cause of abnormal result
Inflammatory changes and later calcification around the insertion of soft tissue to bone.

BONE SCINTIGRAPHY
Advantages/Disadvantages
ADVANTAGES:
- Bone scan may show increased uptake of radionuclide in inflamed joints
- Bone scans may identify stress fractures that are not obvious on plain radiography
- In cases where the physician considers disseminated malignancy to be a differential diagnosis, a bone scan may be helpful in detecting clinically occult bony neoplastic lesions

DISADVANTAGES:
- Technetium bone scans are neither sensitive nor specific for inflammatory spinal disease
- A normal scan does not exclude ankylosing spondylitis
- Bone scans seldom add significantly to clinical diagnostic decisions regarding ankylosing spondylitis
- The scan carries significant radiation dose

Abnormal
Bone scan 'lights up' over sacroiliac joints and probably around spinal ligaments and is supportive of diagnosis ankylosing spondylitis.

Cause of abnormal result
There are two phases to a bone scan:
- The first (perfusion) phase is positive where there is increased blood flow around a lesion (inflammatory or neoplastic)
- The second (bone) phase at about 3h after administration of technetium reveals increased metabolic activity in bone (inflammatory, degenerative, neoplastic, or fracture)

TREATMENT

CONSIDER CONSULT

Physical therapy and nonsteroidal anti-inflammatory drug (NSAID) treatment should be under specialist direction and review.

IMMEDIATE ACTION

- Send for X-ray
- Relieve pain and discomfort by prescribing an NSAID and/or an analgesic
- Early, accurate diagnosis and therapy may minimize years of pain and disability
- Patients with eye pain and redness should be referred to an ophthalmologist

PATIENT AND CAREGIVER ISSUES
Patient or caregiver request

- There are numerous sources of advice on back pain, and a bewildering range of practitioners claiming cures or therapies
- Patients may have misconceptions gleaned from these sources; they may think back pain is something they have to endure, or in desperation, find obscure or unproven remedies
- There are widespread misunderstandings about its causality, and many sufferers feel hopeless about getting adequate treatment

Health-seeking behavior

For back pain, many therapies, diets, programs, and remedies may have been sought and tried.

MANAGEMENT ISSUES
Goals

- Back pain and stiffness must first be relieved with NSAIDs; treatment plans must address prevention, delay, or correction of the deformity and psychosocial and rehabilitation needs
- Physical therapy to ensure that fusion of the apophyseal joints of the spine will form a straight line in order to reduce late postural defects and respiratory problems
- Educate patient about exercises and posture for prevention of advanced spinal deformity
- Treat inflammation in other organs (e.g. iritis)
- Treat heart disease as appropriate
- Advise strongly against smoking

Management in special circumstances

- Older patients with osteoporosis may already be prone to fractures
- Patients with other forms of arthritis may already be in considerable pain

COEXISTING DISEASE

- GI inflammatory disease, cardiovascular problems such as aortitis and aortic insufficiency require specific therapies from consultant
- Other conditions such as osteoporosis may be present which would add to risk of fracture, pain, and deformity

COEXISTING MEDICATION

- Patient may already be on OTC analgesics or a NSAID
- Patient may be taking complementary medication

SPECIAL PATIENT GROUPS

Elderly AS patients may suffer severe deformity, pain, and disability and a selected few may need surgery. Cervical surgery carries significant risk.

PATIENT SATISFACTION/LIFESTYLE PRIORITIES

- If diagnosed early, patients can benefit from physical therapy and an exercise program, which must be continued on a permanent basis. Patients must be reassured that, although the condition can't be cured, physical therapies and anti-inflammatory drugs can minimize pain and disability. The patient must be fully involved in management of their own condition
- Sometimes rest from work is necessary when AS is in a very active state, but bed rest kept to an absolute minimum. Decisions regarding those with manual work and aggressive disease are best made in conjunction with the patient after they have been reviewed by a rheumatologist
- In more severe and advanced cases loss of function and disability may be considerable. Some forms of surgery such as hip replacement may be indicated; rehabilitation post arthroplasty may be difficult because of spinal deformity

SUMMARY OF THERAPEUTIC OPTIONS
Choices
Nonsteroidal anti-inflammatory drugs (NSAIDs)

- First choice: indomethacin
- Second choice: naproxen
- Third choice: diclofenac
- Fourth choice: (one of several new NSAIDs, referred to as 'coxibs' because they selectively inhibit cyclo-oxygenase (COX)-2, show promise of providing equal effectiveness to drugs that inhibit COX-1 and COX-2 with less chance of adverse effects on the gastric mucosa); this is an off-label indication
- NSAIDs facilitate exercise and other supportive measures by suppressing articular inflammation, pain, and muscle spasm. Most NSAIDs are of proven value in AS, but tolerance and toxicity, rather than marginal differences in efficacy, dictate drug choice
- It is impossible to predict which NSAID will be best tolerated by a particular patient; no particular NSAID has demonstrated superiority over others for pain relief. Once a NSAID has been selected, the dose should be increased until pain has been relieved or the maximal tolerated dose has been achieved
- The response of the patient should guide the clinician in selecting dosing intervals of these agents
- Because NSAIDs and adjuvant analgesics have ceiling effects to their efficacy, if a patient does not respond to the maximal dose of one NSAID, another should be tried before discontinuation of NSAID therapy
- Patients should be monitored and warned of potential adverse reactions especially in those with gastrointestinal inflammation. The daily dose of NSAIDs should be as low as possible, but maximum doses may be necessary in active disease
- Drug withdrawal should be attempted only slowly, after systemic and articular signs of active disease have been suppressed for several months

Disease-modifying antirheumatic drugs (DMARDs)

- Sulfasalazine may benefit those with more severe involvement, particularly when the peripheral joints are involved; this is an off-label indication
- Methotrexate is often successful at relieving symptoms; this is an off-label indication
- Corticosteroid preparations are used for persistent enthesitis, peripheral synovitis, and uveitis; local injections of corticosteroid preparations into large joints and/or ocular corticosteroids may be extremely effective, but long-term use is associated with many serious adverse effects, including osteoporosis
- Narcotics and muscle relaxants lack anti-inflammatory properties, although some patients may find them useful to relieve pain in joints that have secondary degenerative changes
- Anti-tumor necrosis factor monoclonal antibody (infliximab) has been reported to be effective in ankylosing spondylitis but there is little clinical experience in its use for this condition at present

Physical therapy

- A course of physical therapy to reduce future disability and occupational therapy is important to prevent the patient from fusing in a less functional flexed position and to advise on home and workplace modifications that can minimize discomfort and handicap
- An exercise and posture program to encourage proper sleep and walking positions, coupled with abdominal and back exercises, can help to maintain posture. Exercises help maintain joint flexibility. Breathing exercises optimize lung capacity, and swimming provides aerobic exercise

Occupational therapy

Occupational therapy is important to advise the patient on home and workplace modifications that can minimize discomfort and handicap

Surgery

Joint replacement surgery may be required in advanced cases

Lifestyle changes

Smoking should be vigorously discouraged.

Guidelines

Guidelines on the management of adult patients with low back pain have been formulated and published by the Institute for Clinical Systems Improvement [2].

Clinical pearls

- NSAIDs and physical therapy are the cornerstones of treatment
- Consider prescribing 2-week courses of different NSAIDs to enable the patient to decide which works best for them and involve the patient in decision making
- Smoking in a patient with reduced ability to expectorate (because of restricted ribcage movement) predisposes to serious lung infection. Advise strongly against smoking

FOLLOW UP
Plan for review

While long-term management of ankylosing spondylitis will probably be conducted by a rheumatology specialist, the patient will need regular reviews if medication and other therapies are at PCP level.

Information for patient or caregiver

- Patients who have early or less severe ankylosing spondylitis and are mobile will need to persevere with exercises and maintain good posture
- Self-help measures are for life and patients will need regular guidance from a physiotherapist, as exercises will change in line with activity cycles of the disease

DRUGS AND OTHER THERAPIES: DETAILS
Drugs
INDOMETHACIN
Nonsteroidal anti-inflammatory drug.

Dose

- Adult: 75mg slow release every day; may increase to twice a day (maximum 200mg a day)
- Child: oral dose 1.5–2.5mg/kg a day in divided doses three or four times a day (maximum 4mg/kg/day or 150–200mg a day)

Efficacy
Considered the strongest NSAID by many patients with AS.

Risks/Benefits
- Risk: use caution in hepatic and cardiac failure, epilepsy, psychiatric disorders and parkinsonism
- Benefit: faster onset of action than colchicines

Side-effects and adverse reactions
- Gastrointestinal: anorexia, nausea, dyspepsia, peptic ulceration
- Central nervous system: headache, dizziness, tinnitus
- Hypersensitivity: rashes, bronchospasm, angioedema
- Thrombocytopenia

Interactions (other drugs)
- Aminoglycosides ■ Anticoagulants ■ Antihypertensives ■ Corticosteroids
- Cyclosporine ■ Digoxin ■ Lithium ■ Methotrexate ■ Phenylpropanolamine
- Triamterene

Contraindications
- Severe renal, hepatic or cardiac disease ■ Hypertension ■ Peptic ulceration
- Hypersensitivity to NSAIDs ■ Coagulation defects

Acceptability to patient
Gastrointestinal tolerance is usually the main issue that limits acceptability.

Follow up plan
Regular follow up necessary to assess efficacy and adverse effects.

Patient and caregiver information
The patient should be told that gastrointestinal tolerance may be increased if medication is taken with food.

DICLOFENAC
Nonsteroidal anti-inflammatory drug.

Dose
- Adult: oral dose of 100–125mg a day; 25mg four times a day and 25mg at bedtime if needed
- Must take with/after food
- Slow-release preparations effective in reducing morning stiffness

Efficacy
Good.

Risks/Benefits
Risks:
- Use caution in hepatic, renal and cardiac failure, porphyria
- Use caution in bleeding and GI disorders

- Benefit: faster onset of action than colchicines

Side-effects and adverse reactions
- Gastrointestinal: anorexia, nausea, dyspepsia, peptic ulceration, vomiting
- Central nervous system: headache, dizziness, tinnitus

- Hypersensitivity: rashes, bronchospasm, angioedema
- Cardiovascular system: CHF, dysrhythmias, hypertension and hypotension
- Eyes, ears, nose and throat: blurred vision

Interactions (other drugs)
- Aminoglycosides
- Anticoagulants
- Antihypertensives
- Corticosteroids
- Cyclosporine
- Digoxin
- Lithium
- Methotrexate
- Phenylpropanolamine
- Triamterene

Contraindications
- Peptic ulceration
- Hypersensitivity to NSAIDs
- Coagulation defects

Acceptability to patient
Good where effective.

Follow up plan
Regular follow up necessary to assess efficacy and adverse effects.

Patient and caregiver information
The patient should be told that gastrointestinal tolerance may be increased if medication is taken with food.

NAPROXEN
Nonsteroidal anti-inflammatory drug.

Dose
Adult: 250-500mg/day twice daily by mouth.

Efficacy
Generally good.

Risks/Benefits
Risks:
- Use caution in hepatic, renal and cardiac failure, porphyria
- Use caution in bleeding and GI disorders

Benefit: faster onset of action than colchicines

Side-effects and adverse reactions
- Gastrointestinal: anorexia, nausea, dyspepsia, peptic ulceration
- Central nervous system: headache, dizziness, tinnitus
- Cardiovascular system: dysrhythmias, edema, palpitations, congestive heart failure
- Hypersensitivity: rashes, bronchospasm, angioedema
- Thrombocytopenia
- Genitourinary: acute renal failure

Interactions (other drugs)
- Aminoglycosides
- Anticoagulants
- Antihypertensives
- Corticosteroids
- Cyclosporine
- Digoxin
- Lithium
- Methotrexate
- Phenylpropanolamine
- Triamterene

Contraindications
- Peptic ulceration
- Hypersensitivity to NSAIDs
- Coagulation defects

Acceptability to patient
Generally good; the main factor that limits patient acceptance is gastrointestinal disturbance.

Follow up plan
Regular follow up is necessary to assess efficacy and adverse effects.

Patient and caregiver information
Patient should be told that gastrointestinal tolerance may be increased if medication is taken with food.

ETODOLAC
Nonsteroidal anti-inflammatory drug.

Dose
- Adult: 800–1200mg per day in divided doses initially, then adjust dose to 600–1200mg per day in divided doses (maximum 1200mg/day)
- Child: (or patients less than 60kg) maximum 20mg/kg; slow release oral dose 400–1000mg every day

Efficacy
High, but depends on severity of pain and deformity.

Risks/Benefits
Risks:
- Use caution in hepatic, renal and cardiac failure, porphyria
- Use caution in gastrointestinal ulceration and bleeding

Side-effects and adverse reactions
- Gastrointestinal: anorexia, nausea, vomiting, dyspepsia, peptic ulceration
- Central nervous system: headache, dizziness, confusion
- Cardiovascular system: dysrhythmias, edema, palpitations, congestive heart failure
- Hypersensitivity: rashes, bronchospasm, angioedema
- Ears, eyes, nose and throat: tinnitus, blurred vision

Interactions (other drugs)
- Aminoglycosides - Antihypertensives - Anticoagulants (aspirin, warfarin, heparins, other NSAIDs) - Antiplatelets (clopidogrel, ticlopidine) - Antidysrhythmics (cardiac glycosides, calcium channel blockers) - Baclofen - Corticosteroids - Cyclosporine, tacrolimus - Lithium - Methotrexate - Phenylpropanolamine - Phenytoin - Pentoxyfylline - Quinolones - Ritonavir - Sulphonylureas - Triamterene - Zidovudine

Contraindications
- Peptic ulceration - Hypersensitivity to NSAIDs - Coagulation defects

Acceptability to patient
High.

Follow up plan
Regular follow up is necessary to assess efficacy and side-effects.

Patient and caregiver information
Patient should be advised to tell his or her medical practitioner about any adverse effects and progress of symptoms.

SULFASALAZINE
Gastrointestinal anti-inflammatory agent and mild disease-modifying antirheumatic drug.

Dose
- Adult: 500mg/day initially, increased by 500mg/day at weekly intervals to 1g twice a day, or a maximum or 1.5g twice daily
- Child: over 2 years: 40–60mg/kg/day in between three and six divided doses; maintenance 30mg/kg/day in four divided doses

Efficacy
May relieve symptoms but full effect not apparent for about 3 months.

Risks/Benefits
Benefit: concomitant relief of symptoms of coexisting gastrointestinal inflammatory disease.

Side-effects and adverse reactions
- Gastrointestinal: abdominal pain, diarrhea, hepatotoxicity, melena, vomiting
- Genitourinary: renal failure, urinary retention
- Hematologic: blood cell disorders
- Musculoskeletal: arthralgia, myalgia, osteoporosis
- Cardiovascular system: pericarditis, allergic myocarditis
- Central nervous system: dizziness, drowsiness, headache, seizures
- Eyes, ears, nose and throat: blurred vision, tinnitus
- Skin: Stevens-Johnson syndrome

Interactions (other drugs)
- Digoxin Methenamine Phenytoin Tolbutamide Warfarin

Contraindications
- Contraindicated in porphyria and gastrointestinal or urinary tract obstruction
- Cross-hypersensitivy with salicylates Caution required in patients with renal or hepatic impairment, glucose-6-phosphate deficiency

Evidence
There is no evidence that sulfasalazine alters disease progression.
- A small, blinded RCT compared sulfasalazine with placebo in the management of ankylosing spondylitis for a 12-month period. Improvement was noted in pain and stiffness in the treatment group. Improvement in laboratory markers of inflammation were also seen with sulfasalazine. Improvement in sleep disturbance, finger-floor distance and ESR were noted in the treatment and control groups. Disease progression measured by X-ray changes was not altered after treatment, and multiple analysis of variance did not show a difference in disease activity indicators between the 2 groups [3] *Level P*

Acceptability to patient
High.

Follow up plan
May need to review for efficacy and adverse effects. Regular blood monitoring (complete blood count and liver function tests) is advised.

Patient and caregiver information
- The patient should be warned about potential side-effects and the need for regular follow up and monitoring

■ The dye in sulfasalazine stains soft contact lenses and turns urine yellow

METHOTREXATE
Disease-modifying antirheumatic drug.

Dose
■ Adult: 7.5–20mg orally or intramuscularly every week; adjust gradually to achieve optimum response – maximum 20mg per week – then reduce to lowest possible effective dose
■ Child: 5–15mg/m^2 orally or intramuscularly every week as single dose or in three divided doses 12h apart

Efficacy
Often successful in relieving symptoms.

Risks/Benefits
Risks:
■ Use caution with infection and bone marrow depression
■ Use caution with peptic ulceration and ulcerative colitis
■ Use caution with renal and hepatic impairment
■ Use caution with the elderly
■ Use caution in pregnancy

Side-effects and adverse reactions
■ Gastrointestinal: abdominal pain, diarrhea, hepatotoxicity, nausea, vomiting, stomatitis
■ Genitourinary: renal failure, urinary retention, depression of and defective spermatogenesis, hematuria
■ Hematologic: blood cell disorders
■ Musculoskeletal: osteoporosis, muscle pain and wasting
■ Respiratory: pulmonary fibrosis
■ Central nervous system: headache, seizures, dizziness, drowsiness
■ Eyes, ears, nose and throat: visual disturbances, tinnitus
■ Skin: rashes, acne, dermatitis, hyperpigmentation, vasculitis

Interactions (other drugs)
■ Aminoglycosides ■ Antimalarials ■ Binding resins ■ Co-trimoxazole ■ Cyclosporin ■ Ethanol ■ Etretrinate ■ Live vaccines ■ NSAIDS ■ Omeprazole ■ Penicillins ■ Probenicid ■ Salicylates ■ Sulfinpyrazone ■ Vaccines

Contraindications
■ Severe renal and hepatic impairment ■ Profound bone marrow depression ■ Nursing mothers ■ Avoid administering live vaccines due to impaired immune response

Acceptability to patient
Administration of methotrexate requires abstinence from alcohol.

Follow up plan
Complete blood count and hepatic profile should be obtained at least every 2 months.

Patient and caregiver information
■ Patient should be told to avoid alcohol and salicylate
■ Patient should report any adverse effects

GLUCOCORTICOSTEROIDS

Dose
The minimum effective dose should be used. Generally, 5–10mg/day brings substantial relief for most patients.

Efficacy
Often extremely effective.

Risks/Benefits
Risks:

- False-negative skin allergy tests. Overwhelming septicemia if patient has an infection
- Loss of control of blood glucose in those with diabetes
- Use caution in elderly due to risk of diabetes and osteoporosis
- Use caution in patients with psychosis, seizure disorders or myasthenia gravis
- Use caution in congestive heart failure, hypertension
- Use caution in ulcerative colitis, peptic ulcer or esophagitis

Side-effects and adverse reactions
Side-effects are minimized by short duration of therapy.

- Gastrointestinal: dyspepsia, peptic ulceration, esophagitis, oral candidiasis, nausea, vomiting
- Cardiovascular system: hypertension, thromboembolism
- Central nervous system: insomnia, euphoria, depression, psychosis, seizures
- Endocrine: adrenal suppression, impaired glucose tolerance, growth suppression in children
- Musculoskeletal: proximal myopathy, osteoporosis
- Skin: delayed healing, acne, striae
- Eyes, ears, nose and throat: cataract, glaucoma, blurred vision

Interactions (other drugs)

- Adrenergic neurone blockers, alpha blockers, beta blockers, beta 2 agonists
- Aminoglutethamide ■ Anticonvulsants (carbemazepine, phenytoin, barbiturates)
- Antidiabetics ■ Antidysrhythmics (calcium channel blockers, cardiac glycosides)
- Antifungals (amphotericin, ketoconazole) ■ Antihypertensives (ACE inhibitors, diuretics: loop and thiazide, acetazolamide; angiotensin II receptor antagonists, clonidine, diazoxide, hydralazine, methyldopa, minoxidil) ■ Cyclosporine ■ Erythromycin ■ Methotrexate
- NSAIDs ■ Nitrates ■ Nitroprusside ■ Oral contraceptives ■ Rifampin ■ Ritonavir
- Somatropin ■ Vaccines

Contraindications

- Systemic infection ■ Avoid live virus vaccines in those receiving immunosuppressive doses

Follow up plan
Regular follow up necessary to assess efficacy and adverse effects.

Physical therapy
MINIMIZING FUTURE DISABILITY

- All AS patients must be referred for physical therapy to minimize future disability where possible
- Essential to prevent the patient from fusing in a less functional flexed position
- For proper posture and joint motion, a program of physical therapy and other supportive measures under physiotherapist supervision (e.g. postural training, therapeutic exercise) are vital to strengthen muscle groups that oppose the direction of potential deformities (i.e. strengthen the extensor rather than flexor muscle groups)

Efficacy
High.

Risks/Benefits
Benefit: great in helping mobility and reducing further deformity. If under correct supervision, patients should not succumb to injuries from the exercise program.

Evidence
A systematic review found that there is a trend towards benefit for physiotherapy in the management of ankylosing spondylitis. There is currently insufficient evidence to recommend for or against physiotherapy [4] *Level M*

Acceptability to patient
May vary according to level of pain and disability, and adaptation to regular program of exercise. However, as symptoms recede on movement, should be high.

Follow up plan
Physical therapist would conduct continuous assessment of patient's progress and inform the PCP.

Patient and caregiver information
The physical therapist would instruct the patient on exercise programs, breathing exercises, posture.

Occupational therapy
Often useful for patients with chronic disease and impairment.

AIDS TO ASSIST IN ACTIVITIES OF DAILY LIVING
Efficacy
Often excellent.

Risks/Benefits
Risk: often vital to help patients remain at work (e.g. aids for driving – extended mirrors to account for poor neck mobility) and reduce disability at home.

Acceptability to patient
Excellent because the treatment is patient-centered.

Surgical therapy
JOINT REPLACEMENT SURGERY
For advanced hip and knee disease.

Efficacy
Varies with severity of disease. Severe spinal disease may make rehabilitation difficult.

Risks/Benefits
- Risk: heterotopic ossification occurs in 20–40% of hip replacements and is more common with trochanteric osteotomy. This risk may be reduced by perioperative use of NSAIDs
- Benefit: significant pain relief in selected patients with consequent improvement in function

Acceptability to patient
Often high because of success rate in increasing mobility.

Follow up plan
Surgeon/consultant would review postoperative aftercare and physical therapy.

Patient and caregiver information
Depends on physiotherapist's instructions during rehabilitation period.

Other therapies
EXERCISE AND POSTURE PROGRAM
- Exercise program to include breathing exercises
- Exercise should be aimed at maintaining the full spinal range of movement, and should be supervised by an experienced physiotherapist
- A stretch program is essential
- Corsets and braces do not provide any help to the back for patients with AS
- Patients should avoid prolonged sitting, especially driving; if working in a sedentary job, they should get up and walk about every 30 min or so
- Swimming is to be encouraged; aquatherapy is often useful
- A firm bed with one pillow is necessary to avoid neck contractures
- Good seating with appropriate support for the back at home, work, and recreation
- Reading while lying prone and thus extending the neck may help keep the back flexible
- Some PCPs may recommend applying a local anti-inflammatory poultice for temporary relief

Efficacy
High. These measures are essential to improve and maintain posture, maximize mobility, and prevent further deterioration and pain.

Risks/Benefits
Benefits are great; there is a small risk of injury if exercise instructions are not followed correctly.

Acceptability to patient
Should be high if exercise regimen is tailored to the individual patient; but depends on level of disability, age, general fitness, how well patient can fit exercise into their lifestyle, and whether it causes more pain and discomfort at first.

Follow up plan
Regular follow up necessary over a long period – by physical therapist and PCP.

Patient and caregiver information
The patient should be aware that persevering with the exercise program is vital.

LIFESTYLE
Smoking should be discouraged strongly. Lung involvement is aggravated by smoking, and this may shorten the life of the patient.

RISKS/BENEFITS
Benefits are great.

ACCEPTABILITY TO PATIENT
Quitting smoking may be very difficult and patients may need help.

FOLLOW UP PLAN
Ask to review patient's progress during quitting program.

PATIENT AND CAREGIVER INFORMATION
Stress how important it is to quit smoking – that the lungs and heart are badly affected in patients with ankylosing spondylitis.

OUTCOMES

EFFICACY OF THERAPIES

- Proper treatment in many patients results in minimal or no disability and in full, productive lives despite back stiffness
- Most patients have a normal life expectancy
- In severe cases the course is progressive, resulting in pronounced incapacitating deformities

Evidence
PDxMD are unable to cite evidence which meets our criteria for evidence.

Review period
May be for life.

PROGNOSIS

- Prognosis is extremely variable. With suitable treatment, the prognosis is excellent and 85% of patients never lose a day's work
- After the early, painful phase, the back may be stiff but disability is minimal unless hip involvement is present
- Some people advance, while others have disease remissions with minimal deformity
- Advanced hip and knee disease may be surgically treated with joint replacement
- The prognosis is guarded for patients with refractory iritis

Clinical pearls

- Patients often become confused by the similar terms 'spondylosis' (common radiological degenerative condition of the spine) and 'spondylitis' (suggesting the inflammatory component in AS) – take care that you are clear which is the problem in new patients with a history of spinal disease
- Many patients derive huge benefit from joining a self-help organization such as the North American Spinal Society (NASS)

Therapeutic failure

- In cases of persistent AS which is unresponsive to anti-inflammatory medications, agents that suppress body immunity are considered or glucocorticoids may have to be prescribed, though their efficacy in AS is usually minimal
- If advanced, severe deformity correction by surgery may be possible

Deterioration
With no treatment or exercise plan, the result is likely to be increased disability and respiratory compromise. In all cases progressive fusion of the apophyseal joints of the spine cannot be predicted or prevented.

COMPLICATIONS
Extraskeletal problems caused by advanced AS include:
- Pulmonary fibrosis. Therefore, breathing difficulty can be a serious complication
- Aortic insufficiency
- Heart block
- Uveitis
- Amyloidosis

CONSIDER CONSULT

- If cardiovascular or pulmonary complications supervene, refer to appropriate specialist
- If eye complications occur, refer to an ophthalmologist

PREVENTION

It is possible to prevent fusion in a flexed posture, but there is no known way to prevent the disease.

MODIFY RISK FACTORS
Because of the risk of inheriting AS, genetic counseling may be advisable for patients with AS planning a family or for people who are aware of a familial tendency.

Lifestyle and wellness
TOBACCO
Smoking should be discouraged strongly as the lung involvement is aggravated by the smoking, and this may shorten the life of the patient.

ALCOHOL AND DRUGS
Regular alcohol consumption is not compatible with methotrexate therapy.

PHYSICAL ACTIVITY
A daily stretching and strengthening program is essential and should include breathing exercises. Good posture habits and a firm bed and seat are vital to maintaining a straight spine.

ENVIRONMENT
- Features of the workplace must be adjusted. For example, workers can adjust chairs and desks for proper postures
- Patients should try to ensure that supportive seating and/or beds are available when traveling or during sedentary recreation
- Drivers can use wide rear-view mirrors and prism glasses to compensate for the limited motion in the spine

FAMILY HISTORY
- Genetic counseling may be advisable for patients with AS planning a family
- Parents should be advised that if the child develops symptoms such as swollen joints or painful eyes, they should seek medical advice

DRUG HISTORY
Use of nonsteroidal anti-inflammatory drugs (NSAIDs) may be restricted by history of peptic ulcer disease or intolerance of NSAIDs.

PREVENT RECURRENCE
Reassess coexisting disease
Further evaluation will be needed for symptoms and signs of other related spondyloarthropathies, such as psoriasis, sexually transmitted diseases, or dysentery (Reiter's syndrome), and inflammatory bowel disease (ulcerative colitis or Crohn's disease).

RESOURCES

ASSOCIATIONS

American College of Rheumatology
1800 Century Place, Suite 250
Atlanta, GA 30345
Tel: (404) 633 3777
Fax: (404) 633 1870
www.rheumatology.org

Arthritis Foundation
Tel: (800) 283 7800
E-mail: help@arthritis.org
www.arthritis.org

The North American Spine Society
LaGrange Office:
22 Calendar Court, Suite 200
LaGrange, IL 60525
Tel: (708) 588 8080
Fax: (708) 588 1080
Rosemont Office:
6300 North River Rd, Suite 500
Rosemont, IL 60018-4231
Tel: (847) 692 5881
Fax (847) 823 8668

Spondylitis Association of America
14827 Ventura Blvd, Suite 222
Sherman Oaks, CA 91403
Tel: (800) 777 8189 (free)
Tel: (818) 981 1616
www.spine.org

KEY REFERENCES

- Cyriax JH. Cyriax's Illustrated Manual of Orthopaedic Medicine, 2nd ed. Butterworth-Heinemann Medical, 1996
- Brewerton DA, Hart FD, Nicholls A. Ankylosing spondylitis and HL-27. Lancet 1973;i:904–7.
- Brown MA, Pile KD, Kennedy LG, et al. A genome-wide screen for susceptibility loci in ankylosing spondylitis. Arthritis Rheum 1998;41:588–95
- De Blecourt JJ, Polman A, De Blecourt-Meindersma T. Hereditary factors in rheumatoid arthritis and ankylosing spondylitis. Ann Rheum Dis 1961;20:215–20
- Clegg DO, Reda DJ, Abdellatif M. Comparison of sulfasalazine and placebo for the treatment of axial and peripheral articular manifestations of the seronegative spondyloarthropathies: a Department of Veterans Affairs cooperative study. Arthritis Rheum 1999;42:2325–9
- Dougados M, vam der Linden S, Leirisalo-Repo M, et al. Sulfasalazine in the treatment of spondylarthropathy: a randomized, multicenter, double-blind, placebo-controlled study. Arthritis Rheum 1995;38:618–27
- Taylor HG, Beswick EJ, Dawes PT. Sulfasalazine in ankylosing spondylitis: a radiological, clinical, and laboratory assessment. Clin Rheumatol 1991;10:43–8
- Brandt J, Haibel H, Cornely D, et al. Successful treatment of ankylosing spondylitis with the anti- TNF receptor monoclonal antibody infliximab. Arthritis Rheum 2000;43:1346–52
- Bradford DS, Schumacher WL, Lonstein JE, Winter RB. Ankylosing spondylitis: experience in surgical management of 21 patients [published erratum appears in Spine 1987;12:590–2]. Spine 1987;12:238–43
- Forouzesh S, Bluestone R. The clinical spectrum of ankylosing spondylitis. Clin Orthop 1979;143:53–8
- Sunshine A, Olson NZ. Non-narcotic analgesics. In: Wall PD, Melzack R, eds. Textbook of Pain, 2nd ed. New York: Churchill Livingstone; 1989, p670–85

Evidence references and guidelines

1. van der Linden S, Valkenburg HA, Cats A. Evaluation of diagnostic criteria for ankylosing spondylitis. A proposal for modification of the New York criteria. Arthritis Rheum 1984;27:361–8. Medline

2. Guidelines on the management of adult patients with low back pain have been formulated and published by the Institute for Clinical Systems Improvement: Adult low back pain. Guideline Oversight Group, 1998.

3. Taylor HG, Beswick EJ, Dawes PT. Sulfasalazine in ankylosing spondylitis. A radiological, clinical, and laboratory assessment. Clin Rheumatol 1991;10:43–8. Medline

4. Dagfinrud H, Hagen K. Physiotherapy interventions for ankylosing spondylitis (Cochrane Review). In: The Cochrane Library, 4, 2001. Oxford: Update Software

FAQS

Question 1
How do you differentiate between mechanical and inflammatory back pain?

ANSWER 1
The differentiation mainly lies in clinical history. Mechanical back pain is sudden in onset; usually associated with an inciting injury; peak prevalence is 40–59 years; worsens with activity and relieved on rest; usually lasts 1–3 weeks. Inflammatory back pain is insidious in onset, usually greater than 3 months; usually begins in people younger than 40 years; is associated with considerable morning stiffness, gets better with stretching, and may be associated with systemic symptoms.

Question 2
What is the prevalence of HLA-B27 in the general population?

ANSWER 2
Varies with various ethnicities. Caucasians have a prevalence rate of about 8%, Chinese have a rate of 2–9%, and it is virtually absent in African-Americans.

Question 3
In a patient with a complaint of prolonged morning stiffness, would ordering HLA-B27 help in diagnosing inflammatory spondyloarthropathies?

ANSWER 3
No. About 8% of Caucasian population are HLA-B27 positive. The majority of patients with low back pain who carry HLA-B27 will have a mechanical disorder rather than AS. This means that the antigen test is not useful clinically to discriminate the two conditions.
Plain radiographs of sacroiliac joints represent the initial investigation of choice, which may show erosions in lower third of the joints.

Question 4
What are the other causes of sacroiliac joint abnormalities?

ANSWER 4
Unilateral sacroiliitis should raise suspicion of an alternative diagnosis:
- Inflammatory – seronegative spondyloarthropathies, infection
- Traumatic – trauma, osteoarthritis

Sacroiliac joint sclerosis is a frequent finding in child-bearing women but there is no erosive change.

Question 5
What is the natural course of AS?

ANSWER 5

The natural course of AS is variable. Most of the patients can live a normal life with regular physical and occupational therapy. The following features are associated with worse outcome:

- Cervical spine ankylosis
- Hip joint involvement
- Uveitis
- Pulmonary fibrosis
- Persistent elevation of erythrocyte sedimentation rate

CONTRIBUTORS

Shane Clarke
Richard Brasington Jr, MD, FACP
Dinesh Khanna, MD

BACK PAIN

SUMMARY INFORMATION

DESCRIPTION

- Back pain is usually due to benign, mechanical causes
- A small number of cases are due to rare, but serious conditions
- In about half the patients, the symptoms will settle within a week, and the symptoms will settle within a month in more than 90% of patients
- Most common cause of disability in persons aged less than 40 years
- Investigations are only indicated if there is clinical suspicion of underlying serious pathology, or if the symptoms persist in spite of adequate treatment for a reasonable period of time

URGENT ACTION

Spinal cord compression, cauda equina compression (not very common), and significant neurological deficit are surgical emergencies and need to be referred immediately.

KEY! DON'T MISS!

- A full general examination must be performed seeking a systemic cause for the back pain, e.g. leaking abdominal aortic aneurysm, psoriatic lesions, primary malignant lesion, source of infection, etc
- A full neurological examination of the lower limbs and the perineum must be done looking for evidence of neurological deficit

ICD9 CODE
724.5 Back pain (postural)
724.2 Low back pain
307.89 Back pain, psychogenic
847.9 Back strain
724.6 Backache, sacroiliac

SYNONYMS
- Low back pain
- Lumbalgia
- Backache

CARDINAL FEATURES
- Back pain is usually due to benign, mechanical causes
- A small number of cases are due to rare, but serious conditions
- In about half the patients, the symptoms will settle within a week, and the symptoms will settle within a month in more than 90% of patients
- Investigations are only indicated if there is clinical suspicion of underlying serious pathology, or if the symptoms persist in spite of adequate treatment for a significant period of time

CAUSES
Common causes
- Degenerative causes, e.g. osteoarthritis, degenerative disc disease, spondylolisthesis
- Muscular causes, e.g. myofascial pain, paraspinal muscle strain
- Mechanical causes, e.g. prolapsed intervertebral disc
- Referred pain, e.g. endometriosis, hip joint pain, abdominal aortic aneurysm

Rare causes
- Malignancy, e.g. bony metastases, multiple myeloma
- Infection, e.g. vertebral osteomyelitis, tuberculosis of the spine, discitis, epidural abscess
- Vascular, e.g. abdominal aortic aneurysm, epidural hematoma, hemoglobinopathy
- Rheumatological, e.g. rheumatoid arthritis, ankylosing spondylitis, psoriatic arthritis, Reiter's syndrome

Serious causes
- Malignancy
- Infection
- Lesions causing spinal cord or cauda equina compression

Contributory or predisposing factors
- Heavy manual labor
- Obesity
- Psychosocial factors, e.g. job dissatisfaction, pre-existing depression

EPIDEMIOLOGY
Incidence and prevalence
- The second most common affliction of mankind (after the common cold)
- Lifetime prevalence of back pain exceeds 70% in most industrialized nations

INCIDENCE
About half the population will report back pain over a 12-month period.

PREVALENCE
150–200 per 1000 is the average one-year prevalence.

Demographics

AGE
Peak prevalence is between 45 and 59 years, but it is common in the young and the elderly. The first episode of back pain is likely to occur between the age of 20 and 40.

GENDER
Equally prevalent in both sexes; men are more likely to require surgery, whereas women are more likely to be referred to a pain clinic.

RACE
Seen in all races, but the cumulative lifetime prevalence is greater in the Caucasian population.

GENETICS
90% of Caucasians who have ankylosing spondylitis have the tissue type HLA-B27; however, the presence of HLA-B27 is of no diagnostic value in the diagnosis of this condition, and should never be ordered as a diagnostic test.

GEOGRAPHY
Back pain has reached epidemic proportions in all Western societies.

SOCIOECONOMIC STATUS
- There is increased incidence of low back pain and disability with lower social class
- Jobs requiring heavy physical work, a static posture, bending and twisting, lifting, repetitive work, and vibrations such as those resulting from driving a vehicle predispose to low back pain

DIFFERENTIAL DIAGNOSIS

In the majority of patients, low back pain is a benign self-limiting condition. There are, however, several relatively rare, but serious causes that have to be excluded.

Low back strain (and other mechanical causes)

Minor self-limiting injury associated with low back pain.

FEATURES
- Often set off by physical exertion or lifting a heavy weight
- Symptoms usually settle down spontaneously within days or weeks
- There is no indication to investigate unless there are 'red flags' suggesting a possible sinister underlying pathology

Osteoarthritis

Frequent cause of low back pain in the older age group.

FEATURES
- Osteoarthritis involving the facet joints may cause nerve root compression such as sciatica
- Osteoarthritic spurs may result in impingement of the intervertebral foramen with subsequent nerve root compression

Osteoporosis

This is very common in postmenopausal women.

FEATURES
- Smoking, alcohol, and a sedentary lifestyle are contributory factors
- The pain is due to compression fractures or microfractures through the trabeculi of the affected vertebrae

Lumbar disc disease

The levels most commonly involved are L4/5 and L5/S1.

FEATURES
- Compression of the exiting nerve root will present as sciatica, sensory loss in the affected dermatome, and motor weakness in the muscles supplied by the affected nerve root
- Central disc herniation will result in cauda equina compression (saddle anesthesia with bladder and bowel dysfunction), although not that common
- Most cases of disc herniation with minimal or no neurological deficit will resolve spontaneously
- Cases that fail to resolve with conservative management may require surgery
- Patients with significant neurological deficit may require urgent surgery

Spinal stenosis

The spinal canal is narrowed resulting in back and leg pain.

FEATURES
- The pain is induced by walking and exercise
- It is relieved by sitting and/or flexing the spine
- Usually due to degenerative changes superimposed on a congenitally narrow spinal canal
- Surgery is indicated when the symptoms interfere with the activities of daily living

Spondylolisthesis

There is forward slippage of the anterior spinal elements while the posterior elements remain *in situ*.

FEATURES

- Most likely to occur at the lumbosacral junction. The L4/5 level is less frequently involved
- May present acutely in the younger patient, or as part of the picture of degenerative changes in the older patient
- Can present as low back pain, nerve root compression, or cauda equina compression (although not that common)
- Can be diagnosed by good quality oblique X-rays of the lumbosacral spine

Immune disorders

Include disorders such as ankylosing spondylitis, rheumatoid arthritis, psoriatic arthritis, enteropathic arthritis, and Reiter's syndrome.

FEATURES

- The back pain may be associated with other joint involvement
- The erythrocyte sedimentation rate (ESR) is often, but not invariably, raised
- The symptoms are usually insidious in onset, associated with morning stiffness, improve with mild activity, and occur in individuals less than 40 years of age
- There may extraspinal findings such as ocular inflammation, aphthous stomatitis, urethritis, or colitis

Neoplastic disease

This is usually due to metastatic disease, but primary malignancy such as multiple myeloma and benign lesions such as osteoid osteoma will also present with back pain.

FEATURES

- The pain is not relieved by rest, and may be worse at night
- Will often result in rapid neurological deterioration
- Neurological compromise may be due to direct pressure from the neoplastic lesion or as a result of the bony destruction and collapse of the bony elements
- The disc space is usually spared
- Urgent MR scan is indicated in patients with a history of cancer if the back pain is suspected to be due to bony metastasis

Infection

May be due to pyogenic organisms (acute), or due to fungal or tuberculous infection (chronic).

FEATURES

- The pain is not relieved by rest
- There is localized tenderness
- The erythrocyte sedimentation rate is elevated
- The disc space is involved
- Fever may or may not be present
- Should always be suspected in postoperative and immunocompromised patients

Visceral diseases

Pain can be referred to the back from pelvic or abdominal organs.

FEATURES

- May be related to eating or the menstrual cycle
- The pain may be colicky or crampy in nature

- Usually unrelated to back movement
- There may be other findings such as urinary symptoms in addition to the back pain
- Causes include endometriosis, duodenal ulcers, pancreatic disease, renal calculi, pelvic neoplasm, and abdominal aortic aneurysm

Nonspecific back pain
Chronic low back pain with no clear cause.

FEATURES
- May be mechanical in nature, has often been attributed to the lumbar muscles, facet joints, hip, or sacroiliac joint
- There may be a functional or psychological component to the pain
- Often associated with poor posture, job dissatisfaction, anxiety, compensation claims, and depression

SIGNS & SYMPTOMS
Signs
- Limitation of all spinal movements due to pain
- Lateral scoliosis may be present due to spasm of the paraspinal muscles on one side
- Points of localized tenderness may be detected
- Severe limitation of straight leg raising, more pronounced on the affected side. (The leg is raised passively by the examiner with the knee extended. This is normally pain free until at least 70 degrees)
- Positive sciatic stretch test (passive dorsiflexion of the foot while performing straight leg raising reproduces the patient's pain)
- The patient may have dermatomal sensory changes
- Motor weakness due to nerve root compression
- Distended bladder due to urinary retention, saddle anesthesia, and a lax anal sphincter indicate cauda equina syndrome. **This is a surgical emergency (although not that common)**

Symptoms
- Pain in the lumbosacral region
- It is usually in the midline or just off the midline
- The pain may radiate into the buttock, groin, or posterior aspect of the thigh – often described as sciatica as this is the general course of the sciatic nerve
- Often follows an episode of bending, twisting, and lifting
- May have been preceded by a period of aching and stiffness in the back that lasted a few days
- Often associated with numbness and parasthesia in one of the lower limbs

ASSOCIATED DISORDERS
Obesity and depression are often associated with chronic low back pain.

KEY! DON'T MISS!
- A full general examination must be performed seeking a systemic cause for the back pain, e.g. leaking abdominal aortic aneurysm, psoriatic lesions, primary malignant lesion, source of infection, etc
- A full neurological examination of the lower limbs and the perineum must be done looking for evidence of neurological deficit

CONSIDER CONSULT
Referral is required:
- When there is significant neurological deficit or evidence of cauda equina compression
- If the back pain might be due to a serious illness, e.g. malignancy or infection

INVESTIGATION OF THE PATIENT

Direct questions to patient

Q Have you had any serious illness in the past (such as cancer or tuberculosis)? Bony metastases and spinal TB can be the cause of persistent unremitting back pain

Q Have you had a fever recently? Be aware that a bony infection will not always result in pyrexia

Q Have you had any burning, discomfort, or difficulty passing your urine? Dysuria will indicate the possible source of the primary infection, whereas hesitancy and retention could indicate cauda equina compression (although not that common)

Q Have you lost any weight? Another indication of a possible malignant etiology for the back pain

Q Do you have any numb areas in the lower limbs or groin? Areas of sensory disturbance may be indicative of spinal cord or nerve root compression

Q Are you on anticoagulants (blood thinning medications)? Patients who are at risk of bleeding spontaneously may present with back pain from an epidural hematoma

Contributory or predisposing factors

Q What is your job? People who are employed to perform heavy manual labor have a higher incidence of low back pain. There is an exceptionally high incidence amongst nursing auxiliaries, construction workers, garbage collectors, and truck drivers. Job dissatisfaction and monotony have also been implicated

Q Do you smoke? Smoking has been implicated as a risk factor in low back pain. Possible explanations include impaired blood supply to the involved spinal segment, increased coughing or smokers' associated lifestyle and behavior

Family history

There is no reported familial association for back pain.

Examination

Q Is there any abnormality on examination of the abdomen? Abdominal pathology such as abdominal aortic aneurysm must be excluded as the cause of the back pain. A distended bladder due to urinary retention may also be noted on abdominal examination

Q Is there significant neurological deficit? Significant weakness, extensive sensory changes, and decreased anal tone are all indications for urgent referral

Q Is the patient febrile? But be aware that not all patients with spinal osteomyelitis will be pyrexial

Summary of investigative tests

- Full blood count and ESR. The ESR will be elevated in most serious conditions that can present with backache. This test is not ordered on the first visit or when cause of backache is obvious

- Plain X-rays. Not indicated for the majority of cases. Cannot be justified in the absence of 'red flags' unless the condition fails to respond to appropriate treatment for several weeks. In these cases, more sophisticated investigations are required

- Computed tomography (CT) scan. Will reveal bony changes, but without intrathecal contrast will not adequately image the spinal cord and nerve roots; falsely negative in about 10% of cases of spinal stenosis. Not ordered for obvious mechanical injury

- Magnetic resonance imaging (MRI). The investigation of choice for suspected disc prolapse, cord, cauda equina or nerve root compression, spinal canal stenosis, and most of the other conditions that present as back pain

- Isotope bone scan. For suspected bony metastases

- Nerve conduction studies. Not routinely performed for back pain, but may be of benefit when investigating some patients who present with a neurological deficit in the lower limbs

DIAGNOSTIC DECISION

It is imperative to exclude serious causes of back pain before embarking on treatment. The following key signs should be looked out for:

From the history:
- History of cancer
- Predisposition to hemorrhage or infection, especially chronic urinary tract infection
- Weight loss
- Recent onset of pain in an older patient

From the present complaint:
- Radiation to below the knee
- Writhing pain, or pain that is not relieved by rest and is worse at night
- Involvement of more than one nerve root
- Perianal sensory changes
- Change in bladder or bowel function
- Significant lower limb weakness
- Worsening neurological deficit

From the physical examination:
- Pulsatile abdominal mass
- Fever

From the preliminary investigations:
- Elevated erythrocyte sedimentation rate

Other:
- Symptoms not compatible with benign mechanical disease
- Lack of response to appropriate medical treatment

Guidelines

The following guidelines are available at the National Guidelines Clearinghouse.
- American Academy of Orthopaedic Surgeons and the North American Spine Society: Clinical guideline on low back pain. [1]
- The Institute for Clinical Sytems Improvement: Adult low back pain. [2]
- The Veterans Health Administration. Low back pain or sciatica in the primary care setting. [3]

CLINICAL PEARLS

- Radicular pain radiates to below the knee
- Spinal stenosis should be suspected when pain with extension is relieved with flexion ('shopping cart' sign)
- Inflammatory spinal disorders present with insidious symptoms in individuals younger than 40 and morning stiffness
- Weight loss, fever, and nocturnal pain are 'red flags' for a serious cause of back pain

THE TESTS
Body fluids
FULL BLOOD COUNT AND ERYTHROCYTE SEDIMENTATION RATE
Description
Indicated if there is any suspicion that the condition is not 'simple benign' low back pain.

Advantages/Disadvantages
- **Advantages:** simple, straightforward & routine investigation
- **Disadvantages:** invasive procedure

Normal
- Leukocytes 4.5–10.5 x 10^9/L
- Hb: Women, 12–16g/dL; Men, 13–18g/dL
- Platelets: 130–400 x 10^9/L
- ESR: Men under 50, 0–15mm/h; women under 50, 0–20mm/h; Men over 50, 0–20mm/h; Women over 50, 0–30mm/h

Abnormal
- Results outside normal range
- Keep in mind the possibility of a false-positive result

Cause of abnormal result
- A raised white cell count is suggestive of infection
- A low Hb may be a manifestation of malignant disease
- Pancytopenia may be due to bone marrow infiltration
- A raised ESR may be due to malignancy, infection or rheumatological disease

Imaging
PLAIN X-RAYS
Advantages/Disadvantages
Advantage: very basic, relatively cheap and widely available

Disadvantages:
- Involves exposure to ionizing radiation
- Can be normal in many serious conditions
- Abnormalities such as osteoarthritis and degenerative disc disease are frequently present, and may not correlate with symptoms

Normal
- Preservation of disc height
- No evidence of bony erosion, destruction or osteosclerosis
- No evidence of spondylolisthesis

Abnormal
- Loss of disc height
- Areas of bony destruction, collapse, or osteosclerosis
- Spondylolisthesis
- Keep in mind the possibility of a false-positive result

Cause of abnormal result
- Loss of disc height is suggestive of current or previous disc disease
- Bony destruction is usually a sign of metastatic bony disease
- Compression fractures of the vertebral body may be due to or metastatic bony disease
- Spondylolisthesis may be congenital or acquired and is best seen in oblique views

Drugs, disorders and other factors that may alter results
Fecal loading of the bowel may obscure relevant findings in the lumbosacral spine.

COMPUTED TOMOGRAPHY (CT) SCAN
Advantages/Disadvantages
Advantages:
- More informative than plain X-rays
- Provides good information about the bony elements of the spine

Disadvantages:

- Involves the use of ionizing radiation
- Information obtained regarding the soft tissues may be insufficient
- Less informative than magnetic resonance scan
- May be inadequate in imaging the spinal cord and nerve roots without the presence of intrathecal contrast

Normal

- No evidence of bony destruction
- The integrity and dimensions of the spinal canal are maintained

The neural exit foramina are patent and there is no impingement of the nerve roots by disc material or any other elements

Abnormal

- Areas of bony destruction
- Vertebral body collapse
- The spinal canal is narrowed in spinal stenosis
- The exiting nerve roots are compressed by disc material
- Keep in mind the possibility of a false-positive result

Cause of abnormal result

- Bony destruction may be due to metastatic disease
- Compression fractures may be traumatic, pathological, or due to osteoporosis
- Facet joint hypertrophy may result in spinal canal stenosis
- A prolapsed lumbar disc can impinge an exiting nerve root or the cauda equina

Drugs, disorders and other factors that may alter results

Metal prostheses will produce artifacts that will affect the quality of the images. This can make it difficult to interpret the scan results.

MAGNETIC RESONANCE IMAGING (MRI)

Advantages/Disadvantages

Advantages:

- Produces superb quality images with excellent detailed information
- Outstanding diagnostic tool for soft tissue disease

Disadvantages:

- Expensive, time consuming and not available in some settings
- Does not produce detailed information about the bony elements
- Patients need to lie still in an enclosed space for about 40 min. Some claustrophobic individuals, or those in severe pain may be unable to tolerate this
- It is not possible to perform the test on some patients who have metallic implants and those with pacemakers

Normal

- No evidence of cord or nerve root compression
- The integrity and dimensions of the spinal canal are maintained
- The neural exit foramina are patent and there is no impingement of the nerve roots by disc material or any other elements

Abnormal

- Cord or cauda equina compression by a soft tissue lesion

- Abnormal signal from bony structures with or without bony collapse
- The spinal canal is narrowed in spinal stenosis
- The exiting nerve roots are compressed by disc material or a soft tissue lesion
- Keep in mind the possibility of a false-positive result

Cause of abnormal result
- Metastatic lesions can cause bone destruction, pathological fractures and vertebral collapse. Cord or cauda equina compression may result from the mass effect of the neoplastic lesion or as a result of the compromise of the structural integrity of the spine
- Cord or cauda equina compression may also be caused by a hematoma, an abscess or any other space-occupying lesion impinging on the neural elements
- Facet joint hypertrophy may result in spinal canal stenosis
- A lumbar prolapsed disc can impinge on an exiting nerve root or the cauda equina

Drugs, disorders and other factors that may alter results
Some prostheses will produce artifacts that will affect the quality of the images. This can make it difficult to interpret the scan results.

ISOTOPE BONE SCAN
Advantages/Disadvantages
Advantages:
- Sensitive for the detection of infection or malignancy
- Can be used to localize lesions for biopsy or excision
- Three-phase technique can be used to study inflammatory diseases such as osteomyelitis

Disadvantage: findings on bone scan are very nonspecific

Normal
Symmetric, homogeneous distribution of activity throughout skeleton.

Abnormal
- Localized areas of high activity relating to increased metabolic activity
- Keep in mind the possibility of a false-positive result

Cause of abnormal result
- Bony metastases
- Inflammatory lesions

Drugs, disorders and other factors that may alter results
Other recent nuclear medical procedures may lead to anomalous results.

Special tests
NERVE CONDUCTION STUDIES
Description
- Not routinely performed for back pain
- May be of benefit when investigating patients who present with a neurological deficit in the lower limbs

Advantages/Disadvantages
Advantage: can help to differentiate between a neurological deficit due to nerve root compression and other conditions such as a diabetic peripheral neuropathy

Disadvantages:
- Time-consuming, invasive, and expensive
- Not always very helpful

Normal
Motor and sensory latencies unaffected.

Abnormal
- Delayed conduction in the affected nerves
- Keep in mind the possibility of a false-positive result

Cause of abnormal result
- Nerve root compression
- Peripheral neuropathy
- Any other neurological condition that affects nerve conduction

Drugs, disorders and other factors that may alter results
The results of nerve conduction studies can be very difficult to interpret in patients with nerve root compression superimposed on an underlying peripheral neuropathy or any other chronic neurological condition.

TREATMENT

CONSIDER CONSULT
If the symptoms persist after several weeks of adequate treatment, referral is necessary.

IMMEDIATE ACTION
Cauda equina compression, cord compression, and significant neurological deficit are surgical emergencies and should be referred immediately.

PATIENT AND CAREGIVER ISSUES
Patient or caregiver request
- **Will I need an operation?** Only about 1% of patients who present with back patient will require surgery. The symptoms will resolve in more than 90% of patients within a month
- **How long must I be confined to bed?** Studies have shown that there is no benefit from restricting patients to bed for more than 48 h. Prolonged bed rest can predispose to serious consequences such as pulmonary embolus, osteoporosis, and muscle wasting
- **Will I become addicted to pain medications?** Pain medications will be given in adequate doses to relieve pain and encourage early mobilization. Muscles relaxants are tried in case of severe spasm to encourage early healing of injured muscles

Health-seeking behavior
- **Are you working and does your job entail heavy lifting?** Predisposing factors may need to be eliminated in order for the symptoms to settle
- **Are your symptoms as a result of an injury and is there a claim pending for compensation?** Studies have shown that in back pain (as in whiplash injury) symptoms often persist until compensation issues have been resolved

MANAGEMENT ISSUES
Goals
- Patients are screened for potentially serious conditions
- Investigations are requested only when indicated
- Patients with evidence or cord compression, cauda equina compression (not that common), and significant neurological deficit are referred urgently
- The majority of the remaining patients can safely be treated symptomatically until their symptoms resolve

Management in special circumstances
- Patients whose back pain may be due to incorrect lifting and handling techniques can be helped by being 're-educated' when they are referred for a course of physical therapy
- Patients who are likely to develop chronic low back pain (symptoms persisting for more than 12 weeks) will benefit from early referral to a pain clinic

COEXISTING DISEASE
Patients with known cancer who present with back pain should be investigated fully to exclude metastasis to the spine as the cause of their back pain.

PATIENT SATISFACTION/LIFESTYLE PRIORITIES
- Patients may have to consider changing their occupation if it involves heavy lifting
- If there are numerous factors predisposing to chronic low back pain, then early referral to a pain clinic is advisable

SUMMARY OF THERAPEUTIC OPTIONS
Choices

- Analgesics/nonsteroidal anti-inflammatory drugs (NSAIDs) such as acetaminophen, ibuprofen, and diclofenac help to alleviate back pain and reduce swelling in inflamed tissues. Most authorities promote the use of narcotic analgesics and delay the use of NSAIDs up to 48 h until the swelling of muscle goes down
- Physical therapy can be used to alleviate pain and restore function (not encouraged in the early phase of injury)
- Occupational therapy can help the patient regain lost function and prevent further deterioration
- Lumbar microdiscectomy/laminectomy/spinal stabilization are useful in specific indications
- Acupuncture may be useful as adjunctive treatment for low back pain
- Massage appears to have some efficacy in the treatment of low back pain, but very few methodologically sound trials have been published and more research is needed
- Many patients frequently seek help from chiropractors and find the therapy quite acceptable
- Percutaneous arthroscopic discectomy is an experimental therapy for the treatment of a prolapsed intervertebral disc
- Local and epidural injections may alleviate symptoms
- Address relevant lifestyle issues

Guidelines

The following guidelines are available at the National Guidelines Clearinghouse.

- American Academy of Orthopaedic Surgeons and the North American Spine Society [1]
- The Institute for Clinical Systems Improvement [2]
- The Veterans Health Administration [3]

Clinical pearls

- 'Myoanalgesics' such as cyclobenzaprine and methocarbamol are often of benefit for soft tissue back pain
- Surgical treatment for radiculopathy or spinal stenosis is more likely to bring relief of lower extremity pain than back pain
- Symptoms in a patient with job dissatisfaction or pending litigation are unlikely to improve

Never

Never start treatment without investigating further if there is a possibility of the back pain being caused by a potentially serious condition.

FOLLOW UP

Patients who present with back pain must be followed up regularly.

Plan for review

The patient must be reviewed within 12 weeks to ensure that their symptoms have resolved. Those that are still in pain after this period of time in spite of adequate treatment must be investigated further and/or referred on.

Information for patient or caregiver

- Predisposing factors must be addressed, e.g. heavy lifting, obesity
- Exercise is helpful to improve fitness and strengthen the back muscles
- Smoking is a risk factor in back pain

DRUGS AND OTHER THERAPIES: DETAILS
Drugs
ACETAMINOPHEN
Dose
Up to 1g four times daily.

Efficacy
Effective in reducing back pain.

Risks/Benefits
Risks:
- Caution in hepatic and renal impairment
- Overdosage results in hepatic and renal damage unless treated promptly

Benefits: reduces fever and malaise

Side-effects and adverse reactions
Acetaminophen rarely causes side-effects when used intermittantly.

Interactions (other drugs)
- Anticoagulants ■ Anticonvulsants ■ Isoniazid ■ Cholestyramine ■ Colestipol

Contraindications
No absolute contraindications are recorded.

Evidence
There is limited evidence for the use of acetaminophen in the treatment of back pain.
- Two RCTs found no significant difference in pain control when acetaminophen was compared to both meptazinol (an opioid) and diflunisal (an NSAID) for the treatment of acute back pain. A third RCT found that acetaminophen was more effective than mefenamic acid (an NSAID) [4] *Level P*
- A small RCT found acetaminophen was less likely to be rated as good or excellent for the relief of chronic back pain than diflunisal [4] *Level P*
- Another small RCT found that acetaminophen was less effective than electroacupuncture in the management of back pain after 6 weeks [4] *Level P*

Acceptability to patient
- Usually well tolerated by most patients
- Some patients may not consider this a valid treatment, as it is available over the counter

Follow up plan
Patients need to be reassessed regularly to ensure that they are improving.

Patient and caregiver information
Patients need to be informed that this is a safe and very effective pain killer. They should be warned that the maximal daily dose must not be exceeded and that it must not be combined with any other 'over-the-counter' analgesic agent that also contains acetaminophen.

IBUPROFEN
Dose
200–800mg three times a day.

Efficacy
Effective at reducing pain and inflammation.

Risks/Benefits
Risk: use caution in hepatic, renal and cardiac failure

Benefits:
- Faster onset of action than colchicines
- Inexpensive

Side-effects and adverse reactions
- Gastrointestinal: anorexia, nausea, dyspepsia, peptic ulceration
- Central nervous system: headache, dizziness, tinnitus
- Hypersensitivity: rashes, bronchospasm, angioedema

Interactions (other drugs)
- Aminoglycosides ▪ Antihypertensives ▪ Corticosteroids ▪ Cyclosporin ▪ Digoxin ▪ Lithium ▪ Methotrexate ▪ Phenylpropanolamine ▪ Diuretics ▪ Warfarin

Contraindications
- Peptic ulceration ▪ Hypersensitivity to NSAIDs ▪ Coagulation defects

Evidence
There is evidence that NSAIDs are effective for the treatment of back pain.
- Multiple RCTs have shown that NSAIDs are more effective than placebo in the management of acute back pain. More people experienced improvement and a decreased need for additional analgesics with NSAIDs [4] *Level M*
- Multiple RCTs found no significant difference in efficacy between different NSAIDs for the management of acute and chronic back pain [4] *Level M*
- There was no evidence from four RCTs that NSAIDs are effective for sciatica [4] *Level P*
- A systematic review found that NSAIDs were effective for short-term symptomatic relief from acute back pain. There is conflicting evidence that NSAIDs are more effective than acetaminophen for acute low back pain. There is a lack of evidence for NSAIDs in chronic back pain [5] *Level M*
- A RCT found naproxen to be more effective than placebo for the treatment of chronic low back pain. The same RCT found no significant difference in pain relief between diflunisal and placebo [4] *Level P*

Acceptability to patient
Some patients are unable to tolerate NSAIDs.

Follow up plan
Patients need to be seen regularly to ensure that they are responding to treatment.

Patient and caregiver information
Patients should be advised to take the medication after meals to minimize gastrointestinal side-effects.

DICLOFENAC
Diclofenac sodium.

Dose
25–50mg two or three times a day.

Efficacy
Effective in decreasing pain and swelling in soft tissues.

Risks/Benefits
- Risk: use caution in hepatic, renal and cardiac failure, porphyria
- Benefit: faster onset of action than colchicines

Side-effects and adverse reactions
- Gastrointestinal: anorexia, nausea, dyspepsia, peptic ulceration
- Central nervous system: headache, dizziness, tinnitus
- Hypersensitivity: rashes, bronchospasm, angioedema
- Thrombocytopenia

Interactions (other drugs)
- **Aminoglycosides** · **Antihypertensives** · **Corticosteroids** · **Cyclosporin** · **Digoxin** · **Lithium** · **Methotrexate** · **Phenylpropanolamine** · **Diuretics** · **Warfarin**

Contraindications
- **Peptic ulcer** · **Hypersensitivity to NSAIDs** · **Coagulation defects**

Evidence
There is evidence that NSAIDs are effective for the treatment of back pain.
- Multiple RCTs have shown that NSAIDs are more effective than placebo in the management of acute back pain. More people experienced improvement and a decreased need for additional analgesics with NSAIDs [4] *Level M*
- Multiple RCTs found no significant difference in efficacy between different NSAIDs for the management of acute and chronic back pain [4] *Level M*
- There was no evidence from four RCTs that NSAIDs are effective for sciatica [4] *Level P*
- A systematic review found that NSAIDs were effective for short-term symptomatic relief from acute back pain. There is conflicting evidence that NSAIDs are more effective than acetaminophen for acute low back pain. There is a lack of evidence for NSAIDs in chronic back pain [5] *Level M*
- A RCT found naproxen to be more effective than placebo for the treatment of chronic low back pain. The same RCT found no significant difference in pain relief between diflunisal and placebo [4] *Level P*

Acceptability to patient
Some patients are unable to tolerate NSAIDs.

Follow up plan
Patients need to be seen regularly to ensure that they are responding to treatment.

Patient and caregiver information
Patients should be advised to take the medication after meals to minimize its gastrointestinal side-effects.

Physical therapy
A brief period of bed rest is recommended initially to overcome the severe pain of the acute phase. Clinical trials have shown that there is no benefit from extending the period of bed rest beyond 48 h. This should be followed by active exercise.

PHYSICAL THERAPY TO ALLEVIATE PAIN AND RESTORE FUNCTION
The aim is to alleviate pain, restore function, teach and train the patient to compensate for deteriorated function, and, if possible, prevent further deterioration and recurrence.

Efficacy
Studies have shown that an exercise regimen commencing after 6 weeks will yield a superior clinical outcome compared to other forms of treatment.

Risks/Benefits
- Risk: some patients may find it difficult to participate in active exercises while they have ongoing back pain

- Benefit: will diminish the risk of recurrence and reduce the total period of incapacity

Evidence
There is evidence that exercise therapy is effective for chronic back pain.
- A systematic review found no evidence for the benefit of specific exercises in the treatment of acute back pain. Patients with chronic low back pain may benefit from exercise, and be able to increase normal daily activities and return to work [6] *Level M*
- Specific back exercises were compared to conservative treatments in the management of acute back pain in eight RCTs. Back pain was not found to be superior to conservative therapy, and exercise mildy increased pain and disability in seven of the trials. The other RCT found that exercises were more effective than back school [4] *Level M*
- Three systematic reviews found that exercises were more effective than conservative treatments in the short term for the management of pain, disability and physical outcomes in patients with chronic back pain. The effect sizes were small [4] *Level M*

Acceptability to patient
Some patients may be reluctant to participate in active exercises while they have ongoing back pain. They need to be informed that active exercise is likely to decrease their overall pain, improve their fitness, and increase their likelihood of returning to gainful employment.

Follow up plan
Patients need to be reassessed regularly to ensure that they are responding to treatment.

Patient and caregiver information
Patients need to be informed that studies have repeatedly shown that inactivity is detrimental and that symptoms can be significantly improved with physical therapy.

Occupational therapy
An occupational therapist may need to be involved along with the physiotherapist in re-educating the patient on lifting techniques and other maneuvers in order to minimize the risk of symptom recurrence.

In some chronic cases, certain aids may need to be provided to minimize the amount of bending and twisting that the patient performs.

OCCUPATIONAL THERAPY TO MINIMIZE RECURRENCE
Can be provided as part of a package of measures available at a specialized back pain rehabilitation center.

Efficacy
Can help the patient regain lost function and prevent further deterioration.

Risks/Benefits
- Risk: none

- **Benefit:** can help the patients to cope with their daily activities and may enable them to return to gainful employment

Acceptability to patient
Some patients might find it difficult to accept their need to use 'aids' that are usually associated with permanent disability.

Follow up plan
The patient needs to be reassessed fairly regularly to ensure that they are coping well and that no new features have revealed themselves.

Patient and caregiver information
The patient needs to be informed that these new techniques should be adhered to for life in order to decrease the risk of symptom recurrence.

Surgical therapy

The number of patients undergoing surgery for low back pain in the Western world varies immensely from country to country. The number of spinal surgical procedures performed per head of population is much higher in the US than it is in Western Europe. These marked differences are attributed to the different style of health care funding provided in these societies.

Overall, only about 1% of patients presenting with back pain need spinal surgery.

LUMBAR MICRODISCECTOMY/LAMINECTOMY/SPINAL STABILIZATION

A number of different surgical procedures have been recommended to deal with the variety of underlying conditions causing the back pain:

- Lumbar microdiscectomy is the surgical procedure usually undertaken to deal with a unilateral prolapsed disc at a single level
- Lumbar laminectomy is used to widen a narrowed canal in conditions such as spinal stenosis
- Spinal stabilization is undertaken when the cause of the back pain is thought to be due to abnormal spinal movement, e.g. in spondylolisthesis

Efficacy
- When performed for the appropriate indication, good results are reported with spinal surgery. However, the large number of patients with persistent or worse symptoms after surgery is a reflection of the inappropriate choice of patient for surgery
- Up to 25% of asymptomatic persons have been shown to have some degree of disc prolapse on routine imaging. Operating on a patient with back pain where there is a strong psychogenic element and an incidentally found prolapsed disc will not improve their symptoms
- In order to obtain good results, surgery should be offered only to those patients who have definite clinical findings that correlate with the evidence seen on their scans

Risks/Benefits
Risks:
- Persistence of symptoms and failure to improve after surgery
- Nerve root injury with subsequent areas of parasthesia or motor deficit
- Hemorrhage
- Postoperative infection

Benefits: may relieve the patient's symptoms

Acceptability to patient
Some patients may be reluctant to undergo spinal surgery. Others may be too unfit medically to receive a general anesthetic.

Follow up plan
Patients should be seen at least once postoperatively to ensure that their wound has healed nicely, that there is no evidence of postoperative infection, and that their symptoms have improved.

Patient and caregiver information
Patients should be informed that all surgery results in postoperative fibrous tissue formation, and that there will be some degree of stiffness even after successful surgery.

Complementary therapy
ACUPUNCTURE
Efficacy
Acupuncture was shown to be superior to control interventions in a meta-analysis published in 1998. A consensus statement by the NIH in 1997 reviewed the world literature on uses for acupuncture and concluded that acupuncture may be useful as adjunctive treatment for a variety of conditions, specifically including low back pain.

Risks/Benefits
Risks:
- The risks of acupuncture are minimal, but include local hematoma at the needle insertion site
- Reports of pneumothorax when needles are used in the chest area are extremely rare
- Patients may experience an exacerbation of pain when first beginning acupuncture therapy

Benefits:
- Relief of pain and of other symptoms
- Balancing of 'qi' (vital life force), which can result in an improved sense of well-being

Evidence
- A meta-analysis found that acupuncture was superior to control interventions for the treatment of back pain, but there was insufficient evidence that acupuncture was more effective than placebo [7] *Level M*
- Another systematic review did not find evidence that acupuncture is effective for the treatment of back pain [8] *Level M*
- Acupuncture may be useful as an adjunct treatment, or an alternative treatment in the management of low back pain [9] *Level C*

Acceptability to patient
Acupuncture is generally well accepted when procedure is well explained. Some patients are unable to lie on a table for the 20–45min usually required for a treatment.

Follow up plan
Patients should be monitored for response to therapy, signs of new neurologic symptoms, and worsening/changing symptoms that might indicate new or more serious pathology.

Patient and caregiver information
Acupuncture is more commonly a process, than a one-off insertion of needles. In general, the more acute the problem, the fewer the treatments required. Patients should always be evaluated individually; different needle patterns are used for different low back pain scenarios.

MASSAGE THERAPY
Efficacy
Massage appears to have some efficacy in the treatment of low back pain, but very few methodologically sound trials have been published and more research is needed.

Risks/Benefits
There are few risks to massage therapy, unless structural instability pre-exists in the patient. Patients should, however, undergo thorough medical evaluation before massage therapy is begun.

Evidence
Two systematic reviews found no difference in pain, functional status, or mobility when massage was compared with spinal manipulation or electrical stimulation in the management of acute back pain. There is conflicting evidence regarding the use of massage in chronic back pain [10,11] *Level M*

Acceptability to patient
Massage is usually well accepted. Massage tends to feel good, and there are the added benefits of muscle relaxation and an hour of quiet in a relaxing environment. Some people are uncomfortable disrobing for a therapist.

Follow up plan
Regular contact with medical personnel to monitor the response to therapy.

Patient and caregiver information
Acute low back pain patients should expect a course of regular massage therapy – possibly 1–2 sessions per week for 2–3 weeks. Cases of chronic or recurrent low back pain may, however, need to use massage therapy intermittently.

CHIROPRACTIC
Risks/Benefits
Risk: manipulation in the setting of structural instability would be unwise

Evidence
There is conflicting evidence for spinal manipulation in acute and chronic back pain.
- Multiple RCTs found conflicting results when manipulation was compared with placebo in the management of acute back pain [4] *Level M*
- Three systematic reviews found conflicting results on the efficacy of spinal manipulation for chronic back pain [4] *Level M*
- Another systematic review found that spinal manipulation was slightly more effective than placebo for the treatment of chronic back pain [12] *Level M*
- A retrospective, outcome-based analysis of patients with uncomplicated mechanical neck or lower back pain found that chiropractic spinal manipulation significantly reduced disability and pain scores [13] *Level S*

Acceptability to patient
Some patients are reluctant to visit chiropractors, for a variety of reasons. Many, though, frequently seek help from chiropractors and find the therapy quite acceptable.

Follow up plan
Patients should be followed for their response to therapy. Any change in symptoms or development of new symptoms, indicating the need for further evaluation or another course of therapy, should be attended to promptly.

Patient and caregiver information
Patients should be advised to contact their physician if any worsening of or change in symptoms occurs while they are receiving chiropractic treatment. Physicians and chiropractors are encouraged to communicate with one another about a given patient's condition and response to therapy.

Endoscopic therapy

Percutaneous arthroscopic discectomies have been advocated. This technique must still be considered experimental at present.

PERCUTANEOUS ARTHROSCOPIC DISCECTOMY
The procedure is performed endoscopically through a trocar that is inserted endoscopically.

Efficacy
The benefits of this technique have yet to be proven.

Risks/Benefits
Risks:
- Inadequate exposure
- Inability to achieve adequate decompression endoscopically

Benefits:
- Small incision
- Minimal postoperative scarring

Acceptability to patient
The patients may not be keen to undergo an 'experimental' procedure. On the other hand, they may want to have 'minimally invasive' surgery.

Follow up plan
The patient must be reassessed postoperatively to ensure that symptoms have subsided.

Patient and caregiver information
The patients must be informed that this is still a novel procedure and that the results cannot be compared at present with the tried and tested standard surgical procedures advocated for back pain due to prolapsed intervertebral discs.

Other therapies
LOCAL AND EPIDURAL INJECTIONS
Local anesthetic, often combined with steroids, is injected into trigger points or into the epidural space.

Efficacy
Good results have been obtained in a significant number of patients.

Risks/Benefits
Risks:
- Nonresolution or worsening of symptoms
- Inadvertent intrathecal injection of anesthetic agents with possible disastrous consequences (very rare)

Benefits: may alleviate the patient's symptoms

Evidence
Epidural steroid injections may be effective for patients with acute back pain and sciatica. There is conflicting evidence for the efficacy of steroid injections in chronic back pain.
- Several systematic reviews have identified 2 RCTs on the use of epidural steroid injections for acute back pain. One RCT found that epidural steroids are not more effective than subcutaneous lidocaine for pain relief at one month in patients with back pain and sciatica. At

3 months, more patients receiving epidural steroids were pain free [4] *Level P*
- The other RCT found that epidural steroids were no more effective than epidural saline, epidural bupivicane or dry needling [4] *Level P*
- Several systematic reviews found limited and conflicting evidence on the efficacy of epidural steroid injections for chronic back pain [4] *Level M*

Trigger point injections may be effective for chronic back pain.
- A systematic review included one RCT assessing trigger point injections in people with chronic back pain. Steroid plus lidocaine injections were effective in achieving complete pain relief for more people at 3 months compared with lidocaine alone [4] *Level P*

Acceptability to patient
Some patients may be very reluctant to submit to treatment, which involves injections in the vicinity of their spine.

Follow up plan
Regular follow up is recommended to ensure response to treatment.

Patient and caregiver information
Patients need to be informed that the procedure may need to be repeated in order to obtain a sustained response.

LIFESTYLE
The patient's occupation, sporting activities, or lifestyle may be contributing to their back pain. Jobs involving heavy lifting, operating vibrating machinery and driving are associated with recurrent episodes of back pain. Job dissatisfaction is also thought to be a significant predisposing factor.

Risks/Benefits
- Risk: the patient's livelihood may depend on the activity that is contributing to or causing the symptoms

- Benefit: minimizing the predisposing factors may alleviate the patient's symptoms and reduce the likelihood of recurrence

ACCEPTABILITY TO PATIENT
The patient may be unable to give up his/her job even though it is likely to be a significant factor contributing to their condition.

FOLLOW UP PLAN
Reassess the patient to ensure that lifestyle alterations have led to an improvement in the patient's condition.

PATIENT AND CAREGIVER INFORMATION
The patient needs to be informed that their symptoms are likely to persist or recur if they continue to engage in heavy lifting and other activities that are known to predispose to low back pain.

EFFICACY OF THERAPIES

Full recovery occurs in over 90% of cases regardless of type of treatment undertaken.

Evidence

- Multiple RCTs have shown that NSAIDs are more effective than placebo in the management of acute back pain [4] *Level M*
- A systematic review found that NSAIDs were effective for short-term symptomatic relief from acute back pain. There is conflicting evidence that NSAIDs are more effective than acetaminophen for acute low back pain. There is a lack of evidence for NSAIDs in chronic back pain [5] *Level M*
- A systematic review found no evidence for the benefit of specific exercises in the treatment of acute back pain. Patients with chronic low back pain may benefit from exercise, and be able to increase normal daily activities and return to work [6] *Level M*
- A systematic review included one RCT assessing trigger point injections in people with chronic back pain. Steroid plus lidocaine injections were more effective in achieving complete pain relief at 3 months, compared with lidocaine alone [4] *Level P*
- There is no evidence that bed rest, exercise, massage, traction or acupuncture are effective for the treatment of acute back pain [4]

Review period

Patients should be reviewed within 12 weeks. If symptoms persist beyond this period of time, they have by definition developed chronic low back pain.

PROGNOSIS

Over 90% of patients return to their baseline state within a month of the onset of their symptoms.

Clinical pearls

- Persistent neurological symptoms after surgery suggests that decompression might not have been adequate
- Patients with prolonged absence from work are unlikely to improve to the point that they are able to return
- Patients have to be asked early in the treatment what their expectations are concerning returning to work, if they consider workman compensation, or if there is a lawsuit pending. These factors have great implications for recovery and therapeutic alliance with the clinician

Therapeutic failure

The back pain will persist for over 12 weeks in about 7% of patients. These patients need to be investigated adequately and referred to a multidisciplinary pain clinic or similar facility for further management of their condition.

Recurrence

Patients who suffer from back pain are likely to have recurrent episodes. The triggering factors should be identified and avoided if possible. The patient may also need to be re-educated regarding lifting techniques and lifestyle adjustments such as increasing active exercise and weight loss may need to be undertaken.

Deterioration

The patient must be reassessed and investigated if necessary to ensure that there is no serious underlying condition causing the back pain. Patients with nonspecific chronic low back pain are best referred to a multidisciplinary pain clinic or similar facilities for further management of their symptoms.

COMPLICATIONS

If the symptoms fail to resolve within a few weeks, the patient may become fixated on their pain. Their functioning ability diminishes and they become less likely to return to work. This can progress to drug dependence (often to codeine-based analgesics) and depression.

RISK FACTORS
- Lifting heavy objects: leads to straining of the paraspinal muscles, especially if improper lifting techniques are used
- Obesity: increases the forces exerted on the weight-bearing joints
- Sedentary lifestyle and lack of exercise: reduces fitness and results in a weak musculature

MODIFY RISK FACTORS
Lifestyle and wellness
TOBACCO

Tobacco has been implicated as a risk factor in low back pain. Possible explanations include impaired blood supply to the involved spinal segment, increased coughing or smokers' associated lifestyle and behavior. Some spine surgeons believe that smoking is a risk factor for failure of a spine fusion.

ALCOHOL AND DRUGS

A statistical association has been confirmed between low back pain and alcohol consumption. The reason is probably due to the patient's associated lifestyle and behavior.

DIET

Obesity is a definite contributory factor to low back pain and steps should be taken to reduce weight.

PHYSICAL ACTIVITY

Patients should be encouraged to:
- Adjust lifting techniques
- Avoid a sedentary posture for prolonged periods of time
- Exercise regularly

CHEMOPROPHYLAXIS

There are some reports that early use of analgesics and/or NSAIDs at the earliest indication of an impending episode of low back pain may abort a prolonged period of incapacity. These claims have not been confirmed in controlled clinical trials.

PREVENT RECURRENCE
Patients should be 're-educated' on lifting techniques. This can often be incorporated into a comprehensive physical therapy program.

Reassess coexisting disease
Prolonged periods of bed rest can exacerbate pre-existing back pain.

PATIENT SATISFACTION/LIFESTYLE PRIORITIES
- Most patients are very keen to get back to an active lifestyle, free from the burden of low back pain
- Some work and/or lifestyle adjustments may need to be implemented to prevent recurrence of symptoms
- Job dissatisfaction and other psychogenic factors have been implicated in long-standing nonspecific low back pain

RESOURCES

ASSOCIATIONS

American College of Rheumatology/Association of Rheumatology Health Professionals
1800 Century Place, Suite 205
Atlanta, GA 30345-4300
Tel: (404) 633 3777
Fax: (404) 633 1870
www.rheumatology.com

Arthritis Foundation
330 West Peachtree Street
Atlanta, GA
Tel: (800) 283 7800
www.arthritis.org

Canadian Arthritis Network
600 University Avenue, Suite 600
Toronto, Ontario, M5G 1X5
Canada
Tel: (416) 586 4770
Fax: (416) 586 8628
www.arthritis.ca

KEY REFERENCES

- Fauci AS, Braunwald E, Isselbacher KJ, et al. Harrison's Principles of Internal Medicine Companion Handbook, 14th Ed (1998) New York: McGraw Hill
- Maddison PJ, Isenberg DA, Woo P, Glass DN. Oxford Textbook of Rheumatology, 2nd Ed. (1998) Oxford: Oxford University Press
- Swenson R. Lower back pain – differential diagnosis. Neurol Clin 1999; 17:149–66

Evidence references and guidelines

1 American Academy of Orthopaedic Surgeons and the North American Spine Society: Clinical guideline on low back pain. Rosemont and LaGrange (IL): American Academy of Orthopaedic Surgeons, North American Spine Society, 1996.
2 The Institute for Clinical Systems Improvement: Adult low back pain. Guideline Oversight Group. Bloomington, MN: Institute for Clinical Systems Improvement, 1999
3 The Veterans Health Administration. Low back pain or sciatica in the primary care setting. Department of Veterans Affairs (U.S.), 1999
4 van Tulder M, Koes B. Low back pain and sciatica: musculoskeletal disorders. In: Clinical Evidence 2001;6:864–83. London: BMJ Publishing Group
5 van Tulder MW, Scholten RJPM, Koes BW, Deyp RA. Non-steroidal anti-inflammatory drugs for low back pain (Cochrane Review). In: The Cochrane Library, 1, 2002. Oxford: Update Software
6 van Tulder MW, Malmivaara A, Esmail R, Koes BW. Exercise therapy for low back pain (Cochrane Review). In: The Cochrane Library, 1, 2002. Oxford: Update Software
7 Ernst E, White AR. Acupuncture for back pain: a meta-analysis of randomized control trials. Arch Intern Med 1998;158:2235-41. Medline
8 van Tulder MW, Cherkin DC, Berman B, Lao L, Koes BW. Acupuncture for low back pain (Cochrane Review). In: The Cochrane Library, 1, 2002. Oxford: Update Software
9 Acupuncture. NIH Consensus Statement 1997;15:1-34.
10 Ernst E. Massage therapy for low back pain: a systematic review. J Pain Symptom Manage 1999;17:65-9. Reviewed in Clin Evidence 2001;6:864-83
11 Furlan AD, Brosseau L, Welch V, Wong J. Massage for low back pain (Cochrane Review). In: The Cochrane Library, 1, 2002. Oxford: Update Software

12 van Tulder MW, Koes BW, Bouter LM. Conservative treatment of acute and chronic nonspecific low back pain: a systematic review of randomized controlled trials of the most common interventions. Spine 1997;22:2128–56. Reviewed in: Clin Evidence 2001;6:864–83

13 McMorland G, Suter E. Chiropractic management of mechanical neck and low back pain: a retrospective, outcome-based analysis. J Manipulative Physiol Ther 2000;23:307-11. Medline

FAQS
Question 1
How can I differentiate between mechanical and inflammatory back pain?

ANSWER 1
The differentiation mainly lies in clinical history. The mechanical back pain is sudden in onset, usually associated with an inciting injury, peak prevalence is 40–59 years, worsens with activity and relieved on rest, usually lasts 1–3 weeks. Inflammatory back pain is insidious in onset, usually affects people in age group of 20–40 years, associated with morning stiffness, gets better with stretching and associated with systemic symptoms.

Question 2
How do you diagnose sciatica?

ANSWER 2
Sciatica is back pain that radiates down one leg below the knee and the character of the pain is sharp, lancinating, or burning and is suggestive of nerve root irritation and usually associated with lumbar spondylosis. Straight leg raising test detects irritation of the sciatic nerve (L4,5,S1). Pain is maximum between 30° and 70°. Symptoms at greater degrees of elevation are usually due to muscle strain. Dorsiflexion of affected foot usually increases the intensity of pain.

Question 3
Is there a role of low-dose antidepressants in treatment of chronic pain?

ANSWER 3
Tricyclic antidepressants have been used for treatment of chronic pain for patients with or without depression. Double-blinded studies have documented the role of tricyclics for relieving chronic pain. Use of low doses in the range of 10–25mg may be needed to control pain after confirming that the patient doesn't have any serious case of back pain. The drug may have to be continued for a number of weeks before the patient notes decrease in symptoms.

Question 4
In a patient who complains of prolonged morning stiffness, would ordering HLA-B27 help in diagnosing inflammatory arthropathies?

ANSWER 4
No. About 8% of the Caucasian population are HLA-B27 positive, but are unaffected by inflammatory arthropathy. HLA-B27 is confirmatory but not diagnostic. Plain radiographs of sacroiliac joints represent the initial investigation of choice, which may show erosions in the lower third of the joints.

Question 5
What are the indications for obtaining a lumbosacral radiograph in a patient with lower back pain?

ANSWER 5
Indications for obtaining a lumbosacral radiograph are:
- Unimproved or increasing symptoms, especially if lasting more than 1 month and not improved with therapy

- Back pain after significant trauma
- History, physical examination consistent with sacroiliitis
- Constitutional symptoms of fever and weight loss

CONTRIBUTORS

Martin Kabongo, MD, PhD
Richard Brasington Jr, MD, FACP
Jane L Murray, MD
Dinesh Khanna, MD

BEHÇET'S SYNDROME

SUMMARY INFORMATION

DESCRIPTION

- Rare, chronic multisystem disease
- Systemic vasculitis involving both arteries and veins with tendency to form thrombosis
- Painful oral aphthous ulcers
- Genital aphthous ulcers
- Ocular inflammation
- Arthritis
- Skin lesions
- Central nervous system involvement
- Relapsing and remitting course

URGENT ACTION

- Refer immediately if there are signs of eye disease (eye involvement can occasionally progress rapidly to blindness)
- Refer immediately if complications arise, such as meningitis or large vasculitis

KEY! DON'T MISS!

Eye involvement, vasculitis involving major organs, thrombosis/embolic disease: all of these complications require urgent intervention.

ICD9 CODE
136.1 Behçets syndrome.

SYNONYMS
- Behçets disease
- Occulo-oral-genital syndrome
- Aphthosis generalisata
- Malignant aphthosis
- Adamantiades-Behçets disease
- Morbus Behçets-Touraine

CARDINAL FEATURES
- Variable signs and symptoms that spontaneously resolve and recur
- Males and females are equally affected. Males tend to have more severe symptoms
- Most prevalent in people from the Mediterranean basin, Middle East, and Japan, although it may occur with any ethnicity
- Oral aphthous ulcers (>90% of cases)
- Genital aphthous ulcers (>70% cases), most commonly involving the scrotum and vulva
- Eye inflammation (>50% of cases) including anterior and posterior uveitis, optic neuritis, retinal vessel occlusion, conjunctivitis, and keratitis
- Skin lesions (50–80% of cases) including folliculitis, erythema nodosum, and pathergy
- Vasculitis that affects veins or arteries, with tendency toward formation of venous thrombosis
- Peripheral nondeforming, nonerosive, oligoarthritis (knee most commonly affected)
- Central nervous system involvement
- Major vessel thrombosis and aneurysm formation

CAUSES
Common causes
- Etiology is unknown; little is known about pathophysiology
- Basic pathologic mechanism appears to be a combination of cellular and humoral immune mechanisms, including deposition of circulating immune complexes in small vessels. Overall pathogenesis involves vasculitis of small and large arteries and veins
- Research is ongoing into possibility of infection with a slow virus or an altered response to a virus in a susceptible individual

Contributory or predisposing factors
There is a predisposition to the disease in people from the Mediterranean basin and Middle East, and Japan (the so-called Silk Route).

EPIDEMIOLOGY
Incidence and prevalence
Rare; there is little agreement on true incidence and prevalence.

INCIDENCE
No accurate estimates available.

PREVALENCE
- The highest prevalence is in Turkey: figures range from 80 to 300 per 100,000
- In Japan 10–15 per 100,000; however, Behçets disease is rare among Japanese Americans
- 0.2 per 100,000 in Western Europe and North America; the low rate may be a result of underdiagnosis and under-reporting

Demographics

AGE

- The majority of patients present between 15 and 45 years
- Very rare in children
- Age of onset at age under 25 years is associated with higher prevalence of eye disease and total clinical activity

GENDER

- Males and females affected equally, except in North America and Australia where females are in the majority
- Disease is more severe in males
- Males have greater chance of developing ocular disease, aneurysms, folliculitis, and probably neurologic disease
- Females are more likely to develop erythema nodosum

RACE

More prevalent in races native to the Middle East, the Mediterranean basin (particularly Turks), and Japan.

GENETICS

Associations with histocompatibility antigens:

- Strongly associated with HLA-B5 (in particular B51) in association with DR7 and DRw52
- HLA-B51 has been related to ocular lesions
- HLA-B12 has been related to mucocutaneous lesions

GEOGRAPHY

Occurs worldwide, but increased prevalence along the old Silk Road (based on Marco Polo's travels) stretching from Japan along the Middle Mediterranean basin and to Turkey.

DIFFERENTIAL DIAGNOSIS
Inflammatory bowel disease
FEATURES

- Bowel symptoms predominate (pain, diarrhea, sometimes bloody)
- Abdominal tenderness, mass or distension
- Erythrocyte sedimentation rate elevated
- Mouth ulcers, perianal and perirectal ulcers can occur (usually in Crohn's disease)
- Anterior eye inflammation, without posterior involvement
- Extraintestinal manifestations, joint swelling and tenderness, hepatosplenomegaly, erythema nodosum, clubbing

Stevens-Johnson syndrome
The severe form of erythema multiforme, can be fatal.

FEATURES

- As for erythema multiforme
- Fever and prostration
- Pneumonitis
- Renal failure
- Requires hospital admission

Pemphigoid
Uncommon autoimmune disease of the elderly; classically there are widespread bullae developing on areas of urticated erythema.

FEATURES

- Bullae
- Mucosal involvement rare
- More benign course than pemphigus

Pemphigus vulgaris
Chronic disease of unknown etiology that presents with intraepidermal blisters.

FEATURES

- Mainly affects middle-aged people (especially Jews)
- Onset insidious with widespread blisters rupturing to leave weeping erosions
- Nikolsky's sign present (firm pressure applied to normal skin with a shearing strain causes a blister)
- Mucous membranes of the mouth, eyes, anus, and genitalia commonly involved
- Treated with systemic steriods

Reiter's syndrome
A seronegative spondyloarthropathy associated with one or more of the following: urethritis or cervicitis, large joint inflammatory arthritis, sacroiliitis, dysentery, inflammation of the eye, or mucocutaneous lesions.

FEATURES

- Urethritis/cervicitis
- Asymmetric polyarthritis (commonly affecting knee and ankle)
- May occur after dysentery
- Inflammatory eye disease (uveitis or conjunctivitis)

- Hyperkeratotic lesions on soles of feet, toes, penis, hands (kerotoderma blennorrhagicum)
- Heel pain and Achilles' tendonitis/plantar fascitis

Recurrent aphthous ulceration

- Recurrent episodes of painful oral ulcers
- Also known as recurrent aphthous stomatitis (RAS)

FEATURES

- Most common oral mucosal disease in North America
- Ulcers can attain large sizes but are commonly up to 5mm across
- Not occurring in association with other connective tissue disorder

Erythema multiforme

- Erythema multiforme is an inflammatory disease that is believed to be secondary to immune complex formation and deposition in the skin and mucous membranes
- Can occur as a response to infection or drugs

FEATURES

- Target lesion is the hallmark, with a pallid or purple center surrounded by one or more rings
- Usually symmetric skin lesions
- Lesions most common on back of hands and feet and extensor aspect of the forearms and legs
- May appear as urticarial papules, pustules, vesicles, or bullae (hence called multiforme)
- Mucosa of eyes, mouth, and genitalia may be involved
- Lesions occur in crops and last 2–3 weeks (no scarring)
- Subsequent exposure to the presenting stimuli will provoke further attacks

Vogt-Koyanagi-Harada syndrome

- An idiopathic multisystem disorder that typically affects pigmented individuals
- Common in Japan

FEATURES

- Uveitis
- Alopecia occurs in about 60% of patients
- Poliosis (whitening of eyelashes)
- Vitiligo
- Neurologic features (meningeal irritation, encephalopathy, and auditory symptoms)

SIGNS & SYMPTOMS
Signs

- Oral aphthous ulcers (round, 2–10mm in diameter, central yellowish necrotic base, single or in crops)
- Genital ulcers; most commonly in males on the scrotum (may cause scarring) and most commonly in females on the vulva (may be painless)
- Epididymitis occurs in 5% of male patients, with pain and swelling of the scrotum
- Skin lesions (pustules, papules, folliculitis, erythema nodosum, ulcers, necrotic lesions consistent with cutaneous vasculitis, and pathergy)
- Joint signs include a nonerosive, nondeforming peripheral oligoarticular arthritis (knee most commonly involved)
- Eye signs (painful red eye, decreased acuity, occasionally hypopyon, cataract, conjunctivitis and keratitis, retinitis, retinal edema, necrosis and atrophy, and periphlebitis)
- Central nervous system signs (weakness and paresthesia, meningeal irritation, can mimic multiple sclerosis)

- Gastrointestinal signs (ulcerative lesions can occur anywhere in the gastrointestinal tract, causing abdominal tenderness and occasionally signs of perforation)
- Vascular: occlusion or aneurysm of large veins or arteries, thrombosis; vasculitis in other areas (e.g. thrombophlebitis, nail infarcts)

Symptoms

There is a wide range of symptoms, reflecting multisystem disease; symptoms may be chronic or intermittent:

- General: fatigue, lethargy, depression, fever, malaise, myalgia, and arthralgia
- Oral: painful aphthous ulcers in mouth
- Genital: painful genital ulcers (but vaginal ulcers may be painless)
- Ophthalmologic: painful eye, red eye with or without visual impairment
- Skin abnormalities: rashes, ulcers, folliculitis, and pathergy
- Gastrointestinal: diarrhea, abdominal pain, occasionally passage of mucus and blood in stools
- Neurologic: inability to focus, diplopia, numbness, paresthesia, paralysis or weakness, balance problems, difficulty walking, hearing loss, confusion, headache, and stiff neck
- Respiratory: chest pain, breathlessness, wheeze, hemoptysis

ASSOCIATED DISORDERS

- Inflammatory bowel disease: closely mimics Behçets disease
- Crohn's disease: virtually all the features of Behçets can be seen in patients with Crohn's disease. In Crohn's colitis, colonic resection has occasionally ameliorated the other features that mimic Behçets
- Relapsing polychondritis: some patients develop an overlap between Behçets and relapsing polychondritis, which has been designated the MAGIC (mouth and genital ulcers with inflamed cartilage) syndrome; may be associated with any other autoimmune disease

KEY! DON'T MISS!

Eye involvement, vasculitis involving major organs, thrombosis/embolic disease: all of these complications require urgent intervention.

CONSIDER CONSULT

Refer:

- To a rheumatologist for making the diagnosis of Behçets disease and advice on treatment. There are no serologic or pathologic tests that are diagnostic
- To an ophthalmologist immediately if eye involvement is suspected (loss of vision, perilimbal redness, pain), as eye involvement may progress rapidly to blindness
- Immediately if complications arise such as meningitis or vasculitis

INVESTIGATION OF THE PATIENT
Direct questions to patient

Q Do you or have you had any ulcers (oral and/or genital)? Recurrent oral and genital ulcers are cardinal features of Behçets disease, and virtually all patients have oral ulcers

Q Are you generally unwell and in what way (lethargy, fevers, etc.)? Although these symptoms are vague, they can help to identify inflammation and to suggest the frequency and severity of symptoms

Q What problems do you suffer with? Consider each symptom to determine whether they are linked

Q How often are these symptoms occurring and when did they first occur (e.g. for ulcers)?

Q What other diseases have you suffered from in the past and what are you suffering from at present? Perhaps the patient or previous health care professionals have misdiagnosed the patient, and this may provide a clue as the proper diagnosis

Q What prescribed medication are you taking? Allergies to certain types of drugs may cause skin lesions and ulcers that may mimic Behçets disease

Q Are you taking over-the-counter medicines or herbal remedies? These may mimic symptoms or interfere with future therapies

Q Do you/have you had any eye symptoms: pain, redness, blurring of vision etc? Eye inflammation occurs in >50% of cases and necessitates referral to an ophthalmologist

Q Do you/have you had any skin problems (site, frequency, description)? Screen for skin lesions that are common to Behçets disease, including pathergy

Contributory or predisposing factors

What is your family's ethnicity? Although Behçets disease may occur in any population, it is more prevalent in patients from the Middle East, Japan, and Mediterranean basin (principally Turkey).

Family history

Q What is your ancestry? Do you have ancestors from the Middle East, Japan, or the Mediterranean basin? Greater prevalence in people from the Mediterranean basin, Middle and Far East, but this is not exclusive

Q Do members of your family have inflammatory bowel disease or autoimmune disease (e.g. systemic lupus erythematosus)? These questions are important because they may lead to other diagnosis or support a diagnosis of Behçets disease. Remember that Crohn's disease is more prevalent and closely mimics Behçets disease, and should seriously be considered as a diagnosis

Examination

General examination for signs of disease

- Check for anemia
- Check for lymphadenopathy
- Check for mucous membrane ulcers: they may be single or in crops, oral or genital
- Are there skin lesions (pustules, papules, nodules, ulcers, folliculitis, or pathergy)?
- Are there any joint abnormalities (oligoarthritis or joint effusion)? The knee is most commonly involved

General examination, looking for complications

- Check for neurologic deficit (signs of meningitis, headache, fever, stiff neck, etc.)
- Check for organomegaly. Approximately 25% of Behçets patients will have splenomegaly. Also, a minority of patients may develop amyloidosis
- Are there signs of nephrotic syndrome?
- Check for thrombosis or embolic involvement of a major blood vessel (e.g. limb ischemia, superior vena cava obstruction, etc.)
- Are there cardiovascular signs (hypertension, aneurysm, etc.)?
- Ophthalmic evaluation: conjunctivitis, keratitis, anterior and/or posterior chamber disease (specialist assessment advised), hypopyon (white blood cells in anterior chamber)?
- General review of systems to assess for complications from vasculitis. If positive, this should prompt a more urgent referral to a rheumatologist

Summary of investigative tests

- There are no generally accepted diagnostic tests for Behçets disease
- Acute-phase reactants (e.g. erythrocyte sedimentation rate, C-reactive protein, haptoglobin, ferritin, fibrinogen and serum amyloid A) may determine the level of systemic inflammation, but are nonspecific
- Pathergy testing is considered to be a specific test for Behçets disease, but response is variable and insensitive
- Routine blood tests will evaluate general level of health and involvement of major organs

DIAGNOSTIC DECISION

Behçets is a rare diagnosis and should be made in conjunction with a rheumatologist. There are no serologic or pathologic tests that are diagnostic.

In 1990 an International Study Group reported proposed standardized diagnostic criteria for Behçets syndrome as follows:
- Recurrent oral ulceration (at least three times per year)

PLUS two of the following symptoms/signs:
- Recurrent genital ulceration
- Eye lesions (anterior uveitis, posterior uveitis, cells in the vitreous by slit lamp examination, or retinal vasculitis)
- Skin lesions (erythema nodosum, pseudofolliculitis, papulopustular lesions, or acneform nodules)
- Pathergy

International Study Group for Behçets Disease. Criteria for diagnosis of Behçets disease. Lancet 1990; 335:1078–80.

CLINICAL PEARLS
- Virtually all patients with Behçets syndrome have aphthous stomatitis
- One rarely sees the classic triad of oral ulcers-genital ulcers-uveitis simultaneously
- Consider Behçets syndrome in the differential diagnosis of any patient who is evaluated for Crohn's disease
- The hypopyon (a precipitate of white cells in the anterior chamber) is very characteristic of Behçets syndrome

THE TESTS
Body fluids
ERYTHROCYTE SEDIMENTATION RATE
Description
Cuffed venous blood sample.

Advantages/Disadvantages
- Advantage: simple
- Disadvantage: nonspecific

Normal
0–20mm/h (normal laboratory values may vary).

Abnormal
- >20mm/h
- Keep in mind the possibility of a falsely abnormal result

Cause of abnormal result
Erythrocyte sedimentation rate is a nonspecific marker of disease, and frequently rises to high levels in connective tissue diseases.

Drugs, disorders and other factors that may alter results
- Increased levels also caused by malignancy, infection, other inflammatory disorder
- Recent anti-inflammatory treatment may result in false-normal result

Tests of function
C-REACTIVE PROTEIN
Description
Venous blood sample. C-reactive protein (CRP) is an acute-phase reactant that is produced in the liver.

Advantages/Disadvantages
Advantages:
- The CRP rises and declines more rapidly with the development and resolution of inflammation, respectively, than the erythrocyte sedimentation rate
- The CRP is not influenced by anemia, unlike the erythrocyte sedimentation rate

Disadvantage: the CRP is a nonspecific indicator of inflammation

Normal
<1.0mg/dL (depending on the laboratory).

Abnormal
- >1.0mg/dL
- Keep in mind the possibility of a falsely abnormal result

Cause of abnormal result
Any inflammatory disorder.

Drugs, disorders and other factors that may alter results
- Increased levels also caused by malignancy, infection, other inflammatory disorder
- Recent anti-inflammatory treatment may result in false-normal result

Special tests
PATHERGY TEST
Description
- Performed by introducing a sterile 25-gauge needle 5mm obliquely into the forearm
- Results are read 24–48 h after procedure. A positive finding is noted by demonstration of greater than 2mm of erythema at entry site

Advantages/Disadvantages
Advantages:
- Inexpensive
- Safe
- Quick
- Usually acceptable to patient
- Specific for Behçets if positive – specificity approaches 100%

Disadvantages:
- This test requires an experienced observer for interpretation
- False negatives occur (sensitivity 44–70%)
- May introduce infection

Normal
No papule at site of needle insertion (read by physician at 24–48 h).

Abnormal
- Erythematous papule at site of needle insertion greater than 2mm diameter, read by physician at 24–48 hours (positive test)

- A positive pathergy reaction is far more common in Turkish and Japanese Behçet's patients than in those from Northern Europe or the US
- Keep in mind the possibility of a falsely abnormal result

Cause of abnormal result
Abnormal neutrophil chemotaxis occurs in Behçet's disease, resulting in localized inflammatory nodule or ulcer.

Drugs, disorders and other factors that may alter results
Surgical cleansing of the site with povidone iodine or 100% chlorhexidine reduces the sensitivity of the test.

TREATMENT

CONSIDER CONSULT
Emergency referral
- Hemoptysis present
- Neurologic involvement (including meningeal irritation, cerebrovascular accident, diplopia, numbness, confusion)
- Cardiovascular involvement (limb ischemia, coronary ischemia, acute aneurysm, organ-threatening vasculitis)
- Most treatments other than those of symptomatic relief must be managed in conjunction with a specialist

IMMEDIATE ACTION
Life- or sight-threatening complications must be referred urgently to hospital.

PATIENT AND CAREGIVER ISSUES
Patient or caregiver request
- **Is my condition infectious?** Behçets disease is not transmissible by person to person contact
- **Is my condition sexually transmitted?** No
- **Is my condition inherited?** No
- **Will it go away?** It tends to be lifelong, but often comes in a series of remissions and exacerbations
- **Will my sight be affected?** In some cases, yes. Any eye symptoms should be reported immediately, as blindness may occur very quickly and without much warning
- **Is there any threat to my life?** There can be with the involvement of major organs, although many people only suffer with mild symptoms and signs
- **Is there a cure?** No
- **Is it cancerous?** No

MANAGEMENT ISSUES
Goals
- Relieve symptoms by reducing inflammation and pain
- Counsel patient on nature of disease and when to seek immediate attention
- Consider treating immune hyperactivity with medication in conjunction with specialist
- Monitor for complications of disease or therapy, and respond appropriately

SUMMARY OF THERAPEUTIC OPTIONS
Choices
- Treatment is symptomatic and empiric and, in the case of eye disease, aimed at reducing progression of the disease process
- The evidence for the effectiveness of each drug is difficult to evaluate
- The majority of treatment decisions will be taken by a specialist
- Specialists vary in their choice of drugs, and patient response is variable
- Mild cases are often managed without specific treatment

A good review of the therapies commonly used in Behçet's syndrome can be found in the Cochrane Review: Pharmacotherapy for Behçet's Syndrome, 3, 2000. Oxford: Update Software.

The treatments listed below are commonly employed for the various clinical manifestations of Behçet's disease (not exhaustive).

Mouth ulcers:
- Antibacterial mouthwashes (e.g. chlorhexidine gluconate, tetracycline solution)

- Topical steroids (e.g. 0.1% triamcinolone acetonide in dental paste)
- Topical lidocaine
- Prednisone
- Methotrexate
- Azathioprine
- Thalidomide (for refractory cases)

Eye involvement (always treated by ophthalmologist):
- Corticosteroids
- Azathioprine
- Methotrexate
- Chlorambucil
- Cyclosporine
- Cyclophosphamide

Genital ulcers:
- Topical corticosteroids
- Colchicine

Arthritis:
- Nonsteroidal anti-inflammatory drugs
- Azathioprine
- Sulfasalazine

Gastrointestinal ulcers:
- Systemic corticosteroids
- Sulfasalazine

Meningoencephalitis:
- Systemic corticosteroids
- Immunosuppressives

Large vessel disease:
- Corticosteroids
- Immunosuppressives
- Anticoagulants (heparin/warfarin) if thrombosis is present

Major vein thrombosis:
- Prednisone
- Anticoagulants
- Immunosuppressives

Complementary therapy:
- No currently available data support the beneficial use of alternative therapy in Behçet's disease
- Osteopathy, chiropractic, and massage may help arthralgia
- Warnings exist regarding the use of herbal medicines, particularly their interaction with conventional medicines, and therefore it is recommended that such therapies are discussed with a specialist before use

Clinical pearls
- Topical treatment may be adequate for mucocutaneous lesions (oral or genital ulcers)
- Systemic corticosteroids in large doses are necessary for systemic disease with major organ involvement

- Various immunosuppressives are often indicated, always under the supervision of a specialist
- Any eye involvement warrants treatment by an ophthalmologist

FOLLOW UP

Frequency of follow up will depend upon the symptomatology and complexity of the disease, as well as the therapy employed.

Plan for review

Establish appropriate review for active disease and regular review in quiescent times.

Information for patient or caregiver

- Patients must be counseled to promptly report any symptoms of disease that may be life- or sight-threatening
- Patients on disease-modifying drugs must be counseled and told to report adverse effects promptly. Provide patient information sheets relating to the individual drug(s)

DRUGS AND OTHER THERAPIES: DETAILS
Drugs
TETRACYCLINE MOUTHWASH

Tetracycline mouthwashes are used for severe recurrent aphthous ulceration.

Dose

- Prepared by adding the contents of a 250mg tetracycline capsule to a small amount of water
- Solution held in the mouth for 2-3 min three or four times daily usually for 3 days
- It is not to be swallowed

Efficacy

Tetracycline is a broad-spectrum antibiotic. No evidence as to efficacy has been reported.

Risks/Benefits

Risks:

- Tetracycline stains teeth, avoid in children aged under 12 years (dental staining and hypoplasia occasionally)
- May exacerbate renal failure in patients with renal disease (risk greater if solution swallowed)
- Prolonged courses may predispose to oral thrush
- May itself cause ulcers and irritation of mucous membranes and allergic reaction
- Risk of general side-effects (if swallowed)
- Use caution in patients with hepatic impairment
- Use caution with repeated or prolonged doses

Benefits:

- Reduces opportunistic bacterial superinfection
- May possibly shorten duration of ulcers

Side-effects and adverse reactions

- Gastrointestinal: abdominal pain, diarrhea, heartburn, hepatotoxicity, vomiting, nausea, dental staining, anorexia
- Central nervous system: headache, paresthesia, fever
- Genitourinary: polyuria, polydipsia, azotemia
- Hematologic: blood cell dyscrasias
- Cardiovascular system: pericarditis
- Skin: pruritus, rash, photosensitivity, changes in pigmentation, angioedema, stinging

Interactions (other drugs)
- Antacids
- Barbiturates
- Bismuth subsalicyclate
- Calcium, iron, magnesium, zinc
- Cholesytramine, colestipol
- Carbamazepine
- Digoxin
- Ethanol
- Methoxyflurane
- Oral contraceptives
- Penicillins
- Phenytoin
- Warfarin

Contraindications
- Renal impairment
- Children under 8 years
- Pregnant or breast-feeding women

Evidence
No evidence found on efficacy.

Acceptability to patient
Generally acceptable, but patients with sight problems may require solution to be made up for them.

Follow up plan
Follow up to exclude superinfection and the presence of oral thrush.

Patient and caregiver information
Patient should be advised not to swallow mouthwash.

TOPICAL STEROIDS
Topical steroid such as 0.1% triamcinolone acetonide in dental paste for oral ulcers.

Dose
- Apply pea-sized amount to lesion 2–4 times a day
- Do not rub in

Efficacy
Helps to limit local inflammatory response.

Risks/Benefits
Risks:
- Risks are those of steroid use
- Steroids are more readily absorbed from mucous membranes than from skin, increasing the systemic risks
- Risk of contact allergy to steroid molecule
- Use caution with glomerulonephritis, ulcerative colitis, renal disease
- Use caution with AIDS, tuberculosis, ocular herpes simplex, live vaccines, viral and bacterial infections
- Use caution in diabetes mellitus, glaucoma, osteoporosis, hypertension
- Use caution in children and the elderly
- Use caution in recent myocardial infarction
- Use caution in psychosis
- Do not withdraw abruptly

Benefit: helps limit inflammation (most effective in the prodromal phase)

Side-effects and adverse reactions
Short duration of therapy minimizes possible systemic side-effects:
- Gastrointestinal: dyspepsia, peptic ulceration, esophagitis, oral candidiasis, nausea, vomiting
- Cardiovascular system: hypertension, thromboembolism
- Central nervous system: insomnia, euphoria, depression, psychosis, seizures

- Endocrine: adrenal suppression, impaired glucose tolerance, growth suppression in children
- Musculoskeletal: proximal myopathy, osteoporosis
- Skin: delayed healing, acne, striae
- Eyes, ears, nose and throat: cataract, glaucoma, blurred vision

Interactions (other drugs)
No known interactions with topical triamcinolone.

Contraindications
- Untreated oral infections, tuberculosis, or viral lesions   Pregnancy and breast feeding

Acceptability to patient
Usually well tolerated and provides symptomatic relief.

Follow up plan
Follow up to monitor clinical response and to exclude secondary infection.

Patient and caregiver information
Advise patient on steroid use.

CHLORHEXIDINE GLUCONATE
An oral solution that is swished in the mouth, then expectorated.

Dose
- Rinse mouth with 15mL chlorhexidine oral rinse for 30 s twice daily after toothbrushing
- Should not be swallowed

Efficacy
May help healing by preventing superinfection.

Risks/Benefits
Risks:
- Stains teeth (reversible with professional cleaning)
- Use caution in pregnancy and lactation

Benefit: may speed healing of oral lesions

Side-effects and adverse reactions
Ears, eyes, nose and throat: dental staining, taste disturbances, irritation, burning.

Interactions (other drugs)
No known interactions.

Contraindications
No known contraindications.

Acceptability to patient
Leaves a very unpleasant taste in the mouth, which is aggravated by drinking liquids.

Patient and caregiver information
- Do not swallow or dilute
- Expectorate after rinsing

EFFICACY OF THERAPIES

Evidence as to the effectiveness of treatment is hard to evaluate as a result of limited trials with common interventions and outcomes.

PROGNOSIS

- Prognosis is difficult to determine because of the vast spectrum of involvement within the group diagnosed with Behçet's disease
- The major causes of mortality in Behçet's disease are central nervous system involvement, vascular disease, intestinal perforation, and pulmonary involvement
- Severe ocular involvement is an important cause of morbidity

Clinical pearls

- Behçet's syndrome is characterized by remissions and exacerbations, so the intensity of treatment depends on the type and severity of clinical manifestation
- Colchicine is frequently used, although controlled clinical trials do not demonstrate its effectiveness
- Severe visual impairment may occur in up to 20% of patients
- The major causes of mortality are bowel perforation, pulmonary hemorrhage, and central nervous system disease

Recurrence

This is typically a disease of remissions and exacerbations.

COMPLICATIONS

- Complications arise from vasculitis affecting large or small vessels throughout all systems, and are therefore extremely varied
- Patients are particularly prone to thrombosis
- Bowel perforation, pulmonary hemorrhage, and central nervous system disease are the most common causes of mortality

PREVENTION

No preventive strategies are known to be effective.

PREVENT RECURRENCE

- Recurrences of Behçet's syndrome cannot be prevented in any predictable manner
- Systemic corticosteroids and immunosuppressive drugs may reduce severity and frequency of recurrences

ASSOCIATIONS

American Behçet's Disease Association
PO Box 280240
Memphis TN 38168-0240
Tel: 1-800-7Behçet's
www.behcets.com
Behçet's organization worldwide
www.behcets.org

KEY REFERENCES

- International Study Group for Behçets Disease. Criteria for diagnosis of Behçet's Disease. Lancet 1990; 335:1078–80
- Barnes CG. Behçets syndrome. Topical Reviews in Reports on Rheumatic Diseases (series 2), no 18. ARC, 1991
- Koopman WJ (ed). Arthritis and Allied Conditions, 13th ed. Baltimore:Williams & Wilkins, 1997
- Kelley WN, Harris ED, Ruddy S, Sledge CB (eds). Textbook of Rheumatology, 3rd ed. London:WB Saunders, 1989 p1209–12
- Souhami RL, Moxham J (editors). Textbook of Medicine, 3rd ed. Edinburgh:Churchill Livingstone
- Saenz A, Ausejo M, Shea B, et al. Pharmacotherapy for Behçet's syndrome. The Cochrane Library, 3, 2000

FAQS
Question 1
How is the diagnosis of Behçet's made?

ANSWER 1
The diagnosis is strongly suggested by recurrent oral aphthous ulcers and two of the following: recurrent genital ulceration, ocular inflammation, characteristic skin lesions, and pathergy.

Question 2
What is the clinical presentation of pathergy?

ANSWER 2
A pathergic lesion occurs from minimal trauma (such as phlebotomy) and tends to deteriorate when debrided.

Question 3
Does Behçet's occur outside of Japan and the Middle East?

ANSWER 3
Although Behçet's is more common in those regions, it occurs less frequently throughout the world.

Question 4
How is Behçet's treated?

ANSWER 4
Treatment depends upon the particular clinical manifestation, and ranges from topical agents to systemic immunosuppressants. Treatment must always be guided by a specialist.

CONTRIBUTORS

Russell C Jones, MD, MPH
Richard Brasington Jr, MD, FACP
Keith M Hull, MD, PhD

CHRONIC FATIGUE SYNDROME

DESCRIPTION

- Chronic fatigue syndrome (CFS) is clinically defined by severe disabling fatigue and a combination of symptoms that prominently features self-reported impairments in concentration and short-term memory, sleep disturbances, and musculoskeletal pain. Symptoms should be present for at least 6 months, and for 50% of the time
- Diagnosis of CFS can be made only after alternate medical and psychiatric causes of chronic fatiguing illness have been excluded
- No pathognomonic signs or diagnostic tests for this condition have been validated in scientific studies
- No definitive treatments exist for CFS
- Some people affected by CFS improve with time but most remain functionally impaired for several years

URGENT ACTION

No urgent action specific to CFS, but exclude underlying life-threatening illness and complications such as severe depression with suicidal ideations.

KEY! DON'T MISS!

- Physical, endocrine, metabolic, infectious, or malignant underlying causes of fatigue
- In children don't miss child abuse (physical, sexual, emotional, neglect) and serious family distress as a cause of symptoms. Always bear in mind the possibility of bullying and primary school refusal

BACKGROUND

ICD9 CODE
- 780.7 Chronic fatigue syndrome
- 300.8 Neurasthenia

SYNONYMS
- CFS
- ME
- Myalgic encephalitis
- Neurasthenia
- Yuppie flu
- Chronic Epstein-Barr syndrome
- Fibromyalgia overlaps considerably but is usually considered a different entity

CARDINAL FEATURES
- Persistent or relapsing fatigue, lasting at least 6 consecutive months, at least 50% of the time, present in patients with no prior history of such fatigue. Patient reports lack of energy, listlessness, and being too tired to participate in family, work, or even leisure activities
- Patients frequently fear physical activity will make them worse and rest excessively
- Migratory arthralgias and musculoskeletal pains present or fluctuating for >6 months
- Sore throat with tender lymph nodes present or fluctuating for >6 months
- New generalized headache present or fluctuating for >6 months
- Unrefreshing sleep present or fluctuating for >6 months
- Postexertional malaise present or fluctuating for >6 months
- Impaired memory or concentration present or fluctuating for >6 months
- Initial presentation may be flu-like, but persists
- Other symptoms include abdominal pain, alcohol intolerance, bloating, chest pain, chronic cough, diarrhea, dizziness, dry eyes or mouth, earaches, palpitations, jaw pain, morning stiffness, nausea, night sweats, depression, irritability, anxiety, panic attacks, shortness of breath, tingling sensations, and weight loss
- Those affected by chronic fatigue syndrome (CFS) can be severely disabled physically, psychologically, and socially
- There are no reliable clinical signs
- The course may be prolonged for up to 20 years
- Depressive features are commonly associated but may be secondary

CAUSES
Common causes
- Etiology of CFS remains unknown
- The most consistent finding of etiologic studies has been the inconsistency of results
- Early studies suggested Epstein-Barr virus reactivation, immunologic dysfunction, and chronic candidal infection, but subsequent controlled studies did not support this
- Investigators continue to explore the relation between stress, immune modulation, and reactivation of latent viruses, hypothesizing that these conditions trigger neuroendocrine responses
- In the US the current thinking is that the underlying etiology is probably centrally mediated via the hypothalamic-pituitary-adrenal (HPA) axis. Some current reports suggest inappropriate signaling in the raphe nucleus and periaqueductal gray areas
- HPA axis. Multiple studies have suggested that the central nervous system may have a role in CFS. CFS patients often produce lower levels of cortisol than do healthy controls but the altered cortisol levels fall within the accepted range of normal. Hormonal replacement is not an effective treatment

- Neurally mediated hypotension (NMH) occurs with increased frequency in CFS patients; it is not clear whether this is cause or effect. NMH can be induced by using tilt table testing, which involves laying the patient horizontally on a table and then tilting the table upright to 70° for 45min while monitoring blood pressure and heart rate. Persons with NMH will develop lowered blood pressure and other characteristic symptoms, such as lightheadedness, visual dimming, or a slow response to verbal stimuli
- One study observed that 96% of adults with a clinical diagnosis of CFS developed hypotension during tilt table testing, compared with 29% of healthy controls. Tilt table testing also provoked characteristic CFS symptoms in the patients. A subset of CFS patients reported a striking improvement in symptoms with NMH medication, but not all improved
- Some view CFS as predominantly a psychiatric condition
- The central issue is whether the CFS or any subset of it is a pathologically discrete entity, as opposed to a debilitating but nonspecific condition shared by many different entities

Contributory or predisposing factors

- Stress is frequently described as preceding CFS
- CFS may follow viral infections, but there is no evidence of clustering or of infection more commonly in CFS patients
- Conditions that have been proposed to trigger the development of CFS include viral infection or other transient traumatic conditions, stress, and toxins
- An association with fibromyalgia has been noted, but it is unclear whether this represents a common pathophysiology or overlapping diagnostic criteria
- Infectious agents: no firm association between infection with any known human pathogen and CFS has been established. The possibility remains that CFS may have multiple causes leading to a common endpoint, i.e. infectious agents might have a contributory role for a subset of cases
- Immunology/allergy: it has been proposed that CFS may be caused by an immunologic dysfunction, e.g. inappropriate production of cytokines. There are no immune disorders in CFS patients on the scale traditionally associated with disease. Some investigators have observed anti-self antibodies and immune complexes in CFS patients. Some investigators have reported lower numbers or activity of natural killer cells among CFS patients. One hypothesis is that trigger events, such as stress or viral infection, may lead to the chronic expression of cytokines and then to CFS. Administration of some cytokines in therapeutic doses is known to cause fatigue, but no characteristic pattern of chronic cytokine secretion has been identified in CFS patients. Several studies have shown that CFS patients are more likely to have a history of allergies than are healthy controls. Allergy could be a predisposing factor for CFS, but not all CFS patients have it
- Nutritional deficiency: there is no published scientific evidence that CFS is caused by a nutritional deficiency. Whereas evidence is lacking for nutritional defects in CFS patients, a balanced diet would be expected to have beneficial effects in any chronic illness. One study suggested reduced functional vitamin B status, most particularly pyridoxine, in CFS. This is unconfirmed, but there may be justification for a proper clinical trial of pyridoxine
- Iatrogenic: one paper on chronic pain suggests that poor advice, dismissal, over-investigation, and other iatrogenic factors played a part in patients developing long-standing chronic pain and suggests that something similar would be found in a study of CFS

EPIDEMIOLOGY
Incidence and prevalence
PREVALENCE

- Prevalence 2–26/1000, depending on criteria used
- Peak prevalence is among persons aged 20–50 years
- Prevalence of CFS-like illness among adolescents is approx. 0.2/1000

FREQUENCY

- In the US, 24% of the general adult population has experienced fatigue lasting 2 weeks or longer, with 59–64% of these people reporting no medical cause
- 24% of primary care clinic patients reported having had prolonged fatigue (one month). In many persons with prolonged fatigue, fatigue persists beyond 6 months (defined as chronic fatigue)
- CFS accounts for about 5–10% of all cases of chronic fatigue

Demographics
AGE

- Average age at onset is 30 years
- Adolescents can have CFS, but few studies of adolescents have been published. The illness in adolescents has many of the same characteristics as it has in adults
- A recently published Centers for Disease Control and Prevention (CDC) study documented that adolescents 12–18 years of age had CFS significantly less frequently than adults, and did not identify CFS in children under 12 years of age
- CFS-like illness has been reported in children under 12 by some investigators, although the symptom pattern varies somewhat from that seen in adults and adolescents and the diagnosis must be made with caution

GENDER

- CFS affects both sexes
- Women are affected up to 1.5 times more often than men

RACE

Rates of CFS are similar in all ethnic groups.

SOCIOECONOMIC STATUS

- The CDC four-city surveillance study of CFS identified a population of patients of whom >80% had advanced education and one-third were from upper income families. However, these data included only patients who were under a physician's care
- On the other hand, CDC's San Francisco study found that CFS-like disease was most prevalent among persons with household annual incomes of under $40,000
- Conclusion is that CFS affects all socioeconomic groups

DIAGNOSIS

DIFFERENTIAL DIAGNOSIS
Depression
- Fatigue is an important somatic symptom of depression
- Abnormalities of central nervous system neurotransmitter metabolism and function are believed to play a major role in the pathogenesis of depression
- Stress, distress, and socioeconomic difficulty may contribute
- Physical manifestations of chronic fatigue syndrome (CFS) are atypical for depression and anxiety, and the anhedonia, guilt, and low motivation that characterize depression are infrequent in CFS. CFS patients are highly motivated to deal with their illness

FEATURES
- Fatigue
- Low mood
- Early morning wakening
- Appetite disturbance
- Loss of concentration
- Loss of libido
- Headache
- Gastrointestinal upset
- Psychomotor retardation
- Suicidal ideation

Anxiety
Chronic anxiety may result in generalized fatigue, in part because it interferes with obtaining adequate rest. Patients report trouble falling asleep and a host of associated bodily complaints. Many maintain their neck muscles in a constantly tensed state, which gives rise to occipitalnuchal headaches. Seemingly unprovoked episodes of palpitations, difficulty breathing, and chest tightness may occur, especially in those whose anxiety is accompanied by a panic disorder.

FEATURES
- Reports of feeling anxious or nervous all the time
- Social isolation due to fear of panic attacks
- Excessive worry
- Muscle tension
- Difficulty concentrating
- Occipitalnuchal headaches
- Palpitations
- Difficulty breathing
- Chest tightness
- Sweating
- Fatigue
- Low mood
- Appetite disturbance
- Loss of libido
- Headache
- Tiredness
- Gastrointestinal upset

Fibromyalgia
- Numerous physicians prefer to separate CFS from fibromyalgia; however, because of the great overlap between the two, the best approach is to consider both as forms of 'generalized rheumatism' and manage them in the same way

- In an analysis contrasting the pain properties with those of rheumatoid arthritis, the fibromyalgia patients used diverse adjectives to describe their pain, the most common being pricking, pressing, shooting, gnawing, cramping, splitting, and crushing. A majority in both groups defined the pain as aching and exhausting
- Fibromyalgia may represent a subset of patients with CFS characterized by heightened musculoskeletal symptoms

FEATURES

- Distinguished by localized areas of tenderness to palpation. These trigger points are not always reproducible. One study found many children with fibromyalgia to have hypermobile joints
- In fibromyalgia, there is rarely evidence of synovitis
- There are no specific laboratory findings
- Anemia and hypothyroidism should be ruled out. Imaging studies, particularly plain radiographs, may be necessary to rule out fractures or other pathology; magnetic resonance imaging (MRI) studies may be necessary to preclude ligamentous injury. The need for additional tests is individualized, depending on specific symptoms and physical finding
- Fibromyalgia is a complex pain disorder, which may respond to physical therapy, low-dose tricyclic antidepressants, muscle relaxants on a time-limited basis, or spinal manipulations
- Coexisting depression is common
- CFS is much less likely to respond to treatment compared with fibromyalgia

Gulf War syndrome

Chronic, debilitating group of features described by soldiers returning from the Gulf War and thought to be due to a combination of vaccines used against chemical and nerve agents. It has also been postulated that Gulf War syndrome may be due to exposure to one or more unknown agents including sarin, depleted uranium, and biologic agents.

FEATURES

- Joint pain (49%)
- Fatigue (47%)
- Headache (39%)
- Memory loss (34%)
- Sleep disturbance (32%)
- Rash/dermatitis (31%)
- Difficulty concentrating (27%)
- Depression (23%)
- Muscle pain (21%)

Polymyalgia rheumatica

Polymyalgia rheumatica is rare under 50 years of age, average age 70 years. It is a disorder of unknown cause, leading to shoulder and hip stiffness, raised erythrocyte sedimentation rate (ESR), and tiredness.

FEATURES

- Stiff neck, shoulders, and hips
- Pervasive tiredness
- Tender muscles
- Depressive features are common
- ESR is raised
- Duration of at least 6 weeks
- Morning stiffness
- Symptoms of giant cell arteritis often coexist
- ESR is raised in virtually all cases

Connective tissue disease

Marked fatigue may dominate the initial clinical presentation of most rheumatoid diseases before characteristic inflammatory connective tissue manifestations become evident, e.g. rheumatoid arthritis, systemic lupus erythematosus (SLE), vasculitis, polymyositis/dermatomyositis.

FEATURES

- May occur in children and adolescents
- Joint pains with swelling and heat
- Systemic symptoms
- Rash
- Raised ESR
- Fatigue
- Malaise
- Symptoms of eye pain and decreased vision: iritis, episcleritis, uveitis
- Multiple tissue inflammations including pericarditis, splenomegaly, vasculitis
- Some syndromes may underlie malignancy (especially dermatomyositis)

Anemia

Iron deficiency is often blamed for fatigue, although the correlation between iron-deficiency anemia and fatigue is poor, especially when the anemia is mild. Other causes of anemia, e.g. pernicious anemia, aplastic anemia, anemia of chronic disease, may have the same features.

FEATURES

- Tiredness
- Dyspnea
- Ankle swelling
- Palpitations
- Pallor
- Poor wound healing
- Glossitis
- Angular stomatitis
- Pica

Somatization disorder

Believed to be the physical expression of psychologic stress; patients in whom somatization represents an underlying personality disorder may complain of chronic fatigue, often accompanied by a host of other refractory symptoms. There is a high association between somatization disorder and substance abuse and personality disorder.

FEATURES

- Individuals have a lifelong history of bodily complaints that elude diagnosis and treatment
- Symptoms begin before age 30 years and persist over several years
- Patients complain of multiple sites of pain (minimum of four), gastrointestinal symptoms (minimum of two), sexual or reproductive symptoms, and a pseudoneurologic symptom
- These cannot be explained by a medical condition or are in excess of expected disability from a coexisting medical condition

Idiopathic fatigue

Patients who meet many of the criteria for CFS but 6 months of symptoms have not elapsed may have idiopathic fatigue. Prolonged fatigue is defined as self-reported, persistent fatigue of one month or longer. Chronic fatigue is defined as self-reported persistent or relapsing fatigue of 6 or more consecutive months.

FEATURES
Some features of CFS but failing to meet diagnostic criteria, usually because symptoms have not been sufficiently prolonged.

Pregnancy
- Early pregnancy, particularly the first trimester and the first half of the second, commonly causes severe fatigue
- Anemia is also common, and infectious illness may take a particular toll on these patients
- First-time mothers seem particularly prone to severe fatigue, perhaps because they do not expect it

Eating disorders
Anorexia and bulimia nervosa are prolonged illnesses. In anorexia, abnormal body image with self-induced and often extreme weight loss predominates. Patients are often young (<20 years) and will deny their condition vehemently, allowing investigations for tiredness or anemia as they fear confrontation of their condition. In bulimia, binging and vomiting of sometimes huge quantities of food predominates. Patient is often of normal weight and will commonly deny behavior. Tiredness is less of a feature and excessive exercise is common.

FEATURES
Anorexia:
- Emaciated patient, cold and tired
- Hair thinning, brittle nails
- Bradycardia, hypotension
- Loss of female fat distribution pattern
- Axillary and pubic hair is preserved but amenorrhea is common

Bulimia:
- Parotid swelling
- Erosion of tooth enamel
- Petechial hemorrhages of the palate, face, or cornea
- Often no physical signs

Sleep disorders
Disturbed sleep may be the cause of chronic fatigue. Sleep disturbance may be due to sleep apnea, or concurrent physical illness such as chronic rhinitis or esophageal reflux. It may also be due to disturbance by small children, crowded or noisy living conditions, and shift work.

FEATURES
Lack of sleep from any cause leads to:
- Daytime sleepiness
- Irritability
- Tremor
- Nausea
- Headache
- Fatigue

Medication
Many medications have substantial sedating effects:
- Long-term use of hypnotics and withdrawal from them may cause sleep disturbance
- Minor tranquilizers
- Hypnotics

- Antihypertensives that penetrate the blood-brain barrier (e.g. reserpine, methyldopa, clonidine, propranolol) may precipitate depression or fatigue
- Beta-blockers
- Antihistamines
- Antiepileptics
- Antidepressants, especially amitriptyline, doxepin, and trazodone
- Drug abuse and drug withdrawal

Endocrine dysfunction
Dysfunction of the thyroid, adrenal, pituitary, parathyroid, or endocrine pancreas can start out as fatigue, perhaps accompanied by more specific symptoms.

FEATURES
- Abnormalities of relevant biochemical testing
- Tiredness in these conditions is usually associated with more specific features
- Hypothyroidism may present as fatigue, perhaps in association with weight gain, dry skin, mild hoarseness, or cold intolerance
- In the elderly, hyperthyroidism may take an atypical form (apathetic hyperthyroidism), characterized by fatigue, marked weight loss, apathy, and otherwise unexplained atrial fibrillation
- Addison's disease causes fatigue in conjunction with weight loss, vague gastrointestinal upset, postural hypotension, and eventually hyperpigmentation
- Panhypopituitarism from postpartum hemorrhage or a sellar tumor can cause fatigue. The postpartum patient fails to lactate or resume menstruation; lassitude, decreased libido, and loss of axillary and pubic hair ensue. Later, symptoms of hypothyroidism may develop. The patient with a pituitary tumor may note galactorrhea and amenorrhea
- Poorly controlled diabetes mellitus may present as fatigue accompanied by polyuria
- Similarly, fatigue may be the initial symptom of hyperparathyroidism and of hypercalcemia. Dehydration, constipation, bone pain, renal stones, confusion, collapse may be present

Metabolic disturbances
Chronic renal failure, hepatocellullar failure, and hypercalcemia may present with fatigue.

FEATURES
- Chronic renal failure may present with fatigue and few localizing symptoms or signs aside from laboratory findings of azotemia, mild anemia, impaired renal concentrating ability, and an abnormal urinary sediment
- Hepatocellular failure causes lassitude. Jaundice, ascites, petechiae, asterixis, spider angiomata, and other signs of hepatic insufficiency may be seen. In anicteric hepatitis and mild forms of chronic hepatitis, jaundice may be minimal or absent while fatigue is prominent; the same holds for the prodromal phase of acute viral hepatitis
- Hypercalcemia often signifies underlying malignancy. Features include dehydration, constipation, bone pain, renal stones, confusion, and collapse

Occult malignancy
Many patients presenting with CFS will fear they have occult malignancy. It is important to exclude it as far as possible and demonstrate to the patient that you have done so.

FEATURES
- Fatigue and lassitude accompany most cancers
- Pancreatic carcinoma is the archetypal example of a tumor that may present initially as marked fatigue with few localizing symptoms
- Severe weight loss, depression, and apathy may also dominate the clinical picture before other manifestations of the malignancy become evident

- Malignancies causing hypercalcemia (e.g. breast cancer, myeloma) may present with fatigue, although usually the hypercalcemia is a late development
- Examine patient for localizing signs

Cardiopulmonary disease

Fatigue is the earliest complaint of congestive cardiac failure and may be evident before orthopnea or paroxysmal nocturnal dyspnea are seen.

FEATURES

- Fatigue associated with a history of exertional dyspnea
- Fatigue sometimes dominates the clinical presentation of patients with chronic congestive heart failure or chronic lung disease
- Shortness of breath on exercise
- Peripheral or pulmonary edema
- Cough or wheeze
- Cyanosis
- Gallop rhythm
- Heart murmurs
- Chest pains
- Reduced exercise tolerance
- Cardiac enlargement
- Reduced left ventricular ejection fraction on echocardiography

Infectious disease

- Infections that have fatigue as a predominant symptom include mononucleosis (Epstein-Barr virus – EBV), viral hepatitis, tuberculosis, cytomegalovirus, subacute bacterial endocarditis, and HIV
- The CFS is not related specifically to EBV infection. A small group of patients with recurring or persistent symptoms have abnormal serologic test results for EBV, as well as for other viruses

FEATURES

- Profound fatigue, low-grade fever, and lymphadenopathy are common
- Raised ESR is frequent
- Tuberculosis and subacute bacterial endocarditis are important infectious etiologies of fatigue in which few localizing symptoms may be present
- A history of cough, night sweats, HIV infection, or exposure is sometimes seen in tuberculosis
- Recent dental work, a heart murmur, and intravenous drug abuse are risk factors for subacute bacterial endocarditis
- Lyme disease is noteworthy for fatigue accompanied by joint complaints, headache, and low-grade fever
- EBV infections present with fever, exudative pharyngitis, lymphadenopathy, hepatosplenomegaly, atypical lymphocytosis
- The spectrum of diseases is variable, ranging from asymptomatic to fatal infection

Multiple sclerosis

Multiple sclerosis (MS) is a chronic demyelinating disease of unknown etiology with demyelinization plaques scattered through the white matter.

FEATURES

- Weakness
- Difficulties in ambulation
- Extreme fatigue
- Visual disturbance
- Numbness, paresthesiae

- Gait impairment, clumsiness
- Vertigo
- Incontinence
- Sexual dysfunction
- Slurred speech
- Mood alteration – raised or lowered

Seasonal affective disorder

Seasonal affective disorder is depression caused by dysfunction of circadian rhythms, believed to be caused by a decrease in exposure to full-spectrum light.

FEATURES

- Most common in winter
- Feelings of sadness and anxiety, hypersomnia, lethargy, carbohydrate craving, weight gain
- Onset in autumn, remission in spring – diagnosis requires a 2– to 3–year mood disturbance pattern
- More common in women, and people living in the northern latitudes

SIGNS & SYMPTOMS
Signs

No clinical signs are reliably detectable.

Symptoms

- Persistent or relapsing chronic fatigue present for >6 months but of new onset
- Postexertional malaise lasting >24h
- Fatigue not substantially alleviated by rest
- Substantial reduction in occupational, educational, social, or personal activities
- Substantial impairment in short-term memory or concentration
- Sore throat fluctuating or present for >6 months
- Tender lymph nodes fluctuating or present for >6 months
- Muscle pain fluctuating or present for >6 months
- Multi-joint pain without swelling or redness fluctuating or present for >6 months
- Headaches of a new type, pattern, or severity fluctuating or present for >6 months
- Unrefreshing sleep fluctuating or present for >6 months
- Hypotension, dizziness, and muscular aches
- All of these symptoms are chronic, persisting, or recurring during 6 or more consecutive months
- Symptoms in children appear to be similar to those in adolescents and adults
- School absenteeism is a major problem

ASSOCIATED DISORDERS

- There is a high prevalence of concurrent psychiatric disease, particularly somatization disorder, found in CFS patients subjected to detailed psychiatric study (range, 20–70%)
- Anxiety, depression, or both, are commonly associated with severe fatigue of any cause (CFS or other disease)
- One study indicated that over half of patients with CFS experienced depression
- Risk of suicidality and major depression is no higher than that found in patients with other chronic disabling disease
- A number of illnesses have a similar spectrum of symptoms to CFS. These include fibromyalgia syndrome, multiple chemical sensitivities, and chronic mononucleosis. Although these illnesses may present with a primary symptom other than fatigue, chronic fatigue is commonly associated with all of them

KEY! DON'T MISS!

- Physical, endocrine, metabolic, infectious, or malignant underlying causes of fatigue
- In children don't miss child abuse (physical, sexual, emotional, neglect) and serious family distress as a cause of symptoms. Always bear in mind the possibility of bullying and primary school refusal

CONSIDER CONSULT

Refer for further investigation when serious underlying disease is suspected

INVESTIGATION OF THE PATIENT
Direct questions to patient

- Two or three visits may be needed to establish the underlying etiology
- The patient may insist that medical illness be ruled out before agreeing to discuss psychosocial matters
- **Can you describe your tiredness?** To be sure that the patient is not confusing focal neuromuscular disease with generalized lassitude
- **How long have you felt tired like this?** At least 6 months is necessary for diagnosis of CFS
- **How is it affecting your life?** CFS causes a substantial reduction in occupational, educational, social, or personal activities
- **Can you remember what started it?** Patients may occasionally recall severe viral infections and often recall preceding periods of severe stress
- **How quickly did it all start?** Most patients diagnosed with CFS relate an abrupt onset to their symptoms, often as part of an initial virus-like illness characterized by low-grade fever accompanied by sore throat and cough. Less frequently, the initial symptoms indicate gastrointestinal tract involvement with nausea and diarrhea
- **Is it affecting your concentration or memory?** CFS causes substantial impairment in short-term memory or concentration
- **Have you had sore throat, muscle pain, joint pain, unusual headaches over the last few months?** All are CFS symptoms if prolonged over 6 months
- **How well are you sleeping?** Unrefreshing sleep with hypersomnia may be associated with CFS or with depression. However, nocturnal sleeping is not usually changed and does not differ from that in unaffected individuals
- **Are you tired after exercise or mental or social effort?** CFS patients have long-term postexertional malaise lasting >24h
- **Do you feel dizzy?** Dizziness is common in CFS, anxiety, somatoform disorders, and anemia
- **Are you in pain?** If so, locate and consider other pathology. Myalgia is common in CFS and more pronounced in fibromyalgia, where there may be tenderness at specified points. Consider occult malignancy and hypercalcemia where aches and pains predominate, especially in more elderly patients in whom CFS is less common
- **Do you feel depressed?** Because depression underlies many cases of fatigue, it is essential to check for its somatic manifestations
- **Are you more weepy or more sad than usual?** Consider mood disturbance
- **How is your appetite?** May go up or down in depression
- **How is your concentration?** Ask if patients can watch a whole television program, read a newspaper article, function at work
- **Have you ever felt that life was hopeless?**
- **Have you ever felt you could not see a way through or that you would like to end it all?** If either of these are positive it is essential to explore suicidal ideation further, e.g. asking about planning behavior, what stops the impulse
- **Do you feel nervous or uneasy?** Consider anxiety
- **Are you often ill?** Look at the patient's records. A lifelong history of refractory bodily complaints that defy diagnosis and treatment raises suspicion of a personality disturbance or somatization
- **Do you have any fever, sweats, or weight loss?** This may point toward smoldering infection

and occult neoplasm

Q Have you lost weight? Are you thirsty or passing urine excessively? Weight loss, polyuria, polydipsia may suggest diabetes mellitus

Q Have you noticed any change in the color of your skin? This may suggest Addison's disease

Q Do you think your skin and hair have changed at all in texture? Do you feel the cold? Do you feel slow? Have you gained weight? All these may suggest hypothyroidism

Q Are your menstrual cycles normal? Consider menopause and also pituitary insufficiency

Q Do you have joint pains? Symmetric joint pain and morning stiffness are clues to underlying rheumatoid disease. Myalgias and low-grade fever in 50–95% of cases characteristically accompany fatigue

Q Do you snore? Consider sleep apnea

Q Are you sleeping well or are your nights disturbed? Consider esophageal reflux and allergic rhinitis

Q Do you consume much alcohol? Do you take any other non-prescribed drugs? Any abuse of hypnotics or tranquilizers needs to be ascertained and considered as a cause of disturbed sleep and resultant fatigue. Fatigue in the elderly patient should not be ascribed to age; an underlying psychogenic or medical illness is likely

Q Are you taking any prescribed medication? A full listing of all the patient's medications should be obtained. Often overlooked are OTC antihistamines that patients use for sleep, allergies, and colds. Most centrally acting antihypertensive agents are capable of causing fatigue and their use should be noted, as should that of all psychotropic agents

Q What is the worst aspect of your illness? Emphasis on one particular physical symptom other than the constitutional symptoms of malaise and fatigability is somewhat uncommon and should prompt further investigation

Q Have you lost weight? Weight loss does occur but is uncommon in CFS

Q Do you feel muddled or confused? Symptoms of cognitive dysfunction are common and include confusion, difficulty concentrating, impaired thinking, and forgetfulness. Adult patients often judge these as among the most debilitating symptoms. They also occur in hypercalcemia, hypothyroidism, and many other organic disorders

Q What do you think might be the problem? It is always important to elicit the patient's illness beliefs and tailor your explanation of what you believe may be wrong to this

Q What worries you most about it? Patients often feel they have an underlying terminal illness and it is important to offer reassurance that you have or will rule this out, emphasizing that CFS, whilst chronic and sometimes prolonged, is not a terminal illness and recovery is entirely possible with appropriate management

Contributory or predisposing factors

As the true etiology of CFS is unclear, there are no questions specific to CFS. Ask the patient:

Q Do you remember being unwell before this all began? Some patients diagnosed with CFS relate an abrupt onset to their symptoms, often as part of an initial virus-like illness characterized by low-grade fever accompanied by sore throat and cough. Consider recurrent urinary tract infection, proteinuria, liver disease, alcohol and drug abuse, depression, tuberculosis, mononucleosis, hepatitis, and AIDS. A sudden common source outbreak of illness may be associated with travel to areas where parasitic infections are endemic

Examination

Initial examination needs to be very thorough because of the large number of possible underlying causes for fatigue:

Q Are the vital signs normal? Vital signs including postural pulse and blood pressure, temperature, and weight should be determined. If no fever is noted on examination, but it is suggested by history, then a 10 p.m. reading at home is indicated

Q Is the skin normal? Assess for change in pigmentation, purpura, dryness, rash, jaundice, and pallor

Q **Are the nails normal?** Endocarditis may be suggested by splinter hemorrhages or petechiae

Q **Are the fundi normal?** Fundoscopic examination may reveal Roth's spots, diabetic retinopathy, or even in rare instances a tuberculoma

Q **Is the patient jaundiced?** The sclerae are observed for icterus

Q **Are there petechiae on the pharynx?** If examination of the pharynx reveals petechiae at the junction of the hard and soft palate, mononucleosis ought to be considered

Q **Is the thyroid enlarged?** Check for goiter

Q **Is there a heart murmur?** Consider subacute bacterial endocarditis, cardiopulmonary disease

Q **Is there any lymphadenopathy?** Careful examination of all lymph nodes is essential; size, degree of tenderness, and distribution should be noted. Diffuse adenopathy suggests malignancy or infection and is sometimes a sign of HIV infection

Q **Are there any breast lumps?** Breasts should be checked for masses, as breast cancer and its attendant hypercalcemia may present as fatigue

Q **Are there abnormal signs in the chest?** Examine the lungs for rales, consolidation, and effusion, and the heart for murmurs, rubs, gallops, and rhythm disturbances. Unexplained atrial fibrillation in the elderly may be a manifestation of apathetic hyperthyroidism

Q **Is abdominal examination normal?** Check for organomegaly, masses, ascites, and hepatic tenderness

Q **Is rectal examination normal?** If suggested by history of bowel symptoms, the rectal examination includes a look for masses, prostatic pathology, and occult blood. Remember to consider use of a chaperone

Q **Are the genitalia normal?** The genitalia should be checked for masses suggestive of malignancy and tenderness indicative of infection. A pelvic examination should be performed in females. Again, consider chaperone

Q **Are there joint abnormalities?** The joints are assessed for signs of inflammation. A complete neurologic examination is necessary to be sure that the patient's fatigue is not really a manifestation of neuromuscular disease. Any tenderness, atrophy, focal weakness, or fasciculations in the muscles are noted

Q **Are reflexes and power normal?** Deep tendon reflexes that have a slow relaxation phase are suggestive of hypothyroidism

Q **Are the visual fields normal?** Visual field testing is important, a pituitary lesion may produce a bitemporal hemianopia

Q **Is the patient's mental status normal?** Mental status assessment is critical, including observation of affect, thinking, judgment, and memory. Observe appearance, self-care, speech, and movements. Formal testing for suicidality is indicated because of the high prevalence of depression in this patient population

Summary of investigative tests

- Routine screening tests for all patients has no known value
- The use of tests to diagnose the CFS (rather than to exclude other diagnostic possibilities) should be done only in the setting of protocol-based research. The fact that such tests are investigational and do not aid in diagnosis or management should be explained to the patient
- Patients with unusual findings in laboratory tests probably have an underlying disorder
- More than 90% of patients presenting with severe fatigue will have normal levels for the series of tests listed
- Assuming that there is nothing in the physical examination or in the personal history of the patient that suggests a clear direction to the doctor, no further laboratory testing is recommended

Specifically recommended tests for screening of CFS:

- In clinical practice, no additional tests, including laboratory tests or neuroimaging studies, can be recommended for the specific purpose of diagnosing the CFS. Tests should be directed toward confirming or excluding other etiologic possibilities
- In the overtly depressed patient with otherwise normal history and physical examination, an extensive laboratory workup for occult illness is unnecessary
- A complete cell blood count (CBC) and ESR are often ordered
- In the patient with no evidence of depression and unrevealing history and physical examination, calcium, phosphate, albumin, blood urea nitrogen (BUN), creatinine, electrolytes, glucose, and liver function tests (alanine aminotransferase (ALT), total protein, alkaline phosphatase, and globulin) are warranted to help rule out clinically subtle conditions such as hypercalcemia, mild renal failure, early diabetes mellitus, and anicteric hepatitis. A thyrotropin (thyroid-stimulating hormone – TSH) test is worth considering because thyroid disease can have a very subtle presentation, and the assay is very sensitive for detection of most hyperthyroidism and hypothyroidism
- The elderly fatigued patient with weight loss and unexplained atrial fibrillation is a prime candidate for a TSH determination. Other thyroid indices add little and should not be obtained unless the TSH level is abnormal
- Urinalysis may be necessary to assess for renal disease
- Heterophile test for infectious mononucleosis is only indicated in patients with recent onset of persisting fatigue and adenopathy

Tests not routinely recommended:
- Viral titers
- Heterophile test (monospot) for EBV is not indicated unless there is a sudden recent onset of persistent fatigue and lymphadenopathy. Other viral antibody titers (with the exception of testing for viral hepatitis and HIV infection where indicated by the history) are unhelpful for patients with undiagnosed chronic fatigue. Without a proven etiologic role for viruses in CFS, viral titers are sometimes misleading, especially when results are 'positive' in a patient with depression who refuses to accept a psychiatric diagnosis
- The same is true of tests for *Candida*
- Lyme titers are also of little use in the absence of other evidence suggestive of Lyme disease, such as polyarthritis, history of tick bite, or erythema chronicum migrans
- Testing for viral hepatitis is clearly indicated in those with a transaminase elevation
- HIV testing is appropriate when diffuse adenopathy or a history of high-risk behavior is present
- Neuroimaging studies have been used investigationally in CFS to assess regional brain function. Because the significance of these findings remains to be determined, these techniques are not indicated at present for the workup of CFS

DIAGNOSTIC DECISION
DIAGNOSIS OF CFS:
- No test or set of tests is diagnostic for CFS
- The published Centers for Disease Control and Prevention (CDC) diagnostic criteria are a useful guide for diagnosis, especially the diagnoses which must be excluded before making the diagnosis of CFC
- Diagnosis is based on clinical findings and ruling out other etiologies
- A designation of idiopathic chronic fatigue was proposed for the substantial number of persons with unexplained fatigue meeting some but not all of the criteria for CFS

US and UK diagnostic guidelines differ in two ways:
- The UK criteria insist upon the presence of mental fatigue for diagnosis of CFS
- The US criteria include a requirement for several physical symptoms, reflecting belief in immunologic or infective pathology

US diagnostic guidelines

Fukuda K, Straus S, Hickie I, et al. The chronic fatigue syndrome: a comprehensive approach to its definition and study. International Chronic Fatigue Syndrome Study Group. [1]

Thorough medical history, physical examination, mental status examination, and laboratory tests must be conducted to identify underlying or contributing conditions.

Clinically evaluated, unexplained chronic fatigue cases can be classified as CFS if the patient meets both the following criteria.

Clinically evaluated, unexplained persistent or relapsing chronic fatigue that is of at least 6 months duration and:

- Is of new or definite onset (i.e. not lifelong)
- Is not the result of ongoing exertion
- Is not substantially alleviated by rest
- There is a substantial reduction in previous levels of occupational, educational, social, or personal activities; and

The occurrence of four or more of the following symptoms:

- Substantial impairment in short-term memory or concentration
- Sore throat
- Tender lymph nodes
- Muscle pain
- Multi-joint pain without swelling or redness
- Headaches of a new type, pattern, or severity
- Unrefreshing sleep
- Postexertional malaise lasting >24h

These symptoms must have persisted or recurred during 6 or more consecutive months of illness and must not have predated the fatigue; however, diagnosis of CFS is excluded by:

- Any active, unresolved or suspected medical condition that may explain the presence of chronic fatigue, such as untreated hypothyroidism, some types of malignancies, chronic hepatitis B or C infection, and iatrogenic conditions such as side-effects of medication
- Any past or current diagnosis of: major depressive disorder with psychotic or melancholic features; bipolar affective disorders; schizophrenia of any subtype; delusional disorders of any subtype; dementias of any subtype; anorexia or bulimia nervosa; alcohol or other substance abuse, occurring within 2 years of the onset of chronic fatigue and any time afterwards; severe obesity; any unexplained abnormality detected that strongly suggests an exclusionary condition must be resolved before attempting further classification

Conditions that do not exclude a diagnosis of CFS:

- Any condition defined primarily by symptoms that cannot be confirmed by diagnostic laboratory tests, including fibromyalgia, anxiety disorders, somatoform disorders, nonpsychotic or melancholic depression, neurasthenia, and multiple chemical sensitivity disorder
- Any condition under specific treatment sufficient to alleviate all symptoms related to that condition and for which the adequacy of treatment has been documented
- Any condition, such as Lyme disease or syphilis, that was treated with definitive therapy before development of chronic symptoms
- Any isolated and unexplained physical examination finding, or laboratory or imaging test abnormality that is insufficient to strongly suggest the existence of an exclusionary condition. Such conditions include an elevated antinuclear antibody titer that is inadequate, without additional laboratory or clinical evidence, to strongly support a diagnosis of a discrete connective tissue disorder

CLINICAL PEARLS

- The vast majority of patients with 'chronic fatigue' do not have 'CFS'

- CFS is a clinical diagnosis and is a diagnosis of exclusion. CFS can be diagnosed only after a very rigorous and thorough evaluation
- True CFS meeting the above diagnostic criteria is very unusual

THE TESTS
Body fluids
COMPLETE BLOOD COUNT
Description
Blood test.

Advantages/Disadvantages
Advantage: easy, quick, and relatively inexpensive.

Normal
- White blood cells: 3200–9800/mm^3 (3.2–9.8x10^9/L)
- Red blood cells (RBCs): male, 4.3–5.9x10^6/mm^3 (4.3–5.9x10^{12}/L); female, 3.5–5.0x10^6/mm^3 (3.5–5.0x10^{12}/L)
- Hemoglobin: male, 13.6–17.7g/dL (136–177g/L); female, 12–15g/dL (120–150g/L)
- Platelet count: 130–400x10^3/mm^3 (130–400x10^9/L)
- Hematocrit: male, 39–49%; female, 33–43%
- Differential white cell count: 2–6 stabs (early mature neutrophils); 60–70 segs (mature neutrophils); 1–4 eosinophils; 0–1 basophils; 2–8 monocytes; 25–40 lymphocytes

Abnormal
- Results outside normal reference range
- Keep in mind the possibility of a false-positive result

Cause of abnormal result
- CBC will usually be normal in CFS
- The CBC, particularly if accompanied by a look at the peripheral smear and differential, may provide important clues to underlying infection, inflammatory disease, hepatocellular failure, or malignancy
- Abnormal values suggest another physical cause for fatigue: particularly relevant would be anemia or lowered white cell counts
- Differences in the number or appearance of any of the normal blood cell populations might serve as an indication of some underlying illness
- Any finding of raised or lowered hemoglobin, white cell counts, or platelets requires further investigation as to its cause, which may be inflammatory, nutritional, malignant, autoimmune, drug-mediated, congenital

ERYTHROCYTE SEDIMENTATION RATE
Description
- Blood test
- This measure indicates the rate at which RBCs settle out in a tube

Advantages/Disadvantages
- Advantage: easily performed, inexpensive, and quick
- Disadvantage: unfortunately, the ESR has not proved to be sensitive or specific enough to help in detecting or ruling out occult illness. Consequently, many physicians no longer order the ESR, whereas others continue to use it with the intent of acting on it only if the result is markedly elevated (e.g. >75mm/h)

Normal
- Male: 0–15mm/h
- Female: 0–20mm/h

Abnormal
- Results outside normal range
- Keep in mind the possibility of a false-positive result

Cause of abnormal result
- Usually normal in CFS although an abnormal result does not exclude CFS
- An increased rate of sedimentation can serve as a sort of general indicator of inflammation in the body
- Inflammation, malignancy, infection, connective tissue disease, allergy, thyroid disease, myocardial infarction, resolving injury may cause a raised ESR

Drugs, disorders and other factors that may alter results
ESR is lowered in patients on steroids, in hyperviscosity syndromes, and in some genetic red cell abnormalities such as sickle cell disease.

ALANINE AMINOTRANSFERASE
Description
Venous blood sample.

Advantages/Disadvantages
Advantages:
- Inexpensive and quick
- Good screen for underlying hepatic dysfunction

Normal
0–35U/L (0.058mckat/L).

Abnormal
- Raised above normal reference range
- Keep in mind the possibility of a false-positive result

Cause of abnormal result
Elevated levels of this enzyme can be an indication of:
- Viral hepatitis and other forms of liver disease
- Myocardial infarction and congestive heart failure
- Severe muscle trauma

Drugs, disorders and other factors that may alter results
Many drugs may affect liver function including:
- Antibiotics
- Narcotics
- Antihypertensives
- Anticoagulants
- Nonsteroidal anti-inflammatory drugs
- Chlorpromazine
- Phenytoin
- Amiodarone
- Acetaminophen (paracetamol)

TOTAL PROTEIN
Description
- Blood test
- Measurement of the total protein concentration in plasma

Advantages/Disadvantages
Advantage: easy, quick, and relatively inexpensive.

Normal
6–8g/dL (60–80g/L).

Abnormal
- Results outside normal range
- Keep in mind the possibility of a false-positive result

Cause of abnormal result
- Usually normal in CFS
- Elevated concentrations may reflect dehydration, which might be attributable to vomiting, diarrhea, Addison's disease, diabetic acidosis, and other conditions
- Also elevated in multiple myeloma, macroglobulinemias, sarcoidosis, collagen vascular diseases
- Lowered in malnutrition, low protein diet, pregnancy, malabsorption, cirrhosis, nephrosis, malignancy

ALBUMIN
Description
- Blood test
- Albumin is the most abundant protein found in blood plasma, representing 40–60% of the total protein

Advantages/Disadvantages
Advantage: easy, quick, and relatively inexpensive test.

Normal
3.5–5.0g/dL (35–50g/L).

Abnormal
- Results outside normal range
- Keep in mind the possibility of a false-positive result

Cause of abnormal result
- Usually normal in CFS
- Elevated in dehydration
- Reduced levels of albumin may reflect a variety of conditions, including primary liver disease, increased breakdown of macromolecules resulting from tissue damage or inflammation, chronic inflammatory diseases, malabsorption syndromes, malnutrition, lymphoma, and renal diseases

Drugs, disorders and other factors that may alter results
- Oral contraceptives
- Lymphomas
- Elevated in dehydration

GLOBULIN
Description
- Blood test
- Globulins are a diverse group of proteins in the blood, and together represent the second most common proteins (after albumin) in the bloodstream

Advantages/Disadvantages
Advantage: easy, quick, and relatively inexpensive.

Normal
2.0–3.5g/dL (20–35g/L).

Abnormal
- Results outside normal range
- Keep in mind the possibility of a false-positive result

Cause of abnormal result
- An elevation in the level of serum globulin can indicate the presence of cirrhosis of the liver
- Usually normal in CFS

ALKALINE PHOSPHATASE
Description
- Blood test
- Alkaline phosphatases are a family of enzymes that are present throughout the body

Advantages/Disadvantages
Advantage: easy, quick, and relatively inexpensive.

Normal
30–120U/L (0.5–2.0mckat/L).

Abnormal
- Results outside normal range
- Keep in mind the possibility of a false-positive result

Cause of abnormal result
- Elevated levels of alkaline phosphatase are associated with liver and bile duct disorders, and bone diseases such as Paget's disease of bone, rickets, and osteomalacia
- May also be raised in some viral infections, e.g. cytomegalovirus, mononucleosis
- May be raised in malignancy, including leukemia, myelofibrosis, multiple myeloma
- Also raised in pregnancy and at puberty
- Occasionally raised in thyroid disease
- Usually normal in CFS

Drugs, disorders and other factors that may alter results
- Estrogens
- Albumin
- Erythromycin and other antibiotics
- Cholestasis-producing drugs

CALCIUM
Description
Blood test.

Advantages/Disadvantages
Advantage: simple test, inexpensive.

Normal
8.8–10.3mg/dL (2.2–2.58mmol/L).

Abnormal
- Results outside normal range
- Keep in mind the possibility of a false-positive result

Cause of abnormal result
- Increased levels of plasma calcium may indicate the presence of malignant disease, including metastatic disease and multiple myeloma
- Increased levels may indicate hormonal disease such as primary or tertiary or hyperparathyroidism
- Less commonly, it could reflect thyrotoxicosis, vitamin D intoxication, the use of thiazide diuretics, sarcoidosis, Addison's disease, and other disorders
- Reduced levels of calcium may reflect vitamin D deficiency, renal disease, hypoparathyroidism, magnesium deficiency, and other disorders
- Levels are usually normal in CFS

Drugs, disorders and other factors that may alter results
- Lithium may raise levels
- Theophylline may raise levels
- Anticonvulsants, gentamicin, and cimetidine may lower levels

PHOSPHATE
Description
Blood test.

Advantages/Disadvantages
Advantage: easy, quick, and relatively inexpensive.

Normal
2.5–5mg/dL (0.8–1.6mmol/L).

Abnormal
- Results outside normal range
- Keep in mind the possibility of a false-positive result

Cause of abnormal result
- Increased levels of plasma phosphate ion may indicate imminent renal failure, hypoparathyroidism, acromegaly, excessive phosphate intake, and vitamin D intoxication
- Sharply decreased levels of plasma phosphate may reflect vitamin D deficiency, primary hyperparathyroidism, magnesium deficiency, and diabetic ketoacidosis
- Levels are usually normal in CFS

Drugs, disorders and other factors that may alter results
Levels decreased by:
- Alcohol withdrawal
- Antacids
- Glucose given parenterally
- Thiazide diuretic

Levels increased by:
- Antacids containing phosphate

FASTING BLOOD GLUCOSE
Description
- Blood test

▣ Ideally, a fasting blood glucose should be taken (i.e. when patient has not eaten for 14h)

Advantages/Disadvantages
▣ Advantage: simple test, inexpensive
▣ Disadvantage: fasting sample may be more difficult to obtain

Normal
70–110mg/dL (3.9–6.1mmol/L).

Abnormal
▣ Results outside normal range
▣ Keep in mind the possibility of a false-positive result

Cause of abnormal result
▣ Elevated fasting blood glucose levels may be an indication of diabetes mellitus, stress, infections, cerebrovascular accident, Cushing's syndrome, and other metabolic disorders
▣ May also be raised if patient has in fact eaten
▣ Sometimes spuriously raised in conditions causing vomiting, e.g. hyperemesis gravidarum
▣ Lower than normal blood glucose levels (hypoglycemia) can be caused in a variety of ways, often transiently, and must be examined under specific clinical conditions before relating this finding to any clinical disorders
▣ Levels are usually normal in CFS

Drugs, disorders and other factors that may alter results
▣ Thiazides
▣ Loop diuretics
▣ Consumption of food in 14h before test

BLOOD UREA NITROGEN
Description
Blood test.

Advantages/Disadvantages
Advantage: relatively inexpensive, easy, and quick.

Normal
7.0–18.8mg/dL (2.5–6.7mmol/L).

Abnormal
▣ Results outside normal range
▣ Keep in mind the possibility of a false-positive result

Cause of abnormal result
▣ Elevated concentrations may reflect dehydration, which might be attributable to vomiting, diarrhea, Addison's disease, diabetic acidosis, and other conditions
▣ Various renal diseases can lead to an increase in the concentration of urea in blood plasma
▣ Myocardial infarction, shock, congestive cardiac failure
▣ Decreased in liver disease, malnutrition, late pregnancy, overhydration, celiac disease
▣ Level in CFS would usually be normal

Drugs, disorders and other factors that may alter results
May be raised by:
▣ Diuretics

- Lithium
- Corticosteroids
- Aminoglycosides and other antibiotics

ELECTROLYTES
Description
- Blood test
- This test measures the levels of charged ions dissolved in the blood, including sodium and potassium

Advantages/Disadvantages
Advantage: relatively easy, inexpensive, and quick.

Normal
- Sodium: 135–147mEq/L (135–147mmol/L)
- Potassium: 3.5–5mEq/L (3.5–5mmol/L)

Abnormal
- Results outside normal range
- Keep in mind the possibility of a false-positive result
- Virtually all the metabolic processes in the body are dependent on the presence of these charged ions, the concentrations of which are tightly controlled

Cause of abnormal result
- In CFS, levels would usually be normal, so any abnormality may rule out CFS and needs further appropriate investigation
- Sodium is raised in dehydration and salt overdose, and is lowered in sodium and water depletion, including due to Addison's disease, congestive heart failure, cirrhosis, nephrotic syndrome, renal failure
- Sodium is falsely raised in hypertriglyceridemia, hyperproteinemia, and severe hyperglycemia
- Potassium is raised in dehydration, renal failure, excessive use of potassium-sparing diuretics, Addison's disease
- Potassium is lowered in cachexia and any severe illness, prolonged diarrhea, trauma, Cushing's syndrome, and cirrhosis
- Deviations from normal levels of each of these cations can reflect a wide variety of clinical problems

Drugs, disorders and other factors that may alter results
Levels raised by potassium-sparing diuretics (angiotensin-converting enzyme (ACE) inhibitors, amiloride, spironolactone)

CREATININE
Description
Venous blood sample.

Advantages/Disadvantages
Advantage: relatively easy, inexpensive, and quick.

Normal
0.79–1.70mg/dL (70–150mcmol/L).

Abnormal
- Results outside normal range
- Keep in mind the possibility of a false-positive result

Cause of abnormal result

- Elevated levels of plasma creatinine may indicate impaired renal function or dehydration
- Decreased levels are seen in pregnancy, decreased muscle mass (e.g. amputees), and prolonged debilitation
- Levels are usually normal in CFS

Drugs, disorders and other factors that may alter results
Increased by:

- Antibiotics (especially aminoglycosides, cephalosporins)
- Hydantoin
- Diuretics
- Methyldopa

THYROID-STIMULATING HORMONE

Description

- Blood test
- This is a test of thyroid function

Advantages/Disadvantages
Advantage: relatively easy, inexpensive, and quick.

Normal
0.5–5.7mU/mL (0.5–5.7mcU/L).

Abnormal

- Results outside normal range
- Keep in mind the possibility of a false-positive result

Cause of abnormal result

- Higher than normal levels of TSH may indicate hypothyroidism and lower than normal levels may suggest hyperthyroidism
- In rare instances, elevated TSH levels may be caused by pituitary tumors
- Increased levels may also be found in Addison's disease, acute psychiatric illness, and after some contrast media
- Decreased levels may also be seen in Cushing's syndrome, corticosteroid therapy, hyperemesis
- Levels would normally be normal in CFS

Drugs, disorders and other factors that may alter results
Raised by:

- Amphetamines
- Large doses of inorganic iodide (e.g. saturated solution of potassium iodide – SSKI)
- Iodine deficiency
- Lithium
- Amiodarone

Lowered by:

- Overtreatment with thyroxine
- Dopamine
- Glucocorticoids
- Interleukin treatment
- Alpha-interferon

URINALYSIS

Description

- Urine may be examined for a variety of diagnostic indicators, including amylase, bilirubin, creatinine, sugars, gamma-glutamyl transferase, hemoglobin, lactate dehydrogenase, osmolality, electrolytes, myoglobin, protein, urea, and many more
- A basic test would be for red and white blood cells, protein, glucose, nitrites
- Other tests should be requested as appropriate to presenting features

Advantages/Disadvantages

Advantage: simple, inexpensive test.

Normal

- RBCs: 0–5/high-power field
- White blood cells: 0–5/high-power field
- Bacteria: absent
- Casts: 0–4 hyaline (low-power field)
- Nitrites, protein, and glucose should be absent
- Ketones: absent

Abnormal

- Results outside normal range
- Keep in mind the possibility of a false-positive result

Cause of abnormal result

- Urinalysis is usually normal in CFS
- Elevated glucose levels may indicate diabetes mellitus
- Elevated protein or white cells may indicate infection or inflammation or primary renal disease
- Elevated nitrites suggest infection with urea-splitting organisms
- Pure growths of bacteria suggest urinary tract infection or renal infection
- RBCs may indicate stones, infection or neoplasm
- RBCs may also indicate menstruation
- Elevated amylase levels can indicate pancreatic disease
- Elevated ketones suggest prolonged fast or uncontrolled diabetes
- Increased urine bilirubin levels signal liver damage or disease
- Increased lactate dehydrogenase in urine is associated with glomerulonephritis, systemic lupus erythematosus, diabetic nephrosclerosis, and bladder and kidney malignancies

Drugs, disorders and other factors that may alter results

Anticoagulants may cause positive red cells in urine.

HETEROPHILE TEST FOR INFECTIOUS MONONUCLEOSIS

Description

Venous blood sample.

Advantages/Disadvantages

- Advantage: easy, quick, and relatively inexpensive
- Disadvantage: indicated only in patients with recent onset of persisting fatigue and adenopathy

Normal
Negative.

Abnormal
Positive.

Cause of abnormal result
Infectious mononucleosis.

TREATMENT

CONSIDER CONSULT

- Refer if there is a specialist center in your area taking chronic fatigue syndrome (CFS) referrals and offering an integrated service to patients
- Refer on if doctor-patient relationship breaking down – perhaps due to patient's illness beliefs
- Refer worsening depressive features within CFS
- Refer children to specialist pediatrician as the diagnosis is difficult to make in children; the entity may not exist in children and there is a high likelihood of other psychologic, psychiatric, or family difficulties
- Refer to rheumatologist or psychiatrist in advanced and complicated cases
- If a patient says he or she is not sleeping well, refer him/her to sleep laboratory to find out why

IMMEDIATE ACTION

Refer patients with severe associated depression for inpatient treatment.

PATIENT AND CAREGIVER ISSUES
Impact on career, dependants, family, friends

- CFS has a huge impact on patient's social and occupational functioning
- This affects relationships, financial life, sexual function, self-esteem, family life, and activity levels
- The results are far reaching and CFS can have an impact on family life equal to many major disabilities
- A positive but realistic outlook needs to be shared by patient, family, caregivers, and physician. Any sense that the patient's family, carers, or physician finds the patient's case hopeless or emotionally wearing will be deeply detrimental

Patient or caregiver request

- Patients frequently present as a result of articles they have read on the Internet or in books suggesting anecdotal therapies for CFS
- It is important to listen and offer support, while making it clear that anecdotal reports which are not evidence based may at best be unhelpful and at worst dangerous. Emphasize to the patient that the vast majority of patients presenting for evaluation for CFS have another explanation for their symptoms
- Emphasizing to the patient that there are known benefits from the treatments which are evidence based may help
- Patients are often resentful that their doctor is unable to provide a treatment they have read about, and often take the view that conventional medicine is united against them
- These feelings need to be explored as they will swiftly undermine the doctor-patient relationship, and may make it difficult for the doctor to monitor adequately the patient's clinical condition
- Some patients may be looking for an organic cause for their illness. They may attribute psychologic symptoms as being secondary to a physical cause

Health-seeking behavior

- Ask about food supplements, drugs bought over the Internet, special diets, or anything else the patient may have tried. This is particularly important as the patient may inadvertently be using something which is likely to make the condition worse
- Many patients speculate that they have a nutritional deficiency and self-treat first

It is important to discover the patient's attitude to the condition:
- Do they regard it as primarily physical or psychologic?
- What are their fears or concerns?

- What are they expecting you to offer?
- What are they hoping you will offer?
- What are they afraid you will not offer?
- What have they read?
- What understanding do they already have of their condition?
- Have they joined a support group?

MANAGEMENT ISSUES
Goals
- Reduce fatigue and associated symptoms
- Increase levels of activity
- Improve quality of life
- Resumption of normal levels of functioning
- Help the patient learn to cope with the fatigue and the limitations it imposes on his or her life

Management in special circumstances
COEXISTING DISEASE
- Depression that coexists with CFS, perhaps as a result of it, should be treated with appropriate antidepressants. There is good evidence of response of depressive symptoms to treatment with appropriate medication
- Other chronic underlying diseases should be managed appropriately and the impact of the CFS on them treated symptomatically
- Patients whose movement is restricted due to pain or joint/muscle disease may find it particularly difficult to participate in exercise programs. Experienced physiotherapists should be involved to tailor treatment to the individual patient. Emphasize the importance of beginning an exercise program at a very low level, advancing it cautiously, and sticking with it
- Patients with other terminal disease should be supported and treated symptomatically

COEXISTING MEDICATION
- It is important to be aware of any medication the patient is taking
- Many treatments may worsen CFS and if an alternative therapy can be substituted symptoms may improve

SPECIAL PATIENT GROUPS
Children:
- CFS is difficult to diagnose in children, who have trouble describing their symptoms and articulating their concerns
- As with any chronic illness in childhood, careful attention must be directed to the family dynamics to identify and resolve family problems or psychopathology that may be contributing to a child's perceptions of his or her symptoms
- The diagnosis of CFS in a child should be made with a great deal of caution
- The label of CFS may be detrimental in children, where some authors believe all cases of 'CFS' are attributable to other causes
- If the label is felt to imply the child is suffering from some mysterious, progressive viral or immunologic disorder, then eyes can be closed to other distress and attempts to rehabilitate the child in the context of family and school ignored
- Poor prognosis or long illness course can become a self-fulfilling prophecy
- Therapy should be directed toward emotional support for patients and their families, relief of symptoms, and minimizing unnecessary and misleading diagnostic and therapeutic tests
- This may include a combination of restoration of a normal sleep pattern, rehabilitation strategies including exercise for fatigue, and optimism
- Psychologic or psychiatric intervention may be a principal component of supportive treatment
- Patients with severe limitation of activity should be started on a schedule of graded

remobilization, determined by individual tolerance and, if warranted, physical therapy leading to a regular regimen of moderate exercise
- Complete bed rest and lack of exercise only perpetuate immobility and lead to deconditioning; rapid remobilization, for whatever reason, usually exacerbates symptoms and should be avoided
- Return to school should also be initiated gradually but systematically to resume normal attendance
- Home tutoring may be an interim alternative
- Patients and their families should clearly understand that there is no evidence that activity harms patients with CFS
- Continued empathy and support by the treating physician are important in maintaining a physician-patient relationship conducive to identification and resolution of both organic and psychologic illness
- Periodic medical re-evaluation approximately every 3 months is warranted for early detection of other identifiable causes of chronic fatigue, especially with development of new symptoms

Adolescents:
- CFS is clearly present among adolescents, although the prevalence for this group is lower than for most adult age groups

Elderly patients:
- CFS is relatively unusual in this group and organic disease is common, so a particularly thorough workup is necessary
- In particular, exclude occult anemia, malignancy, polymyalgia rheumatica, and myeloma, all of which may present with fatigue

PATIENT SATISFACTION/LIFESTYLE PRIORITIES
- Disability is related to the presence of catastrophic beliefs about the disastrous effect of activity. Effective management involves a collaborative approach to testing these assumptions, but not the physical origin of illness
- A positive diagnosis of CFS can be used in a constructive fashion. CFS can be of use in clinical practice as a structure for patient understanding and a model for treatment
- Patients with CFS usually believe that rest is the best way of controlling activity, and that other than that they are helpless to alter the course of the illness. This needs to be corrected
- Diagnosis must be acceptable to both doctor and patient
- A positive but realistic outlook is essential, and this needs to be shared by patient, family, caregivers, and physician

SUMMARY OF THERAPEUTIC OPTIONS
Choices
Treatment begins with communication of diagnosis:
- Suggestion of diagnosis sometimes comes from patient, sometimes from physician
- CFS is a clinical diagnosis and a diagnosis of exclusion – if the diagnostic criteria are met in the absence of the appropriate exclusions, then the diagnosis of CFS is appropriate
- A patient who presents convinced that he or she has CFS is more likely to be satisfied that the diagnosis of CFS is not correct if another diagnosis can be established
- Telling the patient that the alternative label is that of a psychologic problem may be unacceptable to him or her, and damages the doctor-patient relationship. Such patients have often been told that the problem 'is all in your head', or the patient may conclude that this is the opinion the doctor is inferring. The patient may be more willing to consider depression as a potential diagnosis if this possibility is introduced tactfully
- There is little value in confronting a patient with the diagnosis of somatization disorder with the suggestion that the patient has a psychologic disorder

- Begin the consultation with the diagnosis – 'I recognize that you have chronic fatigue and that this is very distressing to you. Now we must determine what is the cause', in order to gain the confidence of the patient
- A positive diagnosis of CFS should be used in a constructive fashion. CFS can be of use in clinical practice as a structure for patient understanding

Because no cause for CFS has been identified, the therapies for this disorder are directed at relief of symptoms. The physician and patient develop an individually tailored program to provide the greatest perceived benefit, based on some combination of the available treatment.

Management plan for CFS in primary care:
- Establish the diagnosis
- Symptomatic treatment
- Medications for depression: antidepressants
- Medications for anxiety
- Medications for pain: nonsteroidal anti-inflammatory drugs (NSAIDs): ibuprofen, acetaminophen, tramadol
- Medications for sleep: low-dose tricyclic antidepressants, trazodone, other sedating antidepressants
- Avoidance of exotic untested remedies

Provide reassurance and emotional support:
- Acceptance of symptoms
- Avoidance of confrontational approach
- Referral to support groups, psychotherapy and counseling, cognitive behavioral therapy (CBT)

Lifestyle management:
- Apply stress reduction techniques
- Restructure activities
- Make realistic goals
- Rehabilitation

Prevent further disability:
- Graded exercise program
- Physical therapy

Regular follow up:
- Continue to rule out other medical problems
- Physical activity should be gradually increased as tolerated

Other therapeutic options:
- Rest may be of some value temporarily, but the patient should be discouraged from thinking of prolonged rest as the mainstay of treatment
- There is insufficient evidence to support the use of corticosteroids, nicotinamide adenine dinucleotide (NADH), immunoglobulins, prolonged rest, antidepressants, evening primrose oil, or magnesium
- Some experimental therapies are detailed below as patients may ask about them – they are not licensed, not recommended, and generally not based on good evidence
- Alternative therapies sometimes useful for CFS patients include acupuncture, aquatic therapy, chiropractic, cranial-sacral, light exercise, massage, self-hypnosis, stretching, tai chi, therapeutic touch, and yoga. There is no evidence base for them but they may improve patient's self-help and motivation

Clinical pearls

- No treatment has been established as effective in treating CFS. The most one can hope for are therapies which relieve the patient's symptoms while awaiting the spontaneous improvement which sometimes occurs
- The main value in distinguishing between CFS and fibromyalgia is that the latter condition is much more likely to respond to treatment

Never

- Never suggest to the patient that they may have an incurable or hopeless condition
- If the patient expresses certainty that their illness is physical, you may attempt to reassure the patient that your evaluation has excluded such diagnoses rather than denying the patient's concern or expectation that a physical cause might be found. It is important to avoid extensive inappropriate diagnostic evaluations which may reinforce the patient's expectation that a physical cause could be identified. Explain that depression often coexists with CFS and other chronic painful conditions. The patients who did best in trials did not change their views about the physical nature of their illness

FOLLOW UP

- Dependent on patient's clinical condition and on whether any medication is being prescribed
- Also dependent on the prevalence of depressive features

Plan for review

- As the doctor can offer little intervention, follow up will be determined by the need to monitor for new-onset conditions such as depression and to offer support and advice
- It may be helpful to offer regular review of patients having ongoing exercise or CBT – a 3- to 6-monthly review would usually be appropriate
- It is therefore usually appropriate to have review initiated at patient's request
- Patients on prescribed medication or with active depressive or other features of concern will need more frequent physician-initiated review as per clinical status

Information for patient or caregiver

- The physician should emphasize the legitimacy of the patient's symptoms and summarize the workup, its rationale, and findings
- Also useful is a review of the idiopathic nature of the illness, its generally self-limited course, and often favorable response to simple measures
- Establishing a partnership with the patient is the key to successful management
- Beliefs and behaviors known to perpetuate disability and lead to a worse outcome in CFS must be addressed, particularly the view that a disease mechanism is present that is unresponsive to intervention and that exercise is harmful. Such ideation contributes to resignation, anxiety, and depression and exacerbates deconditioning and the feeling of fatigue
- If possible, referral for formal CBT is worth pursuing to achieve the educational and behavioral goals so important to recovery
- It is important that any new symptoms or signs be reported and investigated thoroughly and not simply attributed to CFS

Other information patients may seek or receive:

- Because the cause of CFS has not been identified, periodically new invalidated beliefs about cures and causes of CFS are widely circulated
- These may be based on one or more reports from scientific literature, from the anecdotal remarks of clinicians or scientists at medical meetings, or in some cases the origin is obscure. Even work that is published in the scientific literature is not without limitations and design flaws, and all published work needs to be verified and expanded on by others before it can be applied with confidence in clinical situations

- With regard to some stories currently circulating: there is no evidence that CFS patients lose their fingerprints; there is no scientific evidence of any nutritional deficiency in CFS patients; and suicides of CFS patients have been reported, but there is no evidence that the rate is higher or lower than what would be expected in the general population
- Patients should be advised to be wary of information that points to sure cures or that alludes to pathologic damage as a consequence of CFS
- Patients should inform their physician before self-medicating with any alternative cure. They are more likely to do so if they feel their physician is working with them

DRUGS AND OTHER THERAPIES: DETAILS
Drugs
CORTICOSTEROIDS

- Hydrocortisone, fludrocortisone
- There have been a number of studies suggesting that the output of cortisol is slightly reduced in CFS although it is within the normal range
- The use of fludrocortisone, a mineralocorticoid, was based on the hypothesis that CFS is associated with neurally mediated hypotension
- The use of hydrocortisone in the other trials was based on evidence of underactivity of the hypothalamic-pituitary-adrenocortical axis in some people with the syndrome
- The only indication for treatment with corticosteroids is an established diagnosis of adrenal insufficiency. The potential for harm from this treatment far exceeds its potential value in the treatment of CFS
- This is an off-label indication

Dose
Because low levels of cortisol are associated with fatigue in other illnesses, trials of hydrocortisone 5–10mg/day were used.

Efficacy

- Limited data from RCTs provide insufficient evidence to support the use of corticosteroids in people with CFS; any benefit from low-dose glucocorticoid treatment seems to be short-lived, and higher doses are associated with adverse effects
- Evidence for this therapy remains unclear but trials agreed that benefit attenuated rapidly when treatment was discontinued

Risks/Benefits
Risks:

- The study using the higher doses of hydrocortisone found that 12 people (40%) receiving active treatment experienced adrenal suppression
- Minor adverse effects were reported in up to 10% of people in the other studies

Evidence
There is insufficient evidence for the use of corticosteroids in CFS.

- A crossover RCT found no significant difference in symptomatic severity and functional status when fludrocortisone was compared with placebo over 6 weeks [2] *Level P*
- A RCT compared hydrocortisone (25–35mg/day) with placebo for 12 weeks, and found a greater improvement in a self-rated scale of 'wellness' in the treatment group. However, no significant benefit was noted with other self-rating scales [3] *Level P*
- Another RCT compared hydrocortisone (5 or 10mg/day) with placebo over one month. Short-term improvement in fatigue was achieved in more people taking hydrocortisone than placebo [4] *Level P*

Acceptability to patient
Easy to take but with higher doses side-effects may be substantial, particularly weight gain and adrenal suppression.

Follow up plan
This treatment is not recommended.

Patient and caregiver information
This treatment is not recommended.

LOW-DOSE ANTIDEPRESSANTS
- Tricyclic agents are sometimes prescribed for CFS patients to improve sleep and to relieve mild, generalized pain. Examples include doxepin, amitriptyline. Desipramine HCl is a less sedating tricyclic drug
- Patients with CFS appear particularly sensitive to drugs, especially those that affect the central nervous system. Thus, the usual treatment strategy is to begin with very low doses and to escalate the dosage gradually as necessary

Dose
- Amitriptyline:10–50mg at bedtime
- Doxepin: 25–50mg at bedtime
- Trazodone: 25–100mg at bedtime
- Patients with CFS appear particularly sensitive to drugs, especially those that affect the central nervous system. Thus, the usual treatment strategy is to begin with very low doses and to escalate the dosage gradually as necessary

Efficacy
- Known to be helpful for treatment of neuropathic pain
- Benefit in CFS unclear

Risks/Benefits
Benefit: in a study of patients who had fibromyalgia, amitriptyline in doses of 25mg at bedtime resulted in less fatigue, improved sleep, and decreased myalgias when compared with placebo. Responses were usually seen in 3–4 weeks.

Acceptability to patient
Acceptability will be enhanced by starting at a very low dose which is initially tolerated, and increasing the dose slowly.

FULL-DOSE ANTIDEPRESSANTS
- Recommended in CFS if there are depressive features
- Antidepressants have been used to treat depression in CFS patients
- Anxiolytic agents may be used to treat panic disorder in CFS patients
- Examples include buspirone, alprazolam, and lorazepam
- The choice of antidepressant depends on expected side-effects
- Tricyclic antidepressants are associated with sedative and anticholinergic effects
- Patients who have difficulty sleeping sometimes respond well to agents such as amitriptyline HCl or doxepin HCl taken once a day at bedtime
- Bupropion may be effective in patients who are unable to tolerate a tricyclic agent or selective serotonin reuptake inhibitor (SSRI)
- Sexual dysfunction may be less of a problem with bupropion than with SSRI agents

Dose

- When sedation is not desirable, SSRIs, such as fluoxetine, citalopram, or sertaline can be helpful
- Fluoxetine: initially 20mg/day; may be increased gradually after several weeks to a maximum of 80mg/day
- Citalopram: initially 20mg/day, usually increased to 40mg/day after an interval of at least one week
- Sertaline: initially 50mg/day; may be increased gradually to a maximum of 200mg/day if not responding to lower doses; dose changes should not occur at intervals of less than one week
- Bupropion: start with 100mg twice daily and, based on clinical response, increase to 100mg three times daily no sooner than 3 days after beginning treatment
- Venlafaxine: initially 75mg/day; dose may be increased at increments up to 75mg/day at intervals not less than 4 days; the maximum recommended dose for outpatient is 225mg/day
- These drugs are not licensed for the treatment of CFS (this is an off-label indication)

Efficacy

There is insufficient evidence to support the use of antidepressants in people with CFS, but antidepressants may be useful in treating associated depression. Anecdotal reports suggest that venlafaxine is sometimes effective in treating fibromyalgia, but there are no data to support this.

Risks/Benefits

Risks:

SSRIs:

- Use caution in renal, hepatic, and cardiac disease
- Use caution in bipolar disorder and suicidal tendencies
- Use caution in seizure disorders, anorexia nervosa, and diabetes
- Use caution in the elderly and children
- Use caution in pregnancy and nursing mothers
- Consider long duration of action when adjusting dose
- More expensive than tricyclic antidepressants (although there is evidence of greater cost effectiveness)

Bupropion:

- Dose-related risk of seizures
- Use extreme caution when administered to patients with a history of seizure, cranial trauma, or other predisposition to seizure
- Use extreme caution when prescribed with other agents such as antipsychotics, other antidepressants, theophylline, systemic steroids, or any treatment that lowers seizure threshold
- Use caution in renal or hepatic impairment
- Use caution in suicidal patients
- Use caution with recent myocardial infarction
- Risk of precipitation of manic episodes in manic depression

Venlafaxine:

- Use caution in pregnancy or breast-feeding
- Use caution in renal or hepatic impairment, cardiac disease, or hypertension
- Use caution in history of mania or suicidality
- Use caution in history of seizures
- Use caution in underweight patients or those with anorexia nervosa
- Use caution in the elderly
- Use caution in patients with closed-angle glaucoma
- Use caution in patients predisposed to skin and mucous membrane bleeding
- Advise caution with driving or operating machinery

- Avoid alcohol
- Avoid abrupt discontinuation
- Serious infrequent or rare cardiovascular disorders have been reported

Benefits:
- Treats anxiety and depression associated with CFS
- Sleep may be improved

Side-effects and adverse reactions
SSRIs:
- Cardiovascular system: palpitations, vasodilatation, chest pain
- Central nervous system: headache, nervousness, anxiety, asthenia, drowsiness, dizziness, tremor, convulsions, mania, movement disorders, suicidal ideation, abnormal dreams
- Eyes, ears, nose, and throat: dry mouth, rhinitis, visual disturbances
- Gastrointestinal: nausea, vomiting, diarrhea, constipation, dyspepsia, abdominal pain, anorexia, weight loss, flatulence
- Genitourinary: sexual dysfunction
- Metabolic: hyponatremia
- Musculoskeletal: myalgia
- Skin: sweating, purpura, rash

Bupropion:
- Cardiovascular system: arrythmias, hypertension, hypotension, palpitations, syncope, tachycardia
- Central nervous system: dizziness, confusion, anxiety, akinesia, headache, migraine, insomnia, muscle spasms, tremor, fatigue, chills
- Eyes, ears, nose, and throat: blurred vision
- Gastrointestinal: anorexia, increased appetite, diarrhea, dyspepsia, nausea, vomiting, constipation
- Genitourinary: impotence, menstrual complaints, urinary retention
- Musculoskeletal: arthritis
- Skin: rash, pruritus

Venlafaxine:
- Cardiovascular system: hypertension, postural hypotension, migraine
- Central nervous system: drowsiness, dizziness, anxiety, asthenia, insomnia, nervousness, tremor, seizures, amnesia, somnolence, confusion, depersonalization, emotional lability, hypesthesia, vertigo
- Eyes, ears, nose, and throat: blurred vision, abnormality of accommodation, taste perversion
- Gastrointestinal: nausea, vomiting, weight loss, anorexia, constipation, dry mouth
- Genitourinary: sexual dysfunction, menstrual abnormalities
- Metabolic: hyponatremia
- Musculoskeletal system: arthralgia
- Respiratory: dyspnea
- Skin: sweating, rash, pruritus
- Other: chest pain

Interactions (other drugs)
SSRIs:
- Alcohol ▪ Antihistamines, nonsedating ▪ Azole antifungals ▪ Barbiturates ▪ Benzodiazepines ▪ Beta-blockers ▪ Buspirone ▪ Cimetidine ▪ Cisapride ▪ Carbamazepine ▪ Clozapine ▪ Cyclosporine ▪ Cyproheptadine ▪ Diltiazem ▪ Digoxin

Erythromycin Haloperidol Lithium Methadone L-tryptophan Monoamine oxidase inhibitors (MAOIs) Phenytoin Phenothiazines Pimozide Procyclidine St John's wort Sumatriptan Sympathomimetics Tacrine Theophylline Tolbutamide Tricyclic antidepressants Warfarin

Bupropion:
Drugs that affect the cytochrome P-450 (CYP) 2B6 isoenzyme, such as orphenadrine and cyclophosphamide (may alter drug levels) Drugs that are metabolized by the CYP2D6 isoenzyme, such as nortriptyline, imipramine, desipramine, paroxetine, fluoxetine, sertraline, haloperidol, risperidone, thioridazine, metoprolol, propafenone, flecainide MAOIs (may enhance acute toxicity) Levodopa (increased adverse reactions) Drugs that lower seizure threshold, such as antipyschotics, other antidepressants, theophylline systemic steroids

Venlafaxine:
Amphetamines Antivirals Cimetidine Cocaine Dexfenfluramine, fenfluramine Kava kava, valerian Lithium Nefazodone, trazodone SSRIs St John's wort Tricyclic antidepressants Zolpidem Should not be combined with MAOIs

Contraindications
SSRIs:
Manic phase MAOIs Cisapride

Bupropion:
Seizure disorder Previous or current bulimia or anorexia nervosa Concurrent MAOI use Pregnancy and breast-feeding

Venlafaxine:
Concurrent use of MAOIs Under 18 years old

Evidence
There is insufficient evidence that antidepressants are effective in the management of CFS.
- A RCT compared fluoxetine with placebo in depressed and nondepressed patients with CFS. There was no significant improvement in the Beck Depression Inventory and the sickness impact profile after 8 weeks with fluoxetine [5] *Level P*
- Another RCT compared graded exercise plus fluoxetine, graded exercise plus placebo, general advice to exercise plus fluoxetine, and general advice to exercise plus placebo, over 12 weeks. No significant difference was noted in level of fatigue, although there was a modest improvement in measures of depression at 12 weeks [6] *Level P*
- A RCT compared moclobemide with placebo in CFS patients. Improvement in subjective vigor was noted in the treatment group. A nonsignificant trend was noted towards improved clinician-rated Karnofski scale in people receiving moclobemide [7] *Level P*
- Sertraline and clomipramine were compared in another RCT of people with CFS. No significant difference was found between these medications [8] *Level P*

Acceptability to patient
Up to 15% of participants withdrew from active treatment because of adverse drug effects.

Follow up plan
- Follow up as for treating depression – see patient within 3 weeks of starting treatment to assess for compliance, side-effects, and benefits, then reassess at least monthly
- Ask patient to make contact at any time if things deteriorate

Patient and caregiver information
- Remember that telling the patient that their illness is one that is totally unacceptable to them, a psychologic problem, damages the doctor-patient relationship
- The physician should explain that whilst the drugs are antidepressants they sometimes bring benefit in CFS when there are features of reactive depression, and that you are not labeling the patient as having a primary depressive or psychosomatic illness

ACETAMINOPHEN
Use in CFS is symptomatic for relief of pain.

Dose
- Acetaminophen 325–1000mg every 4–6h, as necessary
- Maximum 4g/day

Efficacy
Symptomatic treatment for headaches, arthralgias, and myalgias.

Risks/Benefits
Risks:
- Use caution in hepatic and renal impairment
- Overdosage results in hepatic and renal damage unless treated promptly
- Overdose may lead to multiorgan failure and may be fatal
- Accidental overdosage can occur if OTC preparations containing acetaminophen are taken with prescribed drugs that contain acetaminophen

Benefits:
- Pain due to myalgia and arthralgia may be improved
- Headache is treated with analgesics

Side-effects and adverse reactions
- Acetaminophen rarely causes side-effects when used intermittently
- Gastrointestinal: nausea, vomiting
- Hematologic: blood disorders
- Metabolic: acute hepatic and renal failure
- Skin: rashes
- Other: acute pancreatitis

Interactions (other drugs)
- Alcohol ■ Anticoagulants ■ Anticonvulsants ■ Isoniazid ■ Cholestyramine ■ Colestipol ■ Domperidone ■ Metoclopromide

Contraindications
- Hypersensitivity to acetaminophen ■ Known liver dysfunction

Follow up plan
Review period determined by symptom severity and patient's needs.

Patient and caregiver information
The patient needs to understand that there is no published evidence which clearly supports use of this agent.

IBUPROFEN

- Use in CFS is symptomatic for relief of pain
- NSAIDs are often used to treat myalgias and arthralgias associated with CFS

Dose
Adult recommended dose: 400mg every 4–6h as necessary.

Efficacy
Symptomatic treatment for headaches, arthralgias, and myalgias.

Risks/Benefits
Risks:

- Use caution in the elderly
- Use caution in hepatic, renal, and cardiac failure
- Use caution in bleeding disorders
- There is no evidence that final outcome is changed by NSAIDs

Benefits:

- Pain due to myalgia and arthralgia may be improved
- Headache is treated with analgesics

Side-effects and adverse reactions

- Cardiovascular system: hypertension, peripheral edema
- Central nervous system: headache, dizziness, tinnitus
- Gastrointestinal: anorexia, nausea, dyspepsia, peptic ulceration, bleeding
- Genitourinary: nephrotoxicity
- Hematologic: blood cell disorders
- Hypersensitivity: rashes, bronchospasm, angioedema

Interactions (other drugs)

- Aminoglycosides ▪ Anticoagulants ▪ Antihypertensives ▪ Baclofen ▪ Corticosteroids
- Cyclosporine, tacrolimus ▪ Digoxin ▪ Diuretics ▪ Lithium ▪ Methotrexate
- Phenylpropanolamine ▪ Warfarin

Contraindications

- Peptic ulceration ▪ Hypersensitivity to any pain reliever or antipyretic (including NSAIDs)
- Coagulation defects ▪ Severe renal or hepatic disease

Follow up plan
Review period determined by symptom severity and patient's needs.

Patient and caregiver information
The patient needs to understand that there is no published evidence which clearly supports use of this agent.

ORAL NICOTINAMIDE ADENINE DINUCLEOTIDE (NADH)

The rationale for this treatment is that NADH facilitates generation of adenosine triphosphate (ATP), which may be depleted in CFS.

Efficacy
Some improvement in one trial in a minority of patients – insufficient evidence for its use.

Risks/Benefits
Benefits: uncertain.

Evidence
A randomized, crossover trial compared NADH vs placebo for 4 weeks in people with CFS. On a symptom rating scale, eight of 26 patients receiving NADH attained a 10% improvement, compared with two of 26 patients receiving placebo [9] *Level P*

Acceptability to patient
Acceptable in the clinical trial.

Follow up plan
Not currently recommended treatment, but follow up in accordance with clinical condition.

Patient and caregiver information
Not recommended treatment for this disorder.

IMMUNOTHERAPY

- Gamma-globulin is pooled human immunoglobulin G (IgG). It contains antibody molecules directed against a broad range of common infectious agents and is ordinarily used as a means for passively immunizing persons whose immune system has been compromised, or who have been exposed to an agent that might cause more serious disease in the absence of immunoglobulin
- Its use with CFS patients is experimental and based on the unsubstantiated hypothesis that CFS is characterized by an underlying immune disorder. Serious adverse reactions are uncommon, although in rare instances gamma-globulin may initiate anaphylactic shock

Dose
In trials, dose was 1–2g/kg of IgG, given as in intravenous infusion every 30 days for 3–6 months.

Efficacy
- There was some evidence for benefit – outweighed by high incidence of adverse effects
- RCTs of IgG in people with CFS found only limited benefit and adverse effects; other forms of immunotherapy have no advantage over placebo

Risks/Benefits
Risks:
- Should be given with caution to patients with a history of prior systemic allergic reactions following the administration of human immunoglobulin preparations
- If anaphylactic or severe anaphylactoid reactions occur, discontinue infusion immediately. Epinephrine should be available for the treatment of any acute anaphylactoid reactions

Benefit:: not clear

Side-effects and adverse reactions
Hematologic: transmission of hepatitis B and C, and HIV

Interactions (other drugs)
May interfere with the response by pediatric patients to live viral vaccines such as measles, mumps, and rubella.

Contraindications
- History of anaphylactic or severe systemic response to immunoglobulin intramuscular or

intravenous preparations ▪ Should not be given to persons with isolated IgA deficiency
▪ Pregnancy category C

Evidence
▪ A RCT compared monthly immunoglobulin injections (1g/kg) with placebo for the treatment of CFS. No significant difference in fatigue or functioning (physical and social) was noted after 6 months in either group [10] *Level P*
▪ Another RCT compared IgG injections (2g/kg) with placebo over 3 months. More people in the treatment group achieved an improvement in physician-rated assessment of symptoms and disability. A repeat of this trial did not replicate these results [11,12] *Level P*

Acceptability to patient
Not recommended treatment for this disorder.

Follow up plan
Not recommended treatment for this disorder.

Patient and caregiver information
Not recommended treatment for this disorder.

Physical therapy
EXERCISE
Exercise and advice/supervision from physical therapists may be beneficial.

Efficacy
▪ Graded exercise programs seem to be the most beneficial treatment for CFS
▪ In general, physicians advise patients with CFS to pace themselves carefully and encourage them to avoid unusual physical or emotional stress
▪ A regular, manageable daily routine helps avoid the 'push-crash' phenomenon characterized by overexertion during periods of better health, followed by a relapse of symptoms perhaps initiated by the excessive activity
▪ Although patients should be as active as possible, clinicians may need to explain the disorder to employers and family members, advising them to make allowances as far as possible
▪ Modest regular exercise to avoid deconditioning is important and should be supervised by a physician or physical therapist
▪ In two trials exercise was of great benefit but there was a high dropout rate from the trials (up to 37%)

Risks/Benefits
Risk: no evidence exists that exercise is harmful in CFS, although experience suggests symptoms may be exacerbated by over-ambitious exercise programs.

Evidence
There is evidence that graded exercise is effective in the treatment of CFS.
▪ A RCT compared graded aerobic exercise (active intervention) with flexibility and relaxation training (control intervention), over 12 weeks. Significantly more people in the active treatment group reported improvements in physical fatigue and functioning [13] *Level P*
▪ Another RCT compared graded exercise plus fluoxetine, graded exercise plus placebo, general advice to exercise plus fluoxetine, and general advice to exercise plus placebo. After 26 weeks, significantly fewer patients in the active exercise groups experienced fatigue [14] *Level P*

Acceptability to patient
- High dropout rate
- Patients find this therapy difficult as it involves being more tired for a time

Follow up plan
Review at patient's request.

Patient and caregiver information
Patients need to be aware that this is a difficult therapy to follow, and that it will involve them feeling more tired than they already do at times. Caregivers should be encouraged to support the patient in the support of this treatment.

Complementary therapy
- Patients often turn to complementary therapy for CFS as conventional medicine does not have a simple answer for them
- Most alternative medicine studies in CFS have not been evaluated very well

EVENING PRIMROSE OIL
Both trials used 4g/day orally.

Efficacy
- Mixed results from available trials
- Limited data from small RCTs provide no clear evidence of benefit from oral evening primrose oil in people with CFS

Risks/Benefits
Benefit: no adverse effects.

Evidence
A RCT compared evening primrose oil with placebo in the management of CFS. At 3 months, no significant difference was found between the groups [15] *Level P*

Acceptability to patient
Usually very acceptable.

Follow up plan
- As indicated by clinical condition
- Not recommended treatment for this disorder

Patient and caregiver information
Not recommended treatment for this disorder: patient and caregiver using this therapy need to understand there is no clear evidence base.

MAGNESIUM INJECTIONS
Efficacy
Limited data from small RCTs provide no clear evidence of benefit from magnesium injections in people with CFS.

Risks/Benefits
Risk: not recommended therapy.

Evidence
A small RCT compared intramuscular magnesium injections with placebo over a 6-week period.

Benefit was found for patients treated with magnesium (energy, pain, and emotional reactions were significantly improved) [16] *Level P*

Acceptability to patient
Not recommended treatment for this disorder.

Follow up plan
Not recommended treatment for this disorder.

Patient and caregiver information
Not recommended treatment for this disorder: patients and caregivers need to be aware of the lack of evidence.

EXPERIMENTAL THERAPIES

These nonrecommended and experimental treatments are briefly detailed as patients have frequently read about them and will seek prescription from their physician.

Antimicrobials:
- An infectious cause for CFS has not been identified, and antimicrobial agents are not commonly prescribed for CFS. A controlled trial of the antiviral drug acyclovir found no benefit for the treatment of patients with CFS

Antiallergy therapy:
- Some CFS patients have histories of allergy, and these symptoms may flare periodically. Nonsedating antihistamines may be helpful for CFS patients for relief of allergic symptoms (not for relief of fatigue)
- Examples include astemizole (Hismanal) and loratadine (Claritin). Some of the more common adverse reactions associated with their use include drowsiness, fatigue, and headache. Sedating antihistamines can also be of benefit to patients at bedtime

Therapy for postural hypotension:
- Fludrocortisone has sometimes been prescribed for CFS patients who have had a positive tilt table test. It is currently being tested in controlled studies for its efficacy in the treatment of CFS patients
- Beta-blockers such as atenolol have also been prescribed for patients with a positive tilt table test
- Increased salt and water intake is also tried for these patients but this is currently not recommended. Adverse reactions include elevated blood pressure and fluid retention

Ampligen:
- A synthetic nucleic acid product that stimulates the production of interferons
- One report of a double-blinded, placebo-controlled study of CFS patients documented modest improvements in cognition and performance among ampligen recipients compared with the placebo group. These preliminary results will need to be confirmed by further study. Ampligen is not approved by the US Food and Drug Administration (FDA) for widespread use, and the administration of this drug in CFS patients should be considered experimental. Some participants experienced reactions that might be attributable to ampligen

Dehydroepiandrosterone (DHEA):
- Reported in preliminary studies to improve symptoms in some patients; however, this finding has not been confirmed and the use of DHEA in patients should be regarded as experimental

High colonic enemas:

- Have no demonstrated value in the treatment of CFS. The procedure can promote intestinal disease

Kutapressin:

- A crude extract from pig's liver. Its use should be regarded as experimental in any clinical circumstance, and there is no scientific evidence that it has any value in the treatment of CFS patients. Kutapressin can elicit allergic reactions

Dietary supplements and herbal preparations:

- A variety of dietary supplements and herbal preparations are claimed to have potential benefits for CFS patients. With a few exceptions, the effectiveness of these remedies for treating CFS patients has not been evaluated in controlled trials
- Contrary to common belief, the 'natural' origin of a product does not ensure safety. Dietary supplements and herbal preparations can have potential side reactions and some can interfere or interact with prescription medications. CFS patients should seek the advice of their physician before using any unprescribed remedy

Vitamins, coenzymes, and minerals:

- Preparations that have been claimed to have benefit for CFS patients include adenosine monophosphate, coenzyme Q-10, germanium, glutathione, iron, melatonin, NADH, selenium, l-tryptophan, vitamins B12, C, and A, and zinc. The therapeutic value of all these preparations has not been validated

Herbal preparations:

- Plants are known sources of pharmacologic materials. However, unrefined plant preparations contain variable levels of the active compound as well as many irrelevant, potentially harmful, substances
- Preparations that have been claimed to have benefit to CFS patients include *Astragalus*, borage seed oil, bromelain, comfrey, echinacea, garlic, *Ginkgo biloba*, ginseng, primrose oil, quercetin, St John's wort, and shiitake mushroom extract. Only primrose oil was evaluated in a controlled study, and the beneficial effects noted in CFS patients have not been independently confirmed
- Some herbal preparations, notably comfrey and high-dose ginseng, have recognized harmful effects

Spa treatments, hypnotherapy, massage, and meditation:

- May be effective, but have been evaluated on the basis of less well-designed studies
- Although not studied in well-designed clinical trials, patients may wish to try spa treatments, massage, hypnotherapy, and meditation as they are generally safe and relatively inexpensive interventions, and the limited studies to date suggest a benefit
- Where evidence is lacking, the cost and potential harm of an alternative therapy must be balanced against uncertain efficacy

Bright light treatment, lasers, selenium, chiropractic, musical tones, and malic acid:

- Not effective

Acupuncture:

- A nonsystematic review article identified seven studies of acupuncture for fibromyalgia rather than CFS. All but one of these studies were small and poorly designed. The exception was a study of 70 fibromyalgia patients who improved significantly more than the control group in five of eight outcome measures

SAMe (S-adenosyl-L-methionine):

- Has been evaluated in several double-blind randomized controlled trials for fibromyalgia.

Although fairly well designed, all were small and had mixed results. Only one used the oral form of the drug
- While the drug appears to be relatively safe, it is expensive, and interactions with antidepressants and other drugs have been reported

Other therapies
SUPPORT GROUPS
A useful support group should include:
- Patients who truly have CFS, and not simply individuals who have self-diagnosed this disorder
- Both newcomers and patients who have had CFS for longer periods of time to provide a balance of perspectives for the group
- People with whom the CFS patient feels comfortable
- Leaders who empathize, gently draw out shy members, and keep others from dominating, and who distill discussion into useful information
- A history indicating the group is stable and meeting the needs of its members

Some support groups may put their own interests before those of the individual patient. Groups that engage in any of the following activities should be avoided:
- Promise sure cures and quick solutions
- Conduct meetings that are mainly 'gripe' sessions
- Urge patients to stop prescribed treatment and recommend a single solution to their problem
- Insist that patients reveal private or sensitive information
- Demand allegiance to a cult-like, charismatic leader
- Charge high fees
- Require patients to purchase products

Efficacy
- CFS patients may find it therapeutic to meet with other people who have this illness, and often this can be accomplished by joining a local CFS support group
- Support groups are not appropriate for everyone, and some CFS patients may find that a support group actually adds to their stress rather than relieving it

Risks/Benefits
Benefit: most support groups are free, collect voluntary donations, or charge modest membership dues to cover basic expenses (e.g. refreshments at meetings or photocopying costs).

Acceptability to patient
Some patients find this form of therapy useful; others do not find it acceptable.

Follow up plan
Patients should be followed depending on their individual needs.

Patient and caregiver information
Information should be provided on which support groups are most useful, and how to contact them.

COGNITIVE BEHAVIORAL THERAPY
- CBT attempts to alter attitudes, perceptions, and beliefs that can contribute to maladaptive behavior
- CBT combined with a graded exercise program may be beneficial in improving functioning
- CBT at the level used in the trials may not be available to the PCP

Efficacy
- CBT appears to be an effective and acceptable treatment for adult outpatients with CFS

- People who get better from CFS as a result of CBT do not change their view of what caused their illness – patients at the end of treatment still accepted their illness was physical and had been caused by a virus
- People improved when they reassessed their views about the best way of dealing with symptoms, and looked for different ways of managing their illness
- Skilled therapists in specialist centers offering CBT achieve good results. In nonspecialist settings, such results may not be replicated

Risks/Benefits
Benefit: no harmful effects.

Evidence
There is evidence that CBT is effective for the treatment of CFS.
- A systematic review found that CBT appears to be an effective treatment for adult outpatients with CFS. Physical functioning was significantly improved, and the treatment was highly acceptable to patients [17] *Level M*
- The above review found no evidence that CBT is effective in mild cases of CFS (patients treated in primary care settings), or in severe disease when patients are unable to attend outpatient clinics due to disability [17] *Level M*
- A subsequent RCT compared CBT (administered by therapists with no previous experience in treating CFS) with both guided support groups and no intervention. CBT was more effective for the reduction of fatigue severity and functional impairment at 14 months' follow up [18] *Level P*

Acceptability to patient
CBT appeared highly acceptable to the patients in these trials.

Follow up plan
Follow up depends on individual patient needs.

PSYCHOTHERAPY AND SUPPORTIVE COUNSELING
- Certain psychotherapies, in addition to CBT, have shown promise for facilitating patient coping with CFS and for alleviating some of the distress associated with CFS
- In addition, any chronic illness can affect the patient, caregivers, and family; in such instances, family therapy may foster good communication and reduce the adverse impact of CFS on the family

Efficacy
- May foster good communication and reduce adverse impact of CFS on family life
- May be particularly useful for family where CFS affects an adolescent, helping them communicate their fears and concerns to other family members

Risks/Benefits
Risk: may cause increased distress as not all family members may wish to participate.

Acceptability to patient
Usually very acceptable.

Patient and caregiver information
Need to be aware that family therapy can be unpredictable, and that all participants have to be willing to be honest and give up prolonged amounts of their time for it to be helpful.

PROLONGED REST
This is the option that many patients choose when they develop CFS, believing that exercising and

inducing post-exertional malaise is positively harmful.

Efficacy
There is no evidence that prolonged rest is an effective treatment for CFS – indirect evidence suggests that prolonged rest may be harmful.

Risks/Benefits
Risk: appears to be harmful in CFS.

Acceptability to patient
Not recommended treatment for this disorder.

Follow up plan
Not recommended treatment for this disorder.

Patient and caregiver information
Not recommended treatment for this disorder.

LIFESTYLE
Graduated return to normal social activities in parallel with the graduated increase in exercise, as agreed between patient and physician, is the most practical approach.

RISKS/BENEFITS
Benefit: lifestyle changes can help the patient to return to normal functioning.

ACCEPTABILITY TO PATIENT
- A careful, stepwise approach to a return 'to life', agreed with and under the control of the patient is more likely to bring benefits, particularly as it places 'ownership' of the condition back with the patient
- If this is followed then it is likely to be very acceptable to the patient
- In CFS it is particularly harmful for the patient to perceive that the doctor 'owns' the condition and is responsible for its course whereas the patient is a passive sufferer with no control over the situation. The opposite view must be reached, where patients join in the responsibility for planning exercise and rehabilitation programs and interpret tiredness as their problem which they must overcome, rather than the doctor's problem which he/she must solve for them

FOLLOW UP PLAN
- Follow up at patient's request or according to clinical condition
- Patients being actively treated by the PCP, particularly where there is associated depression or anxiety, will need more frequent review

PATIENT AND CAREGIVER INFORMATION
- Although overexertion or attempting to do too much may result in apparent setback, the patient and carers need to be aware that, in order to work at the various aspects of rehabilitation to normal life, the patient may have to experience episodes of greater tiredness than if inactivity was maintained constantly
- It is often useful to determine patients' views of their illness before proceeding with patient education so that the explanation will address patient concerns and perspectives
- Patients who have a medical view of their condition are more receptive to a biologic explanation for their symptoms, even if the cause is psychogenic
- One must be careful not to evoke a misleading medical explanation, such as 'viral infection' or 'immune dysfunction', especially in the setting of a suspected or possible psychogenic etiology, because this might cause a patient to delay or refuse psychiatric intervention

- Patients with evidence of underlying psychogenic disease need an especially thorough review of the evidence for their diagnosis and a careful explanation of their symptoms because many come to the physician with the belief that they have a medical problem
- The attention given to CFS in the lay press often necessitates addressing the issue of its likelihood and some of its purported, although unfounded, causes (e.g. Epstein-Barr virus infection, yeast infection, immune dysfunction)
- Many patients with a psychogenic etiology prefer to cling to this diagnosis as an acceptable explanation of their psychophysiologic symptoms rather than face a diagnosis of depression, anxiety, or somatization disorder. In addition to a careful workup, a respectful, sympathetic, open-minded approach is essential

EFFICACY OF THERAPIES

- Outcomes may be difficult to measure. Many studies use self-reported recovery as an endpoint. Various objective rating scales have been devised to measure limitation of physical function by ill health
- The patients who do best in trials do not change their views about the physical nature of their illness
- Beneficial interventions include exercise and cognitive behavioral therapy

Evidence

- Graded aerobic exercise has been shown to result in improvements in physical fatigue and functioning [13] *Level P*
- A RCT compared graded exercise plus fluoxetine, graded exercise plus placebo, general advice to exercise plus fluoxetine, and general advice to exercise plus placebo. After 26 weeks, significantly fewer patients in the active exercise groups experienced fatigue [14] *Level P*
- Cognitive behavioral therapy appears to be an effective treatment for adult outpatients with chronic fatigue syndrome (CFS). Physical functioning is significantly improved, and the treatment is highly acceptable to patients [17] *Level M*
- There is insufficient evidence to support the use of corticosteroids, nicotinamide adenine dinucleotide (NADH), immunoglobulins, prolonged rest or antidepressants in the management of CFS [19]

Review period

- According to clinical condition and also reflecting the presence of any depressive features review may be patient- or doctor-initiated, regular or when required for new symptoms or review of progress
- Children should be reviewed at least 3-monthly

PROGNOSIS

- The clinical course of CFS varies considerably
- The patients who did best in trials did not change their views about the physical nature of their illness
- Children have a better outcome than adults: 54–94% show improvement within 6 years. Children and adolescents typically have an undulating course of gradual but substantial improvement, or complete resolution, 1–4 years after diagnosis
- Some patients recover to the point that they can resume work and other activities, but continue to experience various or periodic CFS symptoms
- Some patients recover completely with time, and some grow progressively worse
- CFS often follows a cyclical course, alternating between periods of illness and relative well-being
- 20–50% of adults show improvement in the medium-term and only 6% return to premorbid levels of functioning. In a recent prospective study, most CFS patients improved with time, but remained functionally impaired for several years
- A period of recovery is more likely in the early years
- There is no evidence of increased mortality
- No characteristics were identified that made one patient more likely to recover than another
- At illness onset, the most commonly reported CFS symptoms were sore throat, fever, muscle pain, and muscle weakness. As the illness progressed, muscle pain and forgetfulness increased and the reporting of depression decreased

Clinical pearls

- Patients who truly have idiopathic CFS do have some potential for spontaneous improvement over time. The lack of any improvement should prompt reconsideration of another diagnosis

- Regularly scheduled visits generally produce better results than waiting to see the patient when problems arise. In fact, this tends to reduce the number of visits
- If the diagnosis is somatization disorder (also known as somatoform pain disorder), there is nothing to be gained by confronting the patient with this diagnosis and insisting upon psychiatric care, because such treatment is seldom effective
- The patient's outcome tends to be better when the patient sees him- or herself as the primary agent for improvement, rather than the physician

Therapeutic failure

- The patient and doctor should meet and attempt to adjust the rehabilitation program, assessing where things have gone wrong and altering the approach or the emphasis of the approach
- The doctor should satisfy themselves again that no other illness has been missed or has arisen meanwhile, rechecking blood tests if appropriate
- For example, if the patient has emphasized exercise then referral for cognitive behavioral therapy may be appropriate, or if the patient has been having psychotherapy adapt a more physically based approach
- With this must come reassurance that the situation is not hopeless just because there has been a backwards step – the often fluctuating course of the illness should be explained

Recurrence
No therapies are reserved for recurrence.

Deterioration
No therapies are reserved for deterioration, although psychiatric referral might be considered if there are concerns about depressive features. Referral may be an option if there is a specialist with an interest available to refer to.

COMPLICATIONS

- Depression is a risk, especially with prolonged periods of fatigue and loss of normal function
- Fibromyalgia (which overlaps with CFS), where pain comes to predominate
- Alcoholism

CONSIDER CONSULT

- Hospitalization may be required for severely depressed and suicidal patients
- Consider referral if patient is losing faith in PCP due to recurrence
- Referral for treatment in hospice setting may be necessary for some patients. Those who have a limited support base and prolonged disease may benefit from a hospice stay
- Before initiating referral, ascertain that the physician to whom you plan to refer the patient actually has interest and expertise in treating CFS (many rheumatologists do not)

PREVENTION

There are no preventive measures that can be taken, as the etiology is unknown.

RISK FACTORS

- There are no known risk factors, despite intensive investigation of viral infections, particularly Epstein-Barr virus
- Stress may be a risk factor, as it is often retrospectively reported by patients as preceding their illness, but clearly there is likely to be reporting bias

MODIFY RISK FACTORS
Lifestyle and wellness

There are no known preventive measures, although a balanced diet and reasonable levels of physical activity would seem sensible.

ALCOHOL AND DRUGS

Where possible, avoid or limit the use of the following, as all may cause or exacerbate fatigue (clearly not all of these drugs can be avoided and some will only be given if essential or benefit outweighs potential harm):

- Long-term use of hypnotics
- Minor tranquilizers
- Antihypertensives that penetrate the blood-brain barrier (e.g. reserpine, methyldopa, clonidine, propranolol)
- Beta-blockers
- Antihistamines
- Antiepileptics
- Antidepressants, especially amitriptyline, doxepin, and trazodone
- Antihypertensives
- Drug abuse and drug withdrawal

PHYSICAL ACTIVITY

Exercise and other activities may be helpful in preventing stress.

SCREENING

There is no appropriate screening test or program.

PREVENT RECURRENCE

- Consider whether new medications have been started which could affect clinical state
- Consider whether new blood tests and re-evaluation of the disorder are necessary

Reassess coexisting disease

Consider whether medication for coexisting disease or under treatment of coexisting disease may affect fatigue.

INTERACTION ALERT

- Minor tranquilizers
- Antihypertensives
- Beta-blockers
- Antihistamines
- Antiepileptics
- Antidepressants, especially amitriptyline, doxepin, and trazodone

PATIENT SATISFACTION/LIFESTYLE PRIORITIES

- Patients want to return to full functioning and usually work very hard to achieve this
- Encourage measurement of small steps of progress

ASSOCIATIONS

National Center for Infectious Diseases
Centers for Disease Control and Prevention
Mailstop A15
Atlanta, GA 30333
Tel: (888) 232 3228 (24-hour voice information system on chronic fatigue syndrome)
www.cdc.gov/ncidod

National Institute of Allergy and Infectious Diseases
National Institutes of Health
Bethesda, MD 20892
www.niaid.nih.gov

KEY REFERENCES

- Bates DW, Schmitt W, Buchwald D, et al. Prevalence of fatigue and chronic fatigue syndrome in a primary care practice. Arch Intern Med 1993;153:2759–65
- Dobbins JG, Randall B, Reyes M, et al. Prevalence of chronic fatiguing illness among adolescents in the United States. J Chron Fatig Syndr 1997;3:15–28
- Holmes GP, Kaplan JE, Schonberger LB, et al. Definition of the chronic fatigue syndrome [letter]. Ann Intern Med 1988;109:512
- Klonoff DC. Chronic fatigue syndrome. Clin Infect Dis 1992;15:812–23
- Kouyanou K, Pither C, Wessely S. Iatrogenic factors and chronic pain. Psychosom Med 1997;59:597–604
- See DM, Tilles JG. Alpha interferon treatment of patients with CFS. Immunol Invest 1996:25:153–64
- Volmer-Conna U, Hickie I, Hadzi-Pavlovic D, et al. Imtravenous immunoglobulin is ineffective in the treatment of patients with CFS. Am J Med 1997;103:38–43
- Wessely S, Powell R. Fatigue syndromes: a comparison of chronic postviral fatigue with neuromuscular and affective disorders. J Neurol Neurosurg Psychiatry 1989;42:940–8
- Wessely S. The epidemiology of chronic fatigue syndrome. Epidemiol Rev 1995;17:1–13

Evidence references and guidelines

1 Fukuda K, Straus S, Hickie I, et al. The chronic fatigue syndrome: a comprehensive approach to its definition and study. International Chronic Fatigue Syndrome Study Group. Ann Intern Med 1994;121:953–9. Available at the Centers for Disease Control and Prevention
2 Peterson PK, Pheley A, Schroeppel J, et al. A preliminary placebo-controlled crossover trial of fludrocortisone for chronic fatigue syndrome. Arch Intern Med 1998:158:908–14. Reviewed in: Clinical Evidence 2001;6:819–30
3 McKenzie R, O'Fallon A, Dale J, et al. Low-dose hydrocortisone for treatment of chronic fatigue syndrome. JAMA 1998;280:1061–66. Reviewed in: Clinical Evidence 2001;6:819–830
4 Cleare AJ, Heap E, Malhi G, et al. Low-dose hydrocortisone in chronic fatigue syndrome: a randomised crossover trial. Lancet 1999;353: 455–8. Reviewed in: Clinical Evidence 2001;6:819–30
5 Vercoulen J, Swanink C, Zitman F. Randomised, double-blind, placebo-controlled study of fluoxetine in chronic fatigue syndrome. Lancet 1996;347:858–61. Reviewed in: Clinical Evidence 2001;6:819–30
6 Wearden AJ, Morriss RK, Mullis R, et al. Randomized, double-blind, placebo-controlled treatment trial of fluoxetine and a graded exercise programme for chronic fatigue syndrome. Br J Psychiatry 1998:172:485–90. Reviewed in: Clinical Evidence 2001;6:819–30
7 Hickie IB, Wilson AJ, Murray Wright J, et al. A randomized, double-blind, placebo-controlled trials of moclobemide in patients with chronic fatigue syndrome. J Clin Psychiatry 2000;61:643–8. Reviewed in: Clinical Evidence 2001;6:819–30
8 Behan PO, Hannifah H. 5-HT reuptake inhibitors in CFS. J Immunol Immunopharmacol 1995;15:66–69. Reviewed in: Clinical Evidence 2001;6:819–30
9 Forsyth LM, Preuss HG, MacDowell AL, et al. Therapeutic effects of oral NADH on the symptoms of patients with chronic fatigue syndrome. Ann Allergy Asthma Immunol 1999;82:185–91. Reviewed in: Clinical Evidence 2001;6:819–30
10 Peterson PK, Shepard J, Macres M, et al. A controlled trial of intravenous immunoglobulin G in chronic fatigue syndrome. Am J Med 1990;89:554–60. Reviewed in Clinical Evidence 2001;6:819–30

11 Lloyd A, Hickie I, Wakefield D, et al. A double-blind, placebo-controlled trial of intravenous immunoglobulin therapy in patients with chronic fatigue syndrome. Am J Med 1990;89:561–8. Reviewed in Clinical Evidence 2001;6:819–30

12 Vollmer-Conna U, Hickie I, Hadzi-Pavlovic D, et al. Imtraveous immunoglobulin is ineffective in the treatment of patients with chronic fatigue syndrome. Am J Med 1997;103:38–43. Reviewed in Clinical Evidence 2001;6:819–30

13 Fulcher KY, White PD. A randomised controlled trial of graded exercise therapy in patients with the chronic fatigue syndrome. BMJ 1997;314:1647–52. Reviewed in Clinical Evidence 2001;6:819–30

14 Wearden AJ, Morriss RK, Mullis R, et al. Randomised, double-blind, placebo controlled treatment trial of fluoxetine and a graded exercise programme for chronic fatigue syndrome. Br J Psychiatry 1998;172:485–90. Reviewed in Clinical Evidence 2001;6:819–30

15 Warren G, McKendrick M, Peet M. The role of essential fatty acids in chronic fatigue syndrome. Acta Neurol Scand 1999;99:112–6. Reviewed in Clinical Evidence 2001;6:819–30

16 Cox IM, Campbell MJ, Dowson D. Red blood cell magnesium and chronic fatigue syndrome. Lancet 1991;337:757–60. Reviewed in Clinical Evidence 2001;6:819–30

17 Price JR, Couper J. Cognitive behaviour therapy for chronic fatigue syndrome in adults (Cochrane Review). In: The Cochrane Library, 1, 2002. Oxford: Update Software

18 Prins JB, Bleijenberg G, Bazelmans E, et al. Cognitive behaviour therapy for chronic fatigue syndrome: a multicentre randomised controlled trial. Lancet 2001;357:841–7. Reviewed in Clinical Evidence 2001;6:819–30

19 Reid S, Chalder T, Cleare A, Hotopf M, Wessely S. Chronic fatigue syndromes: Musculoskeletal disorders. In: Clinical Evidence 2001;6:819–30. London: BMJ Publishing Group

FAQS
Question 1
How does one make the diagnosis of chronic fatigue syndrome (CFS)?

ANSWER 1
First, the history, physical examination, and laboratory studies must rigorously exclude a long list of endocrine, infectious, and other medical causes of chronic fatigue. Secondly, the patient must display a number of specific symptoms and signs.

Question 2
Do most patients presenting with chronic fatigue have CFS?

ANSWER 2
No. The vast majority of such patients will have diagnoses other than CFS.

Question 3
What is the cause of CFS?

ANSWER 3
There is no recognized specific cause for CFS based on the scientific data.

Question 4
What is the preferred treatment for CFS?

ANSWER 4
Treatment is symptomatic. There is no specific treatment for CFS, as the underlying cause is unknown.

CONTRIBUTORS
Russell C Jones, MD, MPH
Richard Brasington Jr, MD, FACP
Thiruvalam P Indira, MD

COSTOCHRONDRITIS

DESCRIPTION

- Anterior chest wall pain and tenderness, which occurs in the costochondral and costosternal regions
- It may be associated with trauma, overuse, cough, or may develop spontaneously
- Illness is generally self-limited, it is important to exclude more serious sources of anterior chest pain

URGENT ACTION

Rule out life-threatening conditions in the differential diagnosis, i.e. ischemic heart disease.

KEY! DON'T MISS!

- Always ensure that ischemic heart disease is not the cause for the anterior chest pain
- Always check for a vesicular rash consistent with herpes zoster as a possible cause of chest wall pain

BACKGROUND

ICD9 CODE
733.6 Costochondritis.

SYNONYMS
- Costosternal syndrome
- Anterior chest wall syndrome
- Costosternal chondrodynia
- Tietze's syndrome (note – often used interchangeably, however, local swelling over the costosternal joint is found in Tietze's syndrome and not in costochondritis)

CARDINAL FEATURES
- Anterior chest wall pain and tenderness that occurs in the costochondral and costosternal region
- Pain is generally sharp in nature and may be pleuritic or worse with movement
- Pain may radiate to the arms or shoulders
- The costal cartilage of the second and third ribs are most often the site of pain
- Pain is usually intermittent, lasting minutes or hours, unrelated to activity, for days to weeks
- Illness is generally self-limited, it is important to exclude more serious sources of anterior chest pain
- Many patients present because of concern that pain may represent a serious cardiopulmonary condition
- Therapy consists of explanation and reassurance as well as analgesics, anti-inflammatories, and heat
- More difficult cases may respond to injection with long-acting corticosteroid

CAUSES
Common causes
The exact cause of costochondritis is unknown. Exacerbating conditions may include trauma, overuse, or cough.

EPIDEMIOLOGY
Incidence and prevalence
Data are limited although it appears to be fairly common. In one study of 100 patients with negative cardiac angiography, 69 had chest wall tenderness and, in 16 of these cases, pressure on the costochondral area completely reproduced the pain.

Note that true Tietze's syndrome is, in comparison, quite rare.

FREQUENCY
10% of chest pain complaints.

Demographics
AGE
- Tietze's syndrome <40
- Costochondritis any age beyond adolescence

GENDER
Costochondritis more frequent in women.

RACE
May have slightly higher frequency in Hispanics.

DIAGNOSIS

DIFFERENTIAL DIAGNOSIS
Tietze's syndrome
FEATURES
- Differs from costochondritis with the presence of local costochondral swelling
- Age <40 and male=female
- Usually only one site of pain, tenderness, and swelling as opposed to costochondritis in which most cases have multiple sites of pain and tenderness
- Rare compared to costochondritis

Fibromyalgia
FEATURES
- Similar demographics to costochondritis
- Multiple tender spots on palpation in specific locations and not limited to the chest wall; costochondritis definition describes specific trigger spots, which do not include the anterior chest
- Often have an associated non-refreshing sleep
- Symptoms worsen and remit, but can last months to years

Anxiety
FEATURES
- Discomfort often localized over the precordium
- Location is variable; can move from place to place
- Symptoms can be situational
- Pain can be fleeting or of prolonged duration, but tenderness to palpation is usually inconstent
- Laboratory data are normal

Herpes zoster
FEATURES
- Dermatomal distribution
- May be very painful
- Vesicular rash eventually appears over area of discomfort

SAPHO syndrome (Synovitis, Acne, Pustulosis, Hyperostosis, Osteitis)
FEATURES
- Painful swelling of the clavicles and sternum, which progresses to ossification
- Associated with acne and palmoplantar pustulosis
- Vertebral abnormalities may co-exist

Tumor
FEATURES
Benign or malignant, e.g. chondroma, chondrosarcoma, metastasis

Metastatic disease to ribs
FEATURES
- Diagnosis of malignancy can precede rib pain or rib pain can be initial presenting complaint
- Tenderness with palpation over metastasis
- Diagnosis confirmed when rib films reveal metastatic disease

Osteoarthritis
FEATURES
- Mostly affects older patients
- Slowly evolving, characterized by deterioration of articular cartilage and by formation of bony

outgrowths or spurs (osteophytes)

- ▒ May be associated with osteoarthritis of other joints – most often affected are knees, hips, distal interphalangeal joints of the hands, carpometacarpal joints of thumb, and cervical and lumbosacral spine
- ▒ ESR and C-reactive protein not usually raised

Rheumatoid arthritis
FEATURES

- ▒ Likely to be associated with arthritis affecting other joints
- ▒ Joints most commonly affected are the joints of the hands and feet
- ▒ Rheumatoid nodules sometimes present
- ▒ Associated with elevated rheumatoid factor in most cases
- ▒ Mild anemia is common
- ▒ ESR and C-reactive protein usually raised

Ankylosing spondylitis
FEATURES

- ▒ Back pain, associated with stiffness and restriction after inactivity, often nocturnal
- ▒ Loss of chest expansion
- ▒ Progressive fixed spinal deformity, which may gradually ascend from the thoracolumbar spine to the cervical spine. A fixed 'ankylosis' makes it difficult for the patient to stand and look forward
- ▒ Characteristic radiological findings: sacroiliac joints show sclerosis and narrowing; syndesmophytes
- ▒ Most patients are male and the disease begins in the second or third decade
- ▒ Usually milder and, therefore, less frequently diagnosed in women
- ▒ Extraskeletal disorders are present in one-third of patients – they include cardiac (aortic insufficiency, conduction abnormalities), enthesitis, pulmonary (apical fibrosis, restrictive lung disease), and ocular involvement (painful inflammation e.g. iritis/uveitis)

Coronary artery disease
FEATURES

- ▒ Chest pain (and/or tenderness) often radiates to left shoulder, arm, or jaw
- ▒ May be associated with dyspnea
- ▒ Pain often brought on by exercise that does not involve movement of the chest
- ▒ Cardiac enzymes may be elevated if infarction occurs
- ▒ ECG may show ischemic changes. Angiography will be abnormal

Infection
FEATURES

- ▒ May be associated with heroin abuse
- ▒ Constitutional features such as fever may be present
- ▒ Elevated ESR, elevated white blood count with shift
- ▒ Response to antibiotics and needle aspirations

Pericarditis
FEATURES

- ▒ Constant pain over the anterior chest
- ▒ Pain may radiate to the arms or back
- ▒ Pain worsens with inspiration
- ▒ Pain relieved by sitting up and leaning forward
- ▒ Pericardial friction rub may be heard
- ▒ Low-voltage ECG with diffuse ST segment elevation, echocardiogram is diagnostic
- ▒ Usually has elevated sedimentation rate

Gastroesophageal reflux disease
FEATURES
- Heartburn, acid regurgitation
- Pain may be related to eating
- Pain may be relieved by antacids

Pleurisy
FEATURES
- Pleuritic pain worsened by inspiration and expiration
- Pleural rub may be heard
- Cough (dry) is prominent

Pulmonary embolism
FEATURES
- Sudden pleuritic pain
- May be associated with severe dyspnea
- Hypoxia, ECG changes

SIGNS & SYMPTOMS
Signs
Tenderness to palpation must be present.

Symptoms
- Insidious onset
- Pain sharp in nature
- May be worse with movement or respirations
- May occur at multiple rib articulations on either side
- Pain may radiate to arms
- Heat often lessens pain

KEY! DON'T MISS!
- Always ensure that ischemic heart disease is not the cause for the anterior chest pain
- Always check for a vesicular rash consistent with herpes zoster as a possible cause of chest wall pain

CONSIDER CONSULT
- If infectious cause of joint inflammation, immediate treatment with antibiotics is required
- If the diagnosis is unclear and concern of a more serious condition may exist, referral to a pulmonologist or cardiologist may be appropriate

INVESTIGATION OF THE PATIENT
Direct questions to patient
Q **When did the pain start? Was there a precipitating event?** Patients may have a history of overuse or trauma

Q **Have you ever been diagnosed with a malignancy?** Need to exclude metastatic disease to the ribs

Q **Do you have pain, tenderness, or swelling anywhere else? Have you ever been diagnosed with an autoimmune disease?** Inflammation of the costosternal region may be part of an autoimmune disease rather than costochondritis alone

Q **Have you had a recent upper respiratory infection?** Many patients report recent upper respiratory infection with cough

Q **Does the pain radiate to the arm or neck?** This may be a feature of costochondritis, as well as of other chest pain syndromes including myocardial infarction

- **What is the nature of the pain?** Pain may be sharp (indicating possible costochondritis), pleuritic, or tight in nature
- **What are the precipitating factors?** Movement may make the pain of costochondritis worse
- **What are the relieving factors?** Heat often brings relief in costochondritis

Family history

Family history is important, not in diagnosis of costochondritis but in the elimination of other diagnosis in the differential:

Q **Do you have a family history of any autoimmune conditions?** Consider autoimmune diseases

Q **Do you have a family history of heart disease?** Patients frequently seek medical attention because of concerns that the chest pain may be cardiac in origin

Examination

Q **Does the patient appear unwell on general examination?** May indicate an infective cause

Q **Does patient appear clinically unstable?** Suggests cardiac, pulmonary, or other serious and possibly life-threatening source of chest pain

Q **Does patient have significant tenderness over anterior chest wall?** Second to fifth ribs are usually involved and it may be bilateral

Q **Has patient had any rashes or significant erythema?** May suggest herpes zoster or infectious source

Q **Does patient have any other swollen or tender joints?** Would suggest autoimmune disease

Summary of investigative tests

- Costochondritis is a clinical diagnosis based on a patient's history and physical examination
- No laboratory tests are needed to make the diagnosis; ESR is inconsistently elevated
- Laboratory tests such as ESR and complete blood counts should be obtained if there is a suspicion of another clinical entity that needs to be eliminated from the differential diagnosis
- Rib X-rays may be useful if a metastasis to rib is suspected
- ECG is useful in excluding cardiac pathology, it is normal in costochondritis

DIAGNOSTIC DECISION

- There are no absolute diagnostic criteria. However, in general, patients must have anterior chest wall tenderness as identified by digital palpation, applying enough pressure (4kg/cm^2) to induce partial blanching of the examiner's finger
- Pain on palpation should reproduce the patient's typical pain
- Localized swelling occurs in Tietze's syndrome. As opposed to costochondritis, Tietze's syndrome generally affects only one articulation
- Laboratory studies, rib or chest X-rays, and ECG are all generally normal in this diagnosis

CLINICAL PEARL(S)

- Localized swelling over the costosternal articulation is present in Tietze's syndrome, but not costochondritis
- Costochondritis may affect multiple sites bilaterally, whereas Tietze's syndrome usually affects only one articulation
- A sizable percentage of patients with ischemic heart disease also have anterior chest wall tenderness
- Chest wall pain may indicate a more generalized soft tissue disorder such as fibromyalgia

THE TESTS
Body fluids
ERYTHROCYTE SEDIMENTATION RATE AND COMPLETE BLOOD COUNT
Description
Venous blood sample.

Advantages/Disadvantages
Advantages:
- Simple and widely available
- Inexpensive

Disadvantage: not disease-specific

Normal
- Leukocytes: 3.8–9.8x10^9/L
- Hemoglobin: male 13.8–17.2mg/dL (8.56–10.7mmol/l); female 12.1–5.1mg/dL (7.50–9.36mmol/L)
- Platelets: 190–405x10^9/L
- Erythrocyte sedimentation rate: 0–20mm/h

Abnormal
- Results outside of the normal range
- Keep in mind the possibility of a false positive result

Cause of abnormal result
- Elevated leukocyte count may suggest infection or malignancy
- Anemia may suggest malignancy
- Elevated ESR may suggest rheumatological disease, malignancy or infection, but can be elevated in costochondritis

Drugs, disorders and other factors that may alter results
Marked anemia may falsely elevate the erythrocyte sedimentation rate.

Imaging
RIB X-RAY SERIES
Advantages/Disadvantages
Advantages:
- Widely available
- Useful in excluding rib metastasis in a patient with known or suspected malignancy
- May be psychologically reassuring to the patient

Disadvantages:
- Exposes patient to ionizing radiation
- Should only be obtained if sufficient clinical suspicion exists

Normal
Studies are usually normal in patients with costochondritis.

Abnormal
- Study may disclose a metastasis or rib fracture
- Keep in mind the possibility of a falsely abnormal result

Other tests
ECG
Advantages/Disadvantages
Advantages:
- Widely available
- Easily performed
- Can be instantly interpreted

- Non-invasive
- May be psychologically reassuring to the patient

Disadvantages:
- Only indicated if clinical suspicion of cardiac disease exists
- Study is normal in costochondritis

Abnormal
ST changes and T wave inversion are consistent with ischemia.

Cause of abnormal result
Coronary heart disease.

TREATMENT

CONSIDER CONSULT
Patients may benefit from referral to a rheumatologist or orthopedist for injection with long-acting corticosteroid in maximally tender areas if primary care physician is uncomfortable or unfamiliar with the procedure.

PATIENT AND CAREGIVER ISSUES
Patient or caregiver request
Patients with a family history of cardiac disease may have significant anxiety associated with costochondritis. Another family member may have encouraged the patient's visit. Concerns should be addressed to provide adequate reassurance to the patient.

Health-seeking behavior
- **Has patient visited the ER?** Patients with chest pain frequently seek initial medical care in the emergency room
- **Has patient tried self-medication?** Many patients with costochondritis recognize the musculoskeletal origin of their pain and try over the counter anti-inflammatories

MANAGEMENT ISSUES
Goals
- To exclude more serious and potentially life-threatening problems
- To obtain clinical testing only if indicated
- To reduce pain and lessen anxiety
- To reassure patient of the benign nature of the illness

Management in special circumstances
COEXISTING DISEASE
Patients with known malignancy need investigations to exclude the possibility of metastasis.

PATIENT SATISFACTION/LIFESTYLE PRIORITIES
Most patients are extremely relieved to be advised of the benign nature of their condition.

SUMMARY OF THERAPEUTIC OPTIONS
Choices
- Reassurance is key to therapy. Condition is benign and is usually self limited
- Initial therapy with analgesics such as acetaminophen and NSAIDs such as ibuprofen or naproxen may be useful
- Heat packs or heating pads also help relieve pain
- Injections of trigger points with local anesthetic and long-acting corticosteroids are effective and may be necessary in more difficult cases
- Some lifestyle changes may be useful in lessening or avoiding pain, i.e. stretching of the chest wall muscles may help alleviate pain

Clinical pearls
- In older patients or patients with history of gastrointestinal bleed, consider therapy with a selective COX-2 inhibitor (celecoxib or rofecoxib) to reduce the chance of ulcer and ulcer complications
- The patient's greatest concern is often that the symptoms represent cardiac disease, and reassurance to the contrary is quite therapeutic

Never
Never assume a patient with chest wall tenderness is not suffering from coronary ischemia. Cases of chest wall hyperalgesia as a symptom of coronary insufficiency are infrequently seen but do occur.

FOLLOW UP
Plan for review
Needs to be individualized depending on the patient and the medications chosen for the patient.

Information for patient or caregiver
- Patient needs to inform their physician if the nature of the chest pain worsens or changes
- Patient needs to inform their physician if any additional symptoms develop
- Patient needs to understand that he or she may need to try several different types of medication until the most effective is found

DRUGS AND OTHER THERAPIES: DETAILS
Drugs
ACETAMINOPHEN
Dose
Up to1g by mouth four times daily.

Efficacy
Effective in reducing pain in musculoskeletal conditions.

Risks/Benefits
Risks:
- Avoid in chronic hepatic disease, renal disease, or alcoholism
- Pregnancy Category B compatible with pregnancy and breast -eeding
- Caution in hepatic and renal impairment
- Overdosage results in hepatic and renal damage unless treated promptly

Benfit: inexpensive

Side effects and adverse reactions
- Acetaminophen rarely causes side-effects when used intermittently
- Rare: nausea, vomiting, rashes, blood disorders, acute pancreatitis, acute hepatic and renal failure

Interactions (other drugs)
- Alcohol ■ Anticoagulants ■ Anticonvulsants ■ Isoniazid ■ Cholestyramine ■ Colestipol ■ Domperidone ■ Metoclopromide

Contraindications
No absolute contraindications are recorded.

Acceptability to patient
Generally well tolerated.

Follow up plan
Other stronger analgesics should be considered if this is ineffective.

Patient and caregiver information
Patients need to be reminded that many over-the-counter medications contain acetaminophen and they need to check the contents of these medications before combining with acetaminophen to prevent overdosage.

IBUPROFEN
Dose
200–800mg by mouth every 4 hours, not to exceed 3200mg/day.

Efficacy
Effective in reducing pain and inflammation in musculoskeletal conditions.

Risks/Benefits
Risks:
- Use with caution in hepatic, renal or cardiac disease
- Use caution in elderly
- Use caution in bleeding disorders

Benefit: inexpensive

Side-effects and adverse reactions
- Gastrointestinal: anorexia, nausea, dyspepsia, peptic ulceration, bleeding
- Central nervous system: headache, dizziness, tinnitus
- Hypersensitivity: rashes, bronchospasm, angioedema
- Cardiovascular system: hypertension, peripheral edema
- Genitourinary: nephrotoxicity
- Hematological: blood cell disorders

Interactions (other drugs)
- Aminoglycosides ▪ Anticoagulants ▪ Antihypertensives ▪ Baclofen ▪ Corticosteroids
- Cyclosporine, tacrolimus ▪ Digoxin ▪ Diuretics ▪ Lithium ▪ Methotrexate
- Phenylpropanolamine ▪ Warfarin

Contraindications
- Peptic ulceration ▪ Hypersensitivity to NSAIDs ▪ Coagulation defects
- Severe renal or hepatic disease

Evidence
No clinical studies exist for use of this medication in this condition; however, NSAIDs have a well-established role in the treatment of painful musculoskeletal conditions.

Acceptability to patient
Some patients cannot tolerate NSAIDs due to stomach upset.

Follow up plan
Patient should contact their physician in one or 2 weeks to evaluate the effectivenenss of this medication.

Patient and caregiver information
- Avoid concurrent use of alcohol and aspirin
- Take with food, milk or antacids to decrease gastrointestinal upset

NAPROXEN
Dose
250–500mg twice a day by mouth.

Efficacy
Useful for pain and inflammation of musculoskeletal conditions.

Risks/Benefits
Risks:
- Use with caution in hepatic, renal or cardiac disease

- Use caution in elderly
- Use caution in bleeding disorders
- Use caution in porphyria

Benefits:
- Inexpensive
- Propionic acids are effective and better tolerated than most other NSAIDs

Side-effects and adverse reactions
- Gastrointestinal: diarrhea, vomiting, nausea, dyspepsia, peptic ulceration
- Central nervous system: headache, dizziness, drowsiness
- Hypersensitivity: rashes, bronchospasm, angioedema
- Thrombocytopenia
- Cardiovascular system: congestive heart failure, dysrhythmias, edema, palpitations
- Genitourinary: acute renal failure

Interactions (other drugs)
- Aminoglycosides ▪ Anticoagulants ▪ Antihypertensives ▪ Corticosteroids ▪ Cyclosporine
- Digoxin ▪ Diuretics ▪ Lithium ▪ Methotrexate ▪ Phenylpropanolamine
- Probenecid ▪ Triamterene

Contraindications
- Peptic ulceration ▪ Hypersensitivity to NSAIDs ▪ Coagulation defect
- Do not use naproxen and naproxen sodium concomitantly

Evidence
No clinical studies exist for use of this medication in this condition.

Acceptability to patient
Some patients cannot tolerate NSAIDs because of stomach upset.

Follow up plan
Patient should contact their physician in one or 2 weeks to evaluate the effectivenenss of this medication.

Patient and caregiver information
- Avoid concurrent use of alcohol and aspirin
- Take with food, milk, or antacids to decrease gastrointestinal upset

Other therapies
TRIGGER POINT INJECTION WITH CORTICOSTEROID
Injection of long-acting corticosteroid directly into site of maximum pain and tenderness. Some physicians include a local anesthetic in this injection.

Efficacy
70–80% of patients experience substantial relief of symptoms.

Risks/Benefits
Risks:
- May aggravate pain for first 24–48 h
- Contraindicated if bleeding problems or anticoagulation therapy
- Contraindicated if cellulitis is present over involved site
- Fluorinated preparations (such as triamcinolone) may cause subcutaneous atrophy when injected superficially

Benefits:
- Substantial relief of symptoms
- If effective, reinforces diagnosis

Acceptability to patient
Needles may provoke anxiety in some patients.

Follow up plan
May require additional injection in 1–2 weeks if initial injection is ineffective.

Patient and caregiver information
May aggravate pain for first 24–48 h.

HEAT PACKS OR HEATING PADS
Efficacy
- May bring relief
- May avoid or lessen the need for oral medication

Risks/Benefits
Risk: few risks apart from risk of skin burns in the event of overheated packs or pads.

Acceptability to patient
Generally good.

LIFESTYLE
Useful changes to lifestyle may include:
- Not carrying heavy objects across the chest, as this can aggravate chest wall pain
- Not smoking, as a cough will aggravate chest wall pain
- Sleeping with arms below the level of the chest
- Avoiding extension exercises and activities involving the chest wall and spine while pain is present

ACCEPTABILITY TO PATIENT
Patients may find it difficult to cease smoking.

FOLLOW UP PLAN
Follow up in 1–2 weeks to see if there has been any symptomatic improvement.

EFFICACY OF THERAPIES

Disease is self-limited with most cases resolving without therapy within several months. Response to heat and analgesics appear to decrease symptoms, although no controlled trials exist. In anecdotal reports, refractory patients have responded to acupuncture, biofeedback, and surgical removal.

Evidence

Evidence supporting these treatments is lacking. However, clinical experience indicates that one or more of these treatments is helpful for most patients.

Review period

Patient should be instructed to inform their physician if pain changes in nature or severity. Diagnosis should be re-evaluated at that point.

PROGNOSIS

In general, the majority of patients have resolution of their symptoms by one year. In one study, one-third of patients followed up at one year still had costosternal tenderness. This study did not deal with the type of therapy but rather the natural course of the disease.

Clinical pearls

- Costochondritis is likely to resolve without therapy within a year
- For corticosteroid injection, use preparations less likely to cause subcutaneous atrophy (e.g. betamethasone, methylprednisolone, or hydrocortisone), rather than fluorinated preparations (such as triamcinolone)
- In refractory cases, consider depression or somatization as unrecognized causes

Therapeutic failure

- If patient fails to improve despite attempts at therapy, consider a referral to a rheumatologist or orthopedist who specializes in soft tissue rheumatic complaints such as fibromyalgia and costochondritis
- Consider a referral to mental health professional if significant anxiety is present

Recurrence

- Patients should be aware that recurrences may occur and they should be treated with a similar therapeutic regimen
- Patients should be advised to report any changes in their symptoms to their physicians so other life-threatening conditions are not attributed to costochondritis

COMPLICATIONS

- Complications will not arise from costochondritis itself but may arise from lack of attention to the proper diagnosis
- Alternatively, an inappropriate intervention may be performed on a patient suffering from costochondritis but inaccurately diagnosed with a more serious condition

PREVENTION

Costochondritis is not specifically preventable in the general population.

ASSOCIATIONS
American College of Rheumatology
1800 Century Place
Suite 250
Atlanta, GA 30345
Tel: (404) 633 3777
Fax: (404) 633 1870
www.rheumatology.com

American Academy of Family Physicians
11400 Tomahawk Creek Parkway
Leawood, KS 66211-2672
Tel: (913) 906 6000
www.aafp.org

KEY REFERENCES
- Disla E, Rhim HR, Reddy A Karten I, et al. Costochondritis: a prospective analysis in an emergency department setting. Arch Intern Med 1994;154(21):2466–9
- Gorroll AH, Mulley AG, May LA. Primary Care Medicine 3rd edn. Lippincott Ravens 1995, p94
- Koopman WJ (ed). Arthritis and Allied Conditions, 13th edn. Williams and Wilkins 1997, pp1766–7
- Sheon RP, Moskowitz RW, Goldberg VM. Soft tissue rheumatic pain: recognition, management, prevention, 2nd edn. Philadelphia: Lea and Febiger, 1987, 141–50
- Bluestone R.Practical Rheumatology: Diagnosis and Management. Menlo Park; CA: Addison-Wesley Publishing p90
- Wise CM, Semble EL, Dalton CB. Musculoskeletal chest wall syndromes in patients with noncardiac chest pain: a study of 100 patients. Am Phys Med Rehabil 1992;73:147–9
- Aeschlimann A, Kahn MF. Tietze's syndrome: a critical review. Clin Exp Rheum 1990;8:407–12.

CONTRIBUTORS
Dennis F Saver, MD
Richard Brasington Jr, MD, FACP
Maria-Louise Barilla-LaBarca, MD

DUPUYTREN'S CONTRACTURE

SUMMARY INFORMATION

DESCRIPTION

- A relatively common condition affecting the hands
- There is nodular thickening and contraction of the palmar fascia
- The condition may be progressive, resulting in fixed flexion deformities of the small joints of the fingers and hands
- It is usually painless, but may be quite disabling
- It usually affects both hands symmetrically, and the little and ring fingers are usually the worst affected

ICD9 CODE
728.6 Dupuytren's contracture

CARDINAL FEATURES
- Symmetrical, painless thickening or nodules of the palmar fascia
- Slowly progressive, although the rate of progression is very variable in the same patient over time and varies greatly between patients
- Initial palmar fascial thickening may progress to skin tethering, puckering, and pit formation
- Progressive thickening of the fascia leads to contractures of the finger joints
- There is progressive fixed flexion deformity of the metacarpo-phalangeal joints, proximal interphalangeal joints and, more rarely, of the distal interphalangeal joints
- Fascial thickening may extend proximally to the proximal interphalangeal joints and distally to, but rarely beyond, the wrist
- Is refractive to all medical therapy
- Surgical intervention may be helpful in relieving the resulting flexion deformities, but does not prevent progression of the disease. The condition, therefore, recurs in most patients despite surgical intervention
- Has been observed in association with diabetes mellitus, as well as other conditions, including alcohol abuse, epilepsy, hypercholesterolemia, reflex sympathetic dystrophy, and chronic pulmonary disease
- In most cases, effects are mild and produce no symptoms, or minor symptoms with little disability

CAUSES
Common causes
The etiology of Dupuytren's contractures is unknown.

Contributory or predisposing factors
Alcoholism:
- Incidence of Dupuytren's contracture may reach 66% in chronic alcoholism

Diabetes mellitus:
- Rates of Dupuytren's contracture are much higher in diabetics; may approach 66%

Epilepsy:
- Incidence of Dupuytren's contracture in male epileptics may approach 40%
- The association had been linked to antiepileptic medication, including phenytoin and phenobarbitone, but the association is now thought to be independent of the drug treatments used in epilepsy, and is a link of unknown cause between the two disorders themselves

Chronic pulmonary disease:
- Patients with a chronic respiratory disease aged over 40 years, especially tuberculosis, have 30–40% incidence of Dupuytren's
- Postulated mechanism may involve similar cardiopulmonary digitopalmar associations as seen in finger clubbing

Injuries or operations to the hand:
- Dupuytren's contracture can occur within 6 months of hand injury or surgery, especially if there was a period of hand swelling and immobility. This association is more likely in patients with Dupuytren's diathesis

- Repetitive injury and occupational trauma may very occasionally be important factors in the development of Dupuytren's contracture
- There is a weak association with reflex sympathetic dystrophy

Repetitive manual work and hand vibration (unproven association):
- Prevalence rates of Dupuytren's contracture in people who do repetitive manual work is higher than in controls
- There is also a strong association between vibration-exposed workers and Dupuytren's contracture compared with controls

Dupuytren's diathesis is a clinical association of:
- Dupuytren's contracture
- Plantar fasciitis and nodular plantar fibromatosis
- Peyronie's disease
- Knuckle pads (increased nodularity on the dorsum of the interphalangeal joints of the fingers)
- Nodular fasciitis of the popliteal fascia

Acquired immunodeficiency syndrome (AIDS):
- No increased prevalence of the disorder has been found in patients with AIDS, contrary to popular medical opinion

EPIDEMIOLOGY
Incidence and prevalence
INCIDENCE
- The incidence will again vary on the racial mix of the practitioner's population
- Incidence rates may be less than one patient per year per 1000 population to over 20 cases

PREVALENCE
Similarly this figure will vary from very low rates (fewer than five patients per 1000) to over 30% of patients of Swedish or Norwegian origin.

FREQUENCY
- May be seen in 3–5% of adults
- Overall rates of fewer than five to over 100 per 1000 patients can be expected

Demographics
AGE
- Affects patients over the age of 40 years, especially those over the age of 60 years
- Becomes more common with increasing age
- Females are affected later in life than males

GENDER
- Commoner in men
- Overall male:female ratio 5:1
- Women develop disease at a later age and it progresses more slowly
- Male:female ratio for surgery for Dupuytren's contracture is 10:1, for the reasons mentioned above
- Men seem to tolerate this deformity less well

RACE
- Much commoner in Caucasians, especially Nordic and Celtic races
- Virtually unknown in Southern Europeans, African-Americans, Asians, and Hispanics

GENETICS
More common in people of Northern and Western European origin. It may be familial (autosomal-dominant) in some cases.

GEOGRAPHY
- Predominately a disease affecting those of Northern and Western European origin
- Rates high in areas and communities in North America and Australia that had high immigration from Northern and Western Europe; rates are much lower where immigration was predominately from Southern Europe, Africa, or Asia

SOCIOECONOMIC STATUS
- Originally thought to occur more commonly in those who did manual labor. The association is now known to be with repetitive work or vibration
- There is no relationship between socioeconomic status and the likelihood of developing this condition

DIAGNOSIS

DIFFERENTIAL DIAGNOSIS
Tenosynovitis of flexor tendons of the hand
FEATURES

- This may be seen as a fullness in the palm
- Tenosynovitis is usually painful, and often any movement can produce exquisite pain
- There is usually full range of movements of all the joints of the fingers and hands
- If there is any limitation of movement, it is pain rather than mechanical difficulties that limit the movements
- There is no skin tethering over the surface of the tendons in tenosynovitis, unlike in Dupuytren's contracture

SIGNS & SYMPTOMS
Signs

- Nodular thickening and contraction of the palmar fascia leads to slowly progressive flexion deformities of the fingers
- The tendons and joints are not directly involved in this process
- It is usually symmetrical
- The fourth or ring finger is affected earliest, followed by the fifth (little), third (middle), and second (index) fingers
- The thumbs are not usually affected unless the disorder is more severe or chronic
- There are fibrous nodules in the palmar fascia that can be felt, and later seen and felt
- As the aponeurotic thickening extends distally, there will be flexion deformities of the metacarpo-phalangeal joints caused by tight fibrous bands radiating from the plantar fascia
- At this point, the hand cannot be placed flat on a flat surface (the 'table top test')

Symptoms

- Initially there will be no symptoms
- Pain is unusual at any stage
- As the disorder progresses, the patient may notice the lumpiness in the palmar fascia, and be able to see it
- Patients will usually first present only when the flexion contractures of one or more fingers becomes apparent
- Presentation is usually linked to the patient noticing some functional interference or inability to perform certain tasks, such as sewing or lifting
- The first symptom is often difficulty or embarrassment shaking hands, or of the hands catching in trouser pockets, for example when attempting to reach for small change
- Progressive flexion deformity can lead to severe impairment of function, and if the flexion is extreme, there may be palmar ulceration from pressure of the flexed fingers

ASSOCIATED DISORDERS
These are clinical associations of Dupuytren's contracture:

- Plantar fasciitis and nodular plantar fibromatosis
- Peyronie's disease (penile fasciitis)
- Knuckle pads (increased nodularity on the dorsum of the interphalangeal joints of the fingers)
- Nodular fasciitis of the popliteal fossa

CONSIDER CONSULT
Patients who are experiencing functional disability should be referred. This functional disability will often depend not only on the severity of the Dupuytren's contracture, but also on how much the individual patient is troubled by the resulting disability. Functional disability is more important than clinical interpretation of disease severity.

Refer also if there is diagnostic doubt, especially if patients are of non-Northern or Western European origin.

INVESTIGATION OF THE PATIENT
Direct questions to patient

Q How long have you noticed swelling of your palms? Dupuytren's contracture is of slow, insidious onset and progression. If palmar swelling occurs rapidly, exclude tenosynovitis or infection

Q Have you noticed any difficulty straightening your fingers? Dupuytren's contracture is characterized by flexion deformities of the fingers

Q Is the condition painful? Pain would suggest other diagnoses rather than Dupuytren's contracture, which tends to be completely painless

Q Do you have any lumps or thickening elsewhere? (For men) Is your erect penis bent or angulated? Dupuytren's contracture is associated with Peyronie's disease, plantar fasciitis, knuckle pads and nodular fasciitis of the popliteal fossa

Contributory or predisposing factors

Q How much alcohol do you drink? Dupuytren's contracture occurs more commonly in people who are heavy drinkers of alcohol

Q Have you injured your hands during the past 12 months, or had any operations there? Dupuytren's contracture may follow seemingly trivial injuries or apparently unrelated surgery to the hands, wrists or upper limbs – even if contralateral

Q Are you diabetic or epileptic? The incidence of Dupuytren's contracture is higher in patients with these diseases

Family history

Q Do you have a family history of similar complaints? Dupuytren's has a strong familial and especially racial tendency, occurring much more commonly in people of Northern or Western European origin. The disorder may develop earlier and occur more commonly in certain families.

Examination

Q Examine the hands. Can the patient lay his/her hands down on a flat surface? Can they fully extend all the joints of their hands? If there are flexion deformities as a result of Dupuytren's contracture, the patient will be unable to do either of these maneuvers

Q Is there nontender thickening of the palmar fascia, with possible skin tethering, but no direct tendon or joint involvement? If not, carefully reconsider the diagnosis of Dupuytren's contracture

Q Is there evidence of soft tissue thickening over the knuckle pads, soles of the feet, and popliteal fossae? All of these conditions are strongly associated with Dupuytren's contracture

Q Check for signs of chronic alcoholism. Dupuytren's contracture occurs more commonly in heavy drinkers

Summary of investigative tests

There are no specific diagnostic tests for Dupuytren's contracture, and diagnosis is essentially clinical. MRI may be useful to assess degree and extent of cellularity of the lesion, thus, differentiating 'active' from 'less active' disease (normally performed by a specialist).

The associated disorders of diabetes and alcoholism should be excluded:

- Blood glucose test will confirm diabetes mellitus
- Liver function tests may indicate chronic alcohol abuse
- Soft-tissue biopsy should only be performed in cases of persistent diagnostic doubt

DIAGNOSTIC DECISION

- The diagnosis is essentially clinical, and there is usually little diagnostic confusion
- Relatively painless, slowly progressive fixed flexion deformities of both hands affecting the ring and little fingers, at least initially, in patients who have no other signs or symptoms of any rheumatic diseases, are pathognomonic of Dupuytren's contracture
- The patient is otherwise well, or is diabetic, epileptic, or alcoholic
- Most patients are of Northern or Western European origin
- There is no associated arthritis, systemic disease, or malaise

CLINICAL PEARLS

- This is the most common cause of nodules on the palm
- Look for related conditions: plantar fasciitis, knuckle pads, and penile fibrosis
- Family history and alcohol abuse should always be considered

THE TESTS
Body fluids
BLOOD GLUCOSE
Description
Whole venous blood sample is needed.

Advantages/Disadvantages

- Advantage: a high level will confirm diabetes mellitus, which is associated with Dupuytren's contracture
- Disadvantage: is not a test for Dupuytren's contracture per se

Normal
70–110mg/dL (3.9–6.1mmol/L).

Abnormal

- A level of over 126mg/dl (over 7.1mmol/L) is abnormal in the fasting state
- Keep in the mind the possibility of a falsely abnormal result

Cause of abnormal result

- Diabetes
- Stress
- Cushing's syndrome

Drugs, disorders and other factors that may alter results

- Glucocorticoids
- Thiazide or loop diuretics

Tests of function
LIVER FUNCTION TESTS
Description
Venous blood required for assessment of gamma-glutamyl transferase (GGT) and aspartate aminotransferase (AST) levels.

Advantages/Disadvantages
Disadvantages:

- Abnormal liver function tests may indicate chronic alcohol abuse (which is strongly associated with Dupuytren's contracture), but are not diagnostic
- Similarly, normal liver function tests do not rule out chronic alcohol abuse
- Is not a test for Dupuytren's contracture *per se*

Normal
- GGT: 0–30U/L (0–0.50 mckat/L)
- AST: 0–35U/L (0–0.58 mckat/L)

Abnormal
- GGT: above 30 U/L
- AST: above 35 U/L
- Keep in mind the possibility of a falsely abnormal result

Cause of abnormal result
- Alcoholism
- Hepatitis
- Hepatic congestion

Drugs, disorders and other factors that may alter results
- Congestive heart failure
- Sepsis
- Many drugs

Biopsy
SOFT-TISSUE BIOPSY
Description
A soft-tissue biopsy of the hand is indicated only in extremely rare occasions where there is persistent diagnostic doubt.

Advantages/Disadvantages
Disadvantages:
- Invasive procedure
- Requires local anesthesia
- Entails small risks of subsequent infection and bleeding

Abnormal
- The biopsy will show the characteristic fibroblast and myofibroblast proliferation and vascular hyperplasia associated with Dupuytren's contracture
- In more severe cases, there is dense collagen deposition in a disorganized, random deposition
- Keep in mind the possibility of a falsely abnormal result

Cause of abnormal result
There is an increased amount of collagen, with increased cross-links, and infiltration of the collagen with myofibroblasts.

TREATMENT

CONSIDER CONSULT

With regard to treatment:

- Referral should be on the basis of the patient's perceived functional disability
- Referral can be to physical therapists and occupational therapists, or to a hand surgeon if a surgical approach is to be considered
- Patients with Dupuytren's diathesis, or with Dupuytren's contracture at an early age, or with severe disease, or with concomitant diabetes, epilepsy, or alcoholism, may benefit from early intervention and should be considered for referral early

PATIENT AND CAREGIVER ISSUES
Patient or caregiver request

- What happens if I don't have an operation?
- Will I get worse, and if so at what rate and how much worse?
- Will an operation cure me?
- Will I lose the use of my hands altogether?

MANAGEMENT ISSUES
Goals

- To maximize the ability of the patient to use their hands as they wish
- To relieve existing disability
- To prevent future disability

Management in special circumstances

- Specific degrees of flexion deformity will affect the patient's ability to function differently. For example, a patient whose vocation or hobbies require fine manual dexterity may not tolerate a minor degree of flexion deformity
- The aims of management should be to restore or maintain the individual's functionality to the maximum possible, ensuring maximum quality of life

COEXISTING DISEASE

Surgical intervention should be deferred in patients with poorly controlled diabetes, or alcoholism accompanied by severe liver damage, which may in turn affect blood clotting and wound healing.

SPECIAL PATIENT GROUPS

- Dupuytren's contracture is a disease of middle to old age. It is commoner in diabetics and alcoholics. For these reasons, the ability of a patient to endure a surgical procedure should be carefully weighed against the potential benefits of such surgery
- Patients whose quality of life depends heavily on their having full manual dexterity will benefit most from restoring any lost function

PATIENT SATISFACTION/LIFESTYLE PRIORITIES

- Patients are hoping for restoration of function
- The level of function required will be different for each patient
- The aim should be to restore maximum function needed for each patient, irrespective of their age or other disabilities

SUMMARY OF THERAPEUTIC OPTIONS
Choices

- Treatment will depend on the severity and on the rate of progression of the disease
- Patients need to be clear that treatment is based on the patient's functional impairment
- In addition to specific therapies, general lifestyle recomendations can be made

Mild disease:
- Occupational therapies such as aids and protective therapy
- Physical therapy such as stretching exercises, heat therapy

More severe disease (inability to straighten the fingers):
- Intralesional corticosteroids can be tried such as triamcinolone, hydrocortisone

Most severe disease (functional disability, flexion deformity of over 30 degrees, positive table top test):
- Referral for surgical interventions, such as fasciotomy, fasciectomy, by a specialist is indicated
- Amputation can be considered in extreme cases (performed by a specialist)

Guidelines:
Guidelines for the diagnosis and treatment of Dupuytren's contracture have been published by the American Society of Plastic and Reconstructive Surgery. Dupuytren's contracture. (ASPRS), 1998 (www.plasticsurgery.org). Also available from The National Guideline Clearing House.

Clinical pearls
- Often, no treatment is necessary
- It is not clear that any treatment can influence the ultimate outcome of this condition
- In extreme cases, surgery can be considered, with recognition that the condition might yet recur

FOLLOW UP
- All patients should be reassessed periodically (at least annually)
- Interventions should be offered depending on the patient's wishes and degree of disability

Plan for review
- The degree of functional impairment and disability should be noted
- The table top test should be carried out at least annually
- Coexisting disorders should be appropriately managed (e.g. diabetes)

Information for patient or caregiver
The patient should be instructed that difficulty using their hands is the main reason to seek evaluation and treatment.

DRUGS AND OTHER THERAPIES: DETAILS
Drugs
TRIAMCINOLONE INJECTION
A synthetic glucocorticoid that can be injected directly into the thickened palmar fascia for the treatment of Dupuytren's contracture.

Dose
- Acetonide: 2.5–15mg
- Diacetate: 12.5–25mg
- Hexacetonide: 2–6mg

Efficacy
- With varied success, can slow or temporarily arrest progression of the disorder
- Can reduce flexion deformity
- Overall, rarely provides full or lasting effect

Risks/Benefits
Risks:
- Does not provide quick response; may take several hours for relief

- Risk of infection with intra-articular injection
- Use caution with glomerulonephritis, ulcerative colitis, renal disease
- Use caution with AIDS, tuberculosis, ocular herpes simplex, live vaccines, viral and bacterial infections
- Use caution in diabetes mellitus, glaucoma, osteoporosis, hypertension
- Use caution in children and the elderly
- Use caution in recent myocardial infarction
- Use caution in psychosis
- Do not withdraw abruptly

Benefits:
- Temporary or partial benefits are usual, whilst side-effects are unusual
- Useful when active therapy is warranted, but surgery is not so warranted (either the disability is not major or there may be relative contraindications to surgery or anesthesia)

Side-effects and adverse reactions
- Skin: local irritation, changes in pigmentation, subcutaneous and cutaneous atrophy, scarring, paresthesia, tendon damage
- Minimal systemic effects

Interactions (other drugs)
Significant interactions are very unlikely between intralesional triamcinolone and other drugs.

Contraindications
- Local infection
- Previous soft-tisssue atrophy following intralesional corticosteroids

Acceptability to patient
- This can be done with local anesthesia
- The procedure is quick, easy, and safe

Follow up plan
- Patients should be followed up 2–3 weeks after injection to assess efficacy and check for local atrophy
- Subsequent follow up should be as usual, with at least annual checks

Patient and caregiver information
- Intralesional therapy is unlikely to be completely curative
- It should provide temporary and partial improvement
- It is quick, relatively easy, and safe

HYDROCORTISONE INJECTION
A glucocorticoid injection.

Dose
25–50mg.

Efficacy
- Can reduce flexion deformity
- Overall, rarely provides full or lasting effect

Risks/Benefits
Benefits:
- Temporary or partial benefits are usual, whilst side-effects are unusual
- Useful when active therapy is warranted but surgery is not

Side-effects and adverse reactions
- Skin: local irritation, changes in pigmentation, subcutaneous and cutaneous atrophy, scarring, paresthesia, tendon damage
- Minimal systemic effects

Interactions (other drugs)
Significant interactions are very unlikely between intralesional hydrocortisone and other drugs

Contraindications
- Local sepsis ▪ Previous soft-tissue atrophy after intralesional corticosteroids

Acceptability to patient
- Intralesional therapy can be carried out by primary care physicians in the office
- There is no need for regional, local, or general anesthesia
- The procedure is quick, easy, and safe

Follow up plan
Patients should be followed up 2–3 weeks after injection to assess efficacy and check for local atrophy.

Patient and caregiver information
- Intralesional therapy is unlikely to be completely curative
- It should provide temporary and partial improvement
- It is quick, relatively easy, and safe

Physical therapy
PHYSICAL THERAPY
In early Dupuytren's contracture, or mild degrees of impairment, physical therapy may be helpful:
- Stretching and flexing/extending exercises
- Heat therapy

Efficacy
Physical therapies provides symptomatic relief, but there is no evidence that they reduce the functional disability nor slow the rate of any progression of disability in Dupuytren's contracture.

Risks/Benefits
Benefit: the treatment is safe and well tolerated.

Acceptability to patient
Such therapy is usually very acceptable to patients.

Follow up plan
Follow up should be as usual, with at least annual checks.

Patient and caregiver information
- Multiple therapy sessions may be needed
- The lack of long-term efficacy must be made plain before starting a course of therapy

Occupational therapy
OCCUPATIONAL THERAPY

In patients with established disease for whom surgery is not possible, or for patients whose condition is recurrent despite surgery, occupational therapy may be helpful

- Occupational therapists can offer advice to patients and supply aids: specially adapted door handles, electrical appliance adaptation (e.g. electric kettles), jar and bottle openers, and cutlery
- Protective therapy (e.g. using protective gloves for manual work in patients with early disease) may help decrease progression

Efficacy
Occupational therapy can be life-enhancing and can minimize otherwise fairly disabling flexion deformities.

Acceptability to patient
Such therapy is very acceptable to most patients.

Follow up plan
Follow up should be as usual, with at least annual checks.

Patient and caregiver information
Multiple therapy sessions may be needed.

Surgical therapy

- Many patients with Dupuytren's contracture, especially those with advanced or more rapidly progressive disease, will benefit from surgery
- Operative intervention is indicated when the palmar fascial bands cause flexion contractions of the metacarpophalangeal and proximal interphalangeal joints
- The longer the contracture is present, the more difficult it is to correct
- The metacarpophalangeal joint can be released at any stage of the contracture
- The release of an established proximal interphalangeal joint contraction is less predicable

Complications of healing:
A combination of the following factors predisposes to wound and overall hand complications:
- Older age
- Alcoholism
- Diabetes
- The surgical fashioning of extensive thin skin flaps
- Tethering of the skin in the disease process
- Extensive surgical dissection and possible compromise of the blood supply to the healing tissues
- Excision of scar tissue from the flexor tendon sheaths and interphalangeal joints

Complications of surgery:
- Hematoma
- Infection
- Edema
- Ischemia and skin necrosis
- Tendon adhesions
- Joint adhesions and stiffness
- Palmar fasciitis
- Nerve and/or artery damage
- Hypertrophic scars
- Reflex sympathetic dystrophy

FASCIOTOMY

- This is a division of the contracting fascial band
- Both hands can be operated on at the same time, or as two separate procedures

Efficacy

- It is an effective procedure
- Recurrence is likely

Risks/Benefits

Risks:

- The procedure is simple and effective but there is a strong likelihood of recurrence
- There are risks of infection, ischemia, and hematoma

Acceptability to patient

- The procedure is effective, quick, and relatively simple
- Patients must be informed of the high recurrence rate after this procedure

Follow up plan

Patients should receive usual postoperative care and follow up.

Patient and caregiver information

Patients must be made aware of the strong likelihood of recurrence before consent is requested.

FASCIECTOMY

This may be:

- Radical-extensive resection of entire aponeurosis
- Local or regional – this gives best overall results

Both hands can be operated on at the same time, or as two separate procedures.

Efficacy

Local or regional fasciectomy provides the best results.

Risks/Benefits

Risks:

- Skin cover is required after the operation. This can be obtained from local flap repair or Z-plasty; by skin grafting in recurrent disease; or by leaving the wound open and allowing healing to occur
- The risks of wound complications, especially wound hematoma and sloughing, are higher with radical fasciectomy
- There may be some risk of surgically damaging the digital nerves, causing permanent paresthesia and weakness in the relevant digit

Benefits:

- The open wound healing technique is associated with little bleeding or hematoma formation or infection
- Recurrence of the Dupuytren's contracture is less likely after fasciectomy than after fasciotomy

Acceptability to patient

- The procedure is more time-consuming and difficult than fasciotomy but recurrence rates are lower
- There is greater dissection of the tissues of the hand than with fasciotomy. Therefore, the potential for postoperative scarring and tethering is greater

- There is a greater need for postoperative exercises, massage, and splinting
- Complication rates (bleeding, hematoma, infection, digital nerve damage) are higher than after fasciotomy, but are diminished by the open wound technique
- The open wound technique takes longer to heal and may be less acceptable to patients without access to more prolonged postoperative help or care

Follow up plan

- Patients should receive usual postoperative care and follow up (at 1 and 3 months at least)
- Follow up thereafter should be as usual, with at least annual checks
- Aim for early diagnosis and prevention of wound complications by, for example, prompt treatment of edema and suture removal from any area of skin with poor circulation
- Splintage to maintain correction of the flexion deformity
- Physical therapy to regain full flexion and grip strength
- If there are skin grafts, exercise should be delayed for 7–10 days
- Skin grafts should be monitored carefully, at least daily, for vascularity during early healing

Patient and caregiver information

- Patients must be made aware of the risks of recurrence before consent is requested
- Patients should be fully informed of the options of operative skin cover so that the choice can be agreed between surgeon and informed patient

AMPUTATION

In advanced cases of Dupuytren's contracture, where there is marked fixed flexion deformity of one or more finger, there may be palmar ulceration, or pain from pressure of the flexed finger against the palm.

Efficacy

Amputation may improve function of the hand.

Risks/Benefits

Risk: it is a destructive, irreversible procedure

Benefits:
- It relieves pain and pressure symptoms and their complications (e.g. infection and ulceration)
- It allows rapid postoperative recovery

Acceptability to patient

- Amputation is used as an operation of last resort
- Better surgical techniques, especially skin grafting, have led to the operation being performed less often
- Nevertheless, a few patients will prefer amputation as it allows rapid recovery and effects a cure

Follow up plan

- Patients should receive usual postoperative care and follow up (at 1 and 3 months at least)
- Follow up thereafter should be as usual, with at least annual checks
- Physical therapy to regain full flexion and grip strength

Patient and caregiver information

Patients should be made aware of all the other surgical and nonsurgical options before agreeing to amputation.

Radiation therapy
RADIOTHERAPY
Radiotherapy is often forgotten as a possible therapeutic option, especially in the early stages of the disease.

Efficacy
If used at an early stage, may delay or prevent progression of the Dupuytren's contracture.

Risks/Benefits
- Risk: risks of radiation burns (short term) and radiation damage (long term) are both low if the radiotherapy is given by specialists
- Benefit: good efficacy in preventing progression of the disease

Acceptability to patient
Very acceptable as an alternative to surgery.

Follow up plan
- Patients should receive usual post-therapy care and follow up (at 1 and 3 months at least)
- Follow up thereafter should be as usual, with at least annual checks
- Physical therapy to regain full flexion and grip strength

LIFESTYLE
Patients should be encouraged to use their hands in their normal, everyday way, as much as possible.

Risks/Benefits
Benefit: the discomfort and minor degrees of disability will be somewhat offset by maintaining the existing strength and function of the hands.

OUTCOMES

EFFICACY OF THERAPIES

- Dupuytren's contracture is usually progressive and recurrent, and no treatment has been shown consistently to slow its progression
- Nonsurgical intervention aims to maintain function for as long as possible, and surgical intervention aims to correct deformity and restore function. However, no treatment is curative and recurrence occurs in about 60% of patients postoperatively, often several years later
- Sequential or combined nonsurgical and surgical therapy usually restores adequate function, even if temporarily, allowing patients to maintain their quality of life
- Many patients adapt to their disorder, and nonsurgical interventions may preserve some functioning
- For those with severe disease where surgery is indicated, recurrence risk is greatest with active bilateral nodular disease in a young patient, or with a strong family history

Review period

- All patients with Dupuytren's contracture should be reviewed at least annually
- Reviews should be more frequent in more disabling cases
- Reviews should be more frequent after surgery, if rapidly progressive disease, or after any nonsurgical intervention
- Reviews should be more frequent if the patient has diabetes, alcohol dependance, epilepsy, knuckle pads, or Dupuytren's diathesis
- Reviews should continue for life

PROGNOSIS

- Dupuytren's is an incurable disease that invariably progresses, although the rate of progression varies between patients and in the same patient at different times
- Only 20% of patients who had undergone extensive palmar fasciectomies were free of recurrence 10 years later

Clinical pearls

- Treatment decisions must be individualized to the needs of a particular patient
- The patient's hand function is the most important factor guiding treatment
- Surgery should be considered only as a last resort, with the recognition that it is not curative

Therapeutic failure

- In the earliest stages of Dupuytren's contracture, nonoperative measures should be tried first
- Initially patients may require only explanation and reassurance
- As the disease causes greater functional disability, physical therapy, occupational therapy, and protective gloves should all be considered
- If the disease is progressive, or more importantly if the functional disability is increasing, referral to a hand surgeon is advised

Recurrence

Postoperative recurrence is more likely:

- In younger patients
- In patients with a strong family history
- In patients with rapid onset of disease, especially with skin involvement
- In patients who also have diabetes, or epilepsy, or alcoholism
- In patients with knuckle pads
- In patients with Dupuytren's diathesis

Deterioration

As functional disability increases, the following treatments should be considered, in order:

- Reassurance and explanation
- Physical therapy
- Occupational therapy
- Referral to a hand surgeon

COMPLICATIONS

- Severe flexion deformities can result in palmar ulceration, infection, and painful pressure symptoms
- Severe disability can result in secondary depression and social withdrawal

PREVENTION

RISK FACTORS

Diabetes: Dupuytren's may present soon after the diagnosis of diabetes is made. However, there is no good evidence that the severity or rate of progression of Dupuytren's contracture is related to diabetes control

Alcohol: alcoholism is related to increased risk of developing Dupuytren's

Epilepsy: there is no evidence that good epileptic control reduces the risk of developing Dupuytren's contracture

Occupation: there is no good evidence of occupational links to developing Dupuytren's contracture. Minimizing the risks of hand trauma may reduce the risks of developing Dupuytren's contracture

Hand trauma and surgery: minimizing the risks of hand trauma at home will reduce the risk

MODIFY RISK FACTORS

Diabetes: good diabetic control does not reduce inherent increased risk of developing Dupuytren's contracture

Epilepsy: similarly, good epileptic control does not reduce the increased risk of developing Dupuytren's contracture

Lifestyle and wellness

ALCOHOL AND DRUGS

Drugs (therapeutic or recreational) are not implicated at all in the development of Dupuytren's contracture

Identifying the patient at risk of developing alcoholism may reduce the incidence of Dupuytren's contracture

PHYSICAL ACTIVITY

People exposed to a great deal of hand vibration or who do repetitive work are at increased risk of developing Dupuytren's contracture

There is no other association between occupation, hobbies or past-times, or manual practices and increased risk of developing Dupuytren's contracture

ENVIRONMENT

Reducing risk of hand trauma will have a small effect on the risks of developing Dupuytren's contracture. Good home and workplace safety practices and enforcement of health and safety at work rules, and the use of protective clothing and machinery guards should reduce the risks of hand trauma.

FAMILY HISTORY

A strong family history is a definite risk factor for developing Dupuytren's contracture. There is no way of modifying this risk factor.

DRUG HISTORY

There are no drugs implicated in the development of Dupuytren's contracture.

PREVENT RECURRENCE

There is no proven way to prevent recurrence

Good control of concomitant diseases such as diabetes, epilepsy, and alcoholism do not prevent recurrences

It is sensible to advise minimal exposure to hand vibration and repetitive work

KEY REFERENCES

- American Society of Plastic and Reconstructive Surgery. Dupuytren's contracture, Arlington Heights, IL: ASPRS, 1998. (www.plasticsurgery.org)
- Hueston JT. Dupuytren's contracture. In Converse JM, McCartthy JG, Littler JW Eds. Reconstructive plastic surgery, 2nd edition, Philadelphia: WB Saunders,1997, pp4303–27
- Hueston JT. Dupuytren's contracture. In Jupiter JB Ed. Flynn's Hand Surgery, 4th edition, Baltimore:Williams and Wilkins, 1991, pp865–91
- Hurst LC. Nonoperative treatment of Dupuytren's disease. Hand Clin 1999;15:97–107
- Roush TF. Results following surgery for recurrent Dupuytren's disease. J Hand Surg 2000;25:291–6

FAQS
Question 1
Which other diagnoses should be considered in a patient with Dupuytren's contracture?

ANSWER 1
The 'Dupuytren's diathesis' includes other localized fibrosing disorders, such as Peyronie's disease, nodular plantar fibromatosis, and nodular fasciitis of the popliteal fascia.

Question 2
Is any treatment effective in preventing this disorder?

ANSWER 2
No. The treatment is focused on reducing symptoms and improving hand function.

Question 3
What is the role of surgery?

ANSWER 3
In severe cases, surgical fasciotomy or fasciectomy may be helpful in improving hand function, but the contracture may recur.

CONTRIBUTORS
Randolph L Pearson, MD
Richard Brasington Jr, MD, FACP
Rachel Kim, MD

EPICONDYLITIS

DESCRIPTION

- Lateral epicondylitis: inflammation of tendon fibers that attach forearm extensor muscles to outside of the elbow
- Medial epicondylitis: inflammation of tendon fibers that attach forearm extensor muscles (flexor pronator group) to inside of elbow
- Usually no history of trauma; repetitive use seems to make the pain worse
- Pain is felt where tendon fibers are attached to the bone on outside of the elbow or along forearm muscles and is usually more noticeable during or after stressful use of the arm
- Duration of symptoms ranges from 3 weeks to 3–4 years; average 6–12 weeks

URGENT ACTION

- Refer to orthopedic or rheumatology department if symptoms are so disabling that the patient cannot move the arm or lift anything
- Send for X-ray if fracture suspected

KEY! DON'T MISS!

- If the patient, especially if elderly, cannot move the arm and has problems speaking or moving, suspect stroke
- If patient has fallen, suspect fracture
- Loss of function indicates chronic inflammation

ICD9 CODE
- 726.31 Epicondylitis (medial)
- 726.32 Epicondylitis (elbow, lateral)

SYNONYMS
- Lateral: tennis elbow
- Medial: golfer's elbow

CARDINAL FEATURES
- Tendinosis of extensor carpi radialis brevis tendon (ECRB), usually within 1–2cm of its attachment to the lateral epicondyle of the humerus
- Inflammatory signs such as pain and stiffness following rest, relief with mild activity may indicate tendinitis rather than a degenerative process
- Onset of epicondylitis tends to be insidious but may be brought on by acute trauma such as heavy lifting
- Usually no history of trauma; repetitive use seems to make the pain worse
- Forceful wrist flexion and pronation can damage the tendons that attach to the medial epicondyle
- Pain is felt where these fibers are attached to the bone on the outside of the elbow or along the forearm muscles
- Pain is usually more noticeable during or after stressful use of the arm
- In severe cases, lifting and grasping even light things may be painful. Even such activities as pouring a drink, holding a cup, turning a door knob or a key in a door, brushing the teeth, or writing, become difficult or impossible
- Duration of symptoms ranges from 3 weeks to 3–4 years; average 6–12 weeks

CAUSES
Common causes
- Repeated microtrauma and inflammation is caused by overuse
- Repetitive use with weak shoulder and hand muscles greatly increases risk
- Micro tears in tendon are thought to lead to a hypervascular phenomenon resulting in pain
- Routine use of arm or injury to this area may stress or damage the muscle attachment and cause tennis elbow symptoms. Generally, patients have been involved in activities involving motion of the wrist and arm or lifting with the palm side of the hand facing down
- May begin after a sudden, traumatic movement of the elbow or wrist, e.g. carrying a heavy suitcase; poor lifting techniques commonly associated with medial epicondylitis
- Repetitive use of tools can be cause of both types of epicondylitis

Contributory or predisposing factors
- Recently taking up a sport or other physically strenuous activity
- Occupation that presents risk: factory workers; carpenters; musicians; butchers

EPIDEMIOLOGY
Incidence and prevalence
INCIDENCE
1–3% in the general population; work-related cases 59 per 10,000 workers per year; 7.4% of industrial workers in the US.

PREVALENCE
Nine out of 10,000 people.

FREQUENCY

- Not related to tennis in at least 95% of patients
- Tennis players have a reported incidence from 10 to 50%

Demographics

AGE

- The younger group may have a sports-related injury
- The older group tend to have epicondylitis as a result of a work-related injury or overuse syndrome
- Sports-related: most often in Caucasian males between 30 and 60 years of age
- In preadolescents, who still have maturing secondary ossification centers, traction apophysitis of the medial epicondyle is likely

GENDER

- Sports-related: most often in Caucasian males between 30 and 60 years
- Work-related: higher incidence in women between 30 and 60 years

RACE

Sports-related: most often in Caucasian males between 30 and 60 years of age.

DIFFERENTIAL DIAGNOSIS
Osteoarthritis
Most common joint disorder, affecting many people to some degree by age 70 years.

FEATURES
- Slowly evolving, characterized by deterioration of articular cartilage and by formation of bony outgrowths or spurs (osteophytes)
- Joints most often affected are knees, hips, distal interphalangeal (DIP) joints of the hands, carpometacarpal joints of thumb, and cervical and lumbrosacral spine
- Often benign, but severe changes may cause serious disability
- Initial pain may be alleviated with rest and simple analgesics, such as acetaminophen or nonsteroidal anti-inflammatory agents (NSAIDs)

Median nerve entrapment at other sites
FEATURES
- Most common is pronator teres syndrome, producing entrapment at the elbow
- Neurological deficit is not limited to the areas peripheral to the wrist joint
- Seen much less frequently than carpal tunnel syndrome (CTS)
- Can be differentiated from CTS by clinical examination and nerve conduction studies

Ulnar neuropathy
FEATURES
- Pain and paresthesias in forearm and ulnar distribution of hand (4th and 5th digits)
- Weakness of abductor pollicis brevis (5th digit abduction)
- Most often due to entrapment at elbow
- May be exacerbated by elbow flexion

Pseudogout
Rheumatic manifestation of calcium pyrophosphate dihydrate crystal deposition in articular cartilage (chondrocalcinosis), synovium, and periarticular ligaments and tendons.

FEATURES
- Usually affects the knee (50% of cases) but often also the wrist, elbow, shoulder, ankle, and hand joints
- Acute attacks associated with swelling, restricted movement and increased heat in the affected joints, and fever. The intensity of the periarticular inflammation may suggest cellulitis
- Joints in chronic disease may show bony swelling, crepitus, and restricted movement, with varying levels of synovitis
- Most common cause of acute inflammatory monoarthritis in the elderly
- Identification of crystals is the only means of positive diagnosis

Radiocapitellar arthritis
Aggregation of inflammatory cells and their products in the joint space and synovium.

FEATURES
- Joint swelling, warmth, redness, effusion, and tenderness
- Stiffness and swelling in elbow and other joints, especially in the mornings

SIGNS & SYMPTOMS
Signs

- Tenderness over lateral aspect of forearm – lateral epicondyle, extensor tendons, muscle belly, which may radiate into the forearm; decreased grip strength and pain on gripping, decreased strength
- Pain on active wrist extension, pain on stretch of ECRB, pain on resisted radial deviation
- Extension of middle finger may disturb sleep when severe
- Tends to be a loss of end range elbow extension and/or adduction with extension (due to intimate relationship between ECRB and capsule/ligaments of the elbow complex)
- Onset may be insidious or traumatic – gradual or related to a specific incident

Lateral:
- Worst pain is at lateral epicondyle
- Point tenderness over lateral epicondyle
- Reproduction of pain on passive flexion of the wrist and fingers with the elbow extended; supination against resistance; wrist/finger extension against resistance; resisted lifting with forearm in neutral position
- Weakness of wrist extension and/or grip
- Often elbow motion is normal although painful at end range of extension in severe cases

Medial:
- Worst pain is at medial epicondyle
- Usually no visible swelling

Symptoms

Lateral epicondylitis:
- Slow onset of pain and/or immobility, occurring first in the extensor tendons when the wrist is extended against resistance (e.g. using a manual screwdriver)
- Later, constant pain, usually near lateral epicondyle
- Pain in lateral elbow with radiation into the extensor aspect of forearm on extension of wrist or on forearm supination
- Pain along lateral epicondyle when patient tries to use arm
- Pain can extend from lateral epicondyle to wrist
- Burning sensation that may radiate into forearm

Medial epicondylitis:
- Pain in flexor pronator tendons (attached to the medial epicondyle) and in medial epicondyle
- With continued overuse, muscles and tendons hurt even at rest
- Inner forearm usually tender when touched; often uncomfortable or impossible to grip objects (even lifting a light object such as a cup of coffee can be difficult)
- In severe cases, almost any elbow movement can be uncomfortable
- Weak grip

ASSOCIATED DISORDERS
- Carpal tunnel syndrome in work-related cases
- Tendinitis spreading to the tendons of the hand
- Nerve entrapment syndrome creating referred pain from the neck into the arm
- de Quervain's tendinitis, extensor and flexor forearm
- Tendinitis/tendinosis, cubital tunnel syndrome
- Hand-arm vibration syndrome (HAVS)

There appear to be two main groups of soft-tissue disorders:
- Specific soft-tissue syndromes: occur in joints, muscles, or nerves and are associated with

characteristic symptoms and physical signs: epicondylitis at the elbow, tendon disorders at the wrist, and nerve entrapments such as carpal tunnel syndrome

- Nonspecific soft-tissue syndrome: pain symptoms with muscular symptoms such as weakness and cramp, or nerve symptoms such as numbness, pins and needles, and burning. Any one of these problems can be classed as repetitive strain syndrome depending on the causation

KEY! DON'T MISS!
- If the patient, especially if elderly, cannot move the arm and has problems speaking or moving, suspect stroke
- If patient has fallen, suspect fracture
- Loss of function indicates chronic inflammation

CONSIDER CONSULT
In cases where rest, ice, and NSAIDs over 2–4 weeks have not alleviated symptoms.

INVESTIGATION OF THE PATIENT
Direct questions to patient
Q Is the pain mainly in your elbow?
Q Do both arms hurt? In some chronic cases the patient will compensate by using the nonwriting arm and develop bilateral symptoms
Q Is it stiff in the mornings? To check for arthritis
Q Have you had a fall? To check for fracture
Q Do you have pain in any other joints? To check for arthritis
Q Is the pain on the inner ('crazy bone') or outer side? To ascertain if lateral or medial
Q Does it hurt the rest of your arm and wrist to move the arm? To assess severity
Q Does it hurt the elbow or wrist during these movements? If no movement possible, the condition is chronic and will take a long time to recover – months rather than weeks
Q Can you grip or lift a small object (such as a cup) and/or turn a key in the door? To assess severity and possible associated disorders
Q Do you link your symptoms to any sport or activity? To trace the cause(s). In some cases, a patient could play e.g. tennis AND have a job that involves repetitive arm motions
Q Have you taken up a sport or other strenuous activity recently? Often caused by recent adoption of strenuous activity with unpracticed or untrained technique, no warm-up exercises, and poor muscle tone
Q What is your work? Do you use a keyboard or perform any other repetitive task at work using your arms? Many cases, especially in 30-plus age group, are occupational
Q Does the pain stop when you stop performing the repetitive action? If yes, advice will be to cease that activity completely until recovery is complete, and technique has been relearned. If no, the condition is likely to be chronic
Q Have you had similar symptoms before? To confirm if recurring, and therefore needing referral

Contributory or predisposing factors
Q Do you work with a keyboard or carry out repetitive tasks using your arms at work? To ascertain whether direct trauma to the lateral epicondyle caused by repetitive supination of the forearm or dorsiflexion of the wrist against resistance. Jobs that present a risk include factory workers; carpenters; musicians; butchers; cashiers
Q If so, do you take regular breaks and/or have health and ergonomic assessments at work? If the answers are 'no', the patient may be overworked and at increased risk
Q Have you learned how to use computer programs and other systems at work in ways that reduce the risk of this problem developing or recurring? If the answer is no, the patient may be at increased risk, especially as so many occupations necessitate the use of a computer keyboard, while others require heavy lifting

Q Have you recently taken up a sport or exercise program/dug the garden/painted the house or similar, sudden, strenuous activity? Often patients develop symptoms after either adopting a new activity – especially without prior training – or increasing the duration or intensity of an established one

Q Have you recently done an arm-intensive task (such as home improvements or gardening) that you don't normally do? Patients can develop symptoms after either adopting a new activity or increasing the duration or intensity of an established one

Examination

- Examine cervical spine and shoulder: in order to rule out referred causes of lateral elbow pain
- Ask patient to extend fingers against resistance with elbow held straight: pain occurs along the common extensor tendon
- Alternatively, sit the patient on a chair with his/her arm resting on a table. The hand is held palm downward, and the elbow is straight. Place a hand firmly on top of that of the patient and ask them to try to raise the hand by bending the wrist. The same pain occurs
- Gently palpate tendon near to where it attaches to the humerus. Often there will be pain
- With the patient's elbow flexed and held against the side, ask the patient to grasp your hand and perform supination against resistance: Yergason's sign for bicipital tendinitis can also be positive in lateral epicondylitis
- In medial epicondylitis: when the same examination is done pain is felt on the medial epicondyle and in the flexor pronator tendons

Summary of investigative tests

- X-rays are of very little benefit in assessing soft-tissue damage, but may be used as part of the examination to check for arthritis or other bone disorders, or to rule out fractures, or to assess calcific tendinitis in intractable lateral epicondylitis
- MRI: tendon degeneration and degree of tear are well defined on MR images and correlate effectively with surgical and histologic findings. Areas of signal hyperintensity on MR images correlate with findings of neovascularization and/or mucoid degeneration at histopathologic examination

DIAGNOSTIC DECISION

- Passive forearm pronation and wrist flexion typically reproduces the symptoms of lateral epicondylitis
- Chief finding is location and reproducibility of the pain
- Occasionally, pain and immobility radiate to the long and ring fingers
- Resisted wrist extension and radial deviation intensify the pain

CLINICAL PEARLS

Pain in the lateral elbow brought on by making a fist or squeezing suggests lateral epicondylitis.

THE TESTS
Imaging
X-RAY
Advantages/Disadvantages
Advantages:

- Soft-tissue injuries do not show up on X-ray but it may be useful to assess arthritis or other bone disorders, or to rule out fractures, or to assess calcific tendinitis in intractable lateral epicondylitis
- Noninvasive

Disadvantage: additional radiation

Abnormal
Traction spur or soft-tissue calcification may show on X-ray.

Cause of abnormal result
Indicates intractable epicondylitis or calcific tendinitis.

MRI SCAN
Advantages/Disadvantages
- Excellent in revealing soft-tissue damage such as tendon degeneration and microscopic tears
- Noninvasive
- Not always available and extremely expensive

Abnormal
Tendon degeneration.

Cause of abnormal result
- Most likely from chronic tendinitis
- Areas of signal hyperintensity on MR images correlate with findings of neovascularization and/or mucoid degeneration at histopathologic examination

TREATMENT

CONSIDER CONSULT
- Where diagnosis is proving difficult
- In cases of severe disability

IMMEDIATE ACTION
Prescribe rest and ice.

PATIENT AND CAREGIVER ISSUES
Patient or caregiver request
- **Will I recover the full use of my arm(s)?** Reassure the patient, who may be finding ordinary tasks very painful, that they will recover
- **Will physical therapy help?** Most certainly, but it will take time, effort, and patience. Improvements may be gradual (in severe cases, especially if other disorders are also present, where the patient is unable to perform simple tasks)
- **How will I manage at home/shopping for food etc?** In severe cases ask if someone can look after the patient if they live alone and advise the patient on how to perform tasks with both arms. (However, symptoms this severe are extremely unusual)
- **Can I continue to play my chosen sport?** A period of rest and reassessment of technique is appropriate before resumption
- **Will an injection get rid of the pain?** This treatment provides the most immediate relief of pain, but this is often temporary
- **Am I allowed to have more than one elbow injection?** In some cases, a second injection may be given, but repeated injections may be harmful to the tissues
- **Is this repetitive strain injury (RSI)?** It is often hard to determine whether repetitive activity is causative (This question must be answered carefully, as the physician's answer may be pivotal in a legal assessment of this issue)

Health-seeking behavior
- **Have you taken any painkillers or anti-inflammatory treatments yourself?** To check if over-the-counter (OTC) medication has started
- **Have the tablets brought any relief?** It may take some days for NSAIDs to start taking effect
- **Have you put your arm in a sling or splint? For how long?** This should be discouraged
- **Have you carried on working despite the pain?** Some patients may 'soldier on' and make the condition worse, either because they are under pressure not to miss work or because they feel they cannot be absent from work
- **Have you sought advice about your working practices/technique?** Some patients are aware of the problem and may be trying to improve their situation. Others may be totally unaware

MANAGEMENT ISSUES
Goals
- Relieve pain and reduce inflammation
- Physical therapy: the initial aims of physical therapy are to reduce the level of pain experienced, restore flexibility and strength, and prevent recurrence
- Self-care including exercises under supervision by a physical therapist
- Prescribe and advise proper use of anti-inflammatory medication
- Risk factor modification: if patient has no loss of function, advise him/her to avoid repetitive grip, dorsiflexion of the wrist, and supination of the forearm against resistance
- If epicondylitis is work-related and the patient is still able to work, advise about taking breaks, safe working practices and facilities, as far as are reasonably achievable. If patient unable to work, make sure patient appreciates the need to rest the arm(s) and arrange for physical therapy

Management in special circumstances
COEXISTING DISEASE
Other work-related soft-tissue injuries need similar rest and ice measures and possibly physical therapy, plus the same advice regarding prevention.

COEXISTING MEDICATION
Check whether patient has been taking OTC analgesics and/or NSAIDs.

PATIENT SATISFACTION/LIFESTYLE PRIORITIES
- Depends on severity. If pain and disability make certain activities difficult or impossible, the patient's life will be radically affected in the short term. Examples are writing, pouring a drink, making a meal, turning a doorknob or key, pushing open a door, brushing teeth, or shaking hands. Work modification and help from family/partners/friends to cope at home may be essential to enable the patient to rest the affected arm(s) and enable the inflammation to recede
- While the patient needs to rest from the activity that caused the problem, special exercises supervised by the physical therapist are recommended
- If diagnosed early, patients can benefit from physical therapy and an exercise program, which must be continued on a permanent basis. Patients must be reassured that physical therapies and anti-inflammatory drugs can help and that self-help is necessary, thereby involving the patient in the management of their condition. In more severe and advanced cases long periods off work and/or surgery replacement may be necessary, but the patient may be reassured that rest and physical therapy are often highly successful

SUMMARY OF THERAPEUTIC OPTIONS
Choices
Rest and ice:
- Show patient how to do ice massage 4 times/day until acute pain is controlled
- Advise stopping or limiting activities that cause the pain
- Advise avoiding any activity that hurts on extending or pronating the wrist
- Show patient how to apply icepack (or packet of frozen peas), with pressure, directly to the skin over the lateral epicondyle and proximal extensor musculature for 20 min three times daily. Advise against applying chemical cold packs directly to skin as these may cause frostbite
- Advise relative rest - cessation of activity that exacerbates the condition is recommended for 1-2 weeks, depending on severity of symptoms

Physical therapy, occupational therapy and lifestyle:
- Physical therapy usually essential for all but the mildest cases, enabling patient to restore mobility and strength
- Physical therapists are trained to discuss lifestyle issues, rehabilitation, and self-help

Nonsteroidal anti-inflammatory drugs:
- NSAIDs taken by mouth (ibuprofen, diclofenac, naproxen, and others) often provide pain relief
- NSAIDs facilitate exercise and other supportive measures by suppressing articular inflammation, pain, and muscle spasm
- Tolerance and effectiveness for the individual patient dictate drug choice
- Patients should be monitored and warned of potential adverse reactions

Corticosteroid injections:
- Betamethasone sodium phosphate/betamethasone acetate or methylprednisolone acetate
- Have marked effect on inflammation
- No good data to indicate that steroid injections decrease the long-term adverse effects of chronic inflammatory or degenerative diseases, but temporary relief often results

Ultrasonography and surgery:
- Ultrasonography (usually given by the physical therapist) to reduce inflammation
- Surgery may be advised by the specialist in intractable cases but should only be done as a last resort

Clinical pearls
Activity modification, splints, and exercises are often underutilized in treatment.

Never
Prescribe NSAIDs or painkillers without prescribing rest, ice, splinting, and appropriate exercises.

FOLLOW UP
After 4–6 weeks of conservative treatment, reassessment is appropriate.

Plan for review
- In many cases a physical therapist will be the medical professional in direct charge of reviewing the patient's progress and will 'sign off' the patient once they start to improve and regain strength and mobility
- Rehabilitation period will involve the patient in self-help exercises and they will be advised on how to avoid recurrence, how to recognize symptoms, and to apply rest and ice as soon as symptoms recur

Information for patient or caregiver
The patient should be advised on the importance of rest and ice in the early stages, on precautions for taking NSAIDs, and the implications of possible further treatments such as injections – and in all cases, means of preventing recurrence.

DRUGS AND OTHER THERAPIES: DETAILS
Drugs
NONSTEROIDAL ANTI-INFLAMMATORY DRUGS
NSAIDs: Inhibit prostaglandin synthesis thereby reducing inflammatory response and relieving pain.

Dose
The dose depends on the specific agent: e.g. ibuprofen 400–800mg three times daily, naproxen 500mg twice daily, diclofenac 50mg three times a day (immediate release).

Efficacy
Often successful in relieving symptoms.

Risks/Benefits
Risks:
- GI disturbance may be increased
- All currently available NSAIDS have unwanted effects especially in the elderly
- Substantial individual variation in clinical response to NSAIDs
- Use caution in renal, cardiac, and hepatic impairment

Benefits:
- Safer than aspirin
- Have a range of actions: anti-inflammatory, analgesic, antipyretic

Side-effects and adverse reactions
- Gastrointestinal: diarrhea, dyspepsia, nausea, vomiting, gastric bleeding and perforation
- Skin: rashes, urticaria, photosensitivity

- Genitourinary: reversible renal insufficiency, renal disease (high doses over long periods)
- Respiratory: worsening of asthma
- Ears, eyes, nose and throat: tinnitus, decreased hearing
- Central nervous system: headache, dizziness

Interactions (other drugs)
- Antihypertensives (ACE inhibitors, adrenergic neurone blockers, alpha-blockers, angiotensin-II receptor antagonists, beta-blockers, clonidine, diazoxide, diuretics, hydralazine, methyldopa, minoxidil, nitroprusside) Antidysrhythmics (calcium channel blockers, cardiac glycosides) Antiplatelet agents (clopidogrel, ticlopidine) Aspirin Baclofen
- Cyclosporine Corticosteroids Heparins Ketorolac Lithium Methotrexate
- Moclobemide NSAIDs Nitrates Pentoxifylline (oxpentifylline) Phenindione
- Phenytoin Quinolones Ritonavir Sulfonylureas Tacrolimus Zidovudine

Contraindications
- Pregnancy and breast feeding Coagulation defects Active peptic ulceration

Acceptability to patient
Varies according to gastrointestinal tract tolerance.

Follow up plan
Regular follow up necessary to assess efficacy and adverse effects.

Patient and caregiver information
Better tolerated if taken with food.

CORTICOSTEROIDS
No more than three injections should be given within a 9-month period.

Dose
Intra-articular injection of betamethasone sodium phosphate and betamethasone acetate combination:
Adults and children: 0.25–0.5mL/dose at the appropriate site.

Intra-articular injection of methylprednisolone acetate:
Adults: 10–80mg at the appropriate site, depending upon degree of inflammation and size and location of affected area. Due to very slow absorption, repeated doses are not normally required for 1–5 weeks.

Efficacy
Very effective in relieving symptoms immediately but relief may be only temporary.

Risks/Benefits
Risks:
- Limited to 3–4 per year
- Frequent cortisone injections increase the risk for cortisone side-effects that affect areas throughout the body as the medicine is absorbed into the bloodstream
- Subcutaneous atrophy can occur at this site; triamcinolone should never be used
- Slow-acting
- False-negative skin allergy tests
- Overwhelming septicemia if patient has an infection
- Loss of control of blood glucose in those with diabetes
- Use caution in elderly due to risk of diabetes and osteoporosis
- Use caution in patients with psychosis, seizure disorders, or myasthenia gravis

- Use caution in congestive heart failure, hypertension
- Use caution in ulcerative colitis, peptic ulcer, or esophagitis

Side-effects and adverse reactions
- Gastrointestinal: dyspepsia, peptic ulceration, esophagitis, oral candidiasis, nausea, diarrhea
- Cardiovascular system: hypertension, thromboembolism
- Central nervous system: insomnia, euphoria, depression, psychosis
- Endocrine: adrenal suppression, impaired glucose tolerance, growth suppression in children, Cushing's syndrome
- Musculoskeletal: proximal myopathy, osteoporosis
- Skin: delayed healing, acne, striae
- Eyes, ears, nose and throat: cataract, glaucoma, blurred vision

Interactions (other drugs)
- Adrenergic neurone blockers, alpha-blockers, beta-blockers, beta-2-agonists
- Aminoglutethamide ▪ Anticonvulsants (carbemazepine, phenytoin, barbiturates) ▪ Antidiabetics ▪ Antidysrhythmics (calcium channel blockers, cardiac glycosides) ▪ Antifungals (amphotericin, ketoconazole) ▪ Antihypertensives (ACE inhibitors, diuretics: loop and thiazide, acetazolamide; angiotensin II receptor antagonists, clonidine, diazoxide, hydralazine, methyldopa, minoxidil) ▪ Cyclosporine ▪ Erythromycin ▪ Methotrexate ▪ NSAIDs ▪ Nitrates ▪ Nitroprusside ▪ Oral contraceptives ▪ Rifampin ▪ Ritonavir ▪ Somatropin ▪ Vaccines

Contraindications
- Cellulitis or broken skin over the intended entry site for the injection or aspiration ▪ Anticoagulant therapy that is not well controlled ▪ Severe primary coagulopathy ▪ Septic effusion of a bursa or a periarticular structure (for injection) ▪ More than three previous injections in the preceding 12-month period ▪ Lack of response to two or three prior injections ▪ Systemic infection ▪ Avoid live virus vaccines in those receiving immunosuppressive doses

Acceptability to patient
May be very acceptable if all else has failed.

Follow up plan
Review after 4 weeks as repeat injection may be necessary.

Patient and caregiver information
Crystal irritation can be minimized when the patient applies ice locally following an injection.

Physical therapy
Physical therapy, including self-help exercise program and may also include ultrasonography.

PHYSICAL THERAPY
- Active assisted and nonresisted motion to restore mobility, function, and strength
- In less severe cases (or sports-related cases): initially isokinetic strengthening with light weights and higher repetitions for endurance followed by a strengthening protocol utilizing fewer repetitions and gradually increasing weight
- Ultrasonography applied by the physical therapist to the affected part can reduce inflammation
- Relaxation techniques
- Instruction on healthy hand-use and better posture, and how to make ergonomic improvements to the workplace and home
- Rehabilitation will include strengthening and stretching exercises

Efficacy
High, although further improvements in strength and flexibility are unlikely after one month of adequate physical therapy and treatment may last many months.

Risks/Benefits
If administered correctly with gradual build-up of exercises, there should be no risks and only considerable benefit in restoring strength and mobility and getting the patient back to work.

Acceptability to patient
High, but involves hard work and slow progress can be frustrating.

Follow up plan
6 months to a year, or until the physical therapist feels the patient is ready to be signed off.

Patient and caregiver information
- Must keep up the exercise program and other instructions relating to rest and ice and improved arm mechanisms and/or technique
- In sports-related cases, attention to correct technique is advised
- In work-related cases, attention to ergonomics is important

Occupational therapy
OCCUPATIONAL THERAPY
- Many workplaces run short courses on better working practices to vary tasks, improve keyboard technique, improve posture, and take breaks
- Adjusting workstations and varying tasks
- Training keyboard workers to take breaks and amend their typing methods
- Physical therapy and/or relaxation classes may be available on site in some big organizations

Efficacy
Essential to maintain healthy hand-use in the workplace.

Risks/Benefits
Benefit: maintaining good working practices can prevent future problems in work-related cases.

Acceptability to patient
Usually good.

Patient and caregiver information
Many workplaces regularly produce guidelines on good working practices. In some countries these are mandatory. People who have had epicondylitis will be well served by following the precautions while others can prevent it by following them.

Surgical therapy
Surgery may be indicated if lateral epicondylitis fails to resolve after a 6- to 12- month course of conservative treatment, or if there is no improvement after three steroid injections. The percentage of cases that prove resistant to conservative care or the passage of time ranges from 4% to 10%.

Procedures include:
- Percutaneous release of the tendon off the bone
- Arthroscopic procedures or other procedures involving the joint and resection of a ligament
- The most popular procedure today is a simple excision of diseased tissue from within the tendon

SURGERY
Efficacy
For those with prolonged pain, surgery is generally successful.

Risks/Benefits
Risk: pain may not be alleviated and in all cases rehabilitation is essential to restore function.

Acceptability to patient
If all else has failed, the patient may welcome surgery as a last resort.

Follow up plan
Physical therapy will follow surgery for several weeks.

Patient and caregiver information
A gradual return to normal activity with an appropriate passive and active exercise program is necessary for recovery.

Other therapies
ICE PACK/REST
- Have the patient apply an ice pack (or packet of frozen peas), with pressure, directly to the skin over the lateral epicondyle and proximal extensor musculature for 20 min three times daily
- Advise patients against applying chemical cold packs directly to skin as these may cause frostbite
- Rest (cessation of activity that exacerbates the condition) is recommended for 1–4 weeks, or maybe longer, depending on the severity of symptoms

Efficacy
High.

Risks/Benefits
Benefit: the earlier rest and ice can be applied, the greater the benefits as ice treatment can reduce inflammation and tissue damage and bring relief.

Acceptability to patient
Generally high, but the rest element may be problematic if work-related.

Follow up plan
Review after 4 weeks to see if further measures (physical therapy/referral) are needed.

Patient and caregiver information
Rest and ice is basic advice for early treatment of many sports injuries and can be administered by the patient.

LIFESTYLE
- Lifestyle changes depend on severity. If pain and disability make certain activities difficult or impossible, the patient's life will be radically affected in the short term. Examples are writing, pouring a drink, making a meal, turning a doorknob, pushing open a door, brushing teeth, or shaking hands
- In the long term, patients must realize that the condition can recur and must therefore adjust their lifestyle to prevent recurrence. This may involve sensible precautions about lifting and moving heavy objects and not taking on tasks such as digging the garden or painting the house. Sometimes the sport or other activity has to be curtailed or ceased to guarantee recovery and prevent recurrence

- Time off work and help from family/partners/friends to cope at home may be essential to enable the patient to rest the affected arm(s) and enable the inflammation to recede. The patient should expect 1–8 weeks off work depending on job duties and if modified work is not available
- In less severe cases, absence from work is not anticipated particularly if modified duties are available and advice regarding improved working practices can be taken
- There may be permanent work restrictions following recovery; in some protracted cases patients have to change jobs or career
- Patients must be reassured that self-help is necessary, thereby involving the patient in the management of their condition

RISKS/BENEFITS
The benefits are great, but the risk of deterioration and recurrence is high if lifestyle changes are not made.

ACCEPTABILITY TO PATIENT
- Some patients are reluctant to adapt to change or to accept that they have developed a potentially disabling condition
- Others are unwilling to ask for help or to reduce their activities accordingly for fear of losing their jobs or having to give up (even temporarily) a sport they enjoy
- Some may over-react and become afraid of performing any task they believe will make things worse

FOLLOW UP PLAN
Depends on how long the symptoms last. Lifestyle changes can be moderated once recovery is assured, but many changes, such as improved posture, technique, and working practices, are permanent.

PATIENT AND CAREGIVER INFORMATION
Physical therapists are trained to advise the patient on changes to lifestyle and they will provide guidelines for the patient to follow.

OUTCOMES

EFFICACY OF THERAPIES

- Epicondylitis is often a nagging or chronic condition sometimes requiring many months for healing to occur
- Rest and ice is basic treatment at the onset of symptoms and may reduce symptoms in milder cases without further treatment
- Physical therapy is often essential for recovery
- NSAIDs (and analgesics) alone are insufficient therapies for recovery but bring temporary relief and help to reduce inflammation
- NSAIDs should be combined with physical therapy and retraining
- As the condition improves, there is usually a slow return to normal activities
- Recurrence is common; efficacy and prevention depends on adjusting many activities, sometimes permanently

Review period

4–6 weeks in mild cases; 6 months to 2 years in severe cases.

PROGNOSIS

- Full restoration of function and strength possible in majority of cases, especially younger patients
- Work-related epicondylitis often has less promising prognosis, depending on how long the patient has carried on working with symptoms; how well they respond to physical therapy; and how closely they adhere to the preventive measures, which are for life

Clinical pearls

- A corticosteroid injection provides the most rapid relief of symptoms
- The condition is likely to recur if athletic or ergonomic precipitating factors are not corrected

Recurrence

- Recurrence of this condition is common and preventive measures are important in preventing recurrence
- Some patients ignore all the advice and get worse as a result. They will need referral and advice

Deterioration

- In cases of symptom duration from 6 months to one year, there is evidence of vascular and fibroblastic proliferation accompanied by focal hyaline degeneration of the aponeurotic origin of the ECRB tendon
- This may explain the lack of response to rest and anti-inflammatory medication
- Deterioration often occurs when the patient returns to the causative or other activities before healing is complete, or when they are unable to cease work or other activities (such as housework) in order for recovery to take place

COMPLICATIONS

- Subperiosteal hemorrhage
- Periostitis, spur formation
- Tearing of the medial collateral ligament

PREVENTION

Prevention is essential as this disorder can recur, and includes improved working practices/sports technique; taking breaks and varying tasks; awareness of limitations and adapting lifestyle.

RISK FACTORS

- Overuse during work activities: heavy lifting, improper or excessive keyboard use, or any repetitive arm motion greatly increases risk. Tasks must be varied; breaks should be taken; better keyboard techniques and more 'arm-friendly' software should be used
- Repetitive tasks: any repetitive arm motion at work or at home increases risk
- Poor working conditions: layout of workstations may need adjustment
- Poor technique in racquet and other sports: improved techniques must be adopted to prevent 'tennis elbow' and 'golfer's elbow', particularly in patients with poor muscle tone
- Sudden strenuous activity: taking up a sport without adequate training in good technique or suddenly taking on a task such as home decorating, gardening, or activities involving heavy lifting or screwdriving motions
- Failure to cope with stress: tension as a result of stress response may be an added factor in work-related cases

MODIFY RISK FACTORS

- Education of all parties on preventive measures at work, in sports, or any activity that involves repetitive arm motion
- Modification of tools and/or work activities
- Compliance with limitations and restrictions
- Education related to home, social, and sports activity as well as the work environment
- Education on how to recognize symptoms and advice on rest and ice if symptoms appear
- Knowing when to stop high-risk activities

Lifestyle and wellness

Work and recreation may need radical modification in severe cases. Patients will have to learn when to stop, to take breaks, to do appropriate exercises, to take regular, gentle exercise, to avoid heavy lifting, pushing, pulling, excessive keyboard use for work and recreation.

TOBACCO
As in many disorders where blood circulation and oxygen supply is further impaired by smoking, patients should quit.

ALCOHOL AND DRUGS
Patients should avoid heavy drinking as control over physical well-being is threatened, e.g. there is an increased risk of falling and/or knocking and damaging the affected arm(s).

PHYSICAL ACTIVITY
- Physical therapists can advise patients on rest and ice; on exercise programs to regain and maintain strength and mobility and to relieve stress; on how to modify all relevant activities such as heavy lifting; and how to improve conditions and techniques in the workplace, at home, and at recreation, including sports
- Patients must follow the advice to prevent recurrence
- Patients must be assessed fully before they embark on hard physical activity such as gymnasium exercise and weight-training programs
- Middle-aged patients are at particularly high risk of injury from sudden, untrained activity. Qualified exercise teachers can guide beginners and advise on first taking gentle exercise and doing warm-up exercises
- Many workplaces provide guidance on safe working practices, and in many countries are

legally bound to provide adequate environmental conditions. The total forces exerted on a joint, as well as the cycle time, need to be measured in order to assess workplace injuries to the musculoskeletal system. In one study, strain on the elbow joint was particularly intense for the woman worker because the design of the workplace gave an advantage to taller workers with larger hands

Simple precautions can be followed, such as correct positioning before lifting, healthy hand-use patterns, correct posture, and varying tasks

In tennis, a two-handed backhand stroke will help to prevent a recurrence, as will modifying the duration and intensity of play

ENVIRONMENT

It is often necessary for adaptations to be made to equipment used at work and at home to prevent further injury. Improved seating arrangements; correct height of seat and desk; ease of reach for objects; acquisition and use of lightweight implements; and/or adapted software systems such as voice-recognition programs may be required up to and even beyond recovery.

DRUG HISTORY

Check if patient is already taking NSAIDs, or if they have previously had corticosteroid injections for the same or another disorder.

SCREENING

For previous sufferers, workplace screening is sometimes available to advise high-risk workers on safe practices and make adjustments to workstations and workload.

PREVENT RECURRENCE

All the preventive measures must be followed to prevent recurrence. Often common sense regarding rest, knowing one's limitations, and taking breaks are all that is required.

Reassess coexisting disease

Coexisting orthopedic problems may require similar therapies and preventive measures. Referral is advised for multiple problems.

INTERACTION ALERT

The patient may be taking drugs for arthritis or other orthopedic or nonorthopedic disorders. Check which these are and for how long.

PATIENT SATISFACTION/LIFESTYLE PRIORITIES

This will vary according to severity and how difficult it will be to modify or cease certain activities at work or elsewhere

It is particularly difficult to ease off on essential everyday activities as help is not always available and patients may resume activities before full recovery or try to resume a sport without reassessment and retraining

The pain and disability caused by chronic soft-tissue damage can take a long time to recede and patients often feel frustrated and helpless

RESOURCES

ASSOCIATIONS

American College of Rheumatology
1800 Century Place
Suite 250
Atlanta, GA 30345
Tel: (404) 633 3777
Fax: (404) 633 1870
www.rheumatology.com

Arthritis Foundation
P.O. Box 7669
Atlanta, GA 30357 0669
Tel: 1 800 283 7800
www.arthritis.org

American Society for Surgery of the Hand
6300 North River Road
Suite 600
Rosemont, IL 60018-4256
Tel: (847) 384 8300
Fax: (847) 384 1435
E-mail: info@hand-surg.org
www.hand-surg.org

Southern California Orthopedic Institute
6815 Noble Avenue
Van Nuys, CA 91405
Tel: (818) 901 660
www.scoi.com/teniselb.htm

KEY REFERENCES

- Brukner P, Khan K. Clinical Sports Medicine. Sydney: McGraw-Hill; 1993:220–8.
- Zuluaga M, McMeeken J. Sports Physiotherapy: Applied Science and Practice. Melbourne: Churchill Livingstone; 1995:416–26.
- Ollivierre C, Nirschl R. Tennis elbow: current concepts of treatment and rehabilitation. Sports Med 1996;22(2):133–9.
- Chop WM Jr. Tennis elbow. Postgrad Med 1989;86:301–4/307–8.
- Kivi P. The etiology and conservative treatment of humeral epicondylitis. Scand J Rehabil Med 1983;15:37–41
- Gellman H. Tennis elbow (lateral epicondylitis). Orthop Clin North Am 1992;23:75–82
- Reid DC. Sports Injury Assessment and Rehabilitation. New York: Churchill Livingstone; 1992.
- Potter HG et al. Lateral epicondylitis:correlation of MR imaging, surgical, and histopathological findings. Radiology 1995;196:43–6
- Galloway M et al. Rehabilitative techniques in the treatment of medial and lateral epicondylitis. Orthopaedic Rev 1992;15:1089–96
- Nirschl RP. Elbow tendinosis/tennis elbow. Clin Sports Med 1992;11:851–70
- Hotchkiss RN. Epicondylitis—lateral and medial. A problem-oriented-approach. Hand Clin 2000;16(3):505–8
- Chatigny C, Seifert A M, Messing K. Repetitive strain in nonrepetitive work: a case study. Int J Occup Saf Ergon 1995;1(1):42–50
- Helliwell PS. The elbow, forearm, wrist and hand. Best Pract Res Clin Rheumatol 1999;13(2):311–28
- Piligian G, Herbert R, Hearns M, et al. Evaluation and management of chronic work-related musculoskeletal disorders of the distal upper extremity. 1: Am J Ind Med 2000;37(1):75–93. Mount Sinai School of Medicine, The Mount Sinai Hospital, One Gustave L. Levy Place, New York, NY, USA.
- Sevier TL, Wilson JK. Treating lateral epicondylitis. Sports Med 1999;28(5):375–80. Ball Memorial Sports Medicine Fellowship, Muncie, Indiana

FAQS
Question 1
How do you manage lateral epicondylitis?

ANSWER 1

Management of lateral epicondylitis depends on the duration and severity of the symptoms. For early/mild disease; rest, splinting, and NSAIDs may be adequate. For established disease, local corticosteroid injection or ultrasound therapy may be beneficial. For resistant cases, surgery with 'lateral release,' which is the division of the origin of the common extensor tendon may be beneficial.

Question 2
What are the causes of resistant epicondylitis?

ANSWER 2

Continuing to participate in activities which aggravate this condition (such as carpentry) tend to promote recurrence.

CONTRIBUTORS
Gordon H Baustian, MD
Richard Brasington Jr, MD, FACP
Dinesh Khanna, MD

FIBROMYALGIA

SUMMARY INFORMATION

DESCRIPTION

- May wish to refer patient to a rheumatologist with a special interest in fibromyalgia or experience with fibromyalgia patients to help develop a treatment plan
- If psychopathology appears contributory, a mental health referral may be helpful to help develop a multidisciplinary treatment plan
- Chronic musculoskeletal disorder
- Poorly understood pathophysiology with few, if any, pathognomonic findings (there is controversy even over American College of Rheumatology classification criteria)
- Characterized by widespread pain with distinct tender points (may also be called trigger points in some literature, but tender points is the preferred term) and morning stiffness
- No evidence of inflammatory cause
- Associated problems include sleep disorders and fatigue
- Treatments are symptom-based and finding the right mix for a particular patient can be challenging

KEY! DON'T MISS!

Look for a rash associated with symptoms of pain and fatigue, or a history of a rash that could indicate Lyme disease

ICD9 code
729.1 Fibromyositis
729.0 Rheumatism, unspecified and fibrositis

SYNONYMS
- Fibromyalgia syndrome
- Myofibrositis
- Fibromyositis
- Fibrositis
- Nonarticular rheumatism
- Psychogenic rheumatism
- Myofascial pain syndrome (some experts consider this a synonym; others describe it as a separate disorder)

The 'itis' terms are particularly discouraged, because there is no evidence of inflammation.

CARDINAL FEATURES
Keep in mind that there is great controversy about fibromyalgia (FM) in the medical community. Some experts challenge its very existence, others scoff at the idea that FM can be the basis of disability claims, and other detractors believe it is simply the somatization of psychological illness. There is controversy over the extent to which psychiatric illness, such as depression, is a part of this disorder. Other experts, particularly rheumatologists, fully support the diagnosis of FM as a distinct entity with distinguishing features.

Classification criteria for fibromyalgia from the American College of Rheumatology (ACR):
- History of widespread pain for at least 3 months
- Pain on both sides of the body, above and below the waist
- Axial skeletal pain must be present (cervical spine, anterior chest, thoracic spine, or low back)
- Pain in 11 of 18 tender point sites on digital palpation with an approximate force of 4kg
- Patient must state the palpation is 'painful'; 'tender' does not qualify

In addition to the above ACR classification criteria, most patients (>75%) also describe:
- Awakening from a night of sleep still feeling tired and not refreshed
- Fatigue
- Morning stiffness

Ultimate diagnosis may be one of exclusion after differentials have been ruled out.

CAUSES
Common causes
The cause of FM remains unknown. Hypotheses include:
- Changes in muscle tissue at the cellular level, including changes in blood flow
- Neuroendocrine disorder from abnormal function of the hypothalamic-pituitary-adrenal (HPA) axis resulting in abnormal pain perception via neurohormonal dysfunction
- Immunologic abnormalities (FM has been noted after infections with coxsackievirus, Parvovirus, HIV, and Lyme disease in up to 55% of FM patients)
- Physical injury or tissue trauma such as surgery (between 14% and 23% of FM patients become symptomatic after trauma or surgery)
- Psychological distress (but experts disagree about whether the distress causes the FM symptoms, or the FM symptoms cause the distress)

Contributory or predisposing factors

See Common causes

- Absence of long delta-wave sleep periods, the time during which muscles completely relax and when muscle repair occurs
- In FM, delta-wave sleep is interrupted into alpha-wave sleep, a much lighter sleep phase
- People with FM may not actually wake up, but their sleep is not refreshing, and their muscles do not get the physiological rest needed, resulting in stiffness and pain

EPIDEMIOLOGY

Incidence and prevalence

Because the diagnosis is largely subjective, incidence and prevalence numbers should be interpreted in that context.

INCIDENCE
Unknown.

PREVALENCE
20–30 per 1000.

Demographics

AGE

- Occurs between 18 and 70 years (approximate)
- Most prevalent between 30 and 50 years (approximate)

GENDER
Female:male ratio about 9:1

GENETICS
Appears to be an increased incidence of depression in first-degree relatives of fibromyalgia patients.

Current research funded by NIH is mapping genes in 160 families with a history of fibromyalgia to search for a direct genetic link.

SOCIOECONOMIC STATUS
More commonly diagnosed in middle and upper socioeconomic classes; however, this may be because people in lower socioeconomic groups do not seek medical care for typical fibromyalgia symptoms due to overall poor access to care.

DIFFERENTIAL DIAGNOSIS
Myofascial syndromes
FEATURES

- Due to overuse
- Tender points in one area, rather than all over the body in discrete locations
- Symptoms are focal rather than diffuse
- Associated with increased activity or muscle strain
- No associated sleep problems or fatigue

Rheumatoid arthritis
FEATURES

- In early phases, may have widespread musculoskeletal pain, as with fibromyalgia, but then pain localized in joints rather than muscles
- Serologic studies and other blood tests are abnormal

Polymyalgia rheumatica
FEATURES

- Due to overuse
- Tender points in one area, rather than all over the body in discrete locations
- Symptoms are focal rather than diffuse
- Associated with increased activity or muscle strain
- No associated sleep problems or fatigue

Hypothyroidism
FEATURES

- May see widespread muscle pain and fatigue as in fibromyalgia
- Weight gain
- Goiter
- Abnormal thyroid function tests

Lyme disease
FEATURES

- Pain and fatigue is common; however, pain may be more joint-related than muscular
- Positive serology (ELISA-Western blot)
- Characteristic erythema chronicum migrans (ECM), history of deer tick bite
- Geographic distribution with endemic areas
- Possible neurological and cardiac abnormalities
- Fibromyalgia symptoms may appear after a bout of Lyme disease

Chronic fatigue syndrome
FEATURES

- Shares many of the same features as fibromyalgia (FM), and may be difficult to differentiate if fatigue is significant in a particular FM patient
- Pain tends to be less prominent in chronic fatigue than in FM
- Like FM, chronic fatigue has no specific pathognomonic objective tests, so there is great overlap between the two. However, by the Centers for Disease Control criteria, numerous medical illnesses must be excluded before this diagnosis can be made

Depression and somatization disorder
FEATURES

- May present with fatigue and diffuse musculoskeletal pain

- No consistent tender points as in FM
- More significant evidence of underlying psychopathology than is typically seen in FM

SIGNS & SYMPTOMS
Signs
- Pain to digital palpation at a pressure of approximately 4kg at 11 of 18 identified tender point sites
- Abnormal non-rapid eye movement (non-REM) stage IV sleep

Symptoms
Fibromyalgia is characterized by patient description of symptoms; there are essentially no purely objective criteria on which to base the diagnosis. It is a syndrome based on a compatible history and compatible physical findings, and, more importantly, the absence of other physical findings that might suggest an alternative diagnosis.

Findings characteristic of the diagnosis:
- Diffuse musculoskeletal pain that worsens with weather changes, anxiety, physical or mental stress or reduced hours of sleep (note: joint pain is rarely seen)
- Fatigue
- Nonrestorative sleep, either difficulty initiating and maintaining sleep, or feeling unrefreshed after a night of sleep

Less common, but may be present:
- Chronic headache
- Irritable bowel symptoms
- Complaints of numbness not associated with objective examination findings
- Reported lack of physical endurance, leading to physical inactivity and functional disability
- Depression

KEY! DON'T MISS!
Look for a rash associated with symptoms of pain and fatigue, or a history of a rash that could indicate Lyme disease.

CONSIDER CONSULT
- May wish to refer patient to a rheumatologist or chronic pain specialist with a special interest in fibromyalgia or experience with fibromyalgia patients to establish diagnosis if presentation is not clear, or treatments are not improving symptoms
- If psychopathology appears contributory, a mental health referral may be helpful to help distinguish somatization from fibromyalgia and also to provide counseling given the prolonged duration of this disorder

INVESTIGATION OF THE PATIENT
Direct questions to patient
Because there are no pathognomonic 'tests' for fibromyalgia, and the diagnosis is based on symptom pattern and identification of tender points, a detailed history is critical.

Q **Where do you feel the pain?** According to the classification criteria of the American College of Rheumatology, pain must be widespread, on both sides of the body and above and below the waist
Q **For how long have you felt this pain?** According to the classification criteria of the American College of Rheumatology, pain must be present for at least 3 months before the fibromyalgia diagnosis can be made

◻ Do you have pain in your joints or in your muscles? If a patient can distinguish, FM is characterized by widespread musculoskeletal pain, not discrete joint pain, which is more common with other rheumatological diseases

◻ Do you or have you had a fever? Have you measured it with a thermometer? Fever is not characteristic of FM and is more commonly associated with Lyme disease and other rheumatological diseases. Many people 'feel feverish' when their measured body temperature is normal

◻ Do you feel refreshed when you wake up in the morning? Do you have trouble falling asleep or staying asleep? Sleep disorders are common in people with FM

◻ Do you feel particularly stiff when you wake up in the morning? Does the stiffness lessen as the day goes on? This finding is characteristic of FM when other symptoms are present, such as widespread pain lasting more than 3 months, etc

◻ Do you feel fatigued or tired all the time? If the answer is, 'Yes,' ask, Which is worse for you, the pain or the fatigue? If the fatigue is more significant than the pain, a workup for chronic fatigue syndrome may be in order

◻ How do you feel about your life? Do you often feel depressed or unhappy? If the patient is unhappy with life, or answers 'yes' to the second question, additional screening for depression as the underlying disorder is indicated; the pain and fatigue may be somatization of depression. Try to discriminate whether the patient feels quality of life has declined as a result of pain and fatigue, or if physical symptoms followed onset of unhappiness

◻ Have you gained weight? Are you particularly sensitive to the cold? Have you felt trouble swallowing or a lump in your neck? All are screening questions for hypothyroidism, one of the differentials

◻ Have you also had headaches, diarrhea or other bowel symptoms, swelling or numbness, or noticed your physical endurance declining? These are symptoms also associated with FM in some patients, but are not classic characteristics in most patients

◻ Have you consulted other physicians or tried any medications yourself to relieve your symptoms? People with FM often see numerous physicians and are put through batteries of tests, only to have objective tests come up normal. If you know tests have been done, you may not have to repeat them. Some people may try self-medication and use herbal remedies or supplements in an effort to treat themselves

Contributory or predisposing factors

◻ Have you recently had a significant injury (such as a motor vehicle crash), surgery, or an infection (such as Lyme disease, Parvovirus, coxsackievirus, or HIV)? FM symptoms often develop after a physiological stresson

◻ Do you feel worse when the weather changes, when you are under a lot of stress, or when you've had to get up early and didn't get a lot of sleep? All of these 'triggers' are characteristic of FM

Family history

◻ Is there a history of depression in your immediate family? There appears to be increased incidence of depression in first-degree relatives of FM patients.

Examination

Palpate tender points to see if 4kg of pressure (the amount of pressure required to blanch the examiner's nailbed) results in pain. This is the only examination specific to FM.

Perform other examinations as indicated by differential diagnoses and the particular patient's signs and symptoms:

▨ Skin
▨ Nails
▨ Mucous membranes
▨ Fundi

- Joints
- Muscles
- Spine
- Bones
- Thyroid
- Lymph nodes

Physical examinations for the differential diagnoses include those for:

- Depression
- Chronic fatigue syndrome
- Lyme disease
- Hypothyroidism
- Polymyalgia rheumatica
- Rheumatoid arthritis

Summary of investigative tests

Laboratory tests are characteristically normal in patients with fibromyalgia (FM). Initial routine tests to exclude differential diagnoses are:

- Erythrocyte sedimentation rate (ESR): normal in FM; may be elevated in other rheumatic diseases
- Thyroid-stimulating hormone (TSH): normal in FM, but elevated in hypothyroidism
- T3 and T4: normal in FM, but decreased in hypothyroidism
- Complete blood count (CBC): normal in FM, but anemia or thrombocytosis suggest an inflammatory disease
- Rheumatoid factor: non-reactive in FM; can be more highly reactive in other rheumatic diseases

In most cases, further tests are not helpful and not advised because false-positives can lead to unnecessary further investigations; for example:

- Lyme titer, unless signs and symptoms highly suggestive of the disease, and especially in endemic areas
- The antinuclear antibody test (ANA) is not useful in the assessment of FM, because this very sensitive and non-specific test is often false-positive and misleading in clinical situations where the clinical likelihood of lupus is low

DIAGNOSTIC DECISION

Classification criteria for fibromyalgia from the American College of Rheumatology [1]:

- History of widespread pain for at least 3 months
- Pain on both sides of the body; above and below the waist
- Axial skeletal pain must be present (cervical spine, anterior chest, thoracic spine, or low back)
- Pain in 11 of 18 tender point sites on digital palpation with an approximate force of 4kg
- Patient must state the palpation is 'painful'; 'tender' does not qualify

Guidelines for the initial evaluation of the adult patient with acute musculoskeletal symptoms, [2]. These guidelines focus primarily on patients with acute presentations, but they provide helpful algorithms to guide the diagnosis of arthralgia and polyarthralgia. According to these guidelines, FM meets the following criteria:

- Arthralgia (keep in mind patients are often unable to differentiate between joint pain and generalized musculoskeletal pain; these guidelines do not suggest joint involvement in FM – simply the patient presentation of pain)
- No significant trauma or bone pain
- No effusion or signs of inflammation (no synovitis)
- Point tenderness, particularly on tender points

CLINICAL PEARLS

- Associated symptoms of chronic headaches and irritable bowel syndrome are often clues to the presence of fibromyalgia
- In the absence of sleep disturbance or nonrestorative sleep, the diagnosis of fibromyalgia is quite unlikely
- Underlying depression should always be ruled out when considering FM

THE TESTS
Body fluids
ERYTHROCYTE SEDIMENTATION RATE
Description
Venous blood (anticoagulated).

Advantages/Disadvantages
Disadvantage: requires venous phlebotmoy; risk of hematoma or vaso-vagal response

Normal
Westergren method:
- Men: 0–15mm/h
- Women: 0–20mm/h
- Children: 0–10mm/h

Abnormal
Westergren method:
- Men: >15mm/h
- Women: >20mm/h
- Children: >10mm/h

Cause of abnormal result
- Inflammation and necrotic processes after blood proteins
- Red blood cells aggregate
- Red blood cells become heavier; will fall more rapidly when placed in tube
- With anemia, the reduced packed cell volume results in an increased rate of sedimentation of erythrocytes, even in the absence of inflammation
- Keep in mind the possibility of a false-positive result.

Drugs, disorders and other factors that may alter results
- If blood stands more than 24 h before testing, result will be falsely low
- Refrigerated blood will increase sedimentation; bring blood to room temperature before testing

Increased levels:
- Pregnancy >12 weeks through 4 weeks postpartum
- Menstruation
- Heparin
- Oral contraceptives
- Healthy women aged 70–89 years
- Anemia

Decreased levels:
- High blood sugar
- Steroids
- High-dose aspirin

RHEUMATOID FACTOR
Description
Venous blood/serum.

Advantages/Disadvantages
Disadvantage: requires venous phlebotmoy; risk of hematoma or vaso-vagal response

Normal
Nonreactive: 0–39 IU/mL

Abnormal
- Weakly reactive: 40–79 IU/mL
- Reactive: >80 IU/mL

Cause of abnormal result
Positive results can be seen in other diseases such as:
- Rheumatic diseases
- Infectious diseases
- Malignancies
- Miscellaneous diseases such as sarcoidosis, chronic pulmonary disease, chronic liver disease, cryoglobulinemia, Waldenstrom' macroglobulinemia
- Keep in mind the possibility of a false-positive result.

Drugs, disorders and other factors that may alter results
Normally elevated
- Older patients
- Multiple vaccinations
- Multiple transfusions

THYROID-STIMULATING HORMONE (TSH)
Description
Venous blood/serum.

Advantages/Disadvantages
Disadvantage: requires venous phlebotmoy; risk of hematoma or vaso-vagal response

Normal
2–11 mcU/mL.

Abnormal
Values outside the normal range.

Cause of abnormal result
Increased levels:
- Increased TSH is most sensitive test for primary hypothyroidism
- Pituitary-TSH secreting tumor

Decreased levels:
- Hyperthyroidism
- Secondary and tertiary hypothyroidism
- Pituitary insufficiency
- Keep in mind the possibility of a false-positive result.

Drugs, disorders and other factors that may alter results
Values suppressed:
- Treatment with T3
- Aspirin
- Corticosteroids
- Heparin

Values increased:
- Lithium
- Potassium iodide
- Radioisotopes injected within a week before test

T3 (TRIIODOTHYRONINE)
Description
Venous blood.

Advantages/Disadvantages
Disadvantage: requires venous phlebotmoy; risk of hematoma or vaso-vagal response

Normal
75–220 ng/dL (1.2–3.4 nmol/L).

Abnormal
Values outside the normal range.

Cause of abnormal result
Increased values:
- Hyperthyroidism
- T3 thyrotoxicosis
- Acute thyroiditis

Decreased values:
- Hypothyroidism (but some hypothyroid patients will have normal values)
- Starvation, poor nutrition
- Acute illness
- Keep in mind the possibility of a false-positive result.

Drugs, disorders and other factors that may alter results
Increased values:
- Pregnancy
- Estrogen therapy
- Antiovulatory drugs
- Methadone
- Heroin

Decreased values:
- Anabolic steroids
- Androgens
- Large doses of salicylates
- Phenytoin

T4 (THYROXINE)
Description
Venous blood.

Advantages/Disadvantages
Disadvantage: requires venous phlebotmoy; risk of hematoma or vaso-vagal response

Normal
0.8–2.8 ng/dL (10–36 pmol/L).

Abnormal
Values outside the normal range.

Cause of abnormal result
Increased values:
- Hyperthyroidism
- Acute thyroiditis
- Hepatitis and other liver diseases

Decreased values:
- Hypothyroidism
- Hypoproteinemia
- Treatment with triiodothyronine (T3)
- Keep in mind the possibility of a false-positive result.

Drugs, disorders and other factors that may alter results
Increased values:
- Pregnancy
- Estrogen therapy
- Anticonvulsants
- Heroin
- Methadone

Decreased values:
- Salicylates
- Anticoagulants

Radiopaque contrast medium can affect results.

TREATMENT

CONSIDER CONSULT
- May wish to refer patient to a rheumatologist with a special interest in fibromyalgia (FM) or experience with fibromyalgia patients to help develop a treatment plan
- If psychopathology appears contributory, a mental health referral may be helpful to help develop a multidisciplinary treatment plan

IMMEDIATE ACTION
If depression is present, assessment of suicide risk is very important.

PATIENT AND CAREGIVER ISSUES
Patient or caregiver request
- Has FM been in the news recently?
- Has the patient seen another physician who told the patient FM does not exist?
- Has the patient heard horror stories from friends, Internet or other sources about how terrible FM is?

Note that some Internet sites, e-mail lists and so-called support groups do not provide a positive attitude focused on living with FM; instead, they foster dependence and victimization. If a patient has been involved with or exposed to these attitudes, it may be a challenge to get them to think of FM as a disease they can live with, not a disease they only 'suffer from'.

Health-seeking behavior
- **Have you visited other physicians for your symptoms?** Many patients visit many physicians and have multiple workups without an 'answer' for their pain. If these records can be reviewed, money and effort in additional workups can be avoided
- **Have you tried any self-medication? Over-the-counter drugs? Herbal remedies? Supplements? Homeopathic? Used any prescription medications, perhaps those prescribed for other disorders?** People with chronic pain, particularly those whose symptoms are dismissed by health care providers, often resort to self-medication and may not be forthcoming about their actions if they sense the physician will be dismissive or nonsupportive. This is a particular problem in FM

MANAGEMENT ISSUES
Goals
- The most important aspect of FM treatment is developing a positive, trusting, accepting relationship with the patient
- Validate that the patient has 'real' symptoms; just because tests are normal doesn't mean the patient isn't feeling pain, fatigue and discomfort
- Emphasize that people 'live with' FM and a number of self-care strategies can help the patient feel better
- Work with the patient to try various combinations of medications, exercise, stress management, and sleep strategies that result in the best symptom management
- Getting control of the sleep disorder may be the key to reducing other symptoms in many patients
- The ultimate treatment goal is for the patient to have maximum relief from symptoms with the fewest limitations on activities and minimal drug side-effects

Management in special circumstances
- Careful interviews will help the physician determine if mental health evaluation is in order or other concurrent psychotherapy is needed
- Symptoms of FM can be exacerbated by pregnancy; drug therapy would need to be re-evaluated if a woman with FM wishes to become pregnant

- Care of a newborn, including getting up many times during the night, can significantly exacerbate sleep disorders and make symptoms much worse due to lack of sleep

COEXISTING DISEASE
Separating psychopathology from FM may be particularly difficult. If a patient has depressive symptoms, are widespread pain and fatigue somatization of depression, or has the patient become depressed because repeated work ups have resulted in no firm explanation for the symptoms? Do not hesitate to treat FM and depression together.

PATIENT SATISFACTION/LIFESTYLE PRIORITIES

- Patients with FM may have undergone months of repeated workups and visits to many physicians without a diagnosis; they often have had a series of normal lab values and imaging studies
- Some patients may have been told that nothing is wrong with them because there are no positive test results; some physicians do not believe that FM exists. This can lead to poor self-concept, depression and distrust of the medical profession
- Patients need to receive the message from their physician that the physician believes them and takes their symptoms seriously
- Many patients are tremendously relieved to have a 'name' for their condition and a treatment plan to follow
- Some patients are very anxious to participate in their care and want to take positive actions to improve how they feel; this enhances their functioning and their ability to 'get on with their lives'
- Other patients may use their symptoms and diagnosis as an excuse to avoid responsibilities and activities. These patients may need mental health follow up

SUMMARY OF THERAPEUTIC OPTIONS
Choices

- Tricyclic antidepressants such as amitriptyline, or trazodone, for sleep disturbances
- Cyclobenzaprine for fatigue, sleep disturbance and muscle relaxation
- Other medications have been mentioned in the literature, but without the clinical studies that support the use of amitriptyline and cyclobenzaprine
- Selective serotonin reuptake inhibitors (SSRIs) have not been systematically studied in FM, but, anecdotally, may be helpful in the relief of symptoms
- Alprazolam may help treat anxiety and stress associated with chronic pain and FM, and may be helpful in controlling sleep-disturbance. However, this medication has significant potential for physical dependance
- Although there is no evidence supporting the use of zolpidem, anecdotally this hypnotic has been of benefit in controlling the sleep disturbance of FM
- A supportive approach by the primary care physician is invaluable in achieving a good outcome
- Cardiovascular fitness training: primarily walking for exercise, in conjunction with stretching exercises
- Non-narcotic, over-the-counter analgesics (no indication for NSAIDs or other anti-inflammatory medication)
- Cognitive behavioral therapy
- Massage therapy, mind-body therapies, and acupuncture may be of benefit
- Hot packs, hot tubs, heating pads
- Tender point injections (controversial)
- Sleep hygiene and other lifestyle measures should also be instituted

Guidelines
The American Academy of Family Physicians has produced information treating fibromyalgia. [3].

Clinical pearls

- Patients who do not engage in regular exercise are unlikely to improve
- Coexisting depression must be effectively treated

Never

Never dismiss a patient's complaints as 'all in your head' or as insignificant.

FOLLOW UP
Plan for review

- Individualize the plan for review based on each patient's situation; some patients who have been 'through the system' and have low self-esteem may need more frequent follow up, reassurance, and support than patients the physician knows well or patients for whom the primary care physician makes the diagnosis and implements a treatment plan rather quickly
- Follow-up should consist of reviewing whether the treatment plan is relieving symptoms (particularly improving sleep) and if the patient's quality of life has improved as a result of symptom control and improved physical conditioning

Information for patient or caregiver

- It may take a few attempts at combinations of drug therapy to find the right mix for a particular person. The goal is a balance between symptom control and side-effects, such as morning drowsiness
- The patient should communicate with the physician if therapy does not seem to be working or if side-effects are particularly troublesome
- Physical conditioning, including stretching and aerobic exercise (such as walking), is critically important. The person with fibromyalgia (FM) may have to start very slowly and build up. In the beginning, pain and fatigue may be slightly increased by the physical movement. However, sticking with the program will have immeasurable benefits, not only for the FM but for overall health
- FM typically is not a progressive disease. It will not threaten or shorten a person's life, and its symptoms can be reduced with therapy
- The patient must make a commitment to follow the treatment plan, particularly physical conditioning

DRUGS AND OTHER THERAPIES: DETAILS
Drugs
AMITRIPTYLINE

Typically used to treat the underlying sleep abnormality and promote better quality sleep; some experts believe that small doses of tricyclic antidepressants help patients manage their pain better.

Dose

Doses used for fibromyalgia are lower than doses for treatment of depression.

Begin with 10mg 2 h before bedtime (or closer to bedtime if drowsiness is significant); increase 10mg every 2 weeks if needed to enhance sleep (and reduce daytime pain) to a maximum of 100mg per day in a single, nighttime dose. Larger doses may be necessary in individual cases.

Risks/Benefits
Risks:

- Pregnancy category D; excreted in breast milk
- May have withdrawal if stopped abruptly
- May cause significant drowsiness that the patient must adapt to regarding dosing schedule and daytime 'hangover' drowsiness
- Patients often gain significant weight, even on low doses

Benefits: can achieve symptom relief in lower doses than when used to treat depression; this can help reduce side-effects and enhance compliance

Side-effects and adverse reactions
- Drowsiness
- Dizziness
- Orthostatic hypotension
- Constipation
- Dry mouth
- Urinary retention

Interactions (other drugs)
- Enhanced CNS depression when combined with other drugs, such as benzodiazepines, or narcotic analgesics ▪ Monoamine oxidase inhibitors (MAOI): can cause excessive sympathetic response, mania or hyperpyrexia ▪ Can increase the risk for seizures when coadministered with tramadol ▪ Anticholinergics ▪ Antihypertensives ▪ Norepinephrine

Contraindications
- Weigh risk and benefits of use in pregnant women or in women wishing to become pregnant ▪ Acute recovery phase of myocardial infarction ▪ Avoid using together with MAOI

Evidence
A small crossover RCT compared amitriptyline, fluoxetine or both medications together vs placebo in the treatment of patients with fibromyalgia. Both antidepressants were associated with significant improvements in Fibromyalgia Impact Questionnaire scores. Significantly improved scores on visual analogue scales were also noted in treated patients for pain, global wellbeing, and sleep disturbances. Combination therapy was more effective than either medication alone [4]
Level P

Acceptability to patient
- Side-effects of constipation and dry mouth may be very uncomfortable for some patients
- If medication causes daytime drowsiness, may interfere with patient's ability to work, drive, and carry out regular life activities
- Patients find weight gain unacceptable

Follow up plan
Telephone check-in with patient may be acceptable to see if dosing is treating sleep disorder and helping to relieve pain; dose may be increased as needed until symptoms improve.

Patient and caregiver information
- Constipation may be addressed by drinking more water and adding fiber (fiber supplements) to the diet
- Dry mouth can be relieved by drinking more water and sucking on hard sugarless candy
- Patient may need to take medicine for a few weeks before clinical improvement is seen; dosage may need to be increased

CYCLOBENZAPRINE
Typically used to improve sleep patterns; may also reduce muscle tension that can result from and contribute to pain.

Dose
- 10–30mg, typically taken close to bedtime, or in divided doses during the day
- Start low and gradually increase

Efficacy
Generally effective in improving sleep; sometimes effective in reducing muscle tension.

Risks/Benefits
Risks:
- Pregnancy category B
- May cause significant drowsiness that the patient must adapt to regarding dosing schedule and daytime 'hangover' drowsiness
- Use caution in glaucoma, urinary retention, epilepsy, and the elderly

Side-effects and adverse reactions
- Central nervous system: headache, insomnia, confusion, weakness
- Eye: visual disturbance
- Gastrointestinal: constipation, nausea
- Cardiovascular: palpitations, arrythmias, hypotension
- Urological: hesitancy, frequency, retention

These side-effects can be exacerbated when cyclobenzaprine is used in conjunction with amitriptyline; the combination of drugs can result in better symptom relief but can also increase side-effects.

Interactions (other drugs)
- Tricyclic antidepressants ■ MAOIs

Contraindications
- Recent myocardial infartion ■ Arrythmias ■ Child less than 12 years of age ■ Porphyria
- Hypothyroidism, hyperthyroidism

Evidence
A double-blind controlled trial compared cyclobenzaprine with placebo in patients with fibrositis. Patients receiving cyclobenzaprine experienced a significant decrease in pain severity, and a significant increase in the quality of sleep. There was also an associated reduction in the total number of tender points, and in muscle tightness [5] *Level P*

Acceptability to patient
If medication causes daytime drowsiness, may interfere with patient's ability to work, drive and carry out regular life activities.

Follow up plan
Telephone check-in with patient may be acceptable to see if dosing is treating sleep disorder and helping to relieve pain; dose may be increased as needed.

Patient and caregiver information
Be aware that cyclobenzaprine can result in daytime drowsiness; do not drive or operate machinery until the degree of drowsiness is known.

Complementary therapy
ACUPUNCTURE
Efficacy
Extensive review of the world literature on the clinical usefulness of acupuncture for a wide variety of health problems was undertaken in 1997 by the NIH. The Consensus panel concluded that acupuncture might be considered useful in fibromyalgia as an adjunctive treatment, or an acceptable alternative, or be included in a comprehensive management program.

Risks/Benefits
Risks:

- Occasional bleeding can occur at needle insertion sites, and patients occasionally may experience bruising following treatment
- Only a few case reports of severe complications have been published (e.g. lung puncture with a needle placed improperly in the chest wall)
- Patients sometimes report increased pain initially after an acupuncture treatment
- Few risks have been reported with properly applied acupuncture

Evidence

- Acupuncture may be useful as an adjunctive therapy, or as an alternative treatment in FM [6] *Level C*
- A double-blind RCT compared electroacupuncture with sham treatment in patients with FM. Electroacupuncture was significantly more effective for relieving pain symptoms [7] *Level P*

Acceptability to patient
Some patients feel frightened of needle insertion or have a severe phobia to needles. Cost of treatment, which is usually not covered by conventional insurance plans, and availability of properly trained and certified practitioners may also be problematic for some patients.

Follow up plan
Usually acupuncture is used as adjunctive treatment with other interventions for FM. Patients should be under usual care with regular follow up.

Patient and caregiver information
Patients should be informed that acupuncture may not immediately result in benefit. Several weeks of treatment may be necessary before benefit is perceived. In addition, some patients with severe pain or discomfort to even light touch may find acupuncture is too invasive and painful for them, and should defer this intervention until their system is more tolerant of pain and touch.

MIND-BODY THERAPIES
Efficacy
Patients with many chronic health problems, especially those associated with pain, find that relaxation techniques, biofeedback, hypnotherapy, and meditation can all be of help. This also appears to be true for many patients suffering with FM. Cognitive behavior therapy has also shown some success, as have 'energy therapies' such as Qi Gong.

Risks/Benefits
Risk: some hypnosis techniques may unveil deep emotional issues, and the therapist needs to be trained and experienced to handle these issues.

Evidence

- A RCT compared biofeedback/relaxation training, exercise training, combination treatment, and an educational/attention control program in patients witzh fibromyalgia. The exercise and combination groups had a modest improvement in physical activity measures [8] *Level P*
- A small RCT compared hypnotherapy with physical therapy for 12 weeks in patients with refractory FM. Patients in the hypnotherapy group had significant improvements in pain, fatigue on awakening, sleep pattern, and global assessment at 12 and 24 weeks, compared with patients in the physical therapy group [9] *Level P*

Acceptability to patient
As with any technique that requires the person to learn a new skill and then practice it regularly,

the effectiveness of these therapies depends entirely upon the patient actually using them. If a person finds benefit, they are likely to continue the practice.

Follow up plan
Monitor progress via e.g. usual visits, patient diaries. Encouragement and support by the physician for the patient to continue to practice modalities they have found useful is important.

Other therapies
PRIMARY PHYSICIAN PSYCHOTHERAPEUTIC INTERVENTIONS
Efficacy
Reported in the literature to be cornerstone of effective therapy.

Risks/Benefits:
- Risk: no risks
- Benefits: patient's self-esteem will be enhanced, which will enable patient to engage in more effective self-care

Acceptability to patient
Patients almost universally welcome reassurance, encouragement and support from their primary care physician.

Follow up plan
Continue to provide reassurance, encouragement and support in all follow up contacts with the patient, whether on the telephone or during a visit.

Patient and caregiver information
Patients must understand that they can manage FM on their own, with support, encouragement and reassurance from their primary care physician, and prescription medications when indicated. Especially important is the individual commitment to regular exercise.

CARDIOVASCULAR FITNESS TRAINING
Efficacy
- The success of this therapy is completely up to the patient
- Patient must make the commitment and gradually build up to a cardiovascular fitness program
- Cardiovascular fitness training should be done in conjunction with stretching; stretching alone is not effective in reducing symptoms
- Walking is an ideal approach to cardiovascular fitness training
- This should be a lifetime commitment; some studies show improvement only after 12–20 weeks of regular exercise

Risks/Benefits
- Risk: in the beginning, pain and fatigue may transiently increase; patients should be encouraged to start slowly and build up intensity and duration of walk
- Benefit: realized for a lifetime and include cardiovascular health and numerous other benefits of regular aerobic exercise

Evidence
A small RCT compared cardiovascular fitness training vs simple flexibility exercises for 20 weeks in patients with FM. There was a significant improvement in both patient and physician global assessment scores, and in pain threshold scores (measured directly over fibrositic tender points) in patients participating in cardiovascular fitness training [10] *Level P*

Acceptability to patient
- Patients may resist starting an exercise plan – may state they don't have time, they don't feel well enough, etc.
- Patients may be particularly resistant if initial attempts at exercise transiently increase fatigue and pain

Follow up plan
- Physician encouragement can be critical to the success of this therapy
- Physician can act as 'coach' for patients to keep them motivated and help them work through the initial difficulties inherent in beginning an exercise program and working it into a daily routine

Patient and caregiver information
- Not only will cardiovascular fitness training improve the symptoms of FM, it will provide lifetime benefits to reduce the risk of numerous diseases
- Walking is an excellent way to get started: it doesn't require equipment or a financial investment, can be done almost anywhere, and can be started at low intensity and distance, and then gradually increased
- The patient may feel a bit more tired and sore when they first start, but it is very important that they stick with it and work through this short time of discomfort

COGNITIVE BEHAVIORAL THERAPY
Efficacy
Key is to assist patients in developing an active, resourceful, self-management approach to coping with all aspects of FM.

Risks/Benefits
- Risk: patient may not wish to participate or may not cooperate with change in perception of self and illness
- Benefit: measurable positive outcomes of this approach

Acceptability to patient
- Improvements in perceived pain severity
- Improved perceived affective distress
- Sense of control and mastery over life circumstances enhanced
- Improved functional abilities

Follow up plan
- Research primarily done on multidisciplinary inpatient programs; this may present a problem for the patient being away from home, and for getting third-party payment for such therapy
- Continued support, reassurance and encouragement from physician

Patient and caregiver information
- Patients must want to take control of their life and illness
- Patients must practice behaviors learned in the program so that they become automatic responses
- Patients need support from family, friends, and loved ones to enhance success of therapy

TENDER (TRIGGER) POINT INJECTIONS
Efficacy
- Initially, injection may make pain worse, but relief soon follows
- Works best when discrete painful trigger point can be isolated
- Tends to work better in younger patients

Risks/Benefits

Risks:

- Do not perform injections if there is a clear systemic illness (particularly with fever)
- Bleeding problems or anticoagulant therapy
- Cellulitis over involved area
- 'Needle anxiety'

Benefits

- Pain relief
- Response to injection may be helpful diagnostically; pain relief reduces differential diagnoses of nerve root lesions and nerve compression as source of pain

Acceptability to patient

- Some patients may initially be reluctant to have needle injection
- If relief obtained, may be more amenable to this type of therapy

Follow up plan

Follow up to see if patient received relief from needle/injection therapy.

Patient and caregiver information

- May need follow up injections (3–4 days) to evaluate whether this approach is successful treating isolated, distinct tender areas (trigger points)
- More than one injection may be needed to break the pain cycle

LIFESTYLE

Stress management, sleep hygiene and avoidance of alcohol (due to effects on sleep) help reduce fibromyalgia symptoms.

RISKS/BENEFITS

Benefits are potential reduction of symptoms.

ACCEPTABILITY TO PATIENT

Patients may think they 'don't have time' to develop stress management strategies, learn new ways to manage stress, or work on better sleep habits.

FOLLOW UP PLAN

Physician support, encouragement and reassurance can be critical when asking a patient to make a lifestyle change. Follow up will be individualized by patient, based on:

- How motivated the patient is to change
- Support systems available to patient
- Underlying psychopathology

PATIENT AND CAREGIVER INFORMATION

- Patients have the power to make lifestyle changes that can improve how they feel and thus improve quality of life
- Changes are not always easy, but the benefit is worth the effort
- At first, sleep hygiene measures such as avoiding afternoon naps may make symptoms worse, but as the body adapts, benefits will be evident
- Self-care is the most effective aspect of care of fibromyalgia as it also enhances self-esteem and patients' belief in themselves

OUTCOMES

EFFICACY OF THERAPIES
Amitriptyline, cyclobenzaprine, cardiovascular fitness training, and cognitive behavioral therapy are effective in relieving some symptoms of FM, particularly pain. Alprazolam may be effective in patients with an anxiety component.

Evidence
- A meta-analysis found that antidepressants and non-pharmacological treatments improved physical status and self-report of FM symptoms. Non-pharmacological treatments were also associated with significant improvements in psychological status, and daily functioning [11] *Level M*
- Amitriptyline and fluoxetine, alone and in combination, were associated with significant improvements in Fibromyalgia Impact Questionnaire scores in a RCT. Significantly improved scores on visual analogue scales were also noted in treated patients for pain, global well-being, and sleep disturbances. Combination therapy was more effective than either medication alone [4] *Level P*
- Cyclobenzaprine has been shown to decrease pain severity, total number of tender points, and muscle tightness, and significantly increase quality of sleep compared with placebo [5] *Level P*
- Electroacupuncture is significantly more effective than sham treatment for relieving pain symptoms in patients with FM [7] *Level P*
- A small RCT found that cardiovascular fitness training significantly improved patient and physician global assessment scores and pain threshold scores compared with flexibility training [10] *Level P*
- An RCT compared biofeedback/relaxation training, exercise training, combination treatment, and an educational/attention control program in patients with FM. The exercise and combination groups had a modest improvement in physical activity measures [8] *Level P*
- Hypnotherapy has been shown to significantly improve pain, fatigue on awakening, sleep pattern, and global assessment compared with physical therapy [9] *Level P*

PROGNOSIS
With resolution of sleep disturbance and cardiovascular conditioning, symptoms often significantly improve.
- Some patients will not respond to any therapy
- Fibromyalgia is becoming an increasing cause of time lost at work and physical dysfunction
- Treatment strategies should focus on improving functional outcomes
- Overall, prognosis is uncertain with regard to symptoms: most patients will see significant relief with initial therapies; other patients may need more intensive treatment to achieve significant symptom relief; a small percentage will not experience any relief at all
- Patients can be reassured that fibromyalgia does not appear to be a progressive disease; it is not disfiguring or life-threatening

Therapeutic failure
If therapy is not successful in improving symptoms, consider referral to a:
- Rheumatologist, preferably one who treats a number of patients with fibromyalgia and has expertise working with these patients
- Mental health professional for examination and potential diagnosis and treatment of underlying psychopathology

PREVENTION

Fibromyalgia is not specifically preventable in the general population.

RESOURCES

ASSOCIATIONS

Be aware that some fibromyalgia organizations that patients can find on the Internet do not promote independence and self-care. These sites may provide lists of symptoms relating every body system to fibromyalgia; this information is not necessarily supported by research or in the literature.

The following organizations were vetted by Healthfinder (www.healthfinder.gov)

National Institutes of Health
One AMS Circle
Bethesda, MD 20892
Tel: (301) 495 4484
Tel: (877) 226 4267 (toll-free)
www.nih.gov/niams
This link also provides links to 5 more organizations.

American College of Rheumatology
Suite 250
1800 Century Place
Atlanta, GA 30345-4300
Tel: (404) 633 3777
www.rheumatology.org

American Fibromyalgia Syndrome Association, Inc
Suite D
6380 East Tanque Verde
Tucson, AZ 85715
Tel: (520) 733 1570
www.afsafund.org
Primary goal of this organization is to fund scientific research

Fibromyalgia Network
PO Box 31750
Tucson, AZ 85751
Tel: (800) 853 2929
www.fmnetnews.com

www.clinicaltrials.gov
A Service of the National Institutes of Health through the National Library of Medicine. Search on 'fibromyalgia' for a list of current clinical trials, and those that are recruiting subjects

KEY REFERENCES

- McCain GA. A cost-effective approach to the diagnosis and treatment of fibromyalgia. Rheum Dis Clin North Am 1996;22:323–49.
- Bradley LA, Alarcon GS. Fibromyalgia. In Koopman WJ (ed): Arthritis and Allied Conditions, 13th edn. Baltimore: Williams & Wilkins, 1997. MD Consult via (www.mdconsult.com).
- Approach to the patient with fibromyalgia. Chapter 159. In Goroll AH, Mulley AG: Primary Care Medicine, 3rd edn. Philadelphia: Lippincott-Raven, 1995. MD Consult via (www.mdconsult.com).
- Bohr T. Problems with myofascial pain syndrome. Neurology 1996;46(3):593–7. (This reference attacks fibromyalgia and states the disease does not exist – it helps provide an understanding of the other perspective.)
- Fischbach FT. A Manual of Laboratory and Diagnostic Tests, 5th edn. Lippincott-Raven, 1996

Evidence references and guidelines

1   Wolfe F, Smythe HA, Yunus MB, et al. The American College of Rheumatology 1990 criteria for the classification of fibromyalgia: report of the multicenter criteria committee. Arthritis Rheum 1990;33:160–72

2   Guidelines for the initial evaluation of the adult patient with acute musculoskeletal symptoms. American College of Rheumatology Ad Hoc Committee on Clinical Guidelines. Arthritis Rheum 1996;39:1–8

3   The American Academy of Family Physicians. Millea PJ, Holloway RL. Treating fibromyalgia. Am Fam Physician 2000;62:1575–82, 1587

4   Goldenberg D, Mayskiy M, Mossey C, et al. A randomized, double-blind crossover trial of fluoxetine and amitriptyline in the treatment of fibromyalgia. Arthritis Rheum 1996;39:1852–9. Medline

5   Bennett RM, Gatter RA, Campbell SM, et al. A comparison of cyclobenzaprine and placebo in the management of fibrositis. A double-blind placebo-controlled study. Arthritis Rheum 1988;31:1535–42. Medline

6   National Institutes of Health Consensus Development Panel on Acupuncture. Acupuncture. NIH Consens Statement 1997;15:1–34. Available at the National Guidelines Clearinghouse

7   Deluze C, Bosia L, Zirbs A, et al. Electroacupuncture in fibromyalgia: result of a controlled trial. BMJ 1992;305:1249–52. Medline

8   Buckelew SP, Conway R, Parker J, et al. Biofeedback/relaxation training and exercise interventions for fibromyalgia: a prospective trial. Arthritis Care Res 1998;11:9196–209. Medline

9   Haanen HC, Hoenderdos HT, van Romunde LK, et al. Controlled trial of hypnotherapy in the treatment of refractory fibromyalgia. J Rheumatol 1991; 18:72–5. Medline

10 McCain GA, Bell DA, Mai FM, Halliday PD. A controlled study of the effects of a supervised cardiovascular fitness training program on the manifestations of primary fibromyalgia. Arthritis Rheum 1988;31:1135–41. Medline

11 Rossy LA, Buckelew SP, Dorr N, et al. A meta-analysis of fibromyalgia treatment interventions. Ann Behav Med 1999;21:180–91. Medline

CONTRIBUTORS

Fred F Ferri, MD, FACP
Jane L Murray, MD
Richard Brasington Jr, MD, FACP

FROZEN SHOULDER

SUMMARY INFORMATION

DESCRIPTION

- Shoulder girdle pain, diffuse, constant, insidious in onset, usually unilateral
- Marked loss of active and passive glenohumeral motion in all directions
- Characteristic course of slow abatement of pain, then gradual return of motion
- Almost never recurs in the same shoulder but may subsequently affect the other
- Diabetes mellitus is a major predisposing factor; may be bilateral, more protracted, and more difficult to treat when associated with diabetes
- Clinical course is usually self-limiting, and symptomatic improvement usually occurs within one year

URGENT ACTION

- Refer to a rheumatologist or orthopedist if the diagnosis is uncertain, to avoid missing a more serious cause of rapid loss of shoulder motion (e.g. infectious arthritis)
- Relieve pain: prescribe a NSAID plus additional analgesics if needed. Pain of frozen shoulder is often quite severe, particularly early in the course of the disease

KEY! DON'T MISS!

- Infectious arthritis: rarely, a subacute presentation of joint infection may mimic frozen shoulder, particularly if typical symptoms such as chills and fever are not elicited
- Posterior dislocation of the shoulder: in contrast to the much more common anterior dislocation, this can be more subtle. It may be missed and become chronic. In addition, standard X-ray views of the shoulder may not detect posterior dislocation ('scapular Y' view or axillary view needed if there is any suspicion of dislocation)
- Apical lung tumor (Pancoast's tumor): rarely the most prominent symptoms and examination findings appear to arise in the shoulder girdle and mimic those of frozen shoulder. Chest X-ray with apical lordotics is needed if there is any suspicion

ICD9 CODE
726.0 Adhesive capsulitis of shoulder

SYNONYMS
Adhesive capsulitis.

CARDINAL FEATURES
- Frozen shoulder is a perplexing problem that is frustrating for patients, therapists, and physicians, but is self-limited and often improves with time and conservative treatment
- It has a characteristic course, comprising a 'freezing' phase, a 'frozen phase,' and a 'thawing phase' (each about 4 months in duration), which may last up to one year
- Characterized by shoulder girdle pain, diffuse and insidious in onset, usually unilateral
- There is marked loss of active and passive glenohumeral motion in all directions, which is contributed to by the patient deliberately limiting motion in response to the pain
- Almost never recurs in the same shoulder but may subsequently affect the other
- High prevalence among diabetic patients; may be bilateral and more protracted
- Symptomatic improvement usually occurs within one year

CAUSES
Common causes
Cause unknown but predisposing or contributory factors are often present. Although the cause is unknown, the underlying pathology has been well characterized and can account for the clinical features:
- Capsule of glenohumeral joint becomes thick and shrunken, markedly constricting joint space and preventing full motion
- Histologic evidence of mild inflammation and fibrosis sometimes seen
- Synovial lining adheres to humeral head, but can be stripped away like adhesive tape; hence alternative name 'adhesive capsulitis'

Contributory or predisposing factors
- Immobility of any cause (shoulder disorder; systemic illness; following surgery, especially neurologic, breast or chest surgery; following invasive cardiac procedures, including catheterization and implantation of devices) may predispose to frozen shoulder
- Trauma to the shoulder, which may be minor
- Diabetes mellitus: prevalence may be 10% or more in diabetic persons; may correlate with other musculoskeletal complications of diabetes (e.g. Dupuytren's contracture, diabetic cheiropathy (decreased hand and finger motion))
- Myocardial infarction: this is seen much less commonly now than in the era when patients were prescribed bed rest for much longer periods
- Thyroid disease, both hyperthyroidism (Graves' disease specifically) and hypothyroidism
- Neurological disease, including stroke and Parkinson's disease
- Pulmonary or chest wall tumor
- Adrenal insufficiency. Also, isolated ACTH deficiency was found in a single case report with bilateral involvement
- Drugs are probably a very rare cause. Case reports have implicated protease inhibitor therapy for AIDS, and a matrix metalloproteinase used to treat gastric carcinoma

EPIDEMIOLOGY
Incidence and prevalence
Incidence and prevalence in the general population not known. Prevalence may be as high as 10% or more among patients with diabetes mellitus.

Demographics

AGE

Most commonly aged 40 years or older.

GENDER

Gender ratio not precisely known, but there is a female preponderance.

RACE

Race-related factors have been suggested, but data are few and inconclusive.

GENETICS

- Genetic associations are unknown, but frozen shoulder occasionally afflicts multiple members of one family
- Possible HLA–B27 association investigated; data inconclusive

SOCIOECONOMIC STATUS

Occupation of a sedentary nature is felt by some authorities to be a contributing factor, but conclusive data are not available.

DIFFERENTIAL DIAGNOSIS
When the history and examination are classic, differentiating from other conditions is usually not problematic.

Rotator cuff disorders
Rotator cuff disorders comprise a wide spectrum, including acute tendinitis (with or without calcium deposits on X-ray); rotator cuff tears; and acute or chronic impingement syndrome. Confusion is most likely to occur when an underlying rotator cuff problem has triggered superimposed frozen shoulder.

FEATURES
- Pain, varying from acute and severe, to chronic
- Tenderness is usually more localized, to subacromial space, and not diffuse
- Restriction of shoulder motion due to pain can occur and mimic frozen shoulder. Patient in extreme pain may hold upper extremity rigidly against chest, permitting no movement by examiner
- Passive range of motion is greater than active range, which is opposite to findings in frozen shoulder, although extreme pain may confound examination
- 'Painful arc' of abduction, with pain most severe in the mid range of motion when patient elevates extremity to the side
- Immediate pain relief may be afforded by subacromial injection of local anesthetic such as xylocaine

Arthritis (or arthropathy)
- Differential is wide. Guidelines have been published by the American College of Rheumatology [1]
- Infectious arthritis uncommonly may mimic frozen shoulder, and has the potential for permanent joint damage if diagnosis is delayed
- Any of the forms of systemic arthritis may occasionally be seen presenting first with monoarticular involvement
- Isolated shoulder joint arthropathy (e.g. osteoarthritis) could present with findings similar to those of frozen shoulder
- Polymyalgia rheumatica may sometimes present as bilateral adhesive capsulitis (which may occur in the setting of diabetes)

FEATURES
- Pain, which may be felt predominantly over deltoid, as in frozen shoulder
- Often joint swelling, effusion present; highly inflammatory forms may cause warmth and/or erythema
- Range of motion is variable but restriction is generally not as marked as in frozen shoulder unless acute, severe, or longstanding

Reflex sympathetic dystrophy
Reflex sympathetic dystrophy (RSD), also called 'shoulder hand syndrome,' involves the shoulder in the same manner as frozen shoulder. It is felt by many authorities to be related to frozen shoulder, or to be a variant of that condition. Predisposing factors are similar in the two conditions.

FEATURES
- Shoulder symptoms and signs the same as those in frozen shoulder, combined with ipsilateral hand involvement
- Hand swelling, diffuse

- Color and temperature changes of the hand are believed to be due to vasomotor instability
- Progressive dystrophic change of the hand with eventual contracture may occur

Posterior dislocation of the shoulder

Posterior shoulder dislocation, in contrast to the much more common anterior dislocation, can be more subtle. It may be missed and become chronic. In addition, standard X-ray views of the shoulder may miss this diagnosis ('scapular Y' view or axillary view needed if any suspicion for dislocation).

FEATURES

- History of trauma may be elicited, not necessarily recent; often an athletic injury
- Loss of shoulder motion may mimic the findings of frozen shoulder
- Younger patients may be affected, as well as middle-aged and elderly persons

Tumor in shoulder girdle region

Very rarely an apical lung tumor may cause symptoms and examination findings that mimic those of frozen shoulder. Even more rarely a locally invasive neoplasm affects shoulder.

SIGNS & SYMPTOMS
Signs

- Decreased active range of motion. On careful inspection when the patient elevates the upper extremity to the side, the entire shoulder girdle rises and the scapula tilts, in an attempt to compensate for loss of motion at the glenohumeral joint itself
- Decreased passive range of motion is more pronounced. With the shoulder girdle/scapula prevented from moving by the examiner's hand on top of the shoulder, motion at glenohumeral joint itself is seen to be much more restricted than apparent on casual inspection
- Tenderness, diffusely about the shoulder girdle, not localizing to the subacromial space nor glenohumeral joint space alone
- Pertinent negative: the hand is normal in frozen shoulder, in contrast to the closely related disorder, reflex sympathetic dystrophy. Hand findings should always be sought to distinguish between the two conditions

Symptoms

- Pain, diffusely about shoulder girdle and over deltoid. Insidious in onset but comes on over a period of days or a few weeks. Constant, present at rest, often particularly severe at night
- Decreased range of motion. This may develop fairly rapidly, within one to several weeks. Patient may or may not be aware of the full extent of loss as elevation and tilting of scapula compensate for loss at the glenohumeral joint itself

This is typically a three-phase illness, with each phase lasting a few months:

- In the first phase (the 'freezing phase'), there are both ever-present pain and marked loss of motion
- In the second phase (the 'frozen phase'), pain has abated although motion is still restricted; pain may occur, but only when patient attempts to move joint beyond what its present state will allow
- In third phase (the 'thawing phase') the range of motion gradually returns and, although residual loss may persist indefinitely, this is generally of a degree that is without significant functional impact

ASSOCIATED DISORDERS

- Reflex sympathetic dystrophy (RSD), also known as 'shoulder hand syndrome':
- The shoulder component of this disorder is indistinguishable from that of frozen shoulder. The latter, however, does not involve the hand as does RSD, which is characterized by swelling, vasomotor instability, progressive dystrophic changes, and contracture

- Some authorities believe the two disorders are related
- Predisposing and contributing factors largely shared

KEY! DON'T MISS!
- Infectious arthritis: rarely, a subacute presentation of joint infection may mimic frozen shoulder, particularly if typical symptoms such as chills and fever are not elicited
- Posterior dislocation of the shoulder: in contrast to the much more common anterior dislocation, this can be more subtle. It may be missed and become chronic. In addition, standard X-ray views of the shoulder may not detect posterior dislocation ('scapular Y' view or axillary view needed if there is any suspicion of dislocation)
- Apical lung tumor (Pancoast's tumor): rarely the most prominent symptoms and examination findings appear to arise in the shoulder girdle and mimic those of frozen shoulder. Chest X-ray with apical lordotics is needed if there is any suspicion

CONSIDER CONSULT
Referral to a rheumatologist is warranted when history and/or examination reveal findings that are atypical for frozen shoulder:
- Patient younger than 40: frozen shoulder usually occurs among middle-aged and elderly patients
- Pain more widespread than over the shoulder girdle: for example, involving neck/trapezius ridge or extending distally beyond the elbow
- Pain present mainly on motion: not constant as in frozen shoulder
- Pain quality suggests neuropathic origin: for example paresthesias, numbness
- Bilateral involvement simultaneously, if no predisposing factor for frozen shoulder apparent: frozen shoulder is usually unilateral
- Tenderness highly localized to one area of shoulder girdle: in contrast to more ill-defined, diffuse tenderness in frozen shoulder

INVESTIGATION OF THE PATIENT
Direct questions to patient
Q Does your arm hurt? Where does it hurt? Patients use the term 'shoulder' in different ways. As pain from the glenohumeral joint and surrounding structures is referred to the deltoid region patients often identify that region as its source. Pain in frozen shoulder is diffuse, but mainly anterolateral. Pain mainly on top of the shoulder and along the trapezius ridge suggests another condition

Q How did it start? Onset is insidious but the condition can come on within a fairly short period, days to a few weeks. Occasionally a triggering event will be elicited

Q When do you have pain, and when is it the worst? Pain of frozen shoulder is present even at rest, with often a strong nocturnal component. Pain only with movement points to another condition, or may characterize the late phase of frozen shoulder, many months after onset

Q Has your pain changed since it first began? If the condition has been present for a few months, the pain may have begun to lessen, with restricted shoulder motion remaining. In the latter case there may be pain only when patient attempts to move the shoulder beyond its limitations (presumably due to stretching the still-constricted joint capsule)

Q Do you have trouble moving your arm? How long has that been a problem? Replies vary. Some patients report being unable to reach a high shelf, or to reach behind to their back, starting just within the last few weeks. Others may be unaware of the full degree of the loss of motion because of compensatory maneuvers

Q Have you injured your shoulder recently? Even minor trauma, with attendant pain and immobility, can trigger frozen shoulder

Q Have you had trouble with your shoulder before? A pre-existing shoulder or rotator cuff disorder may have been the trigger for a superimposed frozen shoulder

Q How has your other shoulder been? Frozen shoulder is usually unilateral, or both shoulders may be involved in sequential fashion

Q **Has your hand bothered you?** There are no hand symptoms in frozen shoulder – but in a related condition, 'reflex sympathetic dystrophy,' also called 'shoulder hand syndrome,' there may be ipsilateral hand swelling along with color and temperature changes due to vasomotor instability

Q **Have any other joints bothered you?** Frozen shoulder is a regional disorder. Other joint symptoms would suggest one of the systemic forms of arthritis and related conditions

Q **How have you been feeling overall?** Except for irritability, fatigue and mildy depressed mood consistent with persistent severe pain, any systemic symptoms point to possible underlying disorder and need for a detailed review of systems

Contributory or predisposing factors

Q **Have you recently suffered a trauma, even minor?** This is a common trigger of frozen shoulder

Q **Do you have diabetes?** There is a high prevalence of frozen shoulder in diabetes

Q **Have you had any recent surgery or invasive diagnostic procedures?** These may trigger frozen shoulder, particularly when the arm has been immobilized for a long period

Q **Do you have any underlying medical or neurologic illness leading to immobility in general, or symptoms relating to the shoulders in particular?** A wide range of underlying disorders including various endocrine disorders and neurologic disorders may predispose to frozen shoulder

Family history

Q **Do you have a family history of diabetes mellitus?** The association with diabetes is very strong and the patient may have undiagnosed diabetes

Q **Has anyone else in your family had a similar condition?** Occasionally, frozen shoulder affects multiple members of one family

Examination

■ **Observe the patient as he or she disrobes:** Restricted shoulder motion and/or compensatory maneuvers are often readily apparent

■ **Check for a cervical origin of the pain:** Have the patient flex and extend, and bend the neck to either side

■ **Inspect the shoulder:** for signs of swelling

■ **Palpate the shoulder girdle area:** including acromioclavicular joint, subacromial space, shoulder joint space, which are accessible by pressing the thumb between the humeral head and the coracoid process. The tenderness of frozen shoulder is diffuse. Highly focal tenderness would suggest another disorder

■ **Observe active movement:** Have the patient raise the arm to the side, observing from the front and behind. Elevation of the whole shoulder girdle and tilting of the scapula will be observed as the patient attempts to compensate for restricted glenohumeral motion

■ **Passively move the shoulder joint:** With the patient's elbow flexed at 90 degrees fix the shoulder girdle in place by one hand placed over the top. Using the other hand, lift the arm to the side very gently by holding the elbow and supporting the patient's forearm with one's own arm. It is essential that this be done very patiently and gently as the examination may be very painful. When the maximum of abduction has been reached, externally and internally rotate the shoulder. It will be found that motion is reduced by at least 50% in all directions, and will feel as though the joint is literally locked. Glenohumeral joint motion is found to be markedly more restricted than apparent from casual inspection

■ **Elicit the reflexes of the upper extremities:** in order to check for a cervical origin of pain

■ **Examine the hand:** for any signs of swelling, color changes or temperature changes, all of which are suggestive of reflex sympathetic dystrophy, a related condition

■ **Repeat the examination for the opposite upper extremity:** findings will usually be unilateral

Summary of investigative tests

- X-rays of the shoulder are needed to help exclude arthritis. Frozen shoulder, a condition primarily of the capsule of the joint, produces minimal or no changes, except possibly for a decrease in bone density from prolonged immobility. Axillary or 'scapular Y view' is needed if there is any suspicion of posterior shoulder dislocation, because this will not be apparent on standard views
- Complete blood count should be normal in frozen shoulder and is needed to help exclude other rheumatic conditions that may affect the shoulder
- Erythrocyte sedimentation rate (ESR) screens for signs of inflammation. Abnormality would point to an alternative diagnosis (or reflect a possible predisposing condition). ESR is normal in frozen shoulder itself
- Fasting blood sugar is prudent in order to screen for undiagnosed diabetes mellitus
- Thyroid function tests should be performed, as frozen shoulder may be associated with Graves' disease and hypothyroidism
- Magnetic resonance imaging (MRI) may be needed only in unusual cases in which there is diagnostic uncertainty. MRI is generally part of a specialist's evaluation and is good for imaging soft tissues, including glenoid labrum, rotator cuff as well as bone (may detect avascular necrosis)
- Other specialized imaging techniques include bone scan, arthrography, and computed tomography with arthrography, which are rarely used now for evaluation of frozen shoulder

DIAGNOSTIC DECISION

The following are indicative of a diagnosis of frozen shoulder:

- Insidious onset of diffuse, persistent anterolateral shoulder girdle pain with significant nocturnal component
- Diffuse shoulder girdle tenderness, not focal
- Restriction of passive range of motion of the glenohumeral joint by 50% or more in all directions
- No swelling of the shoulder
- Exclusion of rotator cuff disorder
- No symptoms or signs of a more generalized musculoskeletal disorder
- Normal or minimal nonspecific findings on shoulder X-rays
- Normal complete blood count and ESR

Guidelines

- The American Academy of Family Physicians has published material on frozen shoulder [2]

CLINICAL PEARL(S)

- **Differentiation between adhesive capsulitis and rotator cuff syndrome.** Passive range of motion is severely affected in all planes in adhesive capsulitis, as opposed to forward flexion, abduction and external rotation in rotator cuff disorders
- **Differentiation between adhesive capsulitis and polymyalgia rheumatica.** Symptoms and signs of frozen shoulder are limited to the shoulder, whereas polymyalgia rheumatica also produces stiffness in the neck and hips, symptoms of fatigue and malaise, and laboratory findings of elevated sedimentation rate and anemia

THE TESTS
Body fluids
COMPLETE BLOOD COUNT
Description
Venous blood sample.

Advantages/Disadvantages
Advantages:

- Simple, inexpensive, useful screen to exclude other conditions; normal in frozen shoulder, but may be abnormal in many other rheumatic disorders that could affect the shoulder

- Helps in evaluation of ESR, because an abnormality of the latter may be of less concern if the complete blood count is normal

Normal
- Hemoglobin: male 13.5–18.0g/dL; female 11.5–16.0g/dL
- White cell count: 4.0–11.0x10^9/L
- Platelets: 150–400x10^9/L

Abnormal
- Blood parameters outside the normal ranges
- Keep in mind the possibility of a falsely abnormal result

Cause of abnormal result
- Inflammatory rheumatic disorders, but not frozen shoulder, may cause anemia, leukocytosis, thrombocytosis. Any abnormalities raise the possibility of an alternative diagnosis
- Leukocytosis raises the possibility of infection
- Keep in mind that an abnormality may be coincidental, particularly among elderly patients who may suffer from multiple unrelated medical problems

Drugs, disorders and other factors that may alter results
Many patients with frozen shoulder are elderly and may have multiple medical disorders that may or may not be related to the frozen shoulder. Although normal results help to confirm a diagnosis of frozen shoulder, the interpretation of abnormal results will require a more extensive clinical and laboratory evaluation.

ERYTHROCYTE SEDIMENTATION RATE
Description
Venous blood sample.

Advantages/Disadvantages
Advantages:
- Simple, inexpensive test
- Normal value helps to exclude other rheumatic disorders that may affect the shoulder, as many cause an elevation in ESR

Disadvantages: abnormal values are nonspecific, however, and only indicate need for further evaluation

Normal
- Men: normal range 0–15mm/h
- Women: normal range 0–20mm/h

Abnormal
- Elevated ESR
- Keep in mind the possibility of a falsely abnormal result

Cause of abnormal result
- Elevation of the ESR raises the possibility of an inflammatory disorder affecting the shoulder (inflammation of any cause elevates the ESR as a result of increased levels of fibrinogen, which is an acute-phase reactant)
- Keep in mind, however, that the finding is nonspecific and may or may not be directly related to the shoulder problem

- If an elevated ESR is accompanied by a mild-to-moderate anemia, then this strongly suggests an infection or inflammatory condition (a bone marrow disorder is also possible, particularly among elderly patients)

Drugs, disorders and other factors that may alter results
The ESR is a sensitive screening test but is very nonspecific. Among elderly patients a common harmless cause of elevation is a monoclonal gammopathy of uncertain significance (MGUS).

THYROID FUNCTION TESTS
Description
Venous blood sample.

Advantages/Disadvantages
Advantages:
- Simple test
- Inexpensive

Disadvantage: nonspecific for cause of thyroid disorder

Normal
- Thyroid stimulating hormone: 0.5–5.7mU/L
- Thyroxine (T4): 70–140nmol/L

Abnormal
- Results outside normal reference range
- Keep in mind the possibility of a false-positive result

Cause of abnormal result
- Thyroid disease
- Thyroid disease may predispose to frozen shoulder

FASTING BLOOD SUGAR
Description
Venous blood sample.

Advantages/Disadvantages
Advantages:
- Simple test
- Widely available, and highly suggestive of diabetes mellitus

Normal
3.5–5.5 mmol/L.

Abnormal
- Results above the normal reference range
- Keep in mind the possibility of a falsely abnormal result

Cause of abnormal result
- Diabetes mellitus causes a raised glucose level
- Diabetes is associated with frozen shoulder

Drugs, disorders and other factors that may alter results
Use of corticosteroids may raise the blood glucose level.

Imaging

X-RAY

Advantages/Disadvantages

Advantages:

- Noninvasive
- Not excessively costly

Abnormal

- Any signs of true glenohumeral joint abnormality
- Nonspecific findings or signs of rotator cuff syndrome (which is a predisposing factor to frozen shoulder) may be present
- Keep in mind the possibility of a falsely abnormal result

Cause of abnormal result

X-ray may help to exclude other disorders that affect the shoulder girdle, because the diagnosis of frozen shoulder is often in part a diagnosis of exclusion. Abnormal findings on X-ray may indicate the following:

- Arthritis, as opposed to frozen shoulder, involves the synovium and/or cartilage within the joint
- Inflammatory synovial conditions may erode bone and cartilage by invasion and release of destructive enzymes
- Osteoarthritis is essentially a disorder of the cartilage itself, leading to progressive loss
- Cartilage is not visible on X-ray, but 'joint space narrowing' is indicative of cartilage loss and suggests a diagnosis other than frozen shoulder (frozen shoulder involves mainly the joint capsule)
- Rotator cuff syndrome may reveal itself on X-ray, as thinning of the tendons results in narrowing of the space between the humeral head and overlying acromioclavicular joint

MAGNETIC RESONANCE IMAGING (MRI)

Advantages/Disadvantages

Advantages:

- Noninvasive
- Ideally suited for imaging of soft musculoskeletal tissues, as marked variations in tissue structure easily delineate articular and periarticular anatomy
- Avascular necrosis of bone may be seen long before abnormalities on X-ray are apparent

Disadvantages:

- Cost is high, and in some cases it is inconvenient
- Access to specialists is needed to optimize clinical usefulness and cost-effectiveness

Special tests

ARTHROGRAPHY

Description

An X-ray is taken of the shoulder joint following injection of contrast.

Advantages/Disadvantages

Advantages:

- May show features associated with frozen shoulder (rather than excluding other pathology)
- Distension of the subcapsular bursa by arthrography may provide some symptomatic relief

Disadvantage: invasive procedure

Abnormal

- The characteristic appearance is a shrunken shoulder capsule

- Contracture of the joint capsule may be seen, and obliteration of the axillary fold
- Decreased amount of contrast dye filling the bicipital sheath
- Keep in mind the possibility of a falsely abnormal result

Cause of abnormal result
Frozen shoulder.

TREATMENT

CONSIDER CONSULT

Referral to a rheumatologist or orthopedist may be needed in the following circumstances:

- Failure to achieve relief of pain within the first few weeks during the first phase (freezing phase) of the illness
- Lack of gradual improvement in range of motion starting within a few months in the second phase (frozen phase) of the illness
- Failure to reach the third, final phase (thawing phase) of illness after roughly a year, when it should have settled
- Note: a refractory picture, often with bilateral/symmetric involvement, is often seen when the disorder is a complication of diabetes.

IMMEDIATE ACTION

- Pain relief is the pressing clinical issue, which requires immediate attention
- Nonsteroidal anti-inflammatory drugs (NSAIDs) are commonly used, in full dose. There are no data to suggest one of these agents is superior to another for this condition
- Stronger analgesics may be needed temporarily, or when NSAIDs cannot be used

PATIENT AND CAREGIVER ISSUES
Patient or caregiver request

What is the long-term outcome of this condition? The prognosis for pain relief is excellent, although there may not be complete a recovery of normal range of motion.

MANAGEMENT ISSUES
Goals

- Relief of pain
- Gradual restoration of shoulder motion
- Help with activities of daily living as needed; this is an especially important consideration for elderly patients
- Reassurance and support over long recovery period

Management in special circumstances
COEXISTING DISEASE

- Patients with diabetes are more likely to have bilateral involvement and a refractory course, requiring specialist evaluation and treatment
- Diabetes may be aggravated by the use of corticosteroids, whether orally or by injection
- Diabetes may predispose to the metabolic and renal complications of NSAIDs, notably elevation of creatinine and hyperkalemia
- Other chronic illnesses, especially renal insufficiency, hepatic disease, and cardiovascular disease - notably congestive heart failure, and gastrointestinal disorders, may all be contraindications to the use of NSAIDs due to potential renal, hepatic, metabolic, and gastrointestinal side-effects

COEXISTING MEDICATION

- Angiotensin-converting enzyme (ACE) inhibitors, often taken by elderly patients, may increase the risk of metabolic complications of NSAIDs, notably hyperkalemia, as both ACE inhibitors and NSAIDs may cause this side-effect
- Anticoagulation therapy may contraindicate the use of NSAIDs

SPECIAL PATIENT GROUPS

- Elderly patients, or those already suffering from a disability, may experience greater functional impairment from the loss of upper extremity mobility

- Elderly patients are at much greater risk from osteoporosis if oral steroid therapy is used (not commonly used, but should be avoided if possible)
- Pregnancy is a relative contraindication to many of the medications that might otherwise be freely used for pain relief; this is not a commonly encountered problem, because the age range of frozen shoulder only slightly overlaps the usual childbearing years

PATIENT SATISFACTION/LIFESTYLE PRIORITIES

- Elderly patients may suffer much greater disability from the loss of use of one upper extremity
- Disability may be compounded by the additional burden of impaired motion of an upper extremity
- Patients who are sedentary, for medical or other reasons, may not regain shoulder motion as easily as those who are more active
- Patients who are engaged in manual labor, or who lead a physically active life, may suffer more from the impaired movement of an upper extremity

SUMMARY OF THERAPEUTIC OPTIONS
Choices

In most cases the mainstay of treatment will be conservative measures including nonsteroidal anti-inflammatory drugs (NSAIDs), analgesics, physical therapy or home exercises, and occupational therapy if needed. Various procedures have been used for pain where medications fail, including corticosteroid injection; suprascapular nerve block; arthroscopic surgery; and manipulation of the joint under anesthesia. In general, surgical intervention for treatment of frozen shoulder should be limited to the very small number of patients suffering a severe and refractory course. Pain relief may be afforded, but critical evidence for change in long-term outcome is lacking, as are evidence-based guidelines comparing therapies.

- NSAIDs in full dosage are useful for analgesia (this is an off-label indication)
- Physical therapy: Various shoulder exercises and physical measures for musculoskeletal pain relief are used in the treatment of frozen shoulder. Supervised therapy may be especially beneficial for this disorder
- Occupational therapy when needed is helpful for patients who are experiencing difficulty functioning, particularly the elderly
- Intra-articular corticosteroid injection may be used to manage pain. It is a widely used therapy (this is an off-label indication)
- Suprascapular nerve block is a new therapy using local anesthetic to provide early pain relief (this is an off-label indication). Arthroscopic release may be a successful intervention for patients with severe and refractory frozen shoulder, particularly patients with diabetes mellitus
- Manipulation is a rarely used therapy for patients who are refractory to other treatments. It involves manipulation of the glenohumeral joint, forcefully, under general anesthesia, in an attempt to mobilize the frozen joint
- Brisement procedure involves distention of the subscapular bursa by arthrography
- Lifestyle measures, ensuring patients remain as active as possible, will help to prevent frozen shoulder

Guidelines

The American Academy of Family Physicians has publised material on frozen shoulder [2]

Clinical pearls

- Avoid prolonged immobilization following shoulder injury, particularly in at-risk individuals, to prevent the occurrence of adhesive capsulitis
- Aggressive physical therapy to restore range of motion is critical. Treatment supervised by the therapist may be particularly valuable, as pain on movement may limit the efforts of the patient

Never

- Never use intra-articular corticosteroid injection if there is any suspicion at all of infectious arthritis (there is rarely diagnostic confusion, but it can occur)
- Manipulation of the shoulder joint under anesthesia is a treatment that has largely fallen into disuse. This should be considered a treatment of last resort, because fracture of the humerus may occur

FOLLOW UP
Plan for review

- Within the first few weeks, sooner if necessary, follow up should ensure satisfactory control of pain
- The patient should be referred to a physical therapist. If supervised therapy demonstrates that the patient has potential for pursuing treatment at home, instruction in home exercises would be appropriate
- Within a few months at most, follow up is needed to assess the beginning of the return of lost shoulder motion
- Frequency of follow up visits and need for laboratory studies to monitor NSAID or other drug therapy will depend on the total clinical picture. Patients who are very old and/or suffer from other chronic illness will need closer follow up
- Within a few months, pain may have abated and no longer require medication. This should be monitored
- Within 6 months to a year (sometimes longer) review should show significant improvement in range of motion, which gradually follows the cessation of pain
- Follow up is not commonly needed for an indefinite period, as the condition is self-limiting in most cases (severe cases associated with diabetes are an exception)

Information for patient or caregiver

- The nature of the problem should be explained. Patients may experience pain as seeming to arise from the deltoid muscle. Some are unaware of lost motion, as compensatory maneuvers disguise it. Patients may feel the problem is not being fully addressed if they have their own ideas about the symptoms (e.g. a muscle disorder)
- Reassurance is essential. Course may be prolonged, roughly for a year, but ultimately frozen shoulder does 'thaw'. Any residual loss of motion is generally not significant
- The course of the illness occurs in three phases. At first there is constant pain with loss of motion ('freezing phase'). Within a few months pain usually abates. Lost motion persists in this second phase ('frozen phase'), but pain occurs only at extremes of the range as the joint capsule is stretched. Gradually motion returns to normal or nearly so in the third phase ('thawing phase')
- Guidance on home exercises should be provided

DRUGS AND OTHER THERAPIES: DETAILS
Drugs
NONSTEROIDAL ANTI-INFLAMMATORY DRUGS (NSAIDS)

- This is an off-label indication
- No data support the superiority of one agent in this class over another for use in frozen shoulder

Dose
Standard doses of the various NSAIDs would be appropriate.

Efficacy
For some patients an NSAID may provide satisfactory relief but there are no data to provide a more quantitative assessment of efficacy in terms of degree of pain relief or proportion of patients who respond.

Risks/Benefits
Risks:

- Use with caution in the elderly
- Use with caution in patients with hepatic, renal, or cardiac failure; bleeding disorders
- There is no evidence that the final outcome will be changed by NSAIDs

Benefit: relief of pain

Side-effects and adverse reactions

- Cardiovascular system: hypertension, peripheral edema, congestive heart failure
- Central nervous system: headache, dizziness, tinnitus, fever
- Gastrointestinal: anorexia, nausea, dyspepsia, peptic ulceration, bleeding
- Genitourinary: nephrotoxicity
- Hematologic: blood cell disorders
- Hypersensitivity: rashes, bronchospasm, angioedema
- Skin: pruritus, rash

Interactions (other drugs)

- Aminoglycosides ■ Anticoagulants ■ Antihypertensives ■ Baclofen ■ Corticosteroids
- Cyclosporine, tacrolimus ■ Digoxin ■ Diuretics ■ Lithium ■ Methotrexate
- Phenylpropanolamine ■ Warfarin

Contraindications

- Peptic ulceration ■ Hypersensitivity to nonsteroidal anti-inflammatory drugs (NSAIDs)
- Coagulation defects ■ Severe renal or hepatic disease

Acceptability to patient

- Some patients may have gastrointestinal intolerance to one or more NSAIDs, but usually one can be found that is tolerated
- Over-the-counter (OTC) gastrointestinal preparations such as antacids, or various prescription medications used as acid-blocking agents, are sometimes used to relieve upper gastrointestinal disorders (some of these are also now OTC). This would be an off-label use for any medication of this type
- Consider the institution of a selective cyclo-oxygenase-2 inhibitor in elderly patients or patients at-risk for gastrointestinal bleeding, realizing that at this time there is no evidence that this will avoid the risk

Follow up plan
Periodic laboratory monitoring, including complete blood count, creatinine, potassium, liver function tests, and urinalysis may be required in some circumstances, but no data are available to provide universal guidelines.

Patient and caregiver information
NSAIDs may cause fewer gastrointestinal symptoms if taken after food.

Physical therapy
PHYSICAL THERAPY

- Various shoulder exercises and physical measures for musculoskeletal pain relief are used in physical therapy departments
- Measures will vary in different institutions, but may include ultrasound, ultrasound along with the use of a topical steroid, or other conservative measures
- Guidelines have been published by the American Physical Therapy Association http://www.apta.org for use in the whole range of conditions that are associated with joint

mobility (Impaired joint mobility, motor function, muscle performance, and range of motion associated with capsular restriction. Physical Therapy 77;11)

Efficacy
Clinical experience suggests that many patients experience pain relief and gradual improvement in range of motion with physical therapy.

Risks/Benefits
- Risks: there are no significant risks
- Benefits: may relieve pain, improve range of motion and functional status, as well as benefit the patient emotionally owing to the personal care and attention

Acceptability to patient
Patients are in general quite pleased to receive the personal care and attention provided by formal treatment in a physical therapy department, as opposed to doing home exercises on their own.

Follow up plan
- Progress will generally be monitored by the therapist
- Therapy will be shifted to home exercises when maximum benefit from supervised therapy appears to have been reached

Patient and caregiver information
- Compliance with the recommendation of the therapist and regular attendance at appointments will maximize the benefits of physical therapy
- Otherwise the gain may be little

Occupational therapy
OCCUPATIONAL THERAPY
- This form of therapy will generally be carried out in an occupational therapy department, and the treatment plan arranged and supervised by the therapists
- Assistance with activities of daily living such as dressing, personal hygiene may be afforded
- Especially important to consider for elderly patients and patients who already are disabled from another cause

Efficacy
Clinical experience suggests that occupational therapy can be very effective for carefully selected patients, by going over the history and carefully addressing any difficulties with activities of daily living.

Risks/Benefits
Benefit: improved functioning in activities of daily living.

Acceptability to patient
Patients are often very appreciative of occupational therapy.

Follow up plan
This will be carried out by the occupational therapist.

Surgical therapy
ARTHROSCOPIC RELEASE
This has been reported as a successful intervention for patients with severe and refractory frozen shoulder, particularly patients with diabetes.

Efficacy
A few case series report excellent results, both in terms of pain relief and improved motion.

Risks/Benefits
- Risk: those attendant to anesthesia and the risk of joint infection; quantitative data on magnitude of risk are not available
- Benefit: pain relief and improved range of motion

Acceptability to patient
As arthroscopy is a far less drastic measure than open joint surgery, it does not involve a prolonged recovery period, and would be offered to those patients suffering intractable symptoms. Acceptability should be good.

Follow up plan
This will be carried out by the orthopedic surgeon.

Patient and caregiver information
This should be provided by the orthopedic surgeon.

MANIPULATION
This therapy involves manipulation of the glenohumeral joint, forcefully, under general anesthesia, in an attempt to mobilize the frozen joint. It is rarely used, and many specialists consider it a therapy of last resort.

Efficacy
There is no consensus among specialists (i.e. rheumatologists and orthopedic surgeons) on the efficacy of this procedure.

Risks/Benefits
- Risk: A major risk is that fracture of the humerus can occur. This might be expected to be even more of a risk in an elderly patient who is likely to have poor bone density, which will have been aggravated in the humerus, specifically due to the prolonged period of immobilization that would have preceded the surgery
- Benefit: release of the frozen shoulder and return of motion after all other measures have failed

Evidence
There is some limited evidence that forced manipulation may be effective in the management of frozen shoulder.
- One randomized controlled trial (RCT) (not placebo-controlled) of 30 patients with frozen shoulder compared intra-articular hydrocortisone injection and manipulation with steroid treatment alone. Complete recovery at 3 months was increased in patients who recieved the combination treatment [3] *Level P*

Acceptability to patient
One would anticipate that only patients who have no relief at all from less drastic measures would find this an acceptable treatment.

Follow up plan
This will be carried out by the orthopedic surgeon.

Patient and caregiver information
Patient should be fully apprised of the risks, which is a responsibility of the orthopedic surgeon, although the referring primary care physician should go over the nature of the procedure and advise that the complication of humeral fracture needs to be considered before pursuing this avenue.

Other therapies
SUPRASCAPULAR NERVE BLOCK
This is a fairly recently described therapy, using long-acting local anesthetic agents, for which there is not yet a great deal of clinical experience or more than a few studies. It does appear to provide early pain relief, but it is not clear where it will fit in among the other treatment options. Use will likely become more widespread and specialist recommendations may change.

Efficacy
- Several studies support the efficacy in terms of pain relief, although it is not clear how this compares to other treatments, as opposed to placebo
- Long-term outcome is not demonstrated to change

Risks/Benefits
- Benefit in terms of pain relief speaks for itself, and the avoidance of drugs with possible side-effects make this a desirable option if the results of early studies are borne out
- No major risks

Evidence
Suprascapular nerve block may be an effective and safe treatment for frozen shoulder, but further studies are required.
- A randomized controlled trial (RCT) compared bupivicane suprascapular nerve block with placebo in the treatment of frozen shoulder. A reduction in pain was noted at one month in the treatment group, although no significant effect on function or range of movement was achieved [4] *Level P*
- A small prospective trial performed in a **primary care setting** (not blinded) compared suprascapular nerve block with a series of intra-articular injections in patients with frozen shoulder. Patients treated with the nerve block had a more rapid and complete resolution of pain and return to normal range of movement over a 12-week period [5] *Level P*

Acceptability to patient
As the procedure is relatively simple and not very invasive, acceptability should be good.

Follow up plan
Injections are carried out in a series over a few weeks and assessment of pain relief made along the way. As with essentially all other therapies, relief of pain is much more easily demonstrated than any change in the course of the disorder in termos of return of motion.

INTRA-ARTICULAR CORTICOSTEROID INJECTION
- The procedure has been in widespread use for decades and is fairly straightforward. However, it may be more critical than was previously thought that the medication actually be injected into the joint and not into the surrounding tissue, which is not easy to ascertain clinically. This can be determined by X-ray if dye is also injected
- This is an off-label indication
- A large number of preparations for intra-articular use are available

Efficacy
Multiple studies have documented improvement in pain, but there is no data to show any improved range of motion or change in long-term outlook.

Risks/Benefits
- Risk: the only significant risk is joint infection, which may occur once in several thousand or more injections of this sort
- Benefit: pain relief

Evidence

Intra-articular corticosteroid injections may have a partial and temporary analgesic effect for patients with frozen shoulder.

- A randomized controlled trial (RCT) of 48 patients with frozen shoulder compared injections into the subacromial bursa and glenohumeral joint with either methylprednisolone and lidocaine, or lidocaine alone. No significant difference was noted with intrabursal vs intra-articular injections. The addition of corticosteroid to the injection had no effect on the restoration of range of motion, but was effective as an anlgesic for two-thirds of patients [6] *Level P*
- A RCT of 42 patients with frozen shoulder compared treatment with intrarticlar steroids, ice, mobilization and no therapy. Pain and movement were improved in the short term in the steroid injection group, but no treatment had significant long-term benefit [7] *Level P*

Acceptability to patient

The procedure can be painful if difficulty is encountered but, providing adequate local anesthesia is carefully provided, the procedure is generally tolerated reasonably well, and most patients will readily accept the procedure if their pain is relentless despite other drug treatments.

Follow up plan

- Pain relief should occur with 24–72h, which is a good time to reassess
- A second injection may be considered if response was partial

Patient and caregiver information

- The risk from infection must be reviewed
- The patient must be warned that local anesthetic may produce some immediate relief (provided it was intra-articular), but that this will wear off before the steroid effect begins (i.e. there will be a 'gap')
- Uncommonly, an acute arthritis similar to a crystal-induced arthritis may occur, but this can be treated with an NSAID and is short-lived
- The patient should promptly report any flare-up following the procedure, which would require urgent evaluation to rule out infection as a complication

LIFESTYLE

The single most important issue is avoidance of immobility in general, and of the shoulders in particular. These are felt to be significant predisposing factors to frozen shoulder. While some problems of this nature are due to conditions beyond the patient's control, it is sound advice to encourage the patient to be as active as possible.

RISKS/BENEFITS

Benefits:

- May lessen the chance of ongoing problems and progressive disability
- May help avoid recurrence in the opposite shoulder, or the extremely uncommon recurrence in the same one

PATIENT AND CAREGIVER INFORMATION

Patient education about the nature of the frozen shoulder should include explaining the role of immobility.

OUTCOMES

EFFICACY OF THERAPIES

- Pain relief: clinical experience suggests that non-steroidal anti-inflammatory drugs (NSAIDs), oral steroid therapy, and physical therapy alleviate pain in many patients; studies and case reports support the efficacy of suprascapular nerve block, intra-articular corticosteroid injection, and arthroscopic release in terms of pain relief
- Range of motion: clinical experience suggests improvement of range of motion with physical therapy and arthroscopic release; occupational therapy is useful in addressing difficulties with activities of daily living
- Relief of pain in the early phase of the illness is relatively easy to assess compared to the difficulty of assessing the effects of any therapy on the long-term outcome
- It should be noted that frozen shoulder is in fact a self-limiting condition, albeit of long duration, and it is not entirely clear how much the course is altered by interventions

Evidence

PDxMD are unable to cite evidence that meets our criteria for evidence for all treatment choices. However, the indicated treatments for frozen shoulder are supported by clinical experience which indicates that they are generally effective in the treatment of this disorder.

- Complete recovery (no disability) at 3 months may be increased in patients with frozen shoulder who receive forced manipulation treatment as well as intra-articular corticosteroids [3] *Level P*
- Intra-articular corticosteroid injections may have a partial and temporary analgesic effect for patients with frozen shoulder [6,7] *Level P*
- Suprascapular nerve block may be an effective analgesic in the short-term treatment of frozen shoulder [4,5] *Level P*

Review period

Improvement occurs slowly over a period of several months. In some cases resolution will have been reached earlier and in some the course may drag out somewhat longer. There will be cases that become virtually chronic, notably the more severe form of the condition that appears to occur among patients with diabetes.

PROGNOSIS

- It should be noted that the condition is essentially self-limiting, although treatment certainly may relieve suffering while the process gradually settles
- Prognosis is generally good for relief of pain and gradual return of motion
- It is typically a three-phase illness, with each phase lasting a few months
- In the first phase (the 'freezing phase'), there are both ever present pain and marked loss of motion
- In the second phase (the 'frozen phase') pain has abated, although motion is still restricted; pain may occur, but only when the patient attempts to move the joint beyond what its present state will allow
- In third phase (the 'thawing phase') the range of motion gradually returns and, while residual loss may persist indefinitely, this is generally of a degree without significant functional impact

Clinical pearls

- Patients can generally expect gradual relief of pain, despite some loss of motion
- Supervised physical therapy can be very valuable in the treatment of this disorder

Therapeutic failure

- Cases of therapeutic failure do occur

- This is most commonly seen among diabetic patients
- Surgical intervention for arthroscopic release or, as a last resort, manipulation may be called for in these uncommon cases

Recurrence
- Recurrence in the same shoulder is so rare that even now it may generate a case report
- Recurrence on the other side is not uncommon; approach to treatment will be the same. Of note, the diagnosis may be easier with the past history

Deterioration
Orthopedic consultation to consider arthroscopic release or in a rare case manipulation may be considered in this instance.

COMPLICATIONS
- The patient who experiences a refractory course, particularly one characterized by unremitting pain, may develop the complications seen in any chronic pain disorder
- These include fatigue, irritability, and depression

CONSIDER CONSULT
Most patients will not need referral in the later phases of the illness, after about 6 months or more, if they have not required it up to that point, but specialist referral will be needed in some circumstances. The following circumstance warrants referral:
- Development of a chronic pain syndrome with attendant psychological features (referral to a chronic pain center, if accessible, may be appropriate)

When sophisticated specialist care is not available, the priorities should be pain relief, including chronic, carefully supervised use of strong analgesic medications in rare cases; and psychological interventions, which may include the pharmacologic treatment of depression. Simple supportive care at a minimum should be possible in the absence of specialty care.

PREVENTION

Avoidance of immobility in general and of the shoulders in particular is the single factor which is amenable to intervention in a preventive way.

RISK FACTORS

Any medical or surgical condition that leads to immobility
Surgical operations or certain invasive procedures

MODIFY RISK FACTORS

Encourage as active a lifestyle as possible; be sure that any medical conditions that impair mobility are being fully treated

During and after any surgical or invasive procedure, ensure that immobilization of the shoulder is avoided to the extent possible. Immediate attention by a physical therapist for passive range-of-motion exercises may be appropriate, even while the patient is still in recovery. Frozen shoulder can develop quite quickly; close observation is prudent

Lifestyle and wellness
PHYSICAL ACTIVITY
This should be encouraged, both in terms of overall activity, and activities that keep the shoulders moving.

PREVENT RECURRENCE
Recurrence on the same side is very rare, but the condition may later afflict the opposite shoulder. The very same considerations apply here as in primary prevention.

Reassess coexisting disease
During and after any surgical or invasive procedure, ensure that immobilization of the shoulder is avoided to the extent possible.

ASSOCIATIONS

American Academy of Orthopedic Surgeons
6300 North River Road
Rosemont, IL 60018-4262
Tel: (847) 823 7186 or (800) 346 AAOS
Fax: (847) 823 8125
www.aaos.org

American Physical Therapy Association
1111 North Fairfax Street
Alexandria, VA 22314-1488
Tel: (703) 684 APTA (2782) or (800) 999 APTA (2782); APTA Membership Department, ext 3124
TDD: (703) 683 6748
Fax: (703) 684 7343
www.apta.org

American College of Rheumatology
1800 Century Place, Suite 250
Atlanta, GA 30345
Tel: (404) 633 3777
Fax: (404) 633 1870
www.rheumatology.org

Arthritis Foundation
Tel: (800) 283-7800
www.arthritis.org

KEY REFERENCES

- Balci N. Shoulder adhesive capsulitis and shoulder range of motion in type II diabetes mellitus: association with diabetic complications. J Diabetes Complications 1999;13:135–40
- Binder AI, Bulgen DY, Hazleman BL, Roberts S. Frozen shoulder: a long term prospective study. Ann Rheum Dis 1984;43:361–4
- Bulgen D, Binder A, Hazleman B, Dutton J et al. Frozen shoulder: prospective clinical study with an evaluation of three treatment regimes. Ann Rheum Dis 1984;43:353–60
- Dahan TH et al. Double blind randomized clinical trial examining the efficacy of bupivicaine suprascapular nerve blocks in frozen shoulder. J Rheumatol 2000;27:1464–9
- Dodenhoff RM. Manipulation of the shoulder under anesthesia for primary frozen shoulder: effect on early recovery and return to activity. J Shoulder Elbow Surg 2000;9:23–6
- Gam AM et al. Treatment of "frozen shoulder" with distension and glucocorticoid compared with glucocorticoid alone. A randomised controlled trial. Scand J Rheumatol 1998;27:425–30
- Jones DS, Chattopadhyay C. Suprascapular nerve block for the treatment of frozen shoulder in primary care: A randomized trial. Br J Gen Pract 1999;49:39–41
- O'Kane JW et al. Simple home program for frozen shoulder to improve patients' assessment of shoulder function and health status. J Am Board Fam Pract 1999;12:270–7
- Pollock RG, Duralde XA, Flatlow EL, Bigliani LU. The use of arthroscopy in the treatment of resistant frozen shoulder. Clin Orthop 1994;304:30–6
- Reichmister JP, Friedman SI. Long-term functional results after manipulation of the frozen shoulder. Md Med J 1999;48:7–11
- Rizk TE, Gavant ML, Pinals RS. Treatment of adhesive capsulitis (frozen shoulder) with arthrographic capsular distension and rupture. Arch Phys Med Rehabil 1994;75:803–7
- Rizk TE, Pinals RS, Talaiver AS. Corticosteroid injections in adhesive capsulitis: investigation of their value and site. Arch Phys Med Rehabil 1991;72:20–2
- Thomas D, Williams R, Smith D. The frozen shoulder. A review of manipulative treatment. Rheumatol Rehab 1980;19:173–179. Reviewed in Clinical Evidence 2001;5:850–64

Evidence references and guidelines

1   American College of Rheumatology. Guidelines for the Initial Circulation of the Adult Patient with Acute musculoskeletal Symptoms. Arthritis Rheum 1996;39:1-8. Available at www.rheumatology.org/research/guideline/musc/musc-dis.html

2   Siegal LB, Cohen NJ, Gall EP. Adhesive Capsulitis: A Sticky Issue. American Academy of Family Physicians

3   Thomas D, Williams R, Smith D. The frozen shoulder. A review of manipulative treatment. Rheumatol Rehab 1980;19:173–179. Reviewed in Clinical Evidence 2001;5:850–64

4   Dahan TH et al. Double blind randomized clinical trial examining the efficacy of bupivicaine suprascapular nerve blocks in frozen shoulder. J Rheumatol 2000;27:1464–9

5   Jones DS, Chattopadhyay C. Suprascapular nerve block for the treatment of frozen shoulder in primary care: A randomized trial. Br J Gen Pract 1999;49:39–41

6   Rizk TE, Pinals RS, Talaiver AS. Corticosteroid injections in adhesive capsulitis: investigation of their value and site. Arch Phys Med Rehabil 1991;72:20–2

7   Bulgen D, Binder A, Hazleman B, Dutton J et al. Frozen shoulder: prospective clinical study with an evaluation of three treatment regimes. Ann Rheum Dis 1984;43:353–60

FAQS

Question 1
What is the prognosis of adhesive capsulitis?

ANSWER 1
Good. Although it can be significantly painful in the early months of the disorder, it is usually self-limiting with resolution at about one year. Cases associated with diabetes, however, may be bilateral and recalcitrant to conservative treatment.

Question 2
What distinguishes adhesive capsulitis from rotator cuff injury?

ANSWER 2
Adhesive capsulitis may occur following rotator cuff injury, especially following prolonged shoulder immobility. Examination of passive range of motion may distinguish between the two. Adhesive capsulitis will characteristically have markedly decreased passive range of motion in all planes, as opposed to rotator cuff pathology which will have decreased passive range of motion in flexion, abduction, and external rotation.

Question 3
Can adhesive capsulitis be prevented?

ANSWER 3
In a patient with known risk factors (e.g. diabetes, traumatic injury), avoiding prolonged, excessive immobilization can prevent adhesive capsulitis.

CONTRIBUTORS
Gordon H Baustian, MD
Richard Brasington Jr, MD, FACP
Maria-Louise Barilla-LaBarca, MD

GIANT CELL ARTERITIS

DESCRIPTION

- A vasculitis of large and medium-sized arteries that affects the elderly
- Predominantly involves arteries of the carotid system, especially the temporal artery
- Common 'classic' symptoms include headache, scalp tenderness, tongue and jaw claudication, and visual loss, although may present with nonspecific constitutional symptoms such as fever and weight loss
- Prompt treatment with corticosteroids can avoid permanent visual loss

URGENT ACTION

Prompt initiation of corticosteroid therapy can avoid permanent visual loss. Thrapy must be started immediately if visual symptoms are thought to be due to giant cell arteritis, and before consideration of temporal lobe biopsy.

KEY! DON'T MISS!

A high index of suspicion is often needed to diagnose giant cell arteritis, especially in elderly patients, in whom the presentation is often nonspecific.

ICD9 CODE

446.5 Giant cell arteritis (including cranial arteritis, Horton's disease and temporal arteritis).

SYNONYMS

- Temporal arteritis
- Cranial arteritis
- Granulomatous arteritis
- GCA

CARDINAL FEATURES

- A vasculitis of large and medium-sized arteries, that affects the aorta and its proximal branches, predominantly arteries of the carotid system
- Affects the elderly: it is rare under the age of 50 years and its incidence increases with age
- Characteristic histological appearance involves disruption of the internal elastic lamina, cellular infiltration of the vessel wall, intimal fibrosis and thrombosis, and multinucleated giant cells
- Common 'classic' symptoms include headache, scalp tenderness, tongue and jaw claudication and visual loss, although the presentation is often with nonspecific constitutional symptoms
- Frequently associated with polymyalgia rheumatica, a clinical syndrome characterized by proximal muscle aching and stiffness
- Prompt treatment with corticosteroids can avoid permanent visual loss and other complications caused by the vasculitis

CAUSES

Common causes

Giant cell arteritis is a vasculitis of unknown etiology.

EPIDEMIOLOGY

Incidence and prevalence

INCIDENCE

- 0.22 new cases per year per 1000 of the population aged over 50 years
- The incidence fluctuates in a cyclical pattern

PREVALENCE

2 cases per 1000 of the population.

Demographics

AGE

- Almost exclusively affects those aged over 50 years
- Incidence increases with age

GENDER

Women are two or three times as likely to be affected as men.

RACE

- Almost exclusively affects Caucasians of northern European origin.
- Rare in African-Americans.

GENETICS

There may be a genetic tendency to giant cell arteritis – familial clusters have been found.

DIFFERENTIAL DIAGNOSIS

The differential diagnosis of giant cell arteritis includes:

- Other causes of headache
- Trigeminal neuralgia, dental pathology, and other causes of facial pain
- Takayasu's arteritis (although this generally affects a younger age group and seldom starts after the age of 40 years) and other cerebral vasculitides
- Osteoarthritis of the temporomandibular joint or the cervical spine
- Polymyalgia rheumatica and other rheumatological disorders
- Cerebrovascular insufficiency, including transient ischemic attack and stroke may be associated with temporary or permanent visual loss and headache
- Retinal detachment and other causes of amaurosis fugax or loss of vision
- Occult neoplasm

Giant cell arteritis should also be considered in the differential diagnosis of an elderly patient who presents with fever of unknown origin.

Other causes of headache
FEATURES

- The headache of giant cell arteritis is often severe. Pain may be localized over one temple, or the occiput. Some patients experience more diffuse pain, which may be sharp, or a dull but constant ache
- Any new headache in a middle-aged or elderly patient should raise suspicion

Other causes of facial pain
FEATURES

- Trigeminal neuralgia is characterized by excruciating paroxysms of pain in the lips, gums, cheek, chin, and rarely in the distribution of the ophthalmic division of the fifth nerve. The pain can be triggered by tactile stimuli applied to certain areas on the face, seldom lasts more than a few seconds or a minute, and is followed by a refractory period of up to 2–3 min
- Dental pain, the most common cause of facial pain, is usually provoked by hot, cold, or sweet foods and it can be repeatedly induced by application of a stimulus without a refractory period

Takayasu's arteritis
FEATURES

- Affects predominantly young women
- Seldom starts after the age of 40 years
- Vasculitis most commonly involves the aortic arch and its larger branches

Osteoarthritis of the temporomandibular joint or cervical spine
FEATURES

- Pain and tenderness radiate from temporomandibular joint, or in soft tissues lateral to the neck. Headache and visual symptoms are not features
- X-ray changes of osteoarthritis may be seen
- Pain likely to be worsened by movement of affected joints
- Does not cause raised erythrocyte sedimentation rate (ESR) or other abnormal laboratory results (although these may coexist with osteoarthritis)

Polymalgia rheumatica (PMR)
FEATURES

- Often occurs in the same patient as giant cell arteritis; the two conditions may coexist. Approximately one-third of patients with PMR develop GCA, and vice versa

- Affects mainly patients aged over 50 years
- Associated with a raised ESR
- Symptoms may be of sudden onset
- Proximal joint and muscle pain and stiffness (neck, shoulder, low back, thigh) are common
- Morning stiffness of muscles, and occasionally joints, common

Cerebral insufficiency
FEATURES
- May cause temporary or permanent visual loss and headache
- Features will depend on the areas of ischemia or infarction
- The classic signs and laboratory findings of giant cell arteritis are not features of cerebral insufficiency, as GCA seldom affect arteries which have penetrated the dura

Retinal detachment
FEATURES
- Often precipitated by trauma
- More common in patients with myopia
- Characteristic fundoscopic findings of retinal tears with elevation of the retina and vessels or subretinal hemorrhage

Septic arteritis
FEATURES
- May cause visual loss or persistent focal headache
- Etiology is generally thrombotic emboli
- Commonly associated with infective endocarditis

Multiple myeloma
FEATURES
- Fatigue and weakness
- Fever (secondary to infection)
- Bone pain (including of the cranium)
- Abnormal laboratory investigations: anemia of normochromic, normocytic type; elevated serum urea and creatinine; hypercalcemia; proteinuria; elevated ESR
- X-ray of painful bony areas may show typical 'punched-out' areas of lysis
- Bone marrow examination usually diagnostic

Occult neoplasm
FEATURES
- Should be considered in any older patient who presents with vague, constitutional symptoms such as fever, weight loss, and malaise, all of which can be the presenting features of GCA
- Other features, if any, and results of investigative tests, will depend on the site/type of neoplasm

SIGNS & SYMPTOMS
Signs
Signs related to inflammation of the temporal artery:
- Tenderness over one or both temporal arteries
- Thickened, dilated, and occasionally erythematous temporal artery
- Reduced or absent temporal artery pulse
- Palpable nodules in the temporal artery; the nodules may be tender

Signs related to arteritis in other arteries:
- Reduced or absent pulses in the upper limbs; Raynaud's phenomenon in the elderly
- Bruits over large arteries

- Tenderness over large arteries (most commonly the subclavian artery, but sometimes the occipital artery or other arteries)

Eye and visual signs:
- Reduced visual fields
- Fundoscopic abnormalities
- Ophthalmoplegia (usually not associated with visual loss)

Nonspecific signs may be the only presenting features, especially in the elderly, e.g.:
- Weight loss
- Fever of unknown origin
- Depression or functional impairment

Symptoms

Symptoms related to arteritis of the temporal artery and other arteries in the carotid system:
- Headache is a common symptom: sometimes severe, not always localized to the temple
- Tenderness of the scalp, which may disturb sleep by being painful when the patient's head is on a pillow or be noticed by the patient when brushing the hair or wearing a hat
- Pain on chewing (claudication of the jaw muscles) or claudication of the tongue

Visual symptoms:
- The classic visual presentation is amaurosis fugax, but diplopia may also occur
- Blindness may be the first symptom, but often follows other symptoms

Nonspecific symptoms:
- Constitutional symptoms (anorexia, weight loss, tiredness)
- Fever of unknown origin
- Depression or functional impairment may be the only presenting symptoms, particularly in the elderly

ASSOCIATED DISORDERS

Polymyalgia rheumatica:
- Up to one-third of patients with giant cell arteritis have symptoms of polymyalgia rheumatica
- Up to one-third of patients with polymyalgia rheumatica have giant cell arteritis

The two conditions may have their onset at the same time, or one may precede the other, sometimes by years.

KEY! DON'T MISS!

A high index of suspicion is often needed to diagnose giant cell arteritis, especially in elderly patients, in whom the presentation is often nonspecific.

CONSIDER CONSULT

- Biopsy of temporal artery is not necessary to make the diagnosis of giant cell arteritis but a biopsy is most useful in patients where the diagnosis is unclear and a positive biopsy may help reduce diagnostic doubts in the face of treatment-related side-effects (surgical referral)
- Ideally, patients with giant cell arteritis should be followed by a rheumatologist or by the primary care physician in close contact with a rheumatologist

INVESTIGATION OF THE PATIENT
Direct questions to patient

Q Have you felt unwell recently? Loss of appetite? Lost weight? Constitutional symptoms such as fatigue, loss of appetite, and weight loss sometimes occur and may be the presenting symptoms

Q **Have you had a fever?** Giant cell arteritis must be considered in any elderly patient with a fever of unknown origin

Q **Have you had a headache recently? Did it start suddenly? Where is the pain?** Headache is the most common symptom. It typically is localized to the temples, although it may occur in any location. A complaint of a new onset or new type of headache should raise suspicion of this disorder

Q **Have you noticed any tenderness over your temples or scalp?** Tenderness over the temporal arteries is common, as is scalp tenderness. The tenderness may make sleeping, brushing the hair, or wearing a hat or glasses uncomfortable

Q **Is it painful to chew?** Aching (claudication) in the jaw muscles or tongue may occur

Q **Have you had any problems with your vision?** Visual disturbances occur in 25–50% of patients and constitute an emergency that require immediate treatment and referral to an ophthalmologist. Symptoms range from vague mistiness of vision to complete loss of vision. Blindness may be the first presentation, but it often follows other symptoms by weeks or even months

Q **Have you ever been diagnosed with polymyalgia rheumatica? Do you currently have any aching or stiffness of the neck, shoulder and upper arms, lower back or thigh? Any morning stiffness? Any other symptoms of 'rheumatism?'** Giant cell arteritis and polymyalgia rheumatica often coexist or occur at different times in the same patient

Contributory or predisposing factors

Polymyalgia rheumatica: up to one-third of patients with giant cell arteritis have symptoms of polymyalgia rheumatica at some time.

Examination

- Examine any signs which suggest infection or malignancy
- **Palpate the temporal arteries** for tenderness and the presence of nodules
- **Look for visual field defects and test for loss of vision:** any visual abnormalities are grounds for immediate treatment and referral to an ophthalmologist
- Fundoscopy may reveal abnormalities, usually optic atrophy resulting from visual loss; this is a late sign of disease
- Examine for general rheumatological symptoms and symptoms of polymyalgia rheumatica. (Guidelines for the intial evaluation of the adult patient with acute musculoskeletal symptoms have been produced by the American College of Rheumatology. These guidelines are published: Guidelines for the initial evaluation of the adult patient with acute musculoskeletal symptoms. Arthritis Rheum 1996; 39: 1–8)
- **The presence of joint swelling and tenderness suggests rheumatoid arthritis,** which can be difficult to distinguish from polymyalgia rheumatica

Summary of investigative tests

- Erythrocyte sedimentation rate (ESR) should be performed in all patients suspected of having giant cell arteritis or any other vasculitis or inflammatory disorder. In giant cell arteritis the ESR is often greatly raised at diagnosis, and it can provide a useful means of monitoring the effectiveness of therapy
- Complete blood count may reveal anemia
- Liver function tests are sometimes mildly abnormal, especially the alkaline phosphatase, which can act as an acute phase reactant
- C-reactive protein levels are typically markedly elevated and are sometimes used to monitor therapy
- Temporal artery biopsy provides histological confirmation of the diagnosis. It may be performed by a general or ophthalmic surgeon and is performed in the majority of patients for whom the diagnosis of giant cell arteritis is entertained. There is a relatively high false-negative rate associated with this investigation. Up to one-third of patients with giant cell arteritis have negative biopsies. This is because the vasculitis affects the arteries discontinuously – so called

'skip lesions.' The false-negative rate may be reduced by sampling a several cm segment of artery. If the first side is negative, consideration should be given to biopsying the other temporal artery.

- Diagnostic biopsy findings can be detected several days after the institution ofr corticosteroid treatment. The characteristic histological appearance includes: disruption of the internal elastic lamina, cellular infiltration of the vessel wall, multinucleated giant cells, and intimal fibrosis and thrombosis.
- Imaging studies generally have no place in the diagnosis of temporal arteritis at present.

DIAGNOSTIC DECISION

Temporal artery biopsy remains the 'gold standard' for confirming the diagnosis of giant cell arteritis.

The American College of Rheumatology has published a classification for the diagnosis of giant cell arteritis, which is designed to help discriminate between the various types of vasculitis [1].

Although the classification is not designed specifically as a diagnostic guideline, the presence of three of the following criteria point to the diagnosis of giant cell arteritis:

- Age 50 years or more at onset
- New onset of localized headache
- Temporal artery tenderness or decreased temporal artery pulse
- ESR of 50mm/h or more
- Abnormal temporal artery biopsy (showing mononuclear infiltration or granulomatous infiltration with giant cells)

CLINICAL PEARLS

- If your patient is less than 50 years old and his or her ESR under 50mm/h, it is highly unlikely giant cell arteritis is the diagnosis
- Arrange a temporal artery biopsy quickly for patients with a suggestive history of giant cell arteritis – but treat immediately anyway if there are ocular symptoms

THE TESTS
Body fluids
ERYTHROCYTE SEDIMENTATION RATE (ESR)
Description
Venous blood sample.

Advantages/Disadvantages
Advantages:

- Simple and universally available test
- Useful for monitoring success of treatment and for titrating dose of corticosteroids
- Provides a useful (but not infallible) assessment of disease relapse or recurrence

Disadvantages:

- A normal ESR does not exclude the diagnosis if other features of giant cell arteritis are present
- A raised ESR can occur in many other conditions, such as infection, malignancy, and anemia
- A slightly raised ESR is occasionally found in otherwise healthy elderly people

Normal

- Males: 1–15mm/h
- Females: 0–20mm/h

Abnormal
- Males: >15mm/h
- Females: >20mm/h
- Keep in mind the possibility of a false-positive result

Cause of abnormal result
- Increased fibrinogen levels in response to inflammation
- Giant cell arteritis often causes a massively increased ESR (to >100mm/h)
- A raised ESR is sometimes found in otherwise healthy elderly people
- Anemia can cause an elevated ESR

Drugs, disorders and other factors that may alter results
- Corticosteroid therapy
- Many inflammatory and autoimmune conditions cause a raised ESR
- A raised ESR is sometimes found in otherwise healthy elderly people

COMPLETE BLOOD COUNT
Description
Venous blood sample.

Advantages/Disadvantages
- Simple, universally available test
- Nonspecific

Normal
Hemoglobin:
- Males: 13.6–17.7g/dL
- Females: 12–15g/dL

White blood cells:
- 3200–9800 cells/mm^3

Platelet count:
130,000–400,000 platelets/mm^3

Abnormal
- Values outside the normal ranges
- Keep in mind the possibility of a false result

Cause of abnormal result
- Giant cell arteritis is usually associated with a mild, normochromic or hypocrhomic, normocytic anemia
- Platelet count may be elevated as an acute phase reactant

C-REACTIVE PROTEIN
Description
Venous blood sample.

Advantages/Disadvantages
Advantages:
- Can be used for monitoring success of treatment and for titrating dose of corticosteroids
- Provides a useful (but not infallible) assessment of disease relapse or recurrence

- Not affected by anemia, unlike the ESR
- Rises and falls rapidly with development and resolution of inflammation

Disadvantage: less readily available than ESR

Normal
6.8-820mcg/dL.

Abnormal
Values outside the normal range.

Cause of abnormal result
Inflammatory reactions of any etiology cause an increase in C-reactive protein levels.

Drugs, disorders and other factors that may alter results
Elevated in many inflammatory and neoplastic conditions.

LIVER FUNCTION TESTS
Description
Venous blood.

Advantages/Disadvantages
- Advantage: simple, readily available test
- Disadvantage: nonspecific

Normal
- Bilirubin: 0-1.0mg/dL
- Alakaline phosphatase: 30-120U/L
- Aspartate aminotransferase: 0-35U/L
- Albumin: 4-6g/L
- Gamma-glutamyl transferase: 0-30U/L
- Prothrombin time: 10-12 s

Abnormal
- Values outside the normal ranges
- Keep in mind the possibility of a false-positive result

Cause of abnormal result
About one-third of patients with giant cell arteritis have abnormal liver function tests, particularly:
- Mild elevation of alkaline phosphatase (the most common abnormality)
- Mild elevation of aspartate aminotransferase

Liver function tests usually return to normal with successful treatment of giant cell arteritis.

Biopsy
TEMPORAL ARTERY BIOPSY
Description
Surgical removal of a segment of the temporal artery

Advantages/Disadvantages
Advantages:
- Simple, generally nonmorbid procedure that can be done in a surgeon's office
- A positive biopsy is useful confirmatory evidence of vasculitis in doubtful cases and may be

invaluable if the patient suffers treatment-related side-effects

Disadvantage: a negative result does not exclude giant cell arteritis. There is an appreciable false-negative rate. One-third of patients with giant cell arteritis may have a negative biopsy

Normal
Normal arterial wall histology without inflammatory infiltrate.

Abnormal
Panarteritis with predominantly lymphomononuclear infiltrate, giant cell granuloma formation, and disruption of the internal elastic lamina, intimal fibrosis, and thrombosis often in short 'skip lesions.'

Cause of abnormal result
Inflammatory changes that spread right through the arterial wall.

Drugs, disorders and other factors that may alter results
- Corticosteroids reduce the inflammatory cell infiltrate so temporal artery biopsy should be performed as soon as possible after the initiation of treatment
- Giant cell arteritis involvement of the temporal artery is patchy and therefore a biopsy should sample at least a 4–6cm segment to maximize the yield

TREATMENT

CONSIDER CONSULT
Patients diagnosed with giant cell arteritis who have visual disturbances should be referred to an ophthalmologist for assessment.

IMMEDIATE ACTION
- Prompt initiation of treatment with corticosteroids can prevent permanent visual loss
- Patients with visual loss should not be delayed in starting corticosteroids if a temporal artery biopsy cannot be readily arranged
- In fact, blindness in the contralateral eye can occur even after corticosteroid treatment has been started

PATIENT AND CAREGIVER ISSUES
Patient or caregiver request
- Patients may be dubious about taking corticosteroids because of information gleaned from the media or from family and friends
- Patients may also confuse corticosteroids with anabolic steroids, thereby adding to their reluctance to comply with medication

Health-seeking behavior
Has the patient delayed consultation? Has the condition been missed by another medical practitioner?
- Headache may have been treated with over-the-counter analgesics
- Rheumatic or constitutional symptoms may have been treated with nonsteroidal anti-inflammatory agents or attributed by the patient to 'rheumatism' or 'old age'
- Vague or fleeting visual disturbances may not have prompted medical assessment, so delaying initiation of corticosteroid therapy

MANAGEMENT ISSUES
Goals
- Prevention of permanent visual loss with prompt initiation of corticosteroids
- Relief of symptoms

SUMMARY OF THERAPEUTIC OPTIONS
Choices
Corticosteroids must be given to patients with giant cell arteritis and are the therapy of first choice. They reduce symptoms and can avoid permanent visual loss if instituted promptly – they should be started immediately in patients with visual symptoms or those with fundoscopic abnormalities who are suspected of having giant cell arteritis:
- Oral prednisone is the usual therapy
- Intravenous methylprednisolone in large doses for a few days may be indicated in very ill patients and in patients with significant eye involvement, especially significant unilateral visual loss; such patients would usually require referral

Other therapies:
- There is little evidence for the use of steroid-sparing agents in the management of giant cell arteritis, but methotrexate is the agent that seems to have the most efficacy
- Nonsteroidal anti-inflammatory drugs help to reduce the painful symptoms of associated polymyalgia rheumatica, but they have no beneficial effects on the vasculitis or on the outcome of the condition. There is therefore little place for them in the short-term or long-term management of giant cell arteritis

Clinical pearls

- Corticosteroids are the standard treatment for giant cell arteritis and should be started immediately in patients with visual symptoms or signs, along with prompt ophthalmologic referral
- Warn patients not to stop treatment just because they feel better in a few days
- Reassure patients that the condition is treatable, but that they should expect to receive corticosteroid treatment for at least 2 years
- The great majority of patients with giant cell arteritis improve rapidly on the correct dosage of prednisone. Failure to improve significantly within a few days should prompt reconsideration of the diagnosis
- Large falls in the dose of prednisone can affect the human lens and cause blurred vision, mimicking a recurrence of giant cell arteritis activity

Never

Never delay treatment with corticosteroids until a specialist referral or temporal artery biopsy can be arranged in a patient with suspected giant cell arteritis if visual symptoms are present.

FOLLOW UP

Patients require frequent follow up for adjustment of medication, assessment for recurrence of symptoms and presence of visual symptoms, and monitoring of erythrocyte sedimentation rate.

Plan for review

- Review patient within 3–4 days of starting corticosteroids. Dramatic improvement in all symptoms, including sense of well-being, should be expected within a few days
- Review patient for clinical features and measurement of erythrocyte sedimentation rate (ESR) before each reduction in corticosteroid dose
- Although the ESR is a reasonable parameter for assessing disease activity, the patient's symptoms should be the major consideration in making a decision about reducing or increasing the corticosteroid dose

Information for patient or caregiver

- The patient must be told not to reduce or stop corticosteroid therapy without medical advice
- The patient should be told to report any deterioration or visual symptoms immediately
- Consider giving some patients instructions about increasing corticosteroid doses if deterioration or visual symptoms occur

DRUGS AND OTHER THERAPIES: DETAILS
Drugs
PREDNISONE (ORAL)
Dose
High initial doses are necessary and patients should be warned to expect to need prednisone treatment for 2 years at least.

- 40–60mg/day or more (1mg/kg/day) for about 4 weeks until symptoms resolve and ESR returns to normal. Ocular symptoms prompt use of the higher doses
- A reducing dose regimen can then be used, as long as symptoms or signs do not recur and ESR remains normal. Advice on how to reduce corticosteroid dose varies and is often conflicting. Preferably use local guidelines in association with a rheumatologist or:
- Reduce by 5mg/day every 4 weeks until 10mg/day is reached. Reduce by 1mg/day every 2 months to 5mg/day. Maintain at 5mg/day for 6–12 months. Attempt to withdraw to zero at 1mg/day every 2 months. Most patients require treatment for 3–4 years

Efficacy
Excellent:
- The response to therapy is usually rapid (within days)
- Helps to avoid permanent visual loss if commenced promptly in patients with visual symptoms

Risks/Benefits
Risks:
- Overwhelming septicemia if patient has an infection. Loss of control of blood glucose in those with diabetes
- Prolonged use causes adrenal suppression

Side-effects and adverse reactions
- Side-effects are minimized by short duration of therapy
- Gastrointestinal: dyspepsia, peptic ulceration, oesophagitis, oral candidiasis
- Cardiovascular system: hypertension, thromboembolism
- Central nervous system: insomnia, euphoria, depression, psychosis
- Endocrine: adrenal suppression, impaired glucose tolerance, growth suppression in children
- Musculoskeletal: proximal myopathy, osteoporosis
- Skin: delayed healing, acne, striae
- Eyes, ears, nose, throat: cataract, glaucoma, blurred vision

Interactions (other drugs)
- Aminoglutethamide ▪ Barbiturates ▪ Cholestyramine ▪ Clarithromycin, erythromycin ▪ Colestipol ▪ Isoniazid ▪ Ketoconazole ▪ NSAIDs ▪ Oral contraceptives ▪ Rifampin ▪ Salicylates ▪ Troleandomycin

Contraindications
- Systemic infection ▪ Avoid live virus vaccines in those receiving immunosuppressive doses

Acceptability to patient
After possible initial resistance to the idea of taking steroids, good acceptability in the short term because of the rapid clinical improvement that usually occurs.
- Tapering dose may cause confusion to some patients
- Patients may be worried about longer-term use because of worries about side-effects. Weight gain is especially distressing to patients

Follow up plan
- Steroids usually need to be continued for up to 2 years, often for longer
- Clinical symptoms and ESR must be monitored regularly, especially when dose is decreased

Patient and caregiver information
- Patient must be warned not to stop treatment suddenly
- Patient should be told to report clinical relapse or visual symptoms promptly
- Consider giving instructions to the patient to increase dose if relapse occurs

METHYLPREDNISOLONE (INTRAVENOUS)
Intravenous prednisolone in large doses for a few days may be indicated in very ill patients and in patients with significant eye involvement (especially significant unilateral visual loss); referral is mandatory in such patients.

Dose
1000mg intravenous daily for 2–3 days.

Efficacy
Good.

Risks/Benefits
Risks:
- Overwhelming septicemia if patient has an infection. Loss of control of blood glucose in those with diabetes
- Prolonged use causes adrenal suppression

Side-effects and adverse reactions
- Side-effects are minimized by short duration of therapy
- Gastrointestinal: dyspepsia, peptic ulceration, oesophagitis, oral candidiasis
- Cardiovascular system: hypertension, thromboembolism
- Central nervous system: insomnia, euphoria, depression, psychosis
- Endocrine: adrenal suppression, impaired glucose tolerance, growth suppression in children
- Musculoskeletal: proximal myopathy, osteoporosis
- Skin: delayed healing, acne, striae
- Eyes, ears, nose, throat: cataract, glaucoma, blurred vision

Interactions (other drugs)
- Aminoglutethamide ▪ Barbiturates ▪ Cholestyramine ▪ Clarithromycin, erythromycin ▪ Colestipol ▪ Isoniazid ▪ Ketoconazole ▪ NSAIDs ▪ Oral contraceptives ▪ Rifampin ▪ Salicylates ▪ Troleandomycin

Contraindications
- Systemic infection ▪ Avoid live virus vaccines in those receiving immunosuppressive doses

Evidence
There is evidence that the development or progression of visual loss in giant cell arteritis is rare after the initiation of intravenous methylprednisolone [2] *Level S*

Acceptability to patient
Usually good if the risk to vision is explained to the patient.

Follow up plan
Patient must be started on oral corticosteroid therapy at the end of the course of intravenous methylprednisolone.

LIFESTYLE
Patients taking high-dose corticosteroids should be advised to adopt strategies to prevent loss of bone:
- Smoking cessation
- Moderation in use of alcohol
- Weight-bearing exercise for 30–60 min each day
- Adequate calcium (1500mg daily) and vitamin D intake (800IU daily)
- Administration of a daily bisphophonate may be considered (see risks/benefits of prednisone).

ACCEPTABILITY TO PATIENT
Lifestyle changes are often poorly acceptable to patients.

EFFICACY OF THERAPIES

- Adequate doses of corticosteroids usually provide relief of symptoms and prevent permanent visual loss
- Treatment usually needs to be continued for 1–2 years, and sometimes for longer

Evidence

- PDxMD are unable to cite evidence which meets our criteria for evidence
- Although there is no good evidence from clinical trials, it is well recognized that adequate doses of corticosteroids started promptly usually relieve the symptoms of giant cell arteritis and prevent permanent visual loss

Review period

Patients should be reviewed regularly for recurrence of symptoms for as long as they remain on corticosteroid therapy and for the first year off corticosteroids.

PROGNOSIS

The prognosis is generally good with adequate corticosteroid treatment.

Clinical pearls

With early recognition and prompt treatment with corticosteroids, patients with giant cell arteritis have an excellent prognosis. Morbidity from corticosteroid therapy however can be substantial in this age group and prophylactic treatment should be considered strongly. With treatment, life expectancy in patients with giant cell arteritis is the same as the general population.

Therapeutic failure

- Ensure that adequate, high doses of corticosteroids are being prescribed and that the patient is taking the medication as prescribed
- Reinstitute higher doses of corticosteroids if disease recurs during decreasing dose regimen
- Patients who fail to respond to adequate doses of corticosteroids should be referred to a rheumatologist for further assessment and management
- Patients who develop visual symptoms should be referred to an ophthalmologist urgently

Recurrence

- Recurrence is most likely in the first 18 months but can occur at any time, even after apparently successful treatment with corticosteroids
- Diagnosis of recurrence should be made primarily on clinical grounds, rather than ESR
- Corticosteroid dose should be started again or increased to the initial high dose or more if necessary to control disease activity

Deterioration

Deterioration should prompt immediate referral to a rheumatologist or ophthalmologist, or both, as appropriate.

COMPLICATIONS

- Permanent visual loss occurs in up to 10% of patients
- Prednisone-related side-effects are frequent

CONSIDER CONSULT

Deterioration should prompt immediate referral to a rheumatologist or ophthalmologist, or both, as appropriate.

PREVENT RECURRENCE

Recurrence can usually be prevented by continuing corticosteroids for up to 2 years and tapering therapy slowly and carefully. The patient will often require reassurance and encouragement to continue therapy.

RESOURCES

ASSOCIATIONS

American College of Rheumatology
1800 Century Place
Suite 250
Atlanta GA 30345
Tel: (404) 633 3777
Fax: (404) 633 1870
www.rheumatology.org

KEY REFERENCES

- American College of Rheumatology Task Force on Osteoporosis Guidelines. Recommendations for the prevention and treatment of glucocorticoid-induced osteoporosis. Arthritis Rheum 1996: 39:1791–801
- Caselli RJ. Giant cell (temporal) arteritis. Neurol Clin 1997; 15: 893–902
- Evans JM, Hunder GG. Geriatric Rheumatology: polymyalgia rheumatica and giant cell arteritis. Rheum Dis Clin North Am 2000:26: 493–515
- Gardner GC. Polymyalgia rheumatica, temporal (giant cell) arteritis, and takayasu's arteritis. In: Weisman MH, Weinblatt ME, eds. Treatment of the Rheumatic Diseases. Philadelphia: W.B. Saunders Company, 1995: 158–71
- Hazleman BL. Polymyalgia rheumatica and giant cell arteritis. In: Klippel J, Dieppe P, eds. Rheumatology, 2nd ed. London: Mosby; 1998: 7.21.1–7.21.8.
- Hunder GG. Giant cell arteritis and polymyalgia rheumatica. Med Clin North Am 1997; 45: 334–447
- Hunder GG, Bloch DA, Michel BA, et al. The American College of Rheumatolgy 1990 criteria for the classification of giant cell arteritis. Arthritis Rheum 1990; 33: 1122–8
- Lee AG. Temporal arteritis: a clinical approach. J Am Geriatr Soc 1999: 47: 1364–70
- Salvarani C. Musculoskeletal manifestation in a population-based cohort of patients with giant cell arteritis. Arthritis Rheum 1999; 42: 1259–66
- Weyand CM, Goronzy JJ. Polymyalgia rheumatica and giant cell arteritis. In: Koopman WJ. Arthritis and allied Conditions: a Textbook of Rheumatology, 13th ed. Baltimore: Williams and Wilkins; 1997; 1605–14

Evidence references

1 Hunder GG, Bloch DA, Michel BA, et al. The American College of Rheumatolgy 1990 criteria for the classification of giant cell arteritis. Arthritis Rheum 1990; 33: 1122–8
2 Aiello PD, Trautman JC, McPhee TJ, Kunselman AS, Hunder GG. Visual prognosis in giant cell arteritis. Opthamology 1993;100:p550

FAQS

Question 1

When should symptoms be expected to resolve after the start of therapy?

ANSWER 1

Fatigue and headache usually subside within one week. The erythrocyte sedimentation rate normalizes in 2–4 weeks. Visual symptoms may or may not resolve; therefore, it is imperative to initiate treatment promptly to prevent visual loss or impairment.

Question 2

What dose of corticosteroids should be started to treat giant cell arteritis?

ANSWER 2

If no visual symptoms are present, the equivalent of 40–60mg of prednisone daily should be give for at least 1 month before reduction of dosage. If visual symptoms are present, intravenous methylprednisolone at 1000mg daily for 3 days is given and then afterwards prednisone 60mg daily is started and maintained for one month before reduction of dosage.

Question 3

Does a temporal artery biopsy need to be performed to diagnose giant cell arteritis? Can a patient have giant cell arteritis with a negative temporal artery biopsy? When should a temporal artery biopsy be obtained?

ANSWER 3

Giant cell arteritis can be diagnosed on clinical grounds alone without a temporal artery biopsy; however, it is recommended that all patients suspected of having giant cell arteritis undergo temporal artery biopsy, especially as patients may be committed to long-term therapy with corticosteroids. Biopsy yields confirmatory histological evidence of vasculitis.

A negative temporal artery biopsy does not rule out the possibility of giant cell arteritis, but makes the diagnosis less likely. Some series suggest one-third of patients with giant cell arteritis have a negative biopsy. The investigation is most useful in those patients whose clinical features are systemic and the clinical diagnosis is in doubt.

Ideally, temporal artery biopsy should be carried out prior to start of therapy; however, if visual symptoms are present, treatment should be instituted without delay. Temporal artery biopsy should then be obtained as soon as possible after the initiation of therapy.

Question 4

What parameter(s) should be followed to monitor for relapse?

ANSWER 4

Monitoring of clinical symptoms and signs are most important in the assessment of potential relapse. The erythrocyte sedimentation rate (ESR) should be followed, and a symptom-free patient who develops an increase in the ESR should be followed more closely for a possible flare of the disease. However, the ESR does not always correspond to disease activity, and adjustment of corticosteroid treatment should be based primarily on clinical grounds.

Question 5

What can I tell my patient with giant cell arteritis about his/her prognosis?

ANSWER 5

The prognosis of giant cell arteritis is good. The condition is curable. If corticosteroids were introduced prior to the start of visual impairment, the risk for permanent visual damage is less than 1%. Most patients can discontinue therapy in 2–3 years, with low risk for relapse. The risk of adverse effects from corticosteroids is, however, substantial. Patients with appropriately managed giant cell arteritis have normal life expectancy.

CONTRIBUTORS

Shane Clarke, MD
Richard Brasington Jr, MD, FACP
Elizabeth C Hsia, MD

ACUTE GOUT

SUMMARY INFORMATION

DESCRIPTION

- An excruciatingly painful arthritis, typically but not exclusively monoarticular and classically affecting first metatarsophalangeal joint. May be difficult to distinguish from septic arthritis or periarticular cellulitis
- Caused by the inflammatory reaction associated with deposition of uric acid (urate) crystals in the joint. Closely linked to hyperuricemia – caused by either overproduction or underexcretion of serum uric acid, a breakdown product of circulating purines
- May recur or progress to chronic tophaceous gout if untreated
- Initial pain and joint swelling resolves over a few days with rest and nonsteroidal anti-inflammatory drugs (NSAIDs) and desquamation of overlying skin

URGENT ACTION

If there is a possibility of septic arthritis or cellulitis (patient systemically unwell, septicemic; predisposition to sepsis; or joint affected is atypical of an acute attack of gout), immediately refer to rheumatologist or orthopedic surgeon for investigation and management. The only definitive test is joint aspiration and culture.

KEY! DON'T MISS!

If patient is generally unwell or has fever, or if the affected joint is atypical of acute gout, refer to rheumatologist immediately as it could be septic arthritis, not gout. Gout is rare in children – any hot, painful joint should be assumed to be septic arthritis until proven otherwise.

BACKGROUND

ICD9 CODE
274.0 Gouty arthritis.

SYNONYMS
Podagra (gout of first metatarsophalangeal joint).

CARDINAL FEATURES
- Inflammatory arthritis principally affecting middle-aged men
- Acute attacks excruciatingly painful with joint swelling, redness, heat, and marked tenderness – any light touch may cause exquisite pain
- More than 50% of attacks affect only the first joint of one great toe
- About 90% of attacks are monoarticular
- Other common sites (descending order): instep, heel, ankle and knee
- Rarely polyarticular except in elderly women taking diuretics
- Initial pain and joint swelling resolves over a few days with rest and NSAIDs and a desquamation of overlying skin

CAUSES
Common causes
- Excess alcohol intake (reduces urate excretion; beer high in purines)
- Family history: genetic predisposition to urate undersecretion is responsible for many cases of gout
- Diuretic use: many drugs reduce renal urate clearance. Thiazide diuretics are most often implicated in acute gout attacks. Low dose aspirin or phenylbutazone, furosemide, ethacrynic acid, ethambutol, pyrazinamide, and nicotinic acid may also precipitate gout
- Renal disease: any cause of renal disease predisposes the individual to gout because clearance of urate is adversely affected. Renal failure may be chronic or acute associated with reduced renal perfusion (e.g. post-myocardial infarction, trauma, sepsis, surgical procedures)
- Hypertension is an independent risk factor for gout
- Obesity (implies high purine intake; decreases urate excretion)
- Increased cell turnover: particularly in hemopoietic malignancies, myeloproliferative disorders, chemotherapy, and extensive psoriasis

Rare causes
- Hypothyroidism
- Hyperparathyroidism
- Inherited hypertriglyceridemias
- Environmental toxins, particularly lead (saturnine gout)

Contributory or predisposing factors
- Inadequately controlled hypertension
- Hypertriglyceridemia

EPIDEMIOLOGY
Incidence and prevalence
INCIDENCE
Men 1–3/1000, women 0–2/1000.

PREVALENCE
Men 5–28/1000, women 1–6/1000.

Demographics

AGE

- Men: peak age of onset 40–50 years
- Women: over-60s, usually associated with diuretic use; in young women very rare and should be referred
- Rare in children

GENDER

- Most commonly affects men but is becoming more common in women
- Male:female ratio about 2–7:1
- Polyarticular gout more common in women

RACE

Less common in ethnic Chinese and Polynesians but higher rates are seen in these populations living in the West.

GENETICS

- Family history of gout common in middle-aged men with gout and mild hyperuricemia
- Hyperuricemia may be due to inherited enzyme abnormalities and urate undersecretion
- Rare genetic causes exist but only consider in atypical/severe disease or very young patients

DIFFERENTIAL DIAGNOSIS

- Most important differential diagnosis is septic arthritis: requires urgent attention to avoid severe and irreversible joint destruction
- If any doubt, refer urgently to rheumatologist or orthopedic surgeon for synovial fluid crystal identification and microbial culture to confirm gout or identify pathogens

Septic arthritis
FEATURES
- Abrupt onset
- Predisposing factors, e.g. diabetes mellitus, immune suppression, prosthetic joints, recent infection, foreign body, risk of endocarditis
- Monoarticular, most commonly in knee, hip or shoulder
- Red, swollen and hot joint; such intense pain that movement often impossible
- Fever and shaking chills common

Pseudogout
FEATURES
- Peak age 65–75 years, predominantly in women
- Monoarticular, most common at the knee, followed by wrist, shoulder, ankle, and elbow (very rarely polyarticular)
- Abrupt onset
- Red swollen joint with acute pain and restricted movement
- Fever common
- Attacks self-limiting

Bursitis of periarticular structures
FEATURES
- Tenderness on bursa, diffuse ache, pain when ligaments or tendons are stretched over it. May have minimal pain with limited passive range of motion of joint
- Local swelling if bursa is near the surface
- Swelling is often infected and red, hot and 'angry' – particularly in olecranon bursitis
- Essentially the soft tissue (bursa) is more affected than joint

Cellulitis of periarticular structures
FEATURES
- Local pain, tenderness, erythema, and induration of soft tissue surrounding the joint
- Malaise and fever
- Lymphangitis, lymphadenopathy in proximal lymph nodes may be present

Atypical presentations of psoriatic arthritis
FEATURES
- Usually associated with features of psoriasis (check the nails, hairline, navel and natal cleft)
- Dactylitis (inflammation of an entire toe or finger) is frequent and may affect more than one digit. Characteristic 'sausage' shape
- Involvement of joints in the upper limb is more likely than in gout

Atypical monoarticular presentations of other arthropathies
More details on arthropathy, unspecified.

Other crystal-related arthropathies
More details on arthropathy, unspecified.

Trauma
FEATURES

- History of trauma likely to be present
- In cases where a good history is impossible to obtain (e.g. in loss of consciousness, cerebrovascular accidents, cognitive or sensory deficit), differentiation is more reliant on investigations
- Redness and heat less likely to be present than in gout, although an acute fracture with hematoma may present like gout

SIGNS & SYMPTOMS
Signs

- Redness over affected joint(s) distinguishes gout from most noninfective arthropathies
- Heat and swelling over affected joint(s)
- Extreme tenderness of affected joint – light touch (e.g. bedsheet or sock) may cause exquisite pain
- Synovial effusion apparent in larger joints
- Possibly periarticular cellulitis
- Occasionally accompanying systemic features with high fever and leukocytosis (uncommon)

Symptoms

- Pain: rapid onset and build-up over a few hours (especially at night) usually affecting a single joint
- Redness: the patient will have noted skin color change in early stages of attack
- Heat and swelling involving the entire region (rare)

ASSOCIATED DISORDERS

- Chronic tophaceous gout
- Hypertension
- Renal failure
- Hypothyroidism
- Hyperparathyroidism
- Hyperlipidemias
- Alcoholism
- Obesity
- High cell turnover states (e.g. psoriasis, polycythemia, leukemia)
- Lead poisoning

KEY! DON'T MISS!
If patient is generally unwell or has fever, or if the affected joint is atypical of acute gout, refer to rheumatologist immediately as it could be septic arthritis, not gout. Gout is rare in children – any hot, painful joint should be assumed to be septic arthritis until proven otherwise.

CONSIDER CONSULT

- Diagnostic uncertainty, especially if it might be septic arthritis (patient systemically unwell, predisposition of sepsis, or joint affected is atypical of attack of acute gout)
- Gout with renal disease
- Gout in the context of organ transplantation (very difficult to control)
- Gout in young women

'Guidelines for Obtaining a Rheumatology Consultation' can be obtained from www.rheumatology.org by the American College of Rheumatology, [1].

INVESTIGATION OF THE PATIENT
Direct questions to patient

Q **Has there been trauma to the joint?** Eliminate trauma as a cause of joint swelling and pain – usually obvious from the patient's history but alcohol intoxication may impair memory of trauma. Cognitive impairment, sensory deficit may limit patient's awareness of trauma. Chronic low-grade trauma (e.g. a standing job with poorly fitting shoes) may precipitate acute gout

Q **How quickly did the pain come on?** Onset of pain is abrupt, increasing within hours to an intense peak that is sustained for 1–3 days then resolves spontaneously but gradually

Q **Were there any warning symptoms?** Tickling/pricking sensations in the affected joint an hour or more before the onset of pain are common in gout

Q **Do any other joints hurt?** Gout is usually monoarticular, but it can be polyarticular or occur in the presence of other arthropathies, which should be investigated separately

Q **Have you had this before?** Pain in gout is so acute that it is unlikely that a patient would suffer an attack without consulting a physician

Q **Are you on any medications?** May reveal a cause of hyperuricemia (e.g. thiazide diuretics)

Q **What is your drinking pattern?** Excess alcohol intake, particularly binge drinking, is associated with hyperuricemia

Q **Do you eat a lot of purine-rich foods?** Red meat, poultry, oily fish, liver, kidney, heart, gizzard, sweetbreads, yeast extracts, meat extracts, peas, beans, spinach, lentils

Contributory or predisposing factors
Is there a history of predisposing factors? Hypothyroidism, hyperparathyroidism, hypertriglyceridemia, inadequately controlled hypertension, obesity, renal disease

Family history
Q **Is there a family history of similar problems?** Family history common in middle-aged men with gout due to mild hyperuricemia and reduced urate excretion

Q **Is there a family history of early ischemic heart disease?** Could alert to hypertriglyceridemia

Examination
- **Is the patient well/unwell?** If systemically unwell, suggests septicemia and septic arthritis
- **Check temperature:** fever suggests infection
- **Obesity:** define by body mass index (BMI)
- **Check for signs of liver disease or alcohol abuse**
- **Check for psoriasis:** skin or nail involvement
- **Check pulse, blood pressure and dipstick urine:** for renal disease
- **Inspect eyes for signs of hypertriglyceridemia:** common in gout
- **Inspect joints** and look for tophi on hands, elbow, ears, Achilles tendons
- **Inspect affected joints** and record skin color, tender effusion, signs of lymphangitis, and local lymphadenopathy

Guidelines for the Initial Evaluation of the Adult Patient with Acute Musculoskeletal Symptoms are available at http://www.rheumatology.org/ from the American College of Rheumatology, [2].

Summary of investigative tests
During acute attacks:
- If any suspicion of septic arthritis, immediate referral to specialist is recommended; if referral is not possible, send synovial fluid for culture for pathogens
- Usually the only investigation indicated is synovial fluid aspiration and identification of urate crystals
- Serum urate hyperuricemia predisposes to acute gout but a normal or low serum uric acid level does not exclude the diagnosis; however, serum urate estimation is a helpful adjunctive test if the level is raised in a relevant clinical situation

- Renal function should be checked if NSAIDs are used in the treatment
- Lipid levels should also be checked
- Radiography is not useful except to eliminate fractures – history usually rules out fracture unless memory impaired due to alcohol, or patient has cognitive or sensory deficit

DIAGNOSTIC DECISION

- Most cases of gout are straightforward. Diagnostic difficulty is a reason for referral to a rheumatologist
- Gout is confirmed only by identifying sodium monourate crystals under polarizing microscopy from a joint aspirate
- Suspect gout if patient's history and examination are suggestive, and take into account patient's age, sex, distribution of joints affected and predisposing factors. You should specifically seek risk factors for sepsis (septic arthritis) and consider other crystal arthropathies such as pseudogout
- In a polyarticular presentation the diagnosis of rheumatoid arthritis or psoriatic arthritis must be considered
- Occasionally, monoarticular presentation of psoriatic arthritis causes diagnostic confusion if joints also affected by gout are involved. Only in patients severely affected by plaque psoriasis is serum urate likely to be significantly raised

Guidelines
The American Academy of Family Physicians have published material on the diagnosis and management of acute gout [3,4].

CLINICAL PEARLS

- Gout and rheumatoid arthritis almost never occur in the same patient
- Gout preferentially attacks damaged joints, so there is often co-existence of gout and underlying osteoarthritis. This is especially true of the distal interphalangeal joints in the fingers
- Gout should never be diagnosed solely on the basis of an elevated serum uric acid level, or excluded by a normal serum uric acid level
- Patients often underestimate their alcohol intake. A high red cell mean corpuscular volume (possible folate deficiency) or raised liver gamma-glutaryl transferase suggest excess alcohol intake
- Acute gout may be a clue to previously undiagnosed alcohol abuse

THE TESTS
Body fluids
IDENTIFICATION OF URATE CRYSTALS
Description
Joint aspiration of big toe is difficult and likely to be painful. Infiltration of local anesthetic makes the procedure more tolerable for patient and physician alike. Aspiration of ankle or knee is more straightforward. Obtain synovial fluid using an aseptic 'no touch' technique. Collect aspirate in a plain container with no additives. Send for analysis immediately: yield declines exponentially with time from collection. Usually even one or two drops of aspirate is enough to make a diagnosis.

Advantages/Disadvantages
Advantage: confirms diagnosis

Disadvantages:
- Can be difficult to aspirate the acutely painful joint
- Fluid has to be examined under polarized light microscopy by a specialist experienced in distinguishing urate (crystals) from other arthropathic crystals

Normal
No crystals identified.

Abnormal
- Crystals located under low-power dark field then confirmed as urate under high-power polarized light by virtue of their strong negative birefringence
- Keep in mind the possibility of false-positive results

Cause of abnormal result
Crystal deposition.

SERUM URATE (AS URIC ACID)
Description
Cuffed venous blood sample; may combine with renal function and fasting lipids.

Advantages/Disadvantages
- Raised uric acid is helpful circumstantial evidence to the diagnosis of gout
- Normal levels do not eliminate gout. In 15% of acute attacks of gout the serum urate falls

Normal
There is considerable overlap between the normal and gouty populations with respect to serum uric acid concentration. Gout relatively uncommon (0.8/1000 annually) below 7.0mg/dL (0.42mmol/L) but incidence rises rapidly at higher concentration.

Abnormal
- Above 7.0mg/dL (0.42mmol/L) but see previous comment
- Keep in mind the possibility of false-positive results

Cause of abnormal result
Hyperuricemia is caused by overproduction or undersecretion of uric acid. Most commonly, patients inherit predisposition to gout by an isolated renal lesion causing undersecretion. A number of environmental and concomitant factors can also result in hyperuricemia.

Imaging
RADIOGRAPHY
Advantages/Disadvantages
- Eliminates suspected fracture when this is not obvious in the history – particularly in the patient with cognitive or sensory deficit
- Established gout is often associated with typical erosive lesions in the hands and feet. This may help in differentiating rheumatoid arthritis and psoriatic arthritis
- Otherwise, radiography has no diagnostic or monitoring role in gout

Normal
In acute gout radiographic appearance reflects soft-tissue swelling. There may be typical gouty erosions if the disease has been present for some months.

Abnormal
- May identify fracture of big toe, instep, heel, or ankle, or the presence of underlying osteoarthritis
- Keep in mind the possibility of false-positive results

Cause of abnormal result
Fracture of big toe, instep, heel, ankle.

TREATMENT

CONSIDER CONSULT

- Severe attacks unresponsive to therapy.

Guidelines for Obtaining a Rheumatology Consultation have been published by the American College of Rheumatology [1]

IMMEDIATE ACTION

See patient with hot, swollen, painful joint immediately to assess whether any suspicion of septic arthritis, which requires urgent referral for investigation and treatment.

PATIENT AND CAREGIVER ISSUES
Patient or caregiver request

- Has gout been in the news recently?
- Patients with family history of gout may request antihyperuricemic therapy, but consider control via addressing lifestyle issues first

Health-seeking behavior

- **Waited too long?** Acute gout so painful that patients are quick to seek help unless socioeconomic factors (e.g. alcoholism) make them unwilling to visit doctor
- **Self-medications?** Self-medication with NSAIDs likely to have been successful and is reason why many do not consult their doctor
- **Visited ER?** Patients who visit ER likely to be given NSAIDs and told to visit their family doctor – as attack likely to settle before the appointment, this can be a lost opportunity to screen

MANAGEMENT ISSUES
Goals

- Relieve pain and swelling
- Follow up to assess hyperuricemia and prevent further acute attacks, tophus formation and joint damage
- Reassess prior diagnosis in uncontrolled disease

Management in special circumstances

Young patients (under 30 years) are likely to have inherited an enzymatic disorder leading to hyperuricemia. These patients are difficult to manage and should be referred for specialist opinion.

Patients with pre-existing renal disease (creatinine clearance <60mL/min) should be treated with NSAIDs only with extreme caution. Gout may be managed in the acute stage by local glucocorticoid injection or oral colchicine, although this will require reduced dose in proportion to renal filtration rate.

COEXISTING DISEASE

- History of acute gout does not exclude coexisting arthropathies: psoriatic arthritis, osteoarthritis
- Renal disease is both predisposing factor to gout and complication of undertreated gouty arthropathy. Renal disease should alert the physician to keep serum uric acid levels low but allopurinol may itself reduce renal function in high doses
- Hypertension is a common causative factor in hyperuricemia; thiazide diuretics for hypertension can be a cause or contributory factor
- Hyperlipidemia, usually hypertriglyceridemia (type IV), uncommon but those with type IV are likely to get gout

COEXISTING MEDICATION

- Thiazide diuretics for hypertension can be a cause or contributory factor
- NSAIDs for coexisting disease can worsen renal failure and hyperuricemia

SPECIAL PATIENT GROUPS

Patients with pre-existing renal disease (creatinine clearance <60mL/min) should be treated with NSAIDs only with extreme caution. Gout may be managed in the acute stage by local glucocorticoid injection or oral colchicines, although this will require reduced dosage in proportion to renal filtration rate.

PATIENT SATISFACTION/LIFESTYLE PRIORITIES

- Pain is significant and likely to stop patient from working or carrying out normal daily activities until it ceases
- Patient must address lifestyle factors to reduce chance of further attacks

SUMMARY OF THERAPEUTIC OPTIONS
Choices

- NSAIDs are first-choice drug therapy and act faster than colchicine
- Indomethacin is first-choice NSAID for those not at risk of either renal disease or gastrointestinal side-effects. (Although aspirin is contraindicated in low doses it is possible in high doses, but there are probably more effective medications)
- Other NSAIDs are also possible but dosage is near or above upper limit of normal therapeutic range. Possible NSAIDs include ibuprofen, diclofenac, naproxen, piroxicam, and sulindac
- Systemic corticosteroids can be used if NSAIDs are contraindicated
- Colchicine is reserved for patients who cannot take NSAIDs and generally only effective if started within 24 h of start of acute attack; best reserved for hyperuricemic control after acute attack has subsided
- Intra-articular/intramuscular corticosteroid injection suitable for patients with one or few joints affected or who cannot take oral medication
- Joint aspiration: large gouty effusions (especially of the knee) may be aspirated to dryness with considerable benefit in terms of pain relief
- Concomitant intra-articular glucocorticoid injection is likely to prevent the effusion recurring in the short term
- Advise all patients on lifestyle measures during the attack and to help prevent recurrence
- Once acute attack has subsided, follow up and institute appropriate measures

Guidelines

The American Academy of Family Physicians have published material on the diagnosis and management of acute gout, [3,4].

Clinical pearls

- Colchicine is associated with diarrhea (most common) and nausea/vomiting, which are to be avoided in the relatively immobile elderly. These side-effects are dose-related and may be reduced or eliminated by dose reduction. Overall, the side-effect profile of colchicine makes it preferable to use an NSAID for prophylaxis between acute attacks of gout
- Treatment of acute gouty arthritis requires maximum doses of NSAIDs
- Never start allopurinol during an acute gout attack

FOLLOW UP
Plan for review

- First attack of acute gout: ask patient to return when attack has subsided for review of prevention of further attacks – effective prevention of recurrences requires partnership between physician and patient to optimize compliance

- Review and revise therapy if not effective within 3 days
- Recurrent gout: monitor renal function annually

Information for patient or caregiver

Adjustment of lifestyle issues (alcohol, obesity) can prevent recurrence of gout in mild hyperuricemia.

DRUGS AND OTHER THERAPIES: DETAILS
Drugs
INDOMETHACIN
Dose

Oral: 50mg four times daily, maximum 300 mg/day for severe attacks. Reduce gradually: 50mg three times daily, then 25mg three times daily for 1–2 days after acute inflammation has ceased.

Efficacy
- Pain begins to ease within 2 h
- Other NSAIDs have not been shown to be more effective than indomethacin

Risks/Benefits
Risks
- Use caution in hepatic and cardiac failure, epilepsy, psychiatric disorders and parkinsonism
- Use caution in pregnancy and breast-feeding
- Use caution in bleeding disorders

Benefits: faster onset of action than colchicines

Side-effects and adverse reactions
- Cardiovascular system: cardiac abnormalities, congestive heart failure
- Central nervous system: headache, dizziness, tinnitus, somnolence
- Gastrointestinal: anorexia, nausea, vomiting, abdominal pain, diarrhea, constipation, dyspepsia, peptic ulceration, gastritis, gastrointestinal bleeding
- Genitourinary: renal dysfunction, hyperuricemia
- Hematologic: blood cell disorders
- Hypersensitivity: rashes, bronchospasm, angioedema

Interactions (other drugs)
- Aminoglycosides ▪ Antihypertensives ▪ Corticosteroids ▪ Cyclosporin ▪ Digoxin ▪ Lithium ▪ Methotrexate ▪ Phenylpropanolamine ▪ Diuretics ▪ Warfarin

Contraindications
- Severe renal, hepatic or cardiac disease ▪ Hypertension ▪ Peptic ulceration, gastrointestinal bleeding, ulcerative colitis ▪ Hypersensitivity to NSAIDs ▪ Coagulation defects ▪ Untreated infection ▪ Thrombocytopenia ▪ Cidofovir

Acceptability to patient
High.

Follow up plan
Ask patient to return for review once acute attack resolved.

Patient and caregiver information
Patients subject to repeat attacks can be trained to recognize and manage attacks themselves.

IBUPROFEN

This is an off-label indication.

Dose
Oral: 200–800mg three times daily after meals, usual dose 400mg four times daily

Efficacy
Pain begins to ease within 2 h.

Risks/Benefits
Risks
- Use caution in elderly
- Use caution in hepatic, renal and cardiac failure
- Use caution in bleeding disorders
- May cause severe allergic reactions including hives, facial swelling, asthma, shock

Benefits
- Faster onset of action than colchicines
- Inexpensive

Side-effects and adverse reactions
- Cardiovascular system: hypertension, peripheral edema
- Central nervous system: headache, dizziness, tinnitus
- Gastrointestinal: anorexia, nausea, dyspepsia, peptic ulceration, bleeding
- Genitourinary: nephrotoxicity
- Hematologic: blood cell disorders
- Hypersensitivity: rashes, bronchospasm, angioedema

Interactions (other drugs)
- Aminoglycosides ▪ Anticoagulants ▪ Antihypertensives ▪ Baclofen ▪ Corticosteroids
- Cyclosporine, tacrolimus ▪ Digoxin ▪ Diuretics ▪ Lithium ▪ Methotrexate
- Phenylpropanolamine ▪ Warfarin

Contraindications
- Peptic ulceration ▪ Hypersensitivity to any pain reliever or antipyretic (including NSAIDs)
- Coagulation defects ▪ Severe renal or hepatic disease

Acceptability to patient
High.

Follow up plan
Ask patient to return for review once acute attack resolved.

Patient and caregiver information
Patients subject to repeat attacks can be trained to recognize and manage attacks themselves.

DICLOFENAC

This is an off-ladel indication.

Dose
Oral: 50mg three times daily reducing to 25mg three times daily, suppositories also available.

Efficacy
Pain begins to ease within 2 h.

Risks/Benefits
Risks:
- Use caution in hepatic or renal failure
- Use caution in cardiac failure
- Use cautin in porphyria
- Use caution in bleeding and gastrointestinal disorders

Benefits: faster onset of action than colchicines

Side-effects and adverse reactions
- Cardiovascular system: congestive heart failure, dysrhythmias, hypertension, hypotension
- Central nervous system: headache, dizziness, tinnitus
- Eyes, ears, nose, and throat: blurred vision
- Gastrointestinal: anorexia, nausea, dyspepsia, peptic ulceration, vomiting
- Hypersensitivity: rashes, bronchospasm, angioedema

Interactions (other drugs)
- Aminoglycosides Antihypertensives Corticosteroids Cyclosporin Digoxin
- Lithium Methotrexate Phenylpropanolamine Diuretics Warfarin

Contraindications
- Peptic ulceration Hypersensitivity to NSAIDs Coagulation defects

Acceptability to patient
High.

Follow up plan
Ask patient to return for review once acute attack resolved.

Patient and caregiver information
Patients subject to repeat attacks can be trained to recognize and manage attacks themselves.

NAPROXEN
Dose
- Oral: 750mg initial dose, then 250mg three times daily, maximum 500mg three times daily
- Suppositories available for patients unable to take oral medication

Efficacy
Pain begins to ease within 2 h.

Risks/Benefits
- Risk: use caution in hepatic, renal and cardiac failure
- Benefit: faster onset of action than colchicines

Side-effects and adverse reactions
- Gastrointestinal: anorexia, nausea, dyspepsia, peptic ulceration
- Central nervous system: headache, dizziness, tinnitus
- Hypersensitivity: rashes, bronchospasm, angioedema
- Thrombocytopenia

Interactions (other drugs)
- Aminoglycosides
- Antihypertensives
- Corticosteroids
- Cyclosporin
- Digoxin
- Lithium
- Methotrexate
- Phenylpropanolamine
- Diuretics
- Warfarin

Contraindications
- Peptic ulceration
- Hypersensitivity to NSAIDs
- Coagulation defects

Acceptability to patient
High.

Follow up plan
Ask patient to return for review once acute attack resolved.

Patient and caregiver information
Patients subject to repeat attacks can be trained to recognize and manage attacks themselves.

PIROXICAM
This is an off-label indication.

Dose
- Oral: 40mg daily
- Suppositories available for patients unable to take oral medication

Efficacy
Pain begins to ease within 2 h.

Risks/Benefits
Risks:
- Use caution in hepatic, renal, and cardiac impairment or disease
- Use caution in children and the elderly
- Use caution in immunosuppression
- Use caution in diabetes mellitus
- Use caution in systemic lupus erythrmatosus
- Use caution in bleeding disorders

Side-effects and adverse reactions
- Gastrointestinal: anorexia, nausea, dyspepsia, peptic ulceration
- Central nervous system: headache, dizziness, tinnitus
- Hypersensitivity: rashes, bronchospasm, angioedema
- Thrombocytopenia

Interactions (other drugs)
- Aminoglycosides
- Antihypertensives
- Corticosteroids
- Cyclosporin
- Digoxin
- Lithium
- Methotrexate
- Phenylpropanolamine
- Diuretics
- Warfarin

Contraindications
- Peptic ulceration
- Hypersensitivity to NSAIDs
- Coagulation defects
- Porphyria

Acceptability to patient
High.

Follow up plan
Ask patient to return for review once acute attack resolved.

Patient and caregiver information
Patients subject to repeat attacks can be trained to recognize and manage attacks themselves.

SULINDAC
Dose
Oral: 200mg initial dose, then 100mg four times daily.

Efficacy
Pain begins to ease within 2 h.

Risks/Benefits
■ Risk: use caution in hepatic, renal and cardiac failure, renal calculi
■ Benefit: faster onset of action than colchicines

Side-effects and adverse reactions
■ Urine discoloration occasionally reported
■ Gastrointestinal: anorexia, nausea, dyspepsia, peptic ulceration
■ Central nervous system: headache, dizziness, tinnitus
■ Hypersensitivity: rashes, bronchospasm, angioedema
■ Thrombocytopenia

Interactions (other drugs)
■ Aminoglycosides ■ Antihypertensives ■ Corticosteroids ■ Cyclosporin ■ Digoxin ■ Lithium ■ Methotrexate ■ Phenylpropanolamine ■ Diuretics ■ Warfarin

Contraindications
■ Peptic ulceration ■ Hypersensitivity to NSAIDs ■ Coagulation defects

Acceptability to patient
High.

Follow up plan
Ask patient to return for review once acute attack resolved.

Patient and caregiver information
Patients subject to repeat attacks can be trained to recognize and manage attacks themselves.

PREDNISONE
Dose
Adult: 30–50mg daily, gradually reducing over 7–9 days.

Efficacy
Excellent.

Risks/Benefits
Risks:
■ Overwhelming septicemia if septic arthritis misdiagnosed as gout. Loss of control of blood glucose in those with diabetes
■ Prolonged use causes adrenal suppression

Benefit: suitable if NSAIDs or colchicine cannot be administered

Side-effects and adverse reactions
Side-effects are minimized by short duration of therapy:
- Gastrointestinal: dyspepsia, peptic ulceration, esophagitis, oral candidiasis
- Cardiovascular system: hypertension, thromboembolism
- Central nervous system: insomnia, euphoria, depression, psychosis
- Endocrine: adrenal suppression, impaired glucose tolerance, growth suppression in children
- Musculoskeletal: proximal myopathy, osteoporosis
- Skin: delayed healing, acne, striae
- Eyes, ears, nose, and throat: cataract, glaucoma, blurred vision

Interactions (other drugs)
- Aminoglutethimide ▪ Barbiturates ▪ Cholestyramine ▪ Clarithromycin, erythromycin ▪ Colestipol ▪ Isoniazid ▪ Ketoconazole ▪ NSAIDs ▪ Oral contraceptives ▪ Rifampin ▪ Salicylates ▪ Troleandomycin

Contraindications
- Systemic infection ▪ Avoid live virus vaccines in those receiving immunosuppressive doses

Acceptability to patient
- Patients are cautious about steroid use (press coverage: anabolic steroid use in athletics, severe side-effects due to misprescription of topical steroids in the 1970s) and the benefits have to be explained
- High-dose glucocorticoids for even short periods may precipitate euphoria or depression in up to one-third of patients, and may precipitate psychosis in some patients, particularly those with pre-existing cognitive impairment

Follow up plan
Ask patient to return for review once acute attack resolved.

Patient and caregiver information
- Warn patients of potential to cause facial flushing and the possibility of headaches, euphoria or irritability and depression
- The prescribing physician should also ask the patient to return if the overall condition deteriorates
- Advise patients on long-term therapy to avoid abrupt withdrawal

COLCHICINE
Dose
- Acute attack, oral: 1.0–1.2mg immediately, then 0.5–0.6mg 1- to 2-hourly until relief or side-effects occur, maximum of 8mg in 24 h
- Prophylaxis, oral: 0.6mg twice daily, maximum dose 0.6mg three times daily

Efficacy
75–80% of patients will have relief by 48 h.

Risks/Benefits
Benefits:
- Effective control of gout
- May be used in patients who cannot tolerate NSAIDs

Side-effects and adverse reactions
- Diarrhea, nausea, vomiting, and abdominal pain are common
- Peripheral neuritis, myopathy
- Alopecia

Interactions (other drugs)
- Cyclosporine ▪ Tacrolimus ▪ Clarithromycin, erythromycin, troleandomycin

Contraindications
- Pregnancy and nursing ▪ Significant renal, hepatic or cardiac impairment
- Blood dyscrasias

Evidence
A controlled trial demonstrated that colchicine may be more effective than placebo in acute gout. All patients taking colchicine developed diarrhea, usually before pain relief was achieved [4]
Level P

Acceptability to patient
Limited by diarrhea, nausea, vomiting.

Follow up plan
If recurrent attacks and hyperuricemia, most patients find allopurinol more acceptable.

Patient and caregiver information
Suggest reduction in dose if diarrhea occurs.

TRIAMCINOLONE
Dose
- Intra-articular injection small joint: 2–6mg
- Intra-articular injection large joint: 10–20mg

Efficacy
- As effective as indomethacin. Joint aspiration prior to injection may provide immediate relief
- Useful when NSAIDs are contraindicated

Risks/Benefits
Risks:
- Full aseptic precautions are essential
- Second-line therapy
- Does not provide quick response; make take several hours for relief
- Risk of infection with intra-articular injection
- Risk of joint destruction and sepsis if septic arthritis is misdiagnosed as gout

Side-effects and adverse reactions
- Pain at injection site
- Flushing

Interactions (other drugs)
- Antidiabetics ▪ Isoniazid ▪ Rifampicin ▪ Salicylates

Contraindications
Local or systemic infection

Acceptability to patient
Fair. Patients must not expect a rapid response.

Follow up plan
Ask patient to return for review once acute attack resolved.

Patient and caregiver information
Patient should expect some relief in several hours but should be instructed to watch for signs of infection at injection site.

Surgical therapy
JOINT ASPIRATION
Efficacy
- Useful to relieve pressure and pain at a large joint with tense effusion (e.g. knee)
- Crystal identification required for definitive diagnosis
- Will help to rule out septic arthritis

Risks/Benefits
Risks:
- Chance of introducing sepsis using 'no touch' technique about 1 in 15,000
- Local pain at injection site

Benefit: rapid pain relief from reduction in tense effusion. Locally directed therapy

Acceptability to patient
High.

Follow up plan
Ask patient to return for review once acute attack resolved (information to be confirmed).

Patient and caregiver information
Patient should be instructed to monitor for signs of infection at aspiration site. Patient should be informed that effusion reduced with aspiration may reaccumulate.

LIFESTYLE
- Rest, with limb raised, during acute attack
- Reduce alcohol intake (no more than two drinks a day)
- Advise on fluid intake: tell patients to make sure they drink enough to keep their urine pale
- Long-term dietary modifications may be useful

RISKS/BENEFITS
Helps speed resolution of attack.

ACCEPTABILITY TO PATIENT
Diet – poor.

FOLLOW UP PLAN
Check patient's weight and alcohol consumption at each visit; advise on lifestyle measures to prevent recurrence.

PATIENT AND CAREGIVER INFORMATION
Patient information leaflets are useful.

EFFICACY OF THERAPIES

- Acute gout relatively easy to manage in primary care
- Most people with hyperuricemia do not need antihyperuricemic therapy
- Most patients will benefit more from a combination of lifestyle interventions than from a single intervention

Review period

Arrange to review patient with acute gout within 7 days. Those not responding to initial therapy may be managed more aggressively and others may wish to discuss medium-term management of the disease.

PROGNOSIS

Most cases of acute gout resolve within a few days of commencing treatment, but recurrences are common.

Clinical pearls

Occasionally, most joints respond to first-line therapy but one or two remain painful and swollen. In this case it may be preferable to administer intra-articular injections to the target joints rather than increase the dose of oral therapy and risk toxicity.

Recurrence

- Majority of patients have a second attack within one or 2 years
- Consider colchicine or antihyperuricemic therapy if attacks are more frequent

Deterioration

- Usually result of noncompliance
- Occasionally necessary to reconsider diagnosis
- Refer to specialist if diagnosis is difficult

COMPLICATIONS

- Recurrent painful gouty episodes with significant impingement on lifestyle
- Untreated may result in renal failure
- Chronic tophaceous gout
- Early osteoarthritis in affected joints

CONSIDER CONSULT

- Refer if the attacks are difficult to control
- Acute gout in patients with renal disease or renal calculi often requires specialist follow up

RISK FACTORS

- Alcohol consumption: keep within recommended level for healthy adult
- Obesity: institute weight-reducing diet
- Hypertension: investigate and institute therapy
- Thiazide or loop diuretics: consider alternatives
- Other medications: salicylates, levodopa or carbidopa, ethambutol, pyrazinamide, niacin, cyclosporine

MODIFY RISK FACTORS
Lifestyle and wellness
ALCOHOL AND DRUGS

- Reduce alcohol intake (to no more than two drinks a day)
- Alcoholism: institute therapy

DIET

- Low-purine diet impractical
- Obesity should be tackled as, among many other negative health effects, it predisposes to gout
- Cholesterol reduction reduces chance of hyperlipidemia which is associated with development of gout, among its other deleterious effects

SCREENING

General population screening for gout is unnecessary, particularly as asymptomatic hyperuricemia should not be treated except in the presence of renal disease or permanently high urate levels.

PREVENT RECURRENCE

Most patients have recurrences within 1–2 years. Lifestyle measures sufficient in many patients. Even when they are not, many patients find NSAID treatment of acute attacks more acceptable than the alternatives. Antihyperuricemic therapy is overprescribed.

If there are recurrences, screen between attacks, screen for hyperuricemia by checking serum uric acid.

In the absence of associated disorders:

- First choice is to try lifestyle measures alone, then try the medications below if this fails
- Reduced-purine diet is probably a waste of time as compliance is very low; not worth advising more than avoidance of liver, sardines and anchovies unless patient has a diet unusually high in purines (foods are red meat, poultry, oily fish, liver, kidney, heart, gizzard, sweetbreads, yeast extracts, meat extracts, peas, beans, spinach, lentils)
- Small daily doses of NSAIDs prevent recurrence if lifestyle measures insufficient
- Colchicine prophylaxis is more effective than NSAIDs in recurrence prevention but often less acceptable to patient because dose required for control is often associated with diarrhea
- Side-effect profiles suggest colchicine is preferred to NSAIDs, but no controlled comparisons exist
- NSAID/colchicine prophylaxis particularly important during introduction of antihyperuricemic therapy to prevent acute attacks as initial response to altered urate levels

Neither NSAIDs nor colchicine prevent urate crystal deposition; tophi may still form
Consider antihyperuricemic therapy only when there are recurrent severe attacks likely to lead to joint damage or progression to chronic tophaceous gout

Reassess coexisting disease
Check fasting lipids for hyperlipidemia – hypertriglyceridemia predisposes to gout
Perform annual check on renal function

ASSOCIATIONS

American College of Rheumatology/Association of Rheumatology Health Professionals
1800 Century Place, Suite 205
Atlanta, GA 30345-4300
Tel: (404) 633 3777
Fax: (404) 633 1870
www.rheumatology.org

Arthritis Foundation
330 West Peachtree Street
Atlanta, GA
Tel: (800) 283 7800
www.arthritis.org

Canadian Arthritis Network
600 University Avenue, Suite 600
Toronto, Ontario M5G 1X5
Canada
Tel: (416) 586 4770
Fax: (416) 586 8628

KEY REFERENCES

- Emmerson BT. Drug therapy: the management of gout. N Engl J Med 1996; 334(7):445–51
- Pittman JR, Bross MH. Diagnosis and management of gout. Am Fam Physician 1999; 59(7): 1799–806
- Pal B, Foxall M, et al. How is gout managed in primary care?. Clin Rheumatol 2000; 19(1):21–5

Evidence references and guidelines

1 American College of Rheumatology. Guidelines for obtaining a Rheumatology Consultation. Available at
www.rheumatology.org
2 American College of Rheumatology. Guidelines for the Initial Evaluation of the Adult Patient with Acute
Musculoskeletal Symptoms. Arthritis Rheum 1996;39:1–8. Available at www.rheumatology.org
3 Harris MD, Siegel LB, Alloway JA. Gout and hyperuricemia. Am Fam Physician, 1999;59:925–34
4 Pittman JR, Bross MH. Diagnosis and management of gout. Am Fam Physician, 1999;59:1799–806, 1810
5 Ahern MJ, Reid C, Gordon TP, et al. Does colchicine work? The results of the first controlled study in acute gout.
Aust NZ J Med 1987;17:301–4. Medline

CONTRIBUTORS

Russell C Jones , MD, MPH
Richard Brasington Jr, MD, FACP

CHRONIC TOPHACEOUS GOUT

DESCRIPTION

- Only develops when acute gout and hyperuricemia have not been controlled for a number of years
- Firm nodular swellings (tophi) form as a result of urate crystal deposition, usually on the digits or over the olecranon bursa or Achilles tendon, less commonly on the helix of the ear or any other site
- There is often chronic destructive arthritis of the joints that have suffered acute gout
- Hyperuricemia results from overproduction or under excretion of urate

KEY! DON'T MISS!

Raised blood pressure may be a sign of underlying renal failure.

BACKGROUND

ICD9 CODE

274.81 Tophaceous gout – ear only
274.82 Tophaceous gout

CARDINAL FEATURES

- Nodules on extensor surfaces (including chronic olecranon bursitis)
- Drainage of white substance ('toothpaste' or 'milk of urate') from tophi
- Characteristic radiographic features: periarticular punched-out erosions with overhanging edges and sclerotic margins
- There is often an extended symptom-free interval, which may last for years, after acute gout attacks

CAUSES

Common causes

- Excess alcohol intake (reduces urate excretion; beer high in purines)
- Diuretic use: many drugs reduce renal urate clearance. Thiazide diuretics are most often implicated in acute gout attacks. Low-dose aspirin or phenylbutazone, furosemide, ethacrynic acid, ethambutol, pyrazinamide, nicotinic acid may also precipitate gout
- Renal disease: any cause of renal disease predisposes the individual to gout because clearance of urate is adversely affected. Renal failure may be chronic or acute associated with reduced renal perfusion (e.g. postmyocardial infarction, trauma, sepsis, surgical procedures)
- Hypertension is an independent risk factor for gout
- Obesity (implies high purine intake; decreases urate excretion)
- Increased cell turnover: particularly in hemopoietic malignancies but also related to chemotherapy and extensive psoriasis
- Excess purine consumption in conjunction with urate undersecretion

Rare causes

- Hypothyroidism
- Hyperparathyroidism
- Inherited hypertriglyceridemias
- Environmental toxins, particularly lead

Serious causes

- Neoplastic disorders and their treatment
- Drugs to prevent transplant rejection

Contributory or predisposing factors

- Inadequately controlled hypertension
- Hypertriglyceridemia

EPIDEMIOLOGY

Incidence and prevalence

INCIDENCE
Males 1–3/1000, females 0–2/1000.

PREVALENCE
Males 5–28/1000, females 1–6/1000.

Demographics

AGE
- Peak age of onset 40–50 years in men, over 60 years in women
- Very rare in children (only seen in malignant conditions and rare metabolic disorders such as Lesch-Nyhan syndrome and PRPP synthetase excess syndrome)

GENDER
- Mainly men
- Rare in premenopausal women but elderly women on diuretics are susceptible

GENETICS
- Hyperuricemia may be due to inherited enzyme abnormalities and urate undersecretion
- Rare genetic causes exist but only consider in atypical/severe disease or very young patients

SOCIOECONOMIC STATUS
Often low: Most patients seek treatment for acute gout and so don't progress to chronic tophaceous gout.

DIFFERENTIAL DIAGNOSIS
Nodular rheumatoid arthritis
FEATURES
- Subcutaneous nodules over pressure points, most commonly at the elbow but also occurring at sacrum, occiput, and Achilles tendon
- Nodules can be early indicators of rheumatoid arthritis

Other destructive arthropathies
FEATURES
Including soft-tissue calcification, other soft-tissue masses

Inflammatory osteoarthritis
FEATURES
- Soft-tissue and bony swelling in typical distribution (gout preferentially attacks joints previously affected by osteoarthritis)
- No tophi

Pseudogout
FEATURES
- Inflammatory symptoms and signs similar to gout but affecting different joints in different patient group
- No tophi

SIGNS & SYMPTOMS
Signs
- Tophus formation common at olecranon, Achilles' tendon, digits. Less frequent on the helix/antihelix of the ear and rarely around eye, heart, spine, and carpal tunnel
- Signs of secondary osteoarthritis in previously affected joints
- Raised blood pressure is sign of renal insufficiency
- There may be ulceration and secondary infection of tophi

Symptoms
- Patient may report history of acute gout attacks but these are less frequent in longstanding gout
- Tophi may be uncomfortable if knocked or painful if they ulcerate and/or become infected

ASSOCIATED DISORDERS
- Acute gout
- Hypertension
- Renal failure
- Hypothyroidism
- Hyperparathyroidism
- Hyperlipidemias
- Alcoholism
- Obesity
- High cell turnover states (e.g. psoriasis, polycythemia, leukemia)

KEY! DON'T MISS!
Raised blood pressure may be a sign of underlying renal failure.

CONSIDER CONSULT
- Chronic gout in the context of organ transplantation (very difficult to control)

- Associated renal disease: refer to rheumatologist and/or nephrologist
- Diagnostic uncertainty: either in acute gout attack, especially if it might be septic arthritis (patient systemically unwell, predisposition to sepsis, joint affected atypical of acute gout), or when cannot be distinguished from rheumatoid arthritis, osteoarthritis or pseudogout

INVESTIGATION OF THE PATIENT
Direct questions to patient
Q **Have you had acute gout?** Usually patient has had many acute gout attacks before tophi form but acute attacks become less frequent or stop in chronic stage

Q **Do any joints hurt now?** Joint damage (often severe) usually occurs before tophi develop

Q **Are you on any medications?** May reveal cause of hyperuricemia, e.g. thiazide diuretics

Q **What is your drinking pattern?** Excess alcohol causes hyperuricemia

Q **Do you eat a lot of purine-rich foods?** Red meat, poultry, oily fish, liver, kidney, heart, gizzard, sweetbreads, yeast extracts, meat extracts, peas, beans, spinach, lentils

Contributory or predisposing factors
Q **Is blood pressure normal?** Inadequately controlled hypertension predisposes to gout

Q **Are there signs of hyperlipidemia?** Hypertriglyceridemia often accompanies gout, and should be assessed and treated as appropriate

Family history
Q **Is there a family history of similar problems?** Family history common in middle-aged men with gout due to mild hyperuricemia and reduced urate excretion

Q **Is there a family history of early ischemic heart disease?** Could alert to hypertriglyceridemia

Examination
- **Check blood pressure.** Hypertension strongly associated with gout (25–50% of patients have hypertension); should be managed appropriately to reduce cardiovascular risk factors
- **Inspect joints and look for tophi**
- **Inspect eyes for signs of hypertriglyceridemia** – common in gout and serum lipid test may be needed
- **Check for signs of liver disease or alcohol abuse**
- **Check blood pressure and dipstick urine for renal disease.** If renal disease suspected, refer for specialist treatment
- **Check for signs of infection if there is concomitant acute attack** – rule out septic arthritis
- **Is the patient obese?** Obesity predisposes to gout

Guidelines for the Initial Evaluation of the Adult Patient with Acute Musculoskeletal Symptoms have been published by the American College of Rheumatology [1].

Summary of investigative tests
- Serum urate: hyperuricemia predisposes to acute and chronic gout but a normal or low serum uric acid does not exclude the diagnosis. Serum urate is a helpful test if raised in relevant clinical situation
- Needle aspiration of tophus and examination of fluid for crystals proves the diagnosis
- Screen for hyperlipidemia by measuring fasting triglycerides
- Check renal function
- Obtain radiographs of hands and feet to determine presence of typical gouty erosions and/or changes of osteoarthritis
- Biopsy/pathology of tophi to demonstrate urate crystals is only ever needed after specialist referral in cases of diagnostic difficulty (to distinguish gout from rheumatoid arthritis)
- If any suspicion of septic arthritis, immediate referral to specialist is recommended; if not possible, send synovial fluid for culture for pathogens

DIAGNOSTIC DECISION

The gouty tophus is pathognomic of chronic gout, as are the punched-out erosions with overhanging sclerotic margins seen on radiography in 50% of patients. Identification of urate crystals is essential in diagnosing chronic gout and is easily achieved in the majority of patients.

Guidelines

The American Academy of Family Physicians have published information on chronic gout [2,3]

CLINICAL PEARL(S)

Subcutaneous tophi have a whitish hue, which can be appreciated on careful inspection, especially in the fingers.

THE TESTS
Body fluids
SERUM URATE (AS URIC ACID)
Description
Cuffed venous blood sample, may combine with renal function and fasting lipids.

Advantages/Disadvantages
- Advantage: raised uric acid helpful circumstantial evidence to diagnosis of gout
- Disadvantage: normal levels do not eliminate gout. In 15% of acute attacks of gout the serum urate falls

Normal
There is considerable overlap between the normal and gouty population with respect to serum uric acid concentration. Gout relatively uncommon (0.8/1000 annually) below 7.0mg/dL (0.42mmol/L) but incidence rises rapidly at higher concentrations.

Abnormal
- Above 7.0mg/dL (0.42mmol/L) but see previous comment
- Keep in mind the possibility of a false-positive result

Cause of abnormal result
Hyperuricemia is caused by overproduction or undersecretion of uric acid. Most commonly, patients inherit predisposition to gout by an isolated renal lesion causing undersecretion. A number of environmental and concomitant factors can also result in hyperuricemia.

Tests of function
RENAL FUNCTION
Description
- Venous blood for creatinine estimation
- Urine dipstick, urine microscopy or 24-h urine for protein and creatinine measurement

Advantages/Disadvantages
Advantages:
- Identifies renal failure where creatinine above normal range
- Provides baseline measurement of renal function

Disadvantages:
- Gives no definite diagnosis of gout or cause of poor renal function
- Renal function (creatinine clearance) may be impaired despite 'normal' result
- A urine dipstick is sensitive to hematuria and proteinuria indicating renal tract abnormality but hematuria should be confirmed on light microscopy

- Measurement of 24 h creatinine and protein excretion allows the best estimate of renal function but is time-consuming and inconvenient for the patient

Normal
- Urea (blood urea nitrogen): 8–18mg/dL
- Serum creatinine: 0.6–1.2mg/dL (normal ranges vary between laboratories and by sex and body mass)
- Serum potassium: 3.5–5mEq/L
- Serum calcium: 8.8–10.3mg/dL
- Serum phosphate: 2.5–5mg/dL
- Creatinine clearance: 75–124ml/min
- Urine protein: <150mg/24 h
- Urine hemoglobin: none
- Keep in mind the possibility of a false-positive result

Abnormal
Elevated blood urea nitrogen, serum creatinine, hyperkalemia, hypercalcemia, hyperphosphatemia, elevated urine proteins and presence of hemoglobin in the urine are indicative of renal failure.

Cause of abnormal result
Chronic renal failure.

Biopsy
IDENTIFICATION OF URATE CRYSTALS IN TOPHI
Description
After needle aspiration of the tophus a small amount of tophaceous material is smeared onto a slide and viewed under polarizing light.

Advantages/Disadvantages
Advantage: presence of negatively birefringent crystals confirms gout and excludes rheumatoid arthritis (almost never occur together)

Disadvantages:
- Fluid has to be examined under polarized light microscopy by a specialist experienced in distinguishing urate crystals from other arthropathic crystals
- Presence of crystals does not exclude septic arthritis

Normal
No crystals found.

Abnormal
- Crystals are found under low-power dark field then identified as urate under high-power polarized light by their strong negative birefringence
- Keep in mind the possibility of a false-positive result

Cause of abnormal result
Crystal deposition.

Imaging
RADIOGRAPHY
Advantages/Disadvantages
- Advantage: usually distinguishes chronic tophaceous gout from rheumatoid arthritis
- Disadvantage: in the earlier stages of chronic tophaceous gout may be hard to distinguish from other arthropathies

Abnormal
- Calcification and eventually ossification of tophi
- Bony erosions of joint and some distance from joint may be seen; classically have 'punched-out' appearance usually with a sclerotic margin
- In 50% of patients, erosions have an 'overhang' margin pathognomic of gout
- Some patients develop intraosseous calcification of tophaceous material near affected joints so the bones appear hyperdense
- Juxta-articular osteoporosis absent and joint space maintained (distinguishing from rheumatoid arthritis) except where gout has affected previously osteoarthritic joints where joint space may be reduced
- Keep in mind the possibility of a false-positive result

Cause of abnormal result
- Deposition of urate crystals in tophi
- Intraosseous calcification

TREATMENT

CONSIDER CONSULT

- Failure of antihyperuricemic therapy, deterioration during antihyperuricemic therapy, or plasma urate control difficult to achieve
- Patient intolerant of allopurinol
- Patient is taking azathioprine but needs allopurinol for gout – specialist supervision needed to co-prescribe these drugs, with adjustment of azathioprine dose
- Gout in the context of organ transplantation (very difficult to control)
- Surgery may be required to relieve tophus pressure on important points such as spinal cord though this is very rare

IMMEDIATE ACTION

See patient with hot swollen painful joint immediately to assess whether any suspicion of septic arthritis, which requires urgent referral for investigation and treatment.

PATIENT AND CAREGIVER ISSUES

Health-seeking behavior

- **Self-medications tried?** Low-dose aspirin can precipitate acute gout attack, by reducing renal excretion of uric acid
- **Waited too long?** Patient who has untreated chronic tophaceous gout but has not visited physician before is rare: likely that socioeconomic status is low or other factors involved (e.g. alcoholism)

MANAGEMENT ISSUES

Goals

- Control hyperuricemia to prevent further tophus formation and joint damage
- Reassess diagnosis in uncontrolled hyperuricemia: adjust therapy, or consider differential diagnoses or coexisting disease
- Institute appropriate therapy if there is an acute gout attack

Management in special circumstances

COEXISTING DISEASE

Consider coexisting disease and institute appropriate therapy

- History of acute gout does not exclude coexisting arthropathies – e.g. psoriatic arthritis, osteoarthritis – but in effect excludes rheumatoid arthritis
- Be alert for chronic renal insufficiency, which complicates the administration of NSAIDs and allopurinol
- Hypertension is a common causative factor in hyperuricemia; thiazide diuretics for hypertension may be causal/contributory factors
- Hyperlipidemia, most commonly hypertriglyceridemia (type IV), is seen in many gout patients

COEXISTING MEDICATION

- Low-dose aspirin for coexisting disease can exacerbate hyperuricemia
- Thiazide diuretics for hypertension may be causal/contributory factors

PATIENT SATISFACTION/LIFESTYLE PRIORITIES

In patients with frequent acute attacks, moderation or elimination of alcohol consumption is important.

SUMMARY OF THERAPEUTIC OPTIONS
Choices
- Antihyperuricemic therapy is usually necessary and allopurinol is by far the first choice
- Probenecid may be used if the patient is unable to tolerate allopurinol
- Sulfinpyrazone may be used if the patient is unable to tolerate allopurinol
- Excision of tophi is only necessary if tophi press on important structures, e.g. spinal cord, or if there is vascular disease associated with infected tophi
- Advise patient on lifestyle changes that will help
- Therapy for acute gout if patient is currently having an attack and is already on antihyperuricemic therapy

With antihyperuricemic therapy:
- Risk of acute gout attacks increased during initiation of antihyperuricemic therapy: co-prescribe colchicine or low-dose NSAIDs for first few months until uric acid level stabilizes
- Monitor uric acid levels: goal is sustained serum urate less than 0.4mmol/L (6.5mg/dL), preferably less than 0.3mmol/L (5mg/dL)
- Monitor renal function

Guidelines
The American Academy of Family Physicians have published information on chronic gout [2,3]

Clinical pearls
- For most patients, the drug of choice to lower serum uric acid is allopurinol
- Never start allopurinol during an acute gout attack
- Once allopurinol has been started, it is not necessary to discontinue it during an acute attack
- Therapy to lower the serum uric acid should not be started unless gouty crystals have been demonstrated or the diagnosis confirmed by a rheumatologist

Never
- Never commence antihyperuricemic therapy during acute gout attacks: can transform simple attack into severe polyarticular attack
- Never commence antihyperuricemic therapy unless diagnosis is certain
- Never withdraw antihyperuricemic therapy during acute gout attack
- Never prescribe allopurinol to patients on azathioprine (can be done with reduced dose of azathioprine but requires specialist referral)

FOLLOW UP
Plan for review
- Review every 3 months in the first year after antihyperuricemic therapy initiated, then every 6–12 months thereafter
- Monitor renal function annually

Information for patient or caregiver
Adjustment of lifestyle can prevent recurrence of gout in mild hyperuricemia.

DRUGS AND OTHER THERAPIES: DETAILS
Drugs
ALLOPURINOL
Dose
Oral: 100–200mg once daily, increase every 2–4 weeks depending on severity usually 300–600mg daily, maximum dose 800mg/day.

Efficacy
- High chance of significantly reduced severity and frequency of attacks
- Tophi regression on long-term therapy and possible healing of bony lesions

Risks/Benefits
Risks:
- Do not initiate treatment during acute attack
- Ensure adequate fluid intake during treatment
- Caution in hepatic and renal impairment

Side-effects and adverse reactions
- Skin: rashes, alopecia, Stevens-Johnson syndrome
- Gastrointestinal: nausea, abdominal pain, peptic ulceration, cholestatic jaundice, diarrhea
- Liver failure
- Renal failure
- Central nervous system: drowsiness, headache
- Musculosceletal: athralgia, myopathy

Interactions (other drugs)
- ACE inhibitors ▪ Antacids ▪ Azathioprine ▪ Cyclophosphamide ▪ Mercaptopurine ▪ Oral anticoagulants ▪ Theophylline

Contraindications
Acute gout: do not commence treatment with allopurinol during acute attack

Acceptability to patient
High: great advantages are efficacy, once-daily dose and infrequency of side-effects.

Follow up plan
- Monitor renal function (high-dose allopurinol may reduce renal function)
- Check serum creatinine and liver function tests at intervals

Patient and caregiver information
Patient should be made aware that therapy is lifelong.

PROBENICID
Dose
Oral: 250mg twice daily, increase after one week to 500mg twice daily, thereafter increase gradually to a 2g/day, maximum dose 3g/day. Once control is achieved reduce for maintainance.

Efficacy
- Relatively effective provided the patient's renal function is well preserved (glomerular filtration rate >60mL/min)
- 75% of patients experience reduction in serum urate level to 6.7mg/dL (0.42mmol/L) on standard 1.5g/day dose probenicid

Risks/Benefits
Risks:
- Do not initiate treatment during acute attack
- Ensure adequate fluid intake during treatment
- Caution renal impairment, peptic ulceration

Side-effects and adverse reactions
- Skin: rashes, flushing
- Gastrointestinal: nausea, vomiting, sore gums
- Aplastic anemia
- Renal: nephrotic syndrome, renal calculi, urinary frequency
- Central nervous system: drowsiness, headache

Interactions (other drugs)
- Dapsone ▪ Dyphylline ▪ Methotrexate ▪ Salicylates ▪ Thiopental ▪ Zidovudine

Contraindications
- Acute gout: do not commence therapy during an attack ▪ Renal calculi ▪ Blood dysrasias
- Moderate to severe renal impairment

Acceptability to patient
Less than allopurinol: must be taken several times a day, and ensure at least 1500ml fluid/day and recommend drugs to alkalinize the urine in the first few weeks of therapy.

Follow up plan
Check efficacy by means of serum urate level after several weeks of therapy. Monitor renal function using serum creatinine.

Patient and caregiver information
Patient must be made aware that therapy is lifelong.

SULFINPYRAZONE
Dose
Oral: 200–400mg daily with food; increase over 2–3 weeks to 600mg daily. Continue until serum urate is below 0.4mmol/L, 6.5mg/dL; preferably below 0.3mmol/L, 5mg/dL then reduce for maintenance once control is achieved.

Efficacy
Sulfinpyrazone is a more potent uricosuric agent than probenecid and is more effective in patients with renal disease.

Risks/Benefits
Risks:
- Renal tract calculi are a significant risk if urine volume is not maintained at 1500ml/day
- Caution in cardiac disease, renal impairment and peptic ulceration

Benefits:
- Sulfinpyrazone is a potent uricosuric which is well tolerated
- There is an antithrombotic effect useful in some patients

Side-effects and adverse reactions
- Gastrointestinal: nausea, anorexia, peptic ulceration
- Fluid retention
- Allergic skin reactions
- Acute renal failure
- Hepatitis
- Agranulocytosis
- Aplastic anemia

- Leukopenia
- Thrombocytopenia

Interactions (other drugs)
- Antidiabetics   Beta-blockers   Methotrexate   Oral anticoagulants   Salicylates

Contraindications
- Peptic ulceration   Blood dyscrasias   Avoid salicylates   Porphyria   Renal calculi
- Acute gout: do not commence treatment with allopurinol during acute attack

Acceptability to patient
Generally well tolerated.

Follow up plan
Monitor efficacy of therapy with serum urate level after several weeks to ensure correct dosage.
Monitor renal function using serum creatinine levels.

Patient and caregiver information
Patient must be made aware that therapy is lifelong.

Surgical therapy
EXCISION OF TOPHI
Surgery may be employed to remove a gouty tophus where it is impinging on a critical organ (e.g. on the spinal cord). Sometimes tophi become infected and require surgical debridement if the infection becomes deep-seated and causes sytemic illness.

Risks/Benefits
Risk: only performed where risk of morbidity is great.

Follow up plan
Patients undergoing surgical procedures for debridement or removal of gouty tophi should be managed with antihyperuricemic therapy to reduce the risk of recurrence.

Patient and caregiver information
The patient should be educated to understand the importance of effective antihyperuricemic therapy postoperatively.

LIFESTYLE
- Advise patient to abstain from alcohol
- Advise on fluid intake: tell patients to make sure they drink enough to keep their urine pale
- Rest, with limb raised, during acute attack
- Tackle obesity
- Reduced-purine diet is probably a waste of time as compliance is very low; not worth advising more than avoidance of liver, sardines and anchovies unless patient has unusually high-purine diet (foods are red meat, poultry, oily fish, liver, kidney, heart, gizzard, sweetbreads, yeast extracts, meat extracts, peas, beans, spinach, lentils)

RISKS/BENEFITS
Benefit: controlling hyperuricemia will prevent further acute gout attacks, prevent further tophus development, and lead to the resolution of tophi and healing of tophaceous damage to joints.

ACCEPTABILITY TO PATIENT
Diet: poor, and reduction in alcohol intake often limited.

FOLLOW UP PLAN

A commitment to follow up patients who have been advised to reduce alcohol intake has been shown to improve compliance rates.

PATIENT AND CAREGIVER INFORMATION

Patients need to know about the link between alcohol consumption and gout and that gout is a lifelong predisposition which may result in premature osteoarthritis and/or kidney disease if untreated.

EFFICACY OF THERAPIES

Allopurinol is extremely effective in controlling gout, provided used correctly: gout may therefore be considered 'curable'. Reduction of the serum urate to 5mg/dL or lower results in:

- Significant reduction in frequency and severity or cessation of acute gouty attacks
- Shrinkage (and perhaps disappearance) of tophi with long-term allopurinol therapy (years)
- Some reversal of joint damage, bony lytic lesions may heal but any periarticular damage caused by acute gout is likely to result in premature secondary osteoarthritis

Evidence

PDxMD are unable to cite evidence which meets our criteria for evidence.

Review period

Every 3 months in the first year after antihyperuricemic therapy initiated, then every 6–12 months thereafter.

PROGNOSIS

Most cases of acute gout will resolve within a few days of commencing treatment, but recurrences are common.

Clinical pearls

Allopurinol is such an effective drug that real failure of therapy is relatively rare. Most patients' serum uric acid falls on a dose of 300mg allopurinol per day or less. Among patients who do not respond, poor compliance is the most frequent explanation.

Therapeutic failure

Failure of antihyperuricemic therapy requires specialist referral.

Deterioration

Recurrent deterioration during antihyperuricemic therapy requires specialist referral.

COMPLICATIONS

- Recurrent attacks of acute arthritis
- Tophaceous deposits which are a nuisance, and might become infected
- Joint damage from tophi which might become irreversible
- Chronic urate nephropathy (unusual)
- Kidney stones: 10 times more frequent in chronic gout patients

RISK FACTORS

- Alcohol consumption: keep within recommended level for healthy adult
- Obesity: institute weight-reducing diet
- Hypertension: investigate and institute therapy
- Thiazide diuretics: consider alternatives

MODIFY RISK FACTORS
Lifestyle and wellness
ALCOHOL AND DRUGS

- Alcohol consumption: keep within recommended level for healthy adult
- Alcoholism: institute therapy

DIET

- Low-purine diet impractical
- Obesity should be tackled as, among many other negative health effects, it predisposes to gout
- Cholesterol reduction reduces chance of hyperlipidemia which leads to development of gout, among its other deleterious effects

SCREENING
General population screening for chronic gout is unnecessary; hyperuricemia should not be treated in the absence of gout.

PREVENT RECURRENCE
The key to recurrence prevention is antihyperuricemic therapy to reduce serum uric acid to around 0.3mmol/L (5mg/dL), and prophylactic medication (colchicine) and NSAIDS to prevent exacerbation of acute attacks in the first 3–12 months after urate-lowering drug therapy is started. Patients should abstain from alcohol.

RESOURCES

ASSOCIATIONS

American College of Rheumatology/Association of Rheumatology Health Professionals
1800 Century Place
Suite 205
Atlanta, GA 30345–4300
Tel: (404) 633 3777
Fax: (404) 633 1870
www.rheumatology.org

Arthritis Foundation
1330 West Peachtree Street
Atlanta, GA
Tel: (800) 283 7800
www.arthritis.org

The Arthritis Society
393 University Avenue
Suite 1700
Toronto, Ontario M5G 1E6
Canada
Tel: (800) 321 1433, (416) 979 7228
Fax: (416) 979 8366
www.arthritis.ca

Canadian Arthritis Network
600 University Avenue
Suite 600
Toronto, Ontario, M5G 1X5
Canada
Tel: (416) 586 4770
Fax: (416) 586 8628
E-mail: CAN@arthritis.ca

KEY REFERENCES

- Conaghan PG, Day RO. Risks and benefits of drugs used in the management and prevention of gout. Drug Saf 1994;11(4):252–8
- Gout. In: Klippel JH Dieppe PA Ferri FF (eds) Primary Care Rheumatology London: Mosby, 1999, p117
- Perez-Ruiz F, Alonso-Ruiz A, Calabozo M, et al. Efficacy of allopurinol and benzbromarone for the control of hyperuricemia. A pathogenic approach to the treatment of primary chronic gout. Ann Rheum Dis 1998;57:545–9
- McCarthy GM, Barthelemy CR, Veum JA, Wortmann RL. Influence of antihyperuricemic therapy on the clinical and radiographic progression of gout. Arthritis Rheum 1991;34:1489–94

Guidelines

1 American College of Rheumatology. Guidelines for the Initial Evaluation of the Adult Patient with Musculoskeletal Symptoms. Arthritis Rheum 1996;39:1–8. Available from www.rheumatology.com
2 Harris MP, Siegel LB, Alloway JA. Gout and hyperuricemia. Am Fam Physician 1999;59:925–34
3 Pittman JR, Bross MH. Diagnosis and management of gout. Am Fam Physician 1999;59:1799–806, 1810

FAQS
Question 1
Does chronic gout inevitably follow acute gouty arthritis?

ANSWER 1
No. Many patients will have only intermittent acute attacks with chronic gouty arthritis.

Question 2
Should allopurinol be discontinued during an acute attack?

ANSWER 2
No, but allopurinol therapy should not be initiated during an acute attack.

Question 3
Is dietary restriction essential in the treatment of chronic gouty arthritis?

ANSWER 3
Diet is relatively unimportant in patients taking allopurinol. However, excessive alcohol consumption can trigger gout attacks in such patients.

CONTRIBUTORS
Shane Clarke MB BS, MRCP

LUMBAR SPONDYLOSIS

DESCRIPTION

- Lumbar spondylosis encompasses lumbar disk bulges, herniations, facet joint degeneration, and vertebral bony overgrowths (osteophytes)
- Degenerative changes, including osteophyte formation, increase with age but are often asymptomatic
- Disk herniation is symptomatic when it causes nerve root compression and spinal stenosis
- Common symptoms include low back pain, sciatica, and restriction in back movement
- Treatment is usually conservative, although surgery is indicated for spinal cord compression or intractable pain
- Relapse is common, with patients experiencing episodic back pain

URGENT ACTION

Cauda equina syndrome requires urgent surgical spinal decompression to prevent permanent neurologic damage.

KEY! DON'T MISS!

Cauda equina syndrome, which requires urgent surgical spinal decompression to prevent permanent neurologic damage.

Lumbar spondylosis – BACKGROUND

ICD9 CODE

- 721.3 Lumbar spondylosis
- 724.02 Lumbar stenosis
- 344.60 Cauda equina syndrome

SYNONYMS
Lumbar stenosis.

CARDINAL FEATURES

- The lumbar spine consists of four to six vertebrae with a disk in between each. Each disk comprises a central nucleus pulposus surrounded by the annulus fibrosis, and has a cartilaginous endplate
- Disease results from degenerative changes in the lumbar disk annulus, vertebral body, and facet joints
- Lumbar disks are those most likely to prolapse and herniate, especially the two most distal disks
- Disk degeneration and osteophyte formation is classified into three phases: phase I is the dysfunctional phase, phase II is the unstable phase, and phase III is the final stabilization phase
- Disks endure micro- and macrotraumas that lead to degenerative changes causing disk bulging and herniation in phases I and II
- Osteophytes form in phase III on anterior, lateral, and posterior aspects of vertebral central bodies caused by stress on the annular ligament
- Osteophyte formation is common, increasing with age; usually it is asymptomatic
- Disk degeneration and osteophyte formation can lead to nerve root compression, spinal stenosis, and spinal instability
- Nerve root compression leads to low back pain, sciatica, and restriction of back movement
- Spinal stenosis and spinal instability can lead to neurologic complications
- Treatment is usually conservative but surgery is indicated for spinal stenosis, spinal instability, and intractable pain
- Cauda equina syndrome can result if the lumbar disk prolapses centrally, affecting multiple lumbar and sacral roots; it leads to saddle anesthesia, urinary incontinence or retention, and paralysis. It requires urgent surgical spinal decompression to prevent permanent neurologic damage
- Relapse is common, with patients experiencing episodic back pain

CAUSES
Common causes
The exact cause of disk degeneration is unknown, although trauma, leading to an acute annular tear, may be the inciting pathologic event. Disk degeneration and osteophyte formation are common with age, in which persistent and recurrent forces can lead to disk microtrauma and macrotrauma, and is classified into three phases:

- Phase I (dysfunctional phase) is caused by trauma leading to tears and fissures in the outer annulus of the disk. Endplate separation causes waste accumulation and impaired disk nutrition
- Phase II (unstable phase) results in multiple annular tears, internal disk disruption, reduced disk-space height, and disk herniation. Zygapophyseal joints exhibit cartilage degeneration and capsular subluxation
- Phase III (final stabilization phase) leads to disk resorption and fibrosis, disk-space narrowing, endplate destruction, and osteophyte formation

Phases I and II cause more back pain than phase III, although an individual may exhibit different phases within different disks.

Disk degeneration is probably multifactorial, with age and acute trauma being the most important causes.

Rare causes
There is a genetic link with the CC genotype of the transforming growth factor-beta1 gene found in Japanese women.

Serious causes
Acute trauma can lead to disk herniation, causing spinal stenosis and neurologic signs.

Contributory or predisposing factors
- Adiposity is seen as a risk factor in UK populations but not in Japanese populations
- Heavy regular exercise that stresses the disk and annular ligament may lead to disk degeneration and osteophyte formation
- A traumatic event such as heavy lifting or a sudden twisting movement can precipitate back pain and other clinical features
- Occupations that require repeated lifting can lead to clinical features of lumbar spondylosis
- Patients with a past medical history of lumbar surgery have changes in lumbar biomechanics that predispose to lumbar spondylosis
- Depression and emotional lability can exacerbate the clinical features perceived by the patient

EPIDEMIOLOGY
Incidence and prevalence
FREQUENCY
- 5% of the population is affected by low back pain per year
- Life-time incidence of low back pain is between 60% and 90% of the population
- 400,000 workplace back injuries resulting in disability occurred in the US during 1990
- Low back pain causes 2.4 million Americans to be disabled, with 50% becoming chronically disabled
- Direct medical cost of low back pain was estimated to be >$25 billion in the US during 1990

Demographics
AGE
- Disk herniation typically occurs between 20 and 40 years of age
- Spinal stenosis usually occurs in those over 40 years of age
- Low back pain is rare in those below 20 years of age

GENDER
Male = female.

RACE
No racial predisposition.

GENETICS
There is a genetic link with the CC genotype of the transforming growth factor-beta1 gene found in Japanese women.

SOCIOECONOMIC STATUS
Occupations that require safe and proper lifting (nursing and removals staff) can lead to back pain. Training with lifting should be given to such employees.

DIFFERENTIAL DIAGNOSIS
Lumbar muscular sprain
Muscular sprain of the back can mimic the clinical features of lumbar spondylosis.

FEATURES
- Muscular sprain is common after exercise or heavy lifting
- Back pain and restriction in movement are the main clinical features
- Clinical features are usually more localized than in lumbar spondylosis
- Analgesic agents, including NSAIDs, are effective
- Clinical features normally resolve rapidly

Neoplastic disease
Spinal tumor is a sinister cause of back pain and must be excluded.

FEATURES
- Tumor may be of the spinal cord, meninges, nerves, or bone
- Metastases are not uncommon
- Clinical features include low back pain (especially at night and at rest), neurologic signs, weight loss, anemia, and bladder dysfunction
- Careful medical history to elicit previous malignancies is important
- A simple radiograph is a good screening test for metastatic malignant disease causing back pain, and will almost always show an abnormality if neurologic findings are present
- Magnetic resonance imaging should be requested if a spinal tumor is suspected
- Urgent neurosurgical referral is required for suspected spinal tumor patients

Hip osteoarthritis
Hip osteoarthritis is caused by degeneration and loss of joint cartilage.

FEATURES
- Common with increasing age
- Clinical features include joint stiffness, pain, and crepitus
- Fixed flexion deformities are common, leading to gait abnormalities
- Pain is typically in the groin, anterior thigh, and buttock
- Back pain can occur due to gait abnormality
- X-ray changes include joint space narrowing, subchondral sclerosis, and cyst and osteophyte formation
- Conservative treatment includes analgesia and physiotherapy
- Orthopedic referral is required for surgical management

Fibromyalgia
Fibromyalgia is a poorly defined disorder that is associated with diffuse musculoskeletal pain.

FEATURES
- Characterized by multiple trigger points and referred widespread pain
- Pain occurs in at least 11 of 18 selected tender spots on digital palpation according to criteria from the American College of Rheumatology
- Patients will have pain in multiple areas, as well as sleep disturbance and fatigue
- Females are nine times more likely than males to be diagnosed with this condition

- Occurs between 30 and 50 years of age
- Treatment consists of self-management, including exercise and explanation
- Mild analgesia and sedatives may be necessary
- Prognosis is uncertain

Osteoporosis
Osteoporosis involves progressive loss of bone, leading to bone fragility.

FEATURES
- Osteoporosis of the trabecular bone affects vertebral bodies
- Females are at 4-fold elevated risk in comparison with men
- Risk factors include age, premature menopause, corticosteroid use, smoking, and inactivity
- Osteoporosis produces back pain only in the setting of acute or previous fractures
- Clinical features result from crush fractures to the vertebral bodies
- Fracture compression leads to back pain and loss of height
- Bone mass density measurement is diagnostic
- X-rays of spine can reveal crush fractures
- Calcium and vitamin D supplementation is recommended in at-risk groups
- Hormone replacement therapy is important to prevent osteoporosis in postmenopausal females
- Bisphosphonates can be used to treat osteoporosis in both men and women

Intermittent claudication
Claudication caused by arterial atheroma produces pain in the lower limbs.

FEATURES
- Clinical features include leg pain brought on by exercise and relieved by rest
- Clinical examination of lower limbs may reveal diminished pulses, pallor, hair loss, and skin ulcers
- Continuous-wave Doppler can measure systolic arterial pressures and the ankle-brachial index (ABI)
- ABI range is 0.5–0.8 in claudication
- Duplex ultrasound locates occluded areas
- Angiography is used to confirm extent of arterial atheroma
- Conservative measures include stopping cigarette smoking and starting exercise
- Medication includes pentoxifylline and cilostazol
- Surgical measures include angioplasty and arterial grafting

Vertebral fracture
Traumatic, compression, or osteoporotic fractures of lumbar vertebrae can present with symptoms similar to those of cauda equina syndrome.

FEATURES
- Neurologic impairment is uncommon with osteoporotic fracture, but may be seen in the setting of trauma or pathologic fracture
- History of falls or trauma to spine may be reported
- Diagnosis is by clinical features, examination, and X-ray findings

SIGNS & SYMPTOMS
Signs
Disk herniation can lead to the following:
- Restricted range of movement in the lumbar spine, with reduced flexion, extension, and lateral flexion
- Local lumbar tenderness

- Neurologic signs resulting from radiculopathy, including paresthesia, lower limb weakness, and loss of tendon reflexes
- With L4–L5 prolapse, hallux extension is weak and sensation is reduced on outer dorsum of foot
- With L5–S1 prolapse, calf pain, weak foot plantar flexion, reduced sensation over sole and back of calf, and reduced ankle jerk all occur
- Gait abnormalities are not common

Lumbar osteophytes are normally asymptomatic but can lead to the following:
- Lumbar stenosis leading to spinal claudication (aching and heaviness in legs while walking, relieved with rest), pain on lumbar extension, and neurologic signs
- Nerve root compression leading to lumbar tenderness and sciatica on the affected side

Disk degeneration occurs in advanced disease as seen in the older population, with loss of height.

Cauda equina syndrome (if lumbar disk prolapses centrally affecting multiple lumbar and sacral roots) has the following signs:
- Anesthesia of the saddle area
- Impaired sphincter function
- Impaired sexual function
- Paralysis

Symptoms
Symptoms of disk herniation include:
- Low back pain, exacerbated by coughing, sneezing, or twisting, all of which transmit pressure to the affected nerve root
- Sciatic pain radiating down the leg of the affected side to below the knee
- Increased pain on bending toward the affected side
- Strange sensations, including 'pins and needles' and numbness of the leg
- Problems with walking are rare

Osteophytes are normally asymptomatic but may lead to:
- Low back pain
- Pseudoclaudication pain and sciatic pain when spinal stenosis is present
- Problems walking and weakness in the lower limbs are rare
- Numbness and loss of feeling in the lower limbs are rare

Cauda equina syndrome is a neurologic emergency and can present with the following symptoms:
- Urinary incontinence
- Sexual dysfunction
- Loss of sensation over the saddle area
- Loss of function of lower limbs with complete paralysis

ASSOCIATED DISORDERS
- Osteoarthritis of the vertebra can be associated with lumbar spondylosis, and can lead to low back pain and sciatica due to nerve root compression and inflammation
- Osteoporosis with crush fractures of the vertebra is associated with lumbar spondylosis, and can lead to low back pain and neurologic signs

KEY! DON'T MISS!
Cauda equina syndrome, which requires urgent surgical spinal decompression to prevent permanent neurologic damage.

CONSIDER CONSULT
- Orthopedic consultation should be sought if pain is intractable for 6 weeks or longer
- Neurosurgical spinal specialist referral should be sought if significant neurologic signs are present, including loss of power, loss of sensation, and loss of reflexes in the lower limb(s)

INVESTIGATION OF THE PATIENT
Direct questions to patient
Q **Do you have back pain or pain radiating down your leg(s)?** These symptoms are common in disk degeneration, causing nerve root compression. Pain normally radiates down the lower limb of the affected side

Q **For how long have you experienced these symptoms?** Patients often have experienced symptoms for a few weeks before seeking medical attention

Q **Have you had these pains before?** It is common for patients to have had episodes of back pain in their past medical history

Q **What type of pain are you experiencing?** Continual aching pain is classically found with disk degeneration

Q **What exacerbates the pain?** Sneezing, coughing, twisting, and moving toward the affected side normally exacerbate pain with disk herniation

Q **Does walking bring on your symptoms?** Spinal claudication is a feature of spinal stenosis, and leads to heaviness and aching of the legs, stopping the patient from walking

Q **Do you have any strange sensations in your legs?** Numbness and 'pins and needles', caused by nerve root compression and inflammation, are commonly described by patients with lumbar spondylosis

Q **Do you have problems walking?** The patient's ability to walk must be fully evaluated because impairment is a sinister feature and may require urgent neurosurgical referral

Q **Do you have any problems with urine incontinence or voiding?** This must be fully evaluated because it is a sinister feature and may require urgent neurosurgical referral, especially if cauda equina syndrome is suspected

Q **Do you have any problems with sexual function?** This must be fully evaluated because it is a sinister feature and may require urgent neurosurgical referral, especially if cauda equina syndrome is suspected

Q **Have you noticed the symptoms getting worse?** Cauda equina syndrome can occur if spinal compression worsens, leading to saddle anesthesia, lower limb paralysis, and sphincter dysfunction

Contributory or predisposing factors
Q **Was there a traumatic event that precipitated your back pain?** Patients with back pain often pinpoint the movement that led to the back pain (e.g. heavy lifting, exercise, or a sudden twisting motion)

Q **What is your occupation?** Workplace injuries caused over 400,000 industrial back injuries in 1990. Occupations involving heavy lifting increase risk of back injury, including healthcare workers lifting patients and manual workers such as builders and laborers. These injuries should be documented for medicolegal reasons

Q **Have you been diagnosed with kyphosis or scoliosis of the back?** Both deformities affect the spine's biomechanics, predisposing the patient to lumbar spondylosis

Q **Have you had previous surgery on your back?** Lumbar surgery changes the biomechanics of the spine, predisposing the patient to lumbar spondylosis

Q **Have you suffered from depression or anxiety?** Depression and emotional lability can cause patients to perceive pain to be more severe. This can have adverse consequences on the success of treatment and prognosis

Q **Have you been diagnosed with a cancer in the past?** Spinal tumor due to metastasis can cause back pain and needs to be excluded

Family history

Q **Does back pain affect other family members?** Genetic factors have been implicated, including the CC genotype of transforming growth factor-beta1 gene found in Japanese women

Examination

- **Measure weight and height of patient:** obesity may produce excess loads on the lumbar spine, leading to disk degeneration and complications
- **Inspect lumbar spine for deformity during flexion and extension:** kyphotic and scoliotic deformity may be revealed
- **Inspect lumbar spine for scars:** previous lumbar surgery can lead to disk degeneration
- **Palpate lumbar spine for tenderness:** tenderness may be revealed at the level of disk degeneration
- **Check range of movement of lumbar spine, including flexion, extension, and lateral flexion:** restriction of these movements is common, especially flexion, in lumbar spondylosis. It is important to record because the affected side has restricted lateral flexion
- **Observe gait:** Usually it is normal
- **Perform full neurologic examination for lower limbs:** includes motor power, sensation, and deep tendon reflexes (knee jerk, ankle jerk) to evaluate level of nerve root inflammation and spinal compression. With L4–L5 prolapse, hallux extension is weak and sensation is reduced on the outer dorsum of the foot
- With L5–S1 prolapse, calf pain, weak foot plantar flexion, reduced sensation over sole and back of calf, and reduced ankle jerk all occur. **Neurologic signs indicate a more sinister prognosis that requires specialist referral:** lumbar spondylosis rarely shows neurologic signs
- **Document straight leg lifting:** lifting the leg to 60° and then lowering at successive 15° stages. Test is positive if increasing low lumbar and buttock pain occurs as leg is lowered at successive stages
- **Check for range of movement in hips, knees and ankles:** all should be normal

Summary of investigative tests

- Lumbar spondylosis is mainly diagnosed on clinical features, and investigations are not indicated in most cases
- Imaging techniques are used to evaluate lumbar spondylosis if neurologic signs are found, and to evaluate intractable back pain
- Magnetic resonance imaging (MRI) is the criterion standard imaging modality for delineating lumbar disk herniations, scar tissue, and other spinal pathology. Cauda equina syndrome needs urgent assessment with MRI
- Computed tomography (CT) scanning is useful to detect bulging of the disk's annulus, endplate degenerative changes, and herniations. Imaging is not as detailed as with MRI, however, because with CT the spinal cord and nerve roots cannot be visualized without intrathecal contrast
- Myelography can be used to assess neural compression, and is often combined with CT scanning
- Plain X-ray of the lumbar spine will show gross anatomic intervertebral disk changes, which are best visualized on lateral views. Bony tumors, instabilities, misalignments, and congenital abnormalities can be identified

DIAGNOSTIC DECISION

Lumbar spondylosis, by definition, is a diagnosis that can be made only with the support of imaging data, which document the presence of degenerative disk disease and associated osteoarthritis. The challenge lies in determining whether the radiographic findings in fact account for the patient's symptoms.

CLINICAL PEARLS

- Radiographic evidence of lumbar spondylosis does not necessarily imply that it is the cause of back pain. Lumbar spondylosis is often asymptomatic
- An imaging procedure is most important if there are 'red flags' that suggest the presence of malignancy, infection, or neurologic compromise. These include pain at night or at rest, fever, loss of bowel or bladder function, and weight loss

THE TESTS
Imaging
MAGNETIC RESONANCE IMAGING (MRI)
Description

- Criterion standard imaging modality for detection of disk pathology
- Uses magnetic field to obtain direct multiplanar image
- Images show superb soft-tissue contrast and resolution
- Accurately details intervertebral disk degeneration
- Suspected cauda equina needs urgent assessment with MRI scan

Advantages/Disadvantages
Advantages:

- The best images are obtained through MRI
- Accurately locates and delineates disk degeneration, especially far lateral disks
- Relatively noninvasive to patient
- Guides neurosurgeon if surgery is contemplated
- Good safety profile in experienced centers
- Low false-negative rate (high sensitivity)

Disadvantages:

- Expensive
- Requires specialist centers to obtain and interpret images
- Magnetic, so all metal must be removed from patient prior to scanning
- Significant false-positive rate; low specificity, with disk degeneration seen in 35% of asymptomatic patients aged 20–39 years and in 100% of patients aged 60–80 years
- Imaging report not always representative of clinical features
- Bony structure outline is inferior to that with computed tomography scans

Normal
No abnormalities of intervertebral disks and vertebral bodies with normal alignments of soft-tissue.

Abnormal

- Diminished signal intensity indicates disk degeneration due to diminished water and glycosaminoglycan content, and increased collagen content
- Cartilaginous endplate changes as classified into type 1 (endplate disruption), type 2 (replacement of hemopoietic elements and sclerosis), and type 3 (combination of 1 and 2)
- Loss of disk height, radial tears to annulus

Cause of abnormal result

- Disk degeneration
- Cauda equina syndrome

Drugs, disorders and other factors that may alter results

- Low specificity: disk degeneration will be present in 100% of patients aged 60–80 years, even with no clinical features
- It is imperative to obtain good clinical history and examination results when interpreting MRI scan, especially if surgery is contemplated

COMPUTED TOMOGRAPHY (CT) SCANNING
Description

- Delineates symmetric uniform degenerative changes of disk, including annular bulge and herniation
- Optimum protocol is overlapping 3–5mm axial section images in 3mm increments with multiplanar reformations
- Loss of disk height can be demonstrated by sagittal reformations
- Can be combined with myelography to evaluate severe lumbar spondylosis and for preoperative assessment

Advantages/Disadvantages
Advantages:

- Demonstrates disk changes, including endplate degeneration, annular bulge, loss of disk height, sclerosis, and cortical changes
- Relatively noninvasive to patient
- Good safety profile in experienced centers
- Low false-negative rate (high sensitivity)

Disadvantages:

- Expensive
- Does not show spinal cord and nerve roots reliably in the absence of intrathecal contrast
- Requires specialist centers to obtain and interpret images
- Significant false-positive rate; low specificity, with disk degeneration seen in 35% of asymptomatic volunteers
- Disk degeneration images not as detailed as that with MRI

Normal
No abnormalities in intervertebral disks and vertebral bodies, with normal alignments of soft tissue.

Abnormal

- Symmetric uniform changes of disk, with diffuse peripheral extension of disk material representing annular bulge
- Cartilaginous endplate degeneration, sclerosis, and cortical changes
- Loss of disk height and narrowing

PLAIN X-RAYS OF LUMBAR SPINE
Description

- Can be useful to delineate gross anatomic intervertebral disk changes
- Disk narrowing and loss of height can be evaluated with lumbar X-rays
- Standing anteroposterior and lateral films should be obtained
- Bony tumors, instabilities, and congenital abnormalities can be identified
- Oblique views of neural foramina delineate degenerative changes with disk narrowing and osteophytes
- Flexion and extension views determine whether excess motion occurs between two vertebral bodies
- All preoperative patients should have plain lumbar spine X-rays

Advantages/Disadvantages
Advantages:

- Inexpensive
- Noninvasive
- Useful in evaluating disk space narrowing and loss of height

- Readily available
- Usually shows an abnormality in setting of metastatic disease of spine causing neurologic symptoms

Disadvantages:
- Detail limited, with only gross anatomical changes demonstrated
- Unable to define spinal stenosis, disk annulus bulges, or herniations
- Radiation dose relatively high to obtain good images
- Not recommended in pregnancy

Normal
No abnormalities seen in vertebral column.

Abnormal
- Disk degeneration, including loss of height, endplate sclerosis, and osteophytes
- Subluxation of vertebral bodies
- Loss of vertebral bone and spinal process outline

Cause of abnormal result
- Spinal tumor
- Occult spina bifida

MYELOGRAPHY
Description
- Useful in patients with nerve impingement on moving or standing
- Intravenous contrast used to delineate spinal nerves
- CT scanning or plain X-ray images are then obtained

Advantages/Disadvantages
Advantages:
- Optimal images obtained of nerve root and spinal cord compression
- Useful when planning surgery

Disadvantages:
- Invasive and expensive, especially for CT images
- MRI has superceded myelography in many situations
- Requires specialized centers and specialist interpretation
- Anaphylaxis and seizure risk due to intravenous contrast

Normal
No nerve root or spinal cord compression.

Abnormal
- Compression of nerve roots
- Spinal stenosis

Cause of abnormal result
Spinal tumor.

CONSIDER CONSULT

- If clinical features of lumbar spondylosis do not respond to nonsurgical approaches, then consultation with a spine surgeon is indicated only if there are signs and symptoms of neurologic compromise
- If neurologic complications develop, referral to a neurosurgeon or orthopedic spine surgeon is indicated for further assessment and treatment

IMMEDIATE ACTION

- Cauda equina syndrome requires immediate neurosurgical consultation for cord decompression
- Severe lumbar stenosis with rapid onset and progression of neurologic signs requires immediate referral to a neurosurgeon or orthopedic spine surgeon

PATIENT AND CAREGIVER ISSUES
Forensic and legal issues

- Patients who show signs of cord compression require immediate evaluation by a neurosurgeon or orthopedic spine surgeon
- Treatment failure is common, and full explanation of the treatment to the patient is required
- Fully informed consent for lumbar spine surgery is imperative to avoid medicolegal issues

Impact on career, dependants, family, friends

- Back pain is a chronic disorder with acute exacerbations and has a huge impact on the family
- Family should be kept fully informed of patient's treatment program and should be able to question the program, especially if little progress is being made
- Family's views should be taken into account when designing the treatment program because their influence will have a major impact on how the patient responds

Patient or caregiver request

- **Will I get better?** 90% of patients do recover with rest and pain relief within 2–6 weeks
- **Will I be able to resume my normal life again?** The majority of patients can resume their lives but will need to protect their back from excessive trauma such as heavy lifting
- **Will I be able to work?** Patients may need to resume work initially on a part-time basis and undertake only light duties, especially if work is manual or involves standing for long periods (nurses, shop tellers, builders)
- **What can I do to prevent back problems in future?** Patients can attend a rehabilitation program for the back that teaches about posture, exercise, and lifting
- **Will the treatment be in the long term?** Long-term therapies with chronic analgesic are often not necessary, and usually the patient makes a good recovery. General lifestyle changes should be long-term
- **Will I become addicted to the painkillers?** Patients will not become addicted to the painkillers prescribed for back pain, if they are under close medical supervision. This issue must be discussed because patient compliance is usually low with prescribed painkillers. Patients with a history of substance abuse, or in whom a specific cause of back pain cannot be identified, are not appropriate candidates for chronic narcotic analgesics

Health-seeking behavior

- **Have you tried health supplements for back pain?** A myriad of health supplements of dubious nature is available – their efficacy is unproven
- **Have you tried natural herbal remedies for back pain?** There is little evidence of an analgesic effect. Patients' ideas and beliefs need to be fully evaluated before dissuading them from using these expensive remedies

- **Have you sought manipulation for back pain?** There is evidence to show that manipulation from a chiropractor or osteopathic physician may improve symptoms of acute back pain. Many patients may have tried this therapy before medical consultation
- **Have you tried holistic therapy for back pain?** Acupuncture, homeopathy, and other alternative therapies can give the patient relief from back pain. Apart from acupuncture, there is little evidence for these therapies

MANAGEMENT ISSUES
Goals

- Aim for conservative treatment of lumbar spondylosis in most patients
- Aim to restore patient to premorbid lifestyle
- Educate and counsel patient and family about back pain to improve treatment success
- Prevent further back pain episodes by recommending patient lifestyle adaptations
- Patient's occupation should allow for preventive measures to stop future back problems

Management in special circumstances
COEXISTING DISEASE

- Osteoarthritis can exacerbate back pain and should be assessed because it can affect the prognosis of lumbar spondylosis. Patients with hip osteoarthritis can have referred back pain, complicating management. These patients are often already taking analgesics; check therapy regimen and compliance
- Obesity may require modification of back exercise program, otherwise compliance may be poor. Stress to the obese patient that exercise will have a positive effect on both back pain and obesity

COEXISTING MEDICATION

- Patients taking analgesics should have their medication regimen and compliance evaluated. Analgesia is the mainstay of conservative therapy for lumbar spondylosis, and optimal compliance is required
- Patients on antidepressants should have a mental health assessment to check whether depression is exacerbating back pain symptoms. Appropriate treatment of depression and anxiety is important to improve back pain symptoms and success of therapy

SPECIAL PATIENT GROUPS

- Pregnant women will be limited in their treatment options. Conservative treatment, including back exercises and posture correction, will be necessary
- The elderly require careful assessment of back pain for other pathology. Other medications and side-effects of any prescribed analgesia (nonsteroidals) will affect back treatment regimen

PATIENT SATISFACTION/LIFESTYLE PRIORITIES
Patients in occupations that involve heavy lifting may find alteration of work practices impossible and may have to consider changing jobs.

SUMMARY OF THERAPEUTIC OPTIONS
Choices

- Most patients with symptomatic lumbar spondylosis require a trial of medical treatment
- Medical treatment consists of analgesia and a rehabilitation program tailored to the individual patient
- Nonsteroidal anti-inflammatory drugs (NSAIDs) that have analgesic and anti-inflammatory properties include ibuprofen and naproxen. Newer cyclo-oxygenase-2-specific NSAIDs with a lower risk of serious gastrointestinal toxicity include celecoxib
- Muscle relaxants, such as diazepam, aid in relieving associated muscle spasm, and their sedative effects help patients to sleep. However, chronic use is problematic
- Acetaminophen is another analgesic that can be taken with NSAIDs to maximize pain relief

- Lifestyle measures, including minimal bed rest, gentle mobilization, and an exercise program tailored to the individual patient, will be beneficial
- Physical therapy can be instituted once the patient has recovered sufficiently
- Occupational therapy can be an important addition to the rehabilitation program to ensure that workplace ergonomics are optimal and, thus, prevent future episodes of back pain
- Percutaneous electrical nerve stimulation (PENS) may be useful in selected patients with chronic back pain
- Epidural anesthetic and steroid injections can be used for subacute and chronic low back pain, although the evidence is inconclusive on their therapeutic benefit
- Corsets can be tailored to the patient to support the lumbar spine. However, patients tolerate them poorly

Surgery:
- Surgical investigations and interventions account for as much as one-third of healthcare costs for spinal disorders
- Scientific evidence for most procedures is still unclear
- Indications for surgery include intractable neurologic symptoms that do not respond to conservative treatment
- The main surgical objective is decompression of the spinal cord and/or nerve roots, usually via laminectomy. Fusion of the vertebral column may be necessary if the extent of decompressive laminectomy produces spinal instability
- The primary rationale for surgery for disk prolapse is to relieve nerve root compression due to herniated disk material
- Various techniques for decompression due to disk herniation include percutaneous, micro- and open diskectomy
- Decompressive lumbar laminectomy is used for spinal stenosis
- Arthrodesis of lumbar spine is used for spinal instability

Clinical pearls
- The role of surgery is to relieve neurologic symptoms due to compression, rather than to relieve back pain
- Surgery does not predictably relieve back pain
- Even after decompressive laminectomy, structural problems causing pain may remain and back pain may persist

Never
- Spinal decompression, performed by a neurosurgeon or orthopedic surgeon, should never be delayed when there are significant and progressive neurologic complications
- Never miss 'red flags' that are suggestive of other spinal pathology (such as infection or neoplasm), including progressive intractable back pain, weight loss, anemia, and history of cancer
- Most patients should be given an adequate trial of conservative treatment, and surgery should not be contemplated until this trial is completed. Surgery can permanently alter back mechanics and strength, and should be reserved for a select few patients
- Patients should not undergo spinal surgery before a complete workup, or if the diagnosis is uncertain

FOLLOW UP
- The patient should be reviewed regularly to check that treatment plan is improving clinical features
- Conservative measures should be instituted for most patients, but there will be a few who will require further treatment. These patients need to be referred to a specialist, such as a neurosurgeon or orthopedic surgeon

Plan for review

- Patients should be reviewed initially every 2–4 weeks to check progress and compliance with prescribed therapy
- As patients resume premorbid lifestyle, regular reviews are no longer indicated, but periodic reviews during the first 12 months are recommended to check for relapse and to reinforce importance of lifestyle changes

Information for patient or caregiver

Patients should be informed that back pain can be effectively treated with conservative measures, but that patient compliance with prescribed therapy is pivotal to success of the treatment.

DRUGS AND OTHER THERAPIES: DETAILS
Drugs
IBUPROFEN

- NSAIDs are a choice for patients with mild-to-moderate back pain
- Mechanism of action for pain relief probably involves inhibiting prostaglandin synthesis in the central nervous system
- Patients respond to certain NSAIDs on an individual basis; a 2-week trial for this NSAID should be undertaken
- Short-acting, up to 6h

Dose
Adult oral dose: 1200–3200mg/day (300mg four times daily; 400, 600, or 800mg three or four times daily). Doses should be individualized.

Efficacy
Improves pain symptoms and mobility.

Risks/Benefits
Risks:

- Use caution in the elderly
- Use caution in hepatic, renal, and cardiac failure, and bleeding disorders
- May cause severe allergic reactions including hives, facial swelling, asthma, shock

Benefits:

- Effective and inexpensive
- Improves pain symptoms and mobility

Side-effects and adverse reactions

- Cardiovascular system: hypertension, peripheral edema
- Central nervous system: headache, dizziness, tinnitus
- Gastrointestinal: anorexia, nausea, dyspepsia, peptic ulceration, bleeding
- Genitourinary: nephrotoxicity
- Hematologic: blood cell disorders
- Hypersensitivity: rashes, bronchospasm, angioedema

Interactions (other drugs)

- Aminoglycosides ▪ Anticoagulants ▪ Antihypertensives ▪ Baclofen ▪ Corticosteroids ▪ Cyclosporine, tacrolimus ▪ Digoxin ▪ Diuretics ▪ Lithium ▪ Methotrexate ▪ Phenylpropanolamine ▪ Warfarin

Contraindications

- Peptic ulceration ▪ Hypersensitivity to any pain reliever or antipyretic (including NSAIDs) ▪ Coagulation defects ▪ Severe renal or hepatic disease

Acceptability to patient

- Ibuprofen is effective for back pain
- The safety profile of this medication needs to be explained
- Treatment should be stopped immediately if abdominal pain or dyspepsia occurs
- Elderly patients are particularly at risk for gastrointestinal hemorrhage

Follow up plan

- Patient should be followed up for side-effects, and to check on patient compliance and treatment success
- NSAIDs should not be used long-term unless under medical supervision

Patient and caregiver information

- Patients should be informed about the risk of gastrointestinal side-effects
- Compliance with drug regimen should be discussed
- Minimum 2-week trial is required
- Long-term use should be under medical supervision

NAPROXEN

- Drug of choice for patients with mild-to-moderate back pain; commonly prescribed
- Mechanism of action for pain relief probably involves inhibiting prostaglandin synthesis in the central nervous system
- Patients respond to certain NSAIDs on an individual basis; a 2-week trial for this NSAID should be undertaken
- Intermediate-acting, up to 12h

Dose
Adult oral dose: 250–500mg orally twice daily.

Efficacy
Improves pain symptoms and mobility.

Risks/Benefits
Risks:

- Risk of gastrointestinal ulceration, bleeding, and perforation
- Use caution with renal impairment
- Use caution with hypertension or cardiac conditions aggravated by fluid retention and edema
- Use caution with history of liver dysfunction, and history of coagulation

Benefits:

- Effective and inexpensive
- Improves pain symptoms and mobility
- Naproxen usage has strong evidence

Side-effects and adverse reactions

- Cardiovascular system: congestive heart failure, dysrhythmias, edema, palpitations, dyspnea
- Central nervous system: headache, dizziness, drowsiness, vertigo
- Gastrointestinal: constipation, heartburn, diarrhea, vomiting, nausea, dyspepsia, peptic ulceration, stomatitis
- Genitourinary: acute renal failure
- Hematologic: thrombocytopenia
- Hypersensitivity: rashes, bronchospasm, angioedema
- Skin: pruritus, ecchymoses, sweating, purpura

Interactions (other drugs)
- Aminoglycosides ▪ Anticoagulants ▪ Antihypertensives ▪ Corticosteroids
- Cyclosporine ▪ Digoxin ▪ Diuretics ▪ Lithium ▪ Methotrexate ▪ Phenylpropanolamine
- Probenecid ▪ Triamterene

Contraindications
- Peptic ulceration ▪ Hypersensitivity to NSAIDs ▪ Coagulation defects
- Do not use naproxen and naproxen sodium concomitantly

Acceptability to patient
- Naproxen is effective for back pain
- Safety profile of this medication needs to be explained
- Treatment should be stopped immediately if abdominal pain or dyspepsia occurs
- Elderly patients are particularly at risk for gastrointestinal hemorrhage

Follow up plan
- Patient should be followed up for side-effects, and to check on patient compliance and treatment success
- NSAIDs should not be used long-term unless under medical supervision

Patient and caregiver information
- Patients should be informed about the risk of gastrointestinal side-effects
- Compliance with drug regimen should be discussed
- Minimum 2-week trial is required
- Long-term use should be under medical supervision

CELECOXIB
- Mechanism of action for pain relief probably involves inhibiting prostaglandin synthesis in the central nervous system
- Selective for cyclo-oxygenase (COX)-2, with less risk of serious gastrointestinal toxicity than nonselective NSAIDs
- Appropriate patients are those at increased risk for gastrointestinal toxicity from NSAIDs, including age over 60 years, history of peptic ulcer disease, prolonged usage, and concurrent use of corticosteroids and anticoagulants
- Evidence limited on efficacy specifically for lumbar spondylosis, but there is evidence of efficacy for relief of pain from osteoarthritis of the knee

Dose
- Adult oral dose: 100–200mg orally twice daily
- This is an off-label indication

Efficacy
Evidence on efficacy specifically for lumbar spondylosis is limited, but there is evidence of efficacy for relief of pain from osteoarthritis of the knee.

Risks/Benefits
Risk: use caution in patients with pre-existing asthma.

Side-effects and adverse reactions
- Central nervous system: dizziness, headache
- Gastrointestinal: abdominal pain, diarrhea, dyspepsia, flatulence, nausea
- Respiratory: respiratory tract infections
- Skin: rash

Interactions (other drugs)
- Angiotensin-converting enzyme (ACE) inhibitors ■ Furosemide ■ Aspirin ■ Fluconazole
- Lithium ■ Warfarin

Contraindications
- Allergic reactions to sulfonamide ■ Allergic reactions to NSAIDs ■ Inflammatory bowel disease ■ Severe congestive heart failure ■ Renal impairment

Acceptability to patient
- Celecoxib has a good side-effect profile, enhancing acceptability
- COX-2 inhibitor usage is rapidly increasing due to their safety profile
- Expensive compared with generic nonselective NSAIDs

Follow up plan
- The medication should be prescribed under medical supervision
- Initial hemogram, then 6- to 12-monthly electrolyte, renal function, and liver function tests in at-risk patients
- Patients should be followed up for compliance, effectiveness, and side-effects

Patient and caregiver information
- Patients should be informed about the safety profile
- Compliance with drug regimen should be discussed
- Minimum 2-week trial is required
- Long-term use should be under medical supervision

DIAZEPAM
- Benzodiazepine that is a skeletal muscle relaxant and has sedative properties
- Useful for patients with muscle spasm due to lumbar spondylosis
- Used with analgesic medications
- Addictive properties limit use of diazepam

Dose
Adult dose: 2–10mg orally three times daily.

Efficacy
Effective in reducing muscle spasm.

Risks/Benefits
Risks:
- Use caution in the elderly and children, pregnancy and nursing mothers
- Use caution in hepatic and renal disease

Side-effects and adverse reactions
- Cardiovascular system: orthostatic hypotension, tachycardia, venous thrombus, electrocardiogram changes, phlebitis
- Central nervous system: depression, drowsiness, withdrawal syndrome, anxiety, headache
- Eyes, ears, nose, and throat: visual and hearing disturbances
- Gastrointestinal: nausea, diarrhea, dry mouth, altered liver function, vomiting
- Respiratory: respiratory depression
- Skin: irritation, rash, dermatitis

Interactions (other drugs)
- Antibiotics (clarithromycin, erythromycin, troleandomycin, quinolones, ciprofloxacin)
- Azole antifungals (fluconazole, itraconazole, ketoconazole) Carbamazepine Cimetidine
- Clozapine Delavidine Disulfiram Ethanol Isoniazid Levodopa Metoprolol
- Omeprazole Phenytoin Rifampin Selective serotonin reuptake inhibitors

Contraindications
- Hypersensitivity to diazepam Narrow-angle glaucoma Psychosis

Acceptability to patient
- Effective for back pain and reduced mobility
- Sedative and addictive properties can make diazepam unacceptable to patients

Follow up plan
- Careful follow up is required because of the addictive properties of diazepam
- Diazepam should be prescribed for only one week initially
- Sedation effects need to be evaluated

Patient and caregiver information
- Addictive properties should be explained
- Sedation properties limit the use of diazepam because care with driving and operating machinery is required
- Avoid alcohol

ACETAMINOPHEN
- Useful analgesic for low back pain
- Can be combined with NSAIDs
- Toxic in overdose

Dose
Adult dose: 500–1000mg orally four times daily.

Efficacy
Effective analgesia for low back pain.

Risks/Benefits
Risks:
- Use caution in hepatic and renal impairment
- Overdosage results in hepatic and renal damage unless treated promptly
- Overdosage may lead to multiorgan failure and may be fatal
- Accidental overdosage can occur if over-the-counter (OTC) preparations containing acetaminophen are taken with prescribed drugs that contain acetaminophen

Benefits:
- Inexpensive and effective analgesic agent
- Available OTC
- Can be combined with NSAIDs

Side-effects and adverse reactions
- Acetaminophen rarely causes side-effects when used intermittently
- Gastrointestinal: nausea, vomiting
- Hematologic: blood disorders

- Metabolic: acute hepatic and renal failure
- Skin: rashes
- Other: acute pancreatitis

Interactions (other drugs)
- Alcohol ▪ Anticoagulants ▪ Anticonvulsants ▪ Isoniazid ▪ Cholestyramine
- Colestipol ▪ Domperidone ▪ Metoclopramide

Contraindications
Known liver dysfunction.

Acceptability to patient
- Acetaminophen is an effective analgesic agent which has good patient acceptability
- Inexpensive agent, available OTC

Follow up plan
Compliance and analgesic effect should be followed up.

Patient and caregiver information
Patients should be warned of risks of overdose, especially as many different preparations contain acetaminophen.

Physical therapy
PHYSICAL THERAPY
- Physical therapy programs can be effective in improving mobility and reducing back pain
- Used in conjunction with other therapies, especially analgesia, and postoperatively
- Educates patients about the back and provides an individual program of back exercises
- Manual techniques used to increase soft-tissue pliability and mobilize the spine

Efficacy
Essential for back rehabilitation, because it provides education and improves back pain symptoms.

Risks/Benefits
Benefits:
- Active dynamic lumbar spine stabilization and rehabilitation can improve clinical features of lumbar spondylosis
- Educates the patient about back pain and teaches exercises and posture improvement

Acceptability to patient
- Patients will need to participate actively in the program of physical therapy if it is to be successful
- If the program is individually tailored to the patient, acceptability will be enhanced

Follow up plan
Patient compliance and back pain relief need to be followed up.

Patient and caregiver information
Patient participation and compliance are the keys to the success of this therapy.

Occupational therapy
OCCUPATIONAL THERAPY
- Important when generalized muscular deconditioning has occurred and gives activity-specific reconditioning

- Provides advice on proper ergonomics in the workplace
- Can provide an individual program to return patient back to employment
- Can prevent further injuries and improvement in activities of daily living
- Can be combined with physiotherapy to give an holistic approach

Efficacy
- Effective in returning patient to his/her premorbid lifestyle
- Effective in educating patient to prevent further injuries

Risks/Benefits
Benefits:
- Provides program to return patient back to work
- Provides education to prevent further injury
- Provides an ergonomic environment to prevent back pain
- Reconditions lumbar musculature to strengthen and improve the back

Acceptability to patient
- Patients will need to participate actively in the program of occupational therapy if it is to be successful
- If program is individually tailored to patient, acceptability will be enhanced

Follow up plan
Patient compliance and back pain relief need to be followed up.

Patient and caregiver information
Patient participation and compliance are the keys to the success of this therapy.

Surgical therapy
DISKECTOMY
- Diskectomy procedures include the standard lumbar microdiskectomy
- Variations on the procedure occur between different surgeons
- Complete patient workup, including imaging of lumbar spondylosis, is necessary
- Procedure is carried out under anesthesia, and patient's age and comorbidity need to be fully documented before surgery
- Disk annulus is incised and disk removed
- Nerve roots are decompressed and loose fragments of disk removed
- Patients rarely remain in hospital for more than 24h because mobilization occurs 4–6h postoperatively

Efficacy
There is strong evidence on the relative effectiveness of surgical diskectomy for carefully selected patients.

Risks/Benefits
Benefits:
- Carefully selected patients with lumbar disk prolapse can benefit from microdiskectomy
- Conservative treatment should be tried before this procedure is done
- 75% of patients show long-term benefits following microdiskectomy

Acceptability to patient
Patients will need to be informed of all the risks and benefits of the procedure.

Follow up plan
- Careful follow up is required for operative success and symptom relief
- Usually, patients are followed up for one month postoperatively, and if they remain symptom-free they can be referred back to their family practitioner

Patient and caregiver information
- Patients need to be informed of the procedure, its risks, and benefits
- Patients should be carefully selected for this procedure to ensure that operative benefits are maximal

LAMINECTOMY
- Spinal laminectomy can be performed in patients with lumbar stenosis
- Usually performed without arthrodesis as spinal instability is uncommon with this procedure
- Relatively safe operation having a medium- to long-term success rate
- Required for treatment of cauda equina syndrome

Efficacy
Effective relief of symptoms in carefully selected patients.

Risks/Benefits
Risk: preoperative work-up important for surgical success

Benefits:
- Spinal arthrodesis not usually necessary as this operation rarely causes lumbar instability
- Effective relief of spinal decompression

Acceptability to patient
Major operation requiring careful patient selection for maximal success.

Follow up plan
- Careful follow up required for operative success and symptom relief
- Usually, patients are followed up for one month postoperatively, and if they remain symptom-free they can be referred back to their family practitioner

Patient and caregiver information
- Patients need to be informed of the procedure, its risks, and benefits
- Patients should be carefully selected for this procedure to ensure that operative benefits are maximal

SPINAL ARTHRODESIS
- Indications for lumbar arthrodesis may arise in lumbar spondylosis
- Surgical fusion of lumbar spine is indicated for spinal instability and spinal stenosis
- Arthrodesis can be combined with laminectomy or microdiskectomy for spinal stenosis
- Several techniques are available for assessment of patients to ensure correct selection
- Patient selection includes cases unresponsive to nonsurgical treatment with clearly established structural pathology producing significant persistent disability

Efficacy
- Lumbar arthrodesis is indicated only for a select group of patients and should not routinely be combined with other spinal surgery
- Trials have shown variable results with between 16 and 95% improvement from spinal fusion
- Some trials have shown patient deterioration after fusion

Risks/Benefits
Benefits:
- Most studies state that careful patient selection for spinal arthrodesis offers the best outcome for spinal stenosis and instability
- Long-term results for spinal arthrodesis are good for multidirectional instabilities of the spine

Acceptability to patient
- Patients need to be fully informed about risks and benefits of the procedure to improve its acceptability
- Patients should have conservative treatment before surgery being considered

Follow up plan
- Careful follow up is required for operative success and symptom relief
- Usually, patients are followed up for one month postoperatively, and if they remain symptom-free they can be referred back to their family practitioner

Patient and caregiver information
- Patients need to be informed of the procedure, its risks, and benefits
- Patients should be carefully selected for this procedure to ensure that operative benefits are maximal

Other therapies
PERCUTANEOUS ELECTRICAL NERVE STIMULATION (PENS)
- Useful in a selected group of patients with chronic back pain
- Nonpharmacologic treatment with no side-effects
- Transmits electrical signals that block pain pathways
- Certain patients obtain analgesia from PENS
- Physical therapists can educate and explain correct positioning and use of PENS

Efficacy
The exact mechanism of pain relief with this procedure has not been defined, but it is beneficial to certain patients.

Risks/Benefits
Benefits:
- Inexpensive, safe mechanism of pain relief
- Can be useful for patients with chronic back pain
- Can be used long-term with no known side-effects

Acceptability to patient
Education about the PENS device and usage will enable patients to use it correctly.

Follow up plan
Pain relief from PENS will need to be monitored, because not all patients will find it effective in relieving their back pain.

Patient and caregiver information
Physical therapists can educate and explain to patients the correct positioning and use of the PENS device.

INJECTION THERAPY
- Injection with anesthetics and/or steroids under X-ray control can be used for chronic back pain

- 40mg prednisolone and 1mL 1% lidocaine injection solution can be used
- Different injection sites include the facet joint, epidural space, and local sites
- The best site for injection for maximal outcome is usually at the site of pathology
- Optimal timing for injection therapy is not known, although generally it is indicated for back pain lasting for more than one month
- Frequency of injections is not known, although a timing of at least 2 weeks is advocated between injections

Efficacy
- Improvement in up to 80% of patients can be obtained
- Less favorable response to injection therapy occurs in patients with longer duration of symptoms, intractable pain, smokers, and those with no neurologic symptoms

Risks/Benefits
Benefits:
- Relief of pain, especially chronic back pain, can be obtained with injection therapy
- Can use repeated injection therapy

Acceptability to patient
Injection therapy may not be acceptable to patients, and a full explanation of the risks and benefits is needed.

Follow up plan
- Regular follow up required to monitor therapy success and complications
- Further injection therapy may be required

Patient and caregiver information
- It is important to inform patients about the risks and benefits of injection therapy
- Fully informed consent is needed

CORSETRY
- Back corsets can be individually tailored for patients with chronic back pain
- Corsets can prevent exaggerating lumbar lordosis of standing
- Corset usage is controversial because patient compliance is poor and benefits are minimal

Efficacy
- Corsets are not highly effective at relieving back pain
- Corsets may be beneficial for vertebral instability

Risks/Benefits
- Risk: patient compliance is imperative
- Benefit: individually tailored corsets may provide lumbar stability and pain relief

Acceptability to patient
Patient compliance is poor because corsets are often uncomfortable to wear.

Follow up plan
Follow up on compliance and pain relief is required.

Patient and caregiver information
It is important to stress to patients that corsets will need to be worn daily and that they can cause discomfort.

LIFESTYLE

- Education is an important component of a back care program, including an explanation of the natural history of lumbar spondylosis
- Back exercises taught by a physical or occupational therapist need to be continued by the patient to prevent relapse and improve muscle tone in the lumbar back

RISKS/BENEFITS
Benefits:

- Education and exercises can improve the patient's posture and mobility
- Back rehabilitation programs may prevent future relapses

ACCEPTABILITY TO PATIENT
Compliance is important to maintain any benefits from the back rehabilitation program.

FOLLOW UP PLAN
Regular follow up to ensure compliance is recommended.

PATIENT AND CAREGIVER INFORMATION
Patients should be informed of the benefits of following a back rehabilitation program.

EFFICACY OF THERAPIES

- Most patients require a trial of medical therapy before surgery is contemplated
- Surgical investigations and interventions account for one-third of the healthcare costs for spinal disorders, but the scientific evidence for most procedures is still unclear

Review period
6 months.

PROGNOSIS

- Natural history of low back pain shows that it is usually a self-limiting condition
- Reports indicate that 50% of patients are better within one week, with up to 90% resolving within 12 weeks
- Conservative management duration is under debate, especially as newer surgical techniques become less invasive
- Surgery for back pain is indicated for intractable chronic back pain or for those patients with progressive neurologic signs or cauda equina
- Referral to a neurosurgeon or orthopedic surgeon should occur for patients with progressive deterioration, relapse, and complications

Clinical pearls

- Most patients do not need surgery
- Surgery is indicated for neuropathic symptoms that do not respond to conservative care
- Surgery can relieve numbness and tingling caused by nerve root compression, but not back pain

Therapeutic failure
Patients who do not improve with conservative medical treatment are candidates for surgical treatment, and should be referred to an orthopedic surgeon.

Recurrence
Patients with recurring back pain following surgery should be referred to a neurosurgeon or orthopedic surgeon.

COMPLICATIONS
Complications include:
- Neural compression
- Lumbar stenosis
- Disk height reduction
- Cauda equina, which needs urgent decompression

CONSIDER CONSULT
Patients who relapse following medical or surgical therapy require referral to a neurosurgeon or orthopedic surgeon.

PREVENTION

Back pain caused by workplace incidents accounts for over 30% of compensation payments

Prevention of back pain is imperative because direct medical costs of spinal disorders were >$20 billion in the US in 1990

Ergonomics in the workplace should be optimal to prevent clinical features and complications of lumbar spondylosis

An education-based back rehabilitation program is inexpensive and can restore the patient back to his/her premorbid status. Information and prevention strategies can enable the patient to understand his/her back symptoms and prevent relapses

RISK FACTORS

Lack of exercise and low fitness levels: increase the risk of lumbar spondylosis

Obesity: can lead to lumbar spondylosis due to altered biomechanics and stresses on the lumbar spine

Smoking: is a risk factor for lumbar spondylosis

Occupational risk factors: should be modified to prevent clinical features and complications of lumbar spondylosis

MODIFY RISK FACTORS
Lifestyle and wellness
TOBACCO

Smoking should be discouraged and smoking cessation advice should be given.

DIET

Obesity should be treated with a weight-reducing diet.

PHYSICAL ACTIVITY

Exercises for the back to improve posture and muscle tone will form part of the back rehabilitation program

Patients will need to maintain the exercise program to prevent future relapses

ENVIRONMENT

The patient's workplace should have optimal ergonomics to prevent clinical features of lumbar spondylosis

Occupations requiring lifting should have training programs for their employees

SCREENING

There is no evidence for screening of lumbar spondylosis.

PREVENT RECURRENCE

Recurrence can be prevented if the patient maintains his/her back rehabilitation with regular exercises and posture correction

Workplace ergonomics are important and need to be optimal to prevent relapses

Occupations requiring lifting should have training programs for their employees, including nurses, porters, and removal staff

ASSOCIATIONS

American Academy of Orthopaedic Surgeons

6300 North River Road

Rosemont, IL 60018-4262

Tel: (847) 823 7186 or (800) 346 2267

Fax: (847) 823 8125

www.aaos.org

KEY REFERENCES

- Bassewitz H, Herkowitz H. Lumbar stenosis with spondylolisthesis: current concepts of surgical treatment. Clin Orthop 2001;384:54–60
- Colliers J, Longmore M, Hodgetts T. Back pain. In: Oxford Handbook of Clinical Specialties, 5th edn. New York: Oxford University Press, 1999
- Colliers J, Longmore M, Hodgetts T. Causes of back pain. In: Oxford Handbook of Clinical Medicine, 3rd edn. New York: Oxford University Press
- Gibson JNA, Waddell G, Grant IC. Surgery for degenerative lumbar spondylosis (Cochrane Review). In: The Cochrane Library, 1, 2002. Oxford: Update Software
- Hilibrand AS, Rand N. Degenerative lumbar stenosis: diagnosis and management. J Am Acad Orthop Surg 1999;7:239–49
- Katz J. Lumbar spinal fusion. Surgical rates, costs, and complications. Spine 1995;20(Suppl):78–83
- Kumar MN, Jacquot F, Hall H. Long-term follow-up of functional outcomes and radiographic changes at adjacent levels following lumbar spinal fusion for degenerative disease. Eur Spine J 2001;10:309–13
- Nelemans PJ, Bie RA de, Vet HCW de, Sturmans F. Injection therapy for subacute and chronic benign low back pain (Cochrane Review). In: The Cochrane Library, 1, 2002. Oxford: Update Software
- Sheehan JM, Shaffrey CI, Jane JA Sr. Degenerative lumbar stenosis: the neurosurgical perspective. Clin Orthop 2001;384:61–74
- Silvers HR, Lewis PJ, Asch HL. Decompressive lumbar laminectomy for spinal stenosis. J Neurosurg 1993;78:695–701
- van Tulder M, Koes B. Low back pain and sciatica. In: Clinical Evidence, vol 5. London: BMJ Publishing Group 2001:772–89
- Turner JA, Ersek M, Herron L, Deyo R. Surgery for lumbar spinal stenosis. Attempted meta-analysis of the literature. Spine 1992;17:1–8
- Yong-Hing Y. Pathophysiology and rationale for treatment in lumbar spondylosis and instability. Chir Organic Mov 1994;79:3–10
- Zdeblick T. The treatment of degenerative lumbar disorders. A critical review of the literature. Spine 1995;20(Suppl):123–37

FAQS

Question 1

What does 'lumbar spondylosis' mean?

ANSWER 1

Lumbar spondylosis refers to the radiographic findings of degenerative disk disease in the lumbar spine and the associated adjacent osteoarthritis.

Question 2

What is the significance of finding lumbar spondylosis on a radiograph, computed tomography, or magnetic resonance imaging?

ANSWER 2

The clinical significance depends entirely on the clinical presentation. It is quite common for the findings of lumbar spondylosis to be apparent radiographically in asymptomatic patients.

Question 3
What is the role for surgical treatment for this disorder?

ANSWER 3
Surgery is indicated not for relief of back pain, but rather for relief of symptoms due to neurologic compromise that do not respond to conservative treatment.

Question 4
How often is surgical treatment necessary?

ANSWER 4
In most cases, the symptoms resulting from lumbar spondylosis will respond to conservative treatment, and surgery is unnecessary.

CONTRIBUTORS
Geraldine N Urse, DO
Richard Brasington Jr, MD, FACP
Thiruvalam P Indira, MD

OSGOOD-SCHLATTER DISEASE

DESCRIPTION

- Juvenile osteochondrosis of tibial tuberosity
- Causes pain, tenderness and swelling below the knee
- Usually benign and self-limiting

URGENT ACTION

Recommend the application of ice, to the anterior surface of the tibia, as for any sprain (15- to 20-min applications of ice pack, with 2-hourly intervals over 48- to 72-h).

KEY! DON'T MISS!

Rarely, tumors can present at the tibial tuberosity. Therefore, patients whose symptoms do not resolve after conservative treatment should be evaluated for tumor (as well as osteomyelitis).

BACKGROUND

ICD9 CODE
732.4 Juvenile osteochondrosis of lower extremity, excluding foot.

SYNONYMS
- Tibial tuberosity apophysitis
- Osteochondrosis
- Apophysitis tibialis adolescentium

CARDINAL FEATURES
- Pain, tenderness and swelling of the proximal tibial apophysis following a vigorous period of exercise in an adolescent
- Occurs in one or both knees
- Most cases resolve spontaneously in weeks or several months
- Tends to resolve with fusion of the tibial tuberosity

CAUSES
Common causes
- Etiology unproven: suspected to be chronic microtrauma secondary to overuse of quadriceps muscle
- May occur after growth spurt, when bone growth has outstripped muscle development with resultant loss of flexibility

Contributory or predisposing factors
- Overzealous training in sport involving running, jumping or any heavy quadriceps loading
- Overweight
- Growth spurt during the previous year

EPIDEMIOLOGY
Incidence and prevalence
FREQUENCY
- The most common osteochondrosis
- Up to 10% of sports clinic diagnoses

Demographics
AGE
Most common in:
- Girls aged 8–16 years
- Boys aged 11–18 years

GENDER
More common in boys, possibly related to greater incidence of male sports participation and/or to more rapid skeletal growth in males.

GENETICS
None known.

DIAGNOSIS

DIFFERENTIAL DIAGNOSIS
Anterior knee pain syndrome
FEATURES
- Occurs in adolescent girls and may be bilateral
- Often associated with athletic activity
- Tends to resolve spontaneously by early adulthood

Patellar dislocation or subluxation
FEATURES
- Occurs intermittently
- Affects adolescents, especially girls

Sinding-Larsen-Johansson syndrome
FEATURES
- A traction apophysitis
- Occurs at the distal pole of the patella rather than at the tibial tuberosity (as in Osgood-Schlatter disease)

Chondromalacia patellae
FEATURES
- A softening of the articular cartilage of the patella
- Diagnosed only by direct inspection during arthoscopy or arthotomy

Septic arthritis
FEATURES
- Inflamed joint effusion – hot, red, swollen joint
- Signs of systemic illness – fever and shaking chills common
- Tends to present with a blood-borne infection or a puncture wound

Osteomyelitis of the proximal tibia
FEATURES
- Usually associated with an elevated white blood count and ESR
- An effusion may be present in the knee joint

Osteochondritis dissecans
FEATURES
- Due to a fragment of cartilage with underlying subchondral bone becoming detached
- Activity-related pain occurs and may be associated with clicking, giving way and limping

SIGNS & SYMPTOMS
Signs
- Pain worse with increasing pressure
- Swollen, warm and tender area below knee directly over the tibial tuberosity
- Visible soft tissue edema over proximal tibial tuberosity
- A firm mass may be palpable
- Bony bump may be apparent on upper edge of tibia
- Pain is reproduced by extension against forced resistance
- Knee joint is normal on examination
- No effusion or condylar tenderness

Symptoms

- Mild to moderate cases: pain worse with activity, minimal at rest
- Severe cases: pain worsens with less vigorous activity such as stair-climbing, doing deep knee bends or weight-lifting

ASSOCIATED DISORDERS

Osgood-Schlatter disease may occur concurrently with other osteochondroses such as Sinding-Larsen-Johansson syndrome (tendonitis with *de novo* calcification at inferior pole patellar) or Sever's syndrome (apophysitis of the heel).

KEY! DON'T MISS!

Rarely, tumors can present at the tibial tuberosity. Therefore, patients whose symptoms do not resolve after conservative treatment should be evaluated for tumor (as well as osteomyelitis)

INVESTIGATION OF THE PATIENT
Direct questions to patient

- Q Was pain first noticeable after an accident or other sporting incident? 50% of Osgood-Schlatter cases will report a precipitating trauma
- Q Has pain been present intermittently for several months? Rest and restriction of exercise may produce faster results in patients without a long history of pain
- Q Which of the following make the pain worse? Running, jumping, deep knee bends, climbing or descending stairs? In mild cases, running and jumping will aggravate the pain. In more severe cases, pain will be triggered by climbing or descending stairs or deep knee bends
- Q Are both knees affected? Osgood-Schlatter disease is bilateral in 25–30% of cases
- Q Does the pain disappear after rest? Most cases of Osgood-Schlatter disease will respond to rest and/or restriction of exercise and will not require further treatment

Contributory or predisposing factors

- Q How much sport do you play? Overzealous training in sport involving running, jumping or any heavy quadriceps loading is often a factor
- Q How much have you grown since last year? Many children with Osgood-Schlatter disease will have experienced a growth spurt during the previous year. Most vulnerable period is at the peak of the secondary growth spurt

Examination

- Q Is the area over the tibial tuberosity tender, swollen and warm? These are features of Osgood-Schlatter disease
- Q Does it appear bruised or reddened? Some patients may have erythema of the tibial tuberosity
- Q Is the quadriceps muscle normal? Some patients may have quadriceps atrophy. However, the presence of quadriceps atrophy should suggest pathology within the knee joint
- Q Are bone fragments present on palpation? Such ossicles are detached in 20% of patients
- Q Does examination reveal effusion or joint line tenderness in the knee joint? There should be no evidence of this
- Q Is there effusion or condylar tenderness? If present, this may indicate an active infection
- Q Can pain be reproduced by extension against forced resistance? This is typical of Osgood-Schlatter disease

Summary of investigative tests

- X-ray of the knee, while not diagnostic, may be useful to eliminate other possible diagnoses such as infection, neoplasia, or stress fracture of the proximal tibia
- Ultrasonography is useful to determine the involvement of the tibial tuberosity and the surrounding soft tissue

DIAGNOSTIC DECISION

Pain and swelling of the area over the tibial tuberosity, following an extended period of vigorous exercise in an adolescent indicates a diagnosis of Osgood-Schlatter disease.

CLINICAL PEARLS

Osgood-Schlatter disease is largely a clinical diagnosis, based on excluding the other relevant possibilities.

THE TESTS

Imaging

X-RAY OF THE KNEE

Advantages/Disadvantages

Advantage: may confirm the diagnosis (fragmentation of the tibial tubercle and sometimes a loose ossicle) or demonstrate an alternative diagnosis.

Abnormal

Osgood-Schlatter lesion is best seen on the lateral view with the knee in slight internal rotation. The following abnormalities may be visible:

- Superficial ossicle in the patellar tendon
- Irregular ossification of the proximal tibial tuberosity
- Calcification within the patellar tendon
- Thickening of the patellar tendon
- Soft-tissue edema proximal to the tibial tuberosity

ULTRASONOGRAPHY

Advantages/Disadvantages

Advantage: high resolution ultrasonography is a relatively rapid risk-free method of examining the involvement of the tibial tuberosity and the surrounding soft tissue and can be used to aid diagnosis.

Abnormal

The following abnormalities may be visible:

- Superficial ossicle in the patellar tendon
- Irregular ossification of the proximal tibial tuberosity
- Calcification within the patellar tendon
- Thickening of the patellar tendon
- Soft-tissue edema proximal to the tibial tuberosity

CONSIDER CONSULT

- After any acute inflammation has subsided, refer to a physical therapist to increase muscle flexibility and speed recovery
- Surgery is necessary only in severe cases when a bone fragment forms and remains painful after growth has ceased

IMMEDIATE ACTION

Treat as for a sprain – 'RICE':

- Rest: an initial period of about 6 weeks of relative rest will allow the injury to heal correctly
- Ice: Cold should be applied to the kneecap during the first 24–72 h after injury, for 20 min with 2 hours between applications
- Compression: an ACE bandage or splint may help the swelling and also remind the adolescent not to overuse the leg
- Elevation: Keeping the leg elevated during the first 24 h after injury may decrease swelling

PATIENT AND CAREGIVER ISSUES
Patient or caregiver request

How much will I be able to exercise? The key issue for most adolescents with Osgood–Schlatter disease is how much exercise they can still do. This is based very much on individual cases. In general, although the patient can be reassured that some discomfort while exercising is normal during the healing process, stress on the afflicted area by jumping, or excessive running may cause further strain and may pull bone fragments loose, with the possibility of surgery being needed in the years ahead.

MANAGEMENT ISSUES
Goals

- Reduce pain and swelling
- Prevent recurrence: a premature return to athletic activity could lead to permanent damage
- Allow normal musculoskeletal maturation to take place: immobilization using casts should be avoided where possible, and while vigorous sports should be avoided, moderate or less stressful sports can be encouraged. Pads or braces can be used for support
- Decrease underlying strain on tendon by quadriceps-stretching exercises, including hip extension for complete stretch of the extensor mechanism. Hamstring-stretches should also be encouraged

Management in special circumstances
PATIENT SATISFACTION/LIFESTYLE PRIORITIES

The teenager should not have to completely stop sports, though avoidance of painful activity is important to avoid permanent damage.

SUMMARY OF THERAPEUTIC OPTIONS
Choices

First treatment of choice is conservative:

- Pain should be managed by RICE (REST, in this case including restriction of painful exercise; ICE; COMPRESSION; ELEVATION)
- Nonsteroidal anti-inflammatory drugs (NSAIDs) such as ibuprofen may be used to manage acute bouts of pain but should NOT be used solely to enable athletic activity to continue
- The use of a neoprene knee sleeve, especially one with an inferior 'horseshoe' pad, may aid compliance. Pads and braces can also be used for support. Crutches can be used to avoid weight loading of the affected knee
- Stretching and isometric strengthening exercises should be recommended

- Longer-term immobilization can be considered if progress is not made in 6 weeks. The use of a knee immobilizer or cast may be used to increase compliance, or in cases of severe pain
- Severe cases may require surgery to remove non-united ossicles, after the tibial plate has closed
- The obese teenager should be encouraged to lose weight

Clinical pearls

Treatment should emphasize physical therapy and NSAIDs.

Never

Cortocosteroid injections for pain relief should be avoided because of the risk of degenerative changes and tissue atrophy.

FOLLOW UP

If ultrasound has been used to aid diagnosis, it will also be useful to follow progress.

Plan for review

- Review at 6 weeks, and at 6-weekly intervals if required: referral to a physical therapist for stretching and isometric strengthening exercises should reduce strain on tubercle and speed recovery
- Mild cases should show progress within 6 weeks with rest and restriction of activities and symptoms should resolve within one year
- If lack of progress within the first weeks is due to noncompliance, then a cast may be considered, especially for more severe cases
- Discomfort when kneeling may persist for 2–3 years until the tibial plate closes
- In severe cases, if pain persists after tibial plate has closed surgery may be required

Information for patient or caregiver

It is useful to remind patients regularly that most cases resolve spontaneously with time and conservative management

DRUGS AND OTHER THERAPIES: DETAILS
Drugs
IBUPROFEN
Dose
- Under 12 years: 20–40mg/kg per day divided three times daily or four times daily
- Over 12 years: adult dosage, 200–400mg four times daily, not to exceed 3.2g/day

Efficacy
- NSAIDs reduce the inflammation of Osgood-Schlatter disease and reduce symptoms
- It is unclear whether they speed healing

Risks/Benefits
- Risk: use caution in hepatic, renal, and cardiac failure

Benefits:
- Faster onset of action than colchicines
- Inexpensive

Side-effects and adverse reactions
- Gastrointestinal: anorexia, nausea, dyspepsia, peptic ulceration
- Central nervous system: headache, dizziness, tinnitus
- Hypersensitivity: rashes, bronchospasm, angioedema

Interactions (other drugs)
- Aminoglycosides
- Antihypertensives
- Corticosteroids
- Cyclosporin
- Digoxin
- Lithium
- Methotrexate
- Phenylpropanolamine
- Diuretics
- Warfarin

Contraindications
- Peptic ulceration
- Hypersensitivity to NSAIDs
- Coagulation defects

Acceptability to patient
Lower dose NSAIDs are generally well tolerated by patients

Follow up plan
Because they can be ulcerogenic over long-term use, patients on NSAIDs should be re-evaluated on a regular basis for continued need.

Patient and caregiver information
NSAIDs should not be used to permit over-exercising.

Physical therapy
STRETCHING AND ISOMETRIC STRENGTHENING EXERCISES
Efficacy
Quadriceps and hamstring stretching exercises speed recovery.

Risks/Benefits
- Risks: may encourage return to over-exercising

Benefits:
- These exercises can be performed at home
- Speed recovery
- Maintain fitness, avoids muscle atrophy

Evidence
Physical therapy is frequently preferable to immobilization of the joint, despite the risk that continued sporting involvement may increase the chance of ossicle detachment [1].

Acceptability to patient
Therapy is to be preferred over immobilization.

Follow up plan
At regular visits (every 6 weeks or so), need for continued therapy should be evaluated. Many patients can continue exercise programs begun under the supervision of a physical therapist on their own after 2–3 weeks of guided therapy.

Patient and caregiver information
Extreme care should be taken not to over-exercise since increasing flexibility and strength will not completely remove the chance of further serious damage.

IMMOBILIZATION
Efficacy
- In rare cases when symptoms do not resolve, the affected leg may be immobilized by a cast or brace until the healing takes place, which typically takes another 6–8 weeks
- As a form of enforcing rest and restriction of activity, immobilization can promote recovery

Risks/Benefits
- Risk: loss in muscle tone, decreased fitness
- Benefit: prevents further damage occurring

Evidence
Immobilization slows the speed of recovery but reduces the chances that ossicle formation will take place and reduces the risk of possible future surgery. It is primarily used to aid compliance [1,2].

Acceptability to patient
Fair; immobilization is unlikely to be popular with most patients with Osgood-Schlatter disease.

Follow up plan
- If a brace is used, it may be removed for the duration of stretching exercises
- Once the cast has been removed, exercising may be initiated

SUPPORT AIDS
Efficacy
In the early stages of recovery, teenagers with mild disease may benefit from support in the form of an infrapatellar strap, or a padded brace to be used during activity.

Risks/Benefits
- Risk: may encourage overuse
- Benefit: support and reduction of pain during exercise

Evidence
There is no evidence as to the effectiveness of patellar sleeves or straps in treating the disease, but they are helpful in relieving symptoms in some patients.

Acceptability to patient
Good.

Follow up plan
At regular visits, continued need for sleeves should be assessed.

Patient and caregiver information
Patients should be reminded that the sleeve is an adjunct for comfort, and does not supplant the need for therapy or exercise.

Surgical therapy
RESECTION OF OSSICLE (TIBIAL SEQUESTRECTOMY)
Avulsion injuries in which the tendon has torn a small fragment of bone away from the tibia may result in these ossicles remaining detached and painful after the other physes have sealed. Surgery is used to excise such ossicles. Sequestrectomy has had better results than drilling of tubercle or reattachment of disunited ossicle.

Efficacy
In the event of symptoms remaining persistent and severely disabling, surgery can afford relief.

Risks/Benefits
Risk:
- Has the risks associated with any minor surgical procedure

Benefits:

- Relieves persistent pain (95% of cases)
- Cosmetic removal of bony prominence in 50–85% of cases
- Surgery may be the only remaining option if painful ossicles remain detached after the growth plate has closed

Evidence
Surgery has good results as a final resort for pain alleviation [3–5].

Acceptability to patient
Surgery is only used when conservative therapies have failed, and at this stage is more likely to be welcomed by the patient

Follow up plan
After surgery, a cylinder walking cast is applied for 2–3 weeks. Exercises are then begun.

LIFESTYLE
Being overweight can increase the risks of developing Osgood-Schlatter disease: overweight adolescents should be encouraged to reach a normal weight.

RISKS/BENEFITS
Losing weight reduces impact of jumping sports.

ACCEPTABILITY TO PATIENT
Losing weight may be difficult for a teenager whose exercise is being restricted. They may find it more acceptable to begin a weight loss regimen when exercise is resumed.

EFFICACY OF THERAPIES

In the normal course of Osgood-Schlatter disease, pain and inflammation will resolve with rest and restriction of exercise in approximately 6 weeks, although some discomfort when kneeling may continue to be felt until the epiphyses have closed.

Review period

The patient should be reassessed at 6 weeks, and at 6-weekly intervals if necessary.

PROGNOSIS

For the majority of patients prognosis is excellent.

Clinical pearls

Patients who are refractory to therapy should be referred to an orthopedist.

Therapeutic failure

Surgery for excision of nonfused ossicles may be necessary in patients who continue to experience severe disabling pain after the growth plate has closed.

Recurrence

If recurrence is due to noncompliance, a cast may be necessary.

COMPLICATIONS

- The most common complication is continued pain with kneeling
- More rarely there may be an increased incidence of tibial tuberosity fracture
- Non-union of bony fragment to the tibia occurs in approximately 10% of cases
- Premature fusion of the anterior part of the epiphysis with resultant genu recurvatum. The risk of genu recurvatum is the main reason for delaying surgery until the apophysis has closed

CONSIDER CONSULT

- In the event of non-union of ossicles to the tibia, referral for surgery should be delayed until after the physes have closed
- Otherwise, patients who do not respond to conservative treatment should be referred to an orthopedist

PREVENTION

Because the small injuries which result in Osgood-Schlatter disease often pass unnoticed, prevention is difficult.

MODIFY RISK FACTORS
Lifestyle and wellness
DIET
Teenagers should be encouraged to achieve a normal weight before embarking on sporting regimens.

PHYSICAL ACTIVITY
Exercise and sporting activities should be carried out in moderation to avoid stressing maturing musculosketal structures.

SCREENING
Screening is unnecessary.

PREVENT RECURRENCE
Because this is an overuse injury, limitation of strenuous exercise that stresses the quadriceps during the period when the growth plate is immature is key to preventing recurrence.

RESOURCES

ASSOCIATIONS

The Pediatric Content Network
Tel: (877) 411 PEDS (7337)
Fax: (301) 231 9827
www.pedsnet.org/support

KEY REFERENCES

- Bergami GD, Barbuti, et al. Ultrasonographic findings in Osgood-Schlatter disease. Radiol Med (Torino) 1994; 88(4):368–72
- Binazzi RL. Felli, et al. Surgical treatment of unresolved Osgood-Schlatter lesion. Clin Orthop 1993; 289:202–4
- Cser I, Lenart G. Surgical management of complaints due to independent bone fragments in Osgood-Schlatter disease (apophysitis of the tuberosity of the tibia). Acta Chir Hung 1986; 27(3):169–70
- D'Ambrosia RD, MacDonald GL. Pitfalls in the diagnosis of Osgood-Schlatter disease. Clin Orthop 1975; 110:206–9
- De Flaviis L, Nessi R, et al. Ultrasonic diagnosis of Osgood-Schlatter and Sinding-Larsen-Johansson diseases of the knee. Skeletal Radiol 1989; 18(3):193–7
- Engel A, Windhager R. Importance of the ossicle and therapy of Osgood-Schlatter disease. Sportverletz Sportschaden 1987; 1(2):100–8
- Flowers MJ, Bhadreshwar DR. Tibial tuberosity excision for symptomatic Osgood-Schlatter disease. J Pediatr Orthop 1995; 15(3):292–7
- Kannus P, Nittymaki S, et al. Athletic overuse injuries in children. A 30-month prospective follow-up study at an outpatient sports clinic. Clin Pediatr (Phila) 1988; 27(7):333–7
- Kujala UM, Kvist M, et al. Osgood-Schlatter's disease in adolescent athletes. Retrospective study of incidence and duration. Am J Sports Med 1985; 13(4):236–41
- Kujala UM, Kvist M, et al. Knee injuries in athletes. Review of exertion injuries and retrospective study of outpatient sports clinic material. Sports Med 1986; 3:447–60
- Lanning P, Heikkinen E. Ultrasonic features of the Osgood-Schlatter lesion. J Pediatr Orthop 1991; 11(4):538–40
- Mital MA, Matza RA, et al. The so-called unresolved Osgood-Schlatter lesion: a concept based on fifteen surgically treated lesions. J Bone Joint Surg [Am] 1980; 62(5):732–9
- Rosenberg ZS, Kawelblum M, et al. Osgood-Schlatter lesion: fracture or tendinitis? Scintigraphic, CT, and MR imaging features. Radiology 1992; 185(3):853–8
- Trail IA. Tibial sequestrectomy in the management of Osgood-Schlatter disease. J Pediatr Orthop 1988; 8(5):554–7
- Traverso A, Baldari A, et al. The coexistence of Osgood-Schlatter's disease with Sinding-Larsen-Johansson's disease. Case report in an adolescent soccer player. J Sports Med Phys Fitness 1990; 30(3):331–3

Evidence references

1 Engel A, Windhager R. Importance of the ossicle and therapy of Osgood-Schlatter disease. Sportverletz Sportschaden 1987; 1(2):100–8
2 Stelnicki TD. Control of Osgood-Sclatter disease with open patellar full knee splint. J Am Pediatr Med Assoc 1985; 75:265–7
3 Binazzi RL. Felli, et al. Surgical treatment of unresolved Osgood-Schlatter lesion. Clin Orthop 1993; 289:202–4
4 Cser I, Lenart G. Surgical management of complaints due to independent bone fragments in Osgood-Schlatter disease (apophysitis of the tibia). Acta Chir Hung 1986; 27(3):169–70
5 Trail IA. Tibial sequestrectomy in the management of Osgood-Schlatter disease. J Pediatr Orthop 1988; 8(5):554–7

FAQS
Question 1
What is the most common setting for Osgood-Schlatter disease?

ANSWER 1
It usually occurs in boys during periods of rapid growth and/or vigorous physical activity.

Question 2
How does Osgood-Schlatter disease present?

ANSWER 2
Pain occurs at the tibial tubercle, especially with climbing stairs or during activities that require quadriceps contraction.

Question 3
What is the usual treatment for Osgood-Schlatter disease?

ANSWER 3
Treatment involves supervised physical therapy and avoidance of contact sports.

CONTRIBUTORS
Randolph L Pearson, MD
Richard Brasington Jr, MD, FACP

OSTEITIS DEFORMANS (PAGET'S DISEASE)

SUMMARY INFORMATION

DESCRIPTION

- Localized metabolic bone condition characterized by excessive breakdown of bone followed by formation of abnormal, weak bone, leading to pain and deformity at affected sites
- Characteristic appearance of affected bone on X-ray, especially patchy lytic and sclerotic changes, and bone enlargement (diagnostic)

URGENT ACTION

- Refer immediately if osteosarcoma or osteomyelitis is suspected
- An uncommon but serious complication from skull and vertebral involvement by Paget's disease includes brain stem or spinal cord compression, which requires prompt referral to a neurosurgeon

KEY! DON'T MISS!

- If osteosarcoma or osteomyelitis is suspected, refer immediately
- Symptoms and signs of spinal cord compression should prompt immediate referral to a neurosurgeon

BACKGROUND

ICD9 CODE
731.0 Paget's disease (osteitis deformans).

SYNONYMS
Paget's disease of bone.

CARDINAL FEATURES
- Localized metabolic bone condition characterized by excessive breakdown of bone followed by formation of abnormal, weak bone, leading to pain and deformity at affected sites
- Characteristic appearance of affected bone on X-ray, especially patchy lytic and sclerotic changes, and bone enlargement
- Serum alkaline phosphatase usually increased, mainly in polyostotic disease
- Bowing of long bones in adulthood can be seen with advanced disease
- Bitemporal skull enlargement may be present in advanced disease
- Disease will progress within a given bone; however, new sites of involvement rarely occur after diagnosis

CAUSES
Common causes
- Causes are unknown
- Viral causes have been hypothesized, including measles, canine distemper, and respiratory syncytial viruses
- A genetic link may also exist

Contributory or predisposing factors
A weak link to dog owning has been shown which may support a role for canine distemper involvement.

EPIDEMIOLOGY
Incidence and prevalence
Difficult to establish because many cases are asymptomatic.

INCIDENCE
- Highly dependent on age and geography
- Incidence doubles each decade from age of 50 onward and can reach about 10% for a 90-year-old in North America or Europe, where the disease is common

PREVALENCE
15–80/1000 depending on patient age, race, and geography.

FREQUENCY
Approx. 3% of individuals will suffer the condition during their lifetime.

Demographics
AGE
- Prevalence increases with age
- Rare in patients under 40 years
- Prevalence 0.3/1000 in patients over 40–50 years

GENDER
- Males may be more susceptible
- Published male:female ratios vary from 1:1 to 2:1

RACE

More common in the UK and countries in which high British immigration occurred.

GENETICS

- Dominant inheritance pattern observed within families
- 10–40% of patients have one other family member affected
- Weak associations seen with HLA Dqw1 and DR-2 (US only) and A8, A9, B-15, and Dpw-4 (UK only) antigens

GEOGRAPHY

- More common in UK, North America, Australia, New Zealand, and South Africa
- Rare in other countries of Africa, Scandinavia, and Asia
- Intermediate prevalence in other European countries

DIFFERENTIAL DIAGNOSIS
Osteitis deformans may be initially difficult to distinguish from the following conditions before radiography.

Osteoarthritis
Osteoarthritis is confused with early or mild osteitis deformans. May also occur secondary to osteitis deformans.

FEATURES
- Aching pain localized to affected joints, typically exacerbated by joint use and is not greater at night
- Affects one or a few joints, typically those that are weight-bearing or have suffered previous injury
- Slowly progressive with occasional exacerbations, which are not usually associated with warmth
- Joint enlargement may occur, but no bowing of long bones or skull enlargement
- X-rays display typical joint-space narrowing, subchondral sclerosis, and osteophytic spurring

Skeletal neoplasm
May mimic secondary osteosarcoma, an uncommon complication of osteitis deformans.

FEATURES
- Most are metastases of prostate, breast, or lung primaries (80% of cases)
- Usually affect vertebrae, femur, ribs, sternum, humerus, and skull
- Most frequent symptom is pain: localized and often more severe at night
- Swelling and tenderness
- Pathologic fractures
- Compression of nerves or the spinal cord
- Hypercalcemia
- Osteolytic lesions best detected by X-ray; osteoblastic lesions best detected by radionuclide bone scanning
- Primary malignant bone tumors are rare and include osteosarcoma, chondrosarcoma, Ewing's sarcoma, or malignant fibrous histiocytoma
- Primary malignant bone tumor presents as pain at rest and at night, and causes swelling and tenderness
- Most primary malignant bone tumors occur in patients under 30 years of age or in the very old, and can result in pathologic fractures
- Raised serum alkaline phosphatase (50% of primary bone tumor cases)
- Positively diagnosed after biopsy and X-ray
- Primary malignant bone tumors have a poor prognosis
- Vertebral hemangioma is a rare, benign tumor of vascular origin that is usually solitary
- End plates and neural arches are rarely affected in vertebral hemangioma cases as opposed to Paget's disease

Multiple myeloma
Myeloma leads to bone swelling, pain and/or fracture may mimic osteitis deformans.

FEATURES
- Malignant monoclonal proliferation of plasma cells
- Rare under the age of 40 years
- Bone pain, usually in back or ribs, and exacerbated by movement (65% of patients)
- Swelling, particularly on the skull, clavicles, ribs, or vertebrae

- Pathologic fracture (30% of patients); vertebral collapse may lead to spinal cord compression
- Susceptibility to bacterial infection, resulting in a raised serum and/or urine M component
- Renal failure
- Hypercalcemia
- Anemia and weight loss
- Bone marrow plasmacytosis (above 10%)
- Hyperviscosity syndrome
- Purpura, epistaxis (often with thrombocytopenia or secondary amyloidosis)

Osteomyelitis
Osteomyelitis leads to bone pain may mimic osteitis deformans. Early diagnosis is essential to avoid bone necrosis.

FEATURES
- Acute or chronic infection of the bone secondary to hematogenous or contiguous infection, or nonsterile puncture
- Usually bacterial
- Localized pain, inflammation, and/or signs of infection
- Fever (not always)
- Source of infection may be readily deducible
- Positive diagnosis provided by culture or histology of biopsy, and radionuclide bone scan and/or magnetic resonance imaging

Vertebral compression fracture
Collapsed osteoporotic vertebrae can cause pain and appear sclerotic on X-rays, creating confusion with Paget's disease. However, in Paget's disease there is commonly expansion, as opposed to compression, of the vertebra.

FEATURES
- Osteoporosis is most often a generalized condition, while Paget's disease is localized
- Typically presents with acute pain after some activity, but may be asymptomatic leading to progressive kyphosis
- Pain generally subsides after 4–6 weeks of fracture
- Bone scan shows increased uptake at site, similar to Paget's disease
- Serum alkaline phosphatase may be transiently elevated, but generally no greater than 1.5 times the upper limit of normal

Hyperparathyroidism
Bone pain, kidney stones, and arthropathy seen in hyperparathyroidism may mimic osteitis deformans.

FEATURES
- Caused by excessive secretion of parathyroid hormone
- Most often seen in postmenopausal women
- Hypercalcemia
- Kidney stones
- Renal failure
- Osteopenia
- Bone pain, muscular weakness and atrophy, and easy fatigability
- Central nervous system signs that may include confusion, obtundation, psychosis, lassitude, depression, and coma
- Vague abdominal complaints and disorders of the stomach and pancreas
- Pseudogout and chondrocalcinosis
- Osteitis fibrosa cystica (uncommon)

Pseudogout

Pseudogout, as an arthropathy, may resemble joint-involved osteitis deformans.

FEATURES

- May present as chronic arthritis involving several joints or acutely involving one or two joints
- Most common cause of acute monoarthritis in the elderly
- Most typically observed in the knee and wrist, but also in the elbow, shoulder, ankle, and hand; very rarely affects spine
- Acute attacks associated with swelling, restricted movement, increased heat in the affected joints, and fever (50% of cases)
- Joints in chronic disease may show bony swelling, crepitus, and restricted movement, with varying levels of synovitis
- X-rays display calcification of articular cartilage and tendon inserts, and often hypertrophic appearance of bone, with exuberant formation of cysts and osteophytes
- Positively diagnosed by presence of synovial calcium pyrophosphate crystals, visible under polarized light microscopy, plus typical calcifications in X-rays

Fibrous dysplasia (McCune-Albright syndrome)

Bone pain, deformities, and/or fractures, and raised levels of serum alkaline phosphatase may mimic osteitis deformans.

FEATURES

- Most often diagnosed between 20 and 30 years of age, but precocious puberty may also lead to a diagnosis
- Cutaneous pigmentation in most patients: few isolated dark- to light-brown macules on one side of the midline, irregular in shape
- Localized pain, deformities, or fractures
- Hypertrophy of facial and cranial bones (leontiasis ossea) may resemble osteitis deformans
- Headache, seizures, cranial nerve abnormalities, hearing loss
- Narrowing of the external ear canal
- High levels of serum alkaline phosphatase and urinary collagen breakdown products (30% of patients)
- High cardiac output in some subjects
- X-rays of lesions typically show a radiolucent area with a well-defined smooth or scalloped border, plus cortical thinning; bone enlargement may also be seen
- Spontaneous scalp hemorrhages (rare)

SIGNS & SYMPTOMS
Signs

- Disease most often affects pelvis, femur, skull, tibia, spinal vertebrae (especially lumbar), clavicle, and humerus
- Increased levels of serum alkaline phosphatase in most but not all patients
- Signs of secondary osteoarthritis; most often occurs in the hip, but also in the knee or other joints
- Bowing or swelling of long bones, perhaps affecting gait
- Curvature of the spine
- Increased skull size
- Enlargement of facial bones
- Affected area may be relatively warm to the touch
- Pathologic fracture after trivial trauma, especially in femur, tibia, or forearm
- Hearing loss
- Loss of vision or results of other cranial lesions (uncommon)

- Signs of spinal cord compression, including cauda equina syndrome or paraplegia (rare)
- Signs of brainstem compression, including gait disturbances and/or dementia (rare)
- Signs of osteosarcoma, congestive heart failure, or associated disorders
- Angioid streaking of the retina

Symptoms
- Most patients are asymptomatic and progress is insidious
- Disease most often affects pelvis, femur, skull, tibia, spinal vertebrae (especially lumbar), clavicle, humerus
- Bone pain most often felt in back or legs, but facial pain may also occur
- Pain usually aching and deep, but may be sharp; may be severe and persistent
- Often most symptomatic at night
- Headaches or other pain
- Pain or stiffness due to secondary osteoarthritis; most often occurs in the hip, but also in the knee or other joints
- Bowing or swelling of long bones, perhaps affecting gait
- Curvature of the spine
- Increased skull size
- Enlargement of facial bones (may lead to loosening of teeth, poorly fitting dentures, or disturbed chewing)
- Pathologic fracture after trivial trauma, especially in femur, tibia, or forearm
- Hearing loss
- Loss of vision or results of other cranial lesions (uncommon)
- Symptoms of spinal cord compression, including cauda equina syndrome or paraplegia (rare)
- Symptoms of brainstem compression, including gait disturbances and/or dementia (rare)
- Signs of osteosarcoma, congestive heart failure, or associated disorders

ASSOCIATED DISORDERS
- Osteoarthritis: secondary to bone deformation
- Hyperparathyroidism: 10–15% of patients; secondary to increased skeletal calcium demands. Note that primary hyperparathyroidism is a common disorder and can be seen in pagetic patients (coincidentally). In this case, the calcium level will be elevated. It is important to correct this disorder as parathyroid hormone (PTH) levels do impact on skeletal remodeling
- Kidney stones: more common in osteitis deformans patients
- Gout
- Pseudogout
- Hypercalcemia and/or hypercalciuria if the patient is immobilized (rare)
- Congestive heart failure may occur in individuals at risk secondary to the high output state

KEY! DON'T MISS!
- If osteosarcoma or osteomyelitis is suspected, refer immediately
- Symptoms and signs of spinal cord compression should prompt immediate referral to a neurosurgeon

CONSIDER CONSULT
- Refer to rheumatology to establish or confirm diagnosis
- Refer to rheumatology to interpret laboratory tests
- Refer to rheumatology to determine need for bone biopsy
- Refer to rheumatology if osteomyelitis is suspected
- Refer to oncology if osteosarcoma is suspected
- Refer to neurosurgery if spinal cord compression is suspected

INVESTIGATION OF THE PATIENT
Direct questions to patient

Q How long have you had these symptoms? Progress is insidious and years may have elapsed between onset and examination

Q Do you feel any pain and, if so, where? The answer will direct the practitioner to some possible sites of involvement

Q Describe the pain. Does it hurt more by day or by night? The condition generally produces deep bone pain that is felt more at night. Secondary osteoarthritis may occur in the hips, knees, or other joints. Pain may also be caused by pathologic fractures or neural compression

Q Do any of your bones seem to be swollen or curved? Bone deformation is a classic sign of the condition

Q Have you had any problems with your teeth/dentures? Facial bone deformation may affect the mouth, and the patient may only think to mention such problems to a dentist

Q Have you noticed an increase in hat size recently? Patients may not notice a gradual increase in skull size except as an increase in hat size

Q Have you suffered headaches recently? Headaches are a symptom of cranial compression

Q Have you or your family noticed that you are not hearing as well as you used to? Hearing loss is a relatively common complication of the condition

Family history

Q Have any members of your family suffered from similar symptoms as yourself? Osteitis deformans has a familial link

Q Have any members of your family been diagnosed with osteitis deformans/Paget's disease? Osteitis deformans has a familial link

Q Have you noticed or heard any member of your family complain of bone or joint pain, or a change in the shape of their bones? Osteitis deformans has a familial link

Examination

Q Is there evident swelling or deformation of the long bones of the limbs, the spine, or the skull? Bone deformation is a classic sign of the condition

Q Is the patient's gait normal? Deformation of the leg or pelvis may affect gait

Q Are any affected areas warm to the touch? Pagetic areas often feel warmer than surrounding areas

Q Does the patient appear to be hard of hearing? Hearing loss sometimes occurs due to cranial nerve compression

Q Is angioid streaking of the retina apparent? This sign is sometimes seen in this condition

Q Are there signs of complications or associated disorders? The result will affect the management plan

Summary of investigative tests

- Serum alkaline phosphatase test provides important diagnostic information (normally interpreted by a specialist)
- Serum calcium level
- Urinary hydroxyproline, type I collagen pyridinoline cross-link or collagen N-telopeptide tests (normally performed by a specialist). Sometimes needed to confirm diagnosis
- General radionuclide bone scan indicates extent of involvement (normally performed by a specialist)
- X-ray of areas indicated by a bone scan: essential for positive diagnosis (normally performed by a specialist)
- Bone biopsy. Performed if osteosarcoma is suspected, or occasionally to confirm diagnosis (normally performed by a specialist)

DIAGNOSTIC DECISION

Characteristic appearance of bone upon X-ray, especially if supported by raised serum alkaline phosphatase levels.

CLINICAL PEARLS

- Although disease will progress within a given bone, sites of new bony involvement rarely occur after diagnosis
- The calcium level is normal unless there is a coexistent hyperparathyroidism or prolonged immobilization

THE TESTS
Body fluids
SERUM ALKALINE PHOSPHATASE
Description
Blood/serum sample for analysis.

Advantages/Disadvantages
Advantages:
- Convenient test that often provides crucial diagnostic information
- Is also used to monitor response to pharmacologic treatment

Disadvantages:
- Analysis and (often) interpretation cannot be performed by PCP
- False-negative results are not uncommon

Normal
30–120 IU.

Abnormal
- Above 120 IU
- Levels 2- to 3-fold the normal range strongly indicate osteitis deformans (highest levels of any disease)

Cause of abnormal result
Action of pagetic bone.

Drugs, disorders and other factors that may alter results
- Hepatic and biliary tract disease
- Bone growth (children and adolescents)
- Metastatic tumor with osteoblastic reaction
- Fracture healing
- Granulation tissue formation
- Pregnancy
- Thyrotoxicosis
- Benign transient hyperphosphatasemia
- Hyperparathyroidism
- Many other rarer conditions
- Some parenteral albumin formulations

TOTAL SERUM CALCIUM
Description
Blood/serum sample.

Advantages/Disadvantages
Advantage: convenient.

Normal
8.4–10.2mg/dL.

Cause of abnormal result
- Primary hyperparathyroidism
- Malignancy
- Thyrotoxicosis and other endocrine disorders
- Sarcoidosis and other granulomatous diseases
- Drug-induced
- Immobilization
- Renal failure
- Hypophosphatasia
- Familial hypocalciuric hypercalcemia
- Total serum calcium levels are normal in Paget's disease
- In a patient with known Paget's disease, hypercalcemia may be due to either immobilization or a coexistent primary hyperparathyroidism

Imaging
RADIOGRAPHY
Description
Conventional X-rays.

Advantages/Disadvantages
Advantage: X-rays needed for positive diagnosis and to assess severity.

Abnormal
- Patchy osteolysis and sclerosis (most common finding)
- Cortical thickening
- Bone enlargement
- Coarse, trabecular pattern
- Increased bone density
- Overgrowth
- Bowing and microfractures in long bones
- Osteoporosis circumscripta
- Blade of grass-, flame-, or V-shaped lesion

Cause of abnormal result
Lysis of normal bone followed by replacement with abnormal, weak bone.

BONE SCAN
Description
- Bone scan detects lesions in bones
- Can document the extent of the disease

Advantages/Disadvantages
- Advantage: bone scans are extremely useful during the initial workup in order to define the extent of Pagetic disease
- Disadvantage: not specific and may be positive in both degenerative and metastatic processes

Normal
No bone lesions.

Abnormal
Bone lesions present.

Cause of abnormal result
- Paget's disease
- Degenerative disease
- Metastatic disease

CONSIDER CONSULT

- Preferably, refer to rheumatology to establish a treatment plan
- Refer to a nutritionist to help an obese patient in a program of weight reduction
- Refer to rheumatology if therapy is effective but drug toxicity or intolerance occurs
- Refer for dental evaluation if there is involvement of the jaws
- Refer to ears, nose, throat (ENT) specialist if there is hearing loss
- Refer for ophthalmic evaluation if there are visual disturbances
- Refer to neurosurgery if neurologic symptoms develop

IMMEDIATE ACTION

- Before treating osteitis deformans, ensure that osteosarcoma and osteomyelitis have been ruled out
- If in doubt over the diagnosis, refer immediately
- If spinal cord compression is suspected, refer to neurosurgery immediately

PATIENT AND CAREGIVER ISSUES
Forensic and legal issues

The PCP may have to institute treatment without the patient's consent if there is a complication that must be treated immediately and the patient is not competent to give consent.

Impact on career, dependants, family, friends

- Low impact
- The condition progresses slowly and can be managed well with medical treatment
- Osteosarcoma, a rare complication, will have a traumatic impact

Patient or caregiver request

- **Can the condition be cured?** No, the condition can only be managed
- **Will my quality of life get worse?** The condition can be managed well with treatment now available to maintain optimal quality of life
- **Will the patient need joint replacement?** Sometimes, if destructive changes cause intractable pain
- **Will nonsteroidal anti-inflammatory drugs (NSAIDs) induce side-effects?** These medications are effective analgesic agents but can lead to side-effects. Symptoms must be reported immediately

Health-seeking behavior

- **How long has the patient waited before consulting a physician?** The answer will indicate how long the condition has been established
- **Has the patient tried to treat any pain using NSAIDs, and have they been effective?** The answer will indicate the severity of the pain
- **Has the patient visited any other physicians for these symptoms?** The condition may already be diagnosed, previous treatments may affect future treatment choices, and information about compliance may be available

MANAGEMENT ISSUES
Goals

- Alleviation of pain
- Normalization of disease activity to prevent complications
- Treatment of complications and secondary disorders

Management in special circumstances
COEXISTING DISEASE
- NSAIDs should be prescribed with great care to patients with, or at risk of, gastrointestinal ulceration or renal, cardiovascular, or hepatic problems
- Patients with history of kidney stones should be carefully monitored if prescribed calcium and vitamin D supplements
- Bisphosphonates should be prescribed with care to patients with gastrointestinal disease or mild renal insufficiency
- Bisphosphonates should be avoided in patients with moderate-to-severe renal insufficiency
- Gallium nitrate should not be prescribed to patients with renal insufficiency. Its use should be reserved for a specialist
- Plicamycin should be prescribed with great care to patients with renal or hepatic insufficiency. Its use should be reserved for a specialist
- Plicamycin should not be prescribed to patients with thrombocytopenia, depressed bone marrow function, coagulation disorders, or increased susceptibility to bleeding from any cause

COEXISTING MEDICATION
- NSAIDs have a wide range of interactions with other drugs; in the elderly, interactions with antihypertensive agents and sulfonylurea antidiabetic compounds may be especially relevant
- Bisphosphonate absorption can be impaired by compounds containing aluminum, calcium, iron, or magnesium, e.g. antacids, mineral supplements, and some oral laxatives; best to avoid these compounds
- Coadministration of NSAIDs and bisphosphonates may lead to increased incidence of gastrointestinal and renal toxicities; careful monitoring is necessary
- Aminoglycosides may have additive hypocalcemic effects with bisphosphonates; careful monitoring is necessary

SPECIAL PATIENT GROUPS
- All listed drugs should not be prescribed to pregnant patients
- Side-effects should be monitored with especial care in the elderly
- Surgical intervention is more problematic in the elderly

PATIENT SATISFACTION/LIFESTYLE PRIORITIES
- The side-effects of NSAIDs may be disadvantages
- Alcohol consumption should be limited when NSAIDs are prescribed
- Calcitonin is the drug that has the least impact on a patient's lifestyle; administration is simple and there are few side-effects or interactions
- Oral bisphosphonates need to be self-administered properly and have problematic interactions
- Intravenous bisphosphonates necessitate in-patient treatment, but the effects of one course may last for several months
- Plicamycin and gallium nitrate are highly toxic and should be used only in rare situations by a specialist
- Surgical intervention may be initially inconvenient, but the long-term benefits may be great

SUMMARY OF THERAPEUTIC OPTIONS
Choices
- NSAIDs may be used to control mild-to-moderate pain
- Alendronate, tiludronate, and risedronate are first-choice US Food and Drug Administration (FDA)-approved bisphosphonate agents to control disease activity
- Intravenous pamidronate (another FDA-approved bisphosphonate) may be used if oral administration is not tolerated/feasible
- Ibandronate and zoledronate are other intravenous bisphosphonate agents that reportedly can control pagetic disease activity. These are not commonly used in clinical practice and should not be used by the PCP

- Etidronate is the least potent FDA-approved bisphosphonate, and should be used only if patients are intolerant of more potent compounds
- Calcitonin (FDA-approved) can be used if patients do not respond to or are intolerant of bisphosphonate therapy, in patients with expanding lytic lesions or lytic lesions of weight-bearing bones, to treat fractures making use of its analgesic effects, or for preoperative therapy before elective surgery
- Plicamycin (mithramycin): this is an off-label indication. It is a potentially toxic therapy that has been largely replaced by pamidronate. Its use is now controversial among specialists in the field
- Gallium nitrate. This is an off-label indication. Used only in patients refractory to other treatments by a specialist
- Calcium combined with thiazide diuretics. This is an off-label indication. Used only in patients refractory to other treatments
- Surgical intervention: total joint replacement may be considered in patients who have severe joint pain that is unrelieved by pharmacologic means
- Surgical intervention may also be used to relieve/prevent neurologic complications and where there is progressive deformity (e.g. bowing of the femur) or delayed union of fractures
- Lifestyle: exercise and gaining/maintaining optimum bodyweight is important for skeletal health and to protect the joints

Clinical pearls
- Levels of alkaline phosphatase usually parallel extent of involvement, with monostotic disease having lower elevations than polyostotic disease and skull involvement
- Deafness is a common finding in patients with Paget's. Treatment is not likely to restore hearing, although progression may be delayed

Never
Never prescribe off-label therapies without first consulting a rheumatologist.

FOLLOW UP
Plan for review
- Monitor serum alkaline phosphatase levels 3–6 months after initiating treatment and review periodically
- Retreatment is suggested when levels rise above normal or 25% above the previous nadir

Information for patient or caregiver
The condition is not curable and disease progression should be monitored throughout life.

DRUGS AND OTHER THERAPIES: DETAILS
Drugs
NONSTEROIDAL ANTI-INFLAMMATORY DRUGS
Used to control mild-to-moderate pain.

Dose
Usual pain relieving doses:
- Ibuprofen: 1200–3200mg/day orally (300mg three times daily; 400, 600, or 800mg 3–4 times daily)
- Naproxen: starting with 500mg (20mL or 4 teaspoons) orally, followed by 250mg (10mL or 2 teaspoons) every 6–8h as required. The total daily dose should not exceed 1250mg (50mL or 10 teaspoons)

Efficacy
Normally effective in controlling mild-to-moderate pain.

Risks/Benefits

Risks:

- Risk of gastrointestinal ulceration, bleeding, and perforation
- Do not use during late pregnancy
- Use caution in pregnancy and nursing mothers
- Do not use in patients with history of drug-related syndrome of asthma, rhinitis, and nasal polyps
- Risk of anaphylactoid reactions and severe allergic reactions
- Risk of renal disease, peripheral edema, aseptic meningitis (ibuprofen)
- Risk of liver enzyme elevations (rare severe reactions have been reported)
- Use caution in renal and hepatic impairment
- Use caution with fluid retention, hypertension, or heart failure
- Use caution in the elderly
- Use caution in bleeding, gastrointestinal disorders, and porphyria
- Antipyretic and anti-inflammatory action may mask infection
- Risk of visual change or disturbance
- Advise caution with driving and operating machinery
- Safety and effectiveness in children below the age of 2 (naproxen) or 6 years (ibuprofen) have not been established

Benefit: these drugs are usually effective and relatively inexpensive

Side-effects and adverse reactions

Ibuprofen:

- Cardiovascular system: hypertension, peripheral edema
- Central nervous system: headache, dizziness, tinnitus
- Gastrointestinal: anorexia, nausea, dyspepsia, peptic ulceration, bleeding
- Genitourinary: nephrotoxicity
- Hematologic: blood cell disorders
- Hypersensitivity: rashes, bronchospasm, angioedema

Naproxen:

- Cardiovascular system: congestive heart failure, dysrhythmias, edema, palpitations, dyspnea
- Central nervous system: headache, dizziness, drowsiness, vertigo
- Gastrointestinal: constipation, heartburn, diarrhea, vomiting, nausea, dyspepsia, peptic ulceration, stomatitis
- Genitourinary: acute renal failure
- Hematolgic: thrombocytopenia
- Hypersensitivity: rashes, bronchospasm, angioedema
- Skin: pruritis, ecchymoses, sweating, purpura

Interactions (other drugs)

Ibuprofen

- Aminoglycosides   Anticoagulants   Antihypertensives   Baclofen   Corticosteroids   Cyclosporine, tacrolimus   Digoxin   Diuretics   Lithium   Methotrexate   Phenylpropanolamine   Warfarin

Naproxen

- Aminoglycosides   Anticoagulants   Antihypertensives   Corticosteroids   Cyclosporine   Digoxin   Diuretics   Lithium   Methotrexate   Phenylpropanolamine   Probenecid   Triamterene

Contraindications
Ibuprofen
- Peptic ulceration Hypersensitivity to any pain reliever or antipyretic (including NSAIDs)
- Coagulation defects Severe renal or hepatic disease

Naproxen
- Peptic ulceration Hypersensitivity to NSAIDs Coagulation defects Do not use naproxen and naproxen sodium concomitantly

Acceptability to patient
Some patients may be unable to tolerate these drugs.

Follow up plan
Regular follow up consultations are vital to detect the emergence of any side-effects.

Patient and caregiver information
Patients should be aware of the possible side-effects and the need to report their occurrence immediately.

ALENDRONATE
- FDA-approved bisphosphonate for patients with at least 2-fold elevation of serum alkaline phosphatase
- Alternative first-choice agent to tiludronate or risedronate
- Calcium 1000mg/day and vitamin D 400 IU are co-prescribed

Dose
- Adult oral dose: 40mg/day orally for 6 months
- Alendronate should be taken at least 30min before the first food, beverage, or medication of the day with plain water only. Patients should not lie down for 30min after taking the medicine, and only lie down after the first food of the day

Efficacy
- Superior to etidronate
- Oral administration: normalization or at least 60% reduction in serum alkaline phosphatase levels in approx. 85% of patients
- One study showed no reduction in bone pain

Risks/Benefits
Risks:
- Use caution in renal disease, enterocolitis, mineral deficiencies
- Use caution with NSAIDs – increased risk of gastric ulcer

Benefits:
- Duration of remission may exceed a year following one course of treatment
- Heals osteolytic lesions
- Newly forming bone after successful treatment is lamellar in appearance, with no clinically significant mineralization abnormality

Side-effects and adverse reactions
- Gastrointestinal: diarrhea, metallic taste, nausea, abdominal pain, esophageal ulcer
- Genitourinary: abnormalities in renal function
- Musculoskeletal: hypocalcemia, bone pain

Interactions (other drugs)
- Aminoglycosides ▪ Antacids ▪ Antiulcer agents ▪ Aspirin ▪ Calcium salts ▪ Iron
- Food (coffee and orange juice) ▪ NSAIDs

Contraindications
- Hypocalcemia ▪ Esophageal abnormalities ▪ Nursing mothers

Acceptability to patient
- Medium
- The instructions for oral administration are complicated, which may hinder compliance

Follow up plan
- Check serum alkaline phosphatase levels 4–6 months after every course of bisphosphonate treatment
- Retreatment is suggested when levels rise above normal or 25% above the previous nadir

Patient and caregiver information
- Must be taken correctly to avoid gastrointestinal side-effects
- Patient/caregiver must be aware of side-effects and to report them if necessary

TILUDRONATE
- FDA-approved bisphosphonate
- Alternative first choice to alendronate or risedronate
- Calcium 1000mg/day and vitamin D 400 IU are usually co-prescribed

Dose
- Adult oral dose: 400mg/day for 3–6 months
- Take with water, and not within 2h of food

Efficacy
- Superior to etidronate
- More than halves serum alkaline phosphatase levels and normalizes values in 35–70% of patients

Risks/Benefits
Risks:
- Risk of upper gastrointestinal disorders (e.g. dysphagia, esophagitis, esophageal ulcer, and gastric ulcer)
- Not recommended in severe renal failure
- Use caution in pregnancy and nursing mothers
- Safety and efficacy have not been established in children

Benefits:
- Reduces bone pain
- Duration of remission may exceed a year following one course of treatment
- Heals osteolytic lesions
- Newly forming bone after successful treatment is lamellar in appearance, with no clinically significant mineralization abnormality

Side-effects and adverse reactions
- Cardiovascular: chest pain and peripheral edema
- Gastrointestinal: diarrhea, dysphagia, nausea, vomiting, flatulence, esophagitis, esophageal ulcer, and gastric ulcer
- Skin: rash

Interactions (other drugs)
- Aspirin - Indomethacin - Food reduces bioavailability by 90% - Antacids reduce bioavailability by 60–80%

Contraindications
- Hypersensitivity to the drug nm - Not recommended in severe renal failure - Pregnancy category C

Acceptability to patient
The instructions for oral administration are complicated, which may hinder compliance.

Follow up plan
- Check serum alkaline phosphatase levels 4–6 months after every course of bisphosphonate treatment
- Retreatment is suggested when levels rise above normal or 25% above the previous nadir

Patient and caregiver information
- Must be taken correctly to avoid gastrointestinal side-effects
- Patient/caregiver must be aware of side-effects and to report them if necessary

RISEDRONATE
- FDA-approved bisphosphonate
- Alternative first choice to alendronate or tiludronate
- May be used to treat etidronate-resistant patients
- Calcium 1000mg/day and vitamin D 400 IU are usually co-prescribed

Dose
- Adult oral dose: 30mg/day for 2 months
- Take with water at least 30min before first food or drink (other than water)
- Do not lie down for 30min after taking risedronate

Efficacy
- Reduces serum alkaline phosphatase levels by 65–86%; normalization in 50–75% of patients
- Superior to etidronate

Risks/Benefits
Risks:
- Risk of upper gastrointestinal disorders (e.g. dysphagia, esophagitis, esophageal ulcer, and gastric ulcer)
- Not recommended in severe renal failure
- Calcium and vitamin D supplements may be required
- Use caution in pregnancy and nursing mothers
- Safety and effectiveness have not been established in children

Benefits:
- Duration of remission may exceed a year following one course of treatment
- Reduces bone pain
- Heals osteolytic lesions
- Newly forming bone after successful treatment is lamellar in appearance, with no clinically significant mineralization abnormality

Side-effects and adverse reactions
- Central nervous system: headache
- Gastrointestinal: diarrhea, metallic taste, nausea, abdominal pain, esophageal ulcer

- Respiratory: apnea, bronchitis
- Eyes, ears, nose, and throat: sinusitis, glossitis, corneal lesion, dry eyes, and tinnitus
- Genitourinary: abnormalities in renal function
- Musculoskeletal: hypocalcemia, bone pain
- Skin: rash

Interactions (other drugs)
- Food reduces bioavailability by 90%   Antacids reduces bioavailability by 60–80%

Contraindications
- Hypocalcemia   Hypersensitivity to the drug   Pregnancy category C   Inability to stand or sit upright for 30min

Acceptability to patient
The instructions for oral administration are complicated, which may hinder compliance.

Follow up plan
- Check serum alkaline phosphatase levels 4–6 months after every course of bisphosphonate treatment
- Retreatment is suggested when levels rise above normal or 25% above the previous nadir

Patient and caregiver information
- Must be taken correctly to avoid gastrointestinal side-effects
- Patient/caregiver must be aware of side-effects and to report them if necessary

PAMIDRONATE
- FDA-approved bisphosphonate for patients with 3-fold or greater elevation of serum alkaline phosphatase levels
- Alternative bisphosphonate for patients intolerant of oral treatment
- Only given intravenously
- Useful in patients with severe disease, when oral administration is not practical, or when patients are refractory to other agents

Dose
- 30mg/day as a 4h infusion on 3 successive days (FDA-approved regimen)
- Alternative regimen: 60mg as a 3h infusion once a week for 1–2 weeks
- One course may be initially sufficient in mild disease; when clinically indicated, patients should be retreated at the dose of initial therapy

Efficacy
- More effective than etidronate
- Serum alkaline phosphatase levels fall 50–70%

Risks/Benefits
Risks:
- Monitor renal function
- Use caution in renal dysfunction
- Use caution in pregnancy and nursing mothers
- Safety and efficacy have not been established in children
- It may prove inconvenient and costly for multiple outpatient intravenous doses

Benefits:
- May produce disease remission for up to 3 years in 90% of patients

- Reduces bone pain
- Heals osteolytic lesions

Side-effects and adverse reactions
- Cardiovascular system: hypertension
- Gastrointestinal: abdominal pain, anorexia, nausea and vomiting
- Central nervous system: headache, seizures
- Eyes, ears, nose, and throat: iritis
- Metabolic: decrease in potassium, magnesium, and phosphate levels

Interactions (other drugs)
- Aminoglycosides ▪ Antacids ▪ Calcium salts ▪ Iron

Contraindications
- Hypersensitivity to the drug ▪ Pregnancy and nursing mothers

Acceptability to patient
- Medium
- Inpatient treatment is inconvenient, but one course of treatment has effects for many months

Follow up plan
- Assess serum alkaline phosphatase 2–3 months after every course
- Retreatment is suggested when levels rise above normal or 25% above the previous nadir

Patient and caregiver information
Patient/caregiver must be aware of side-effects and report them if necessary.

ETIDRONATE
- FDA-approved treatment
- May cause defective mineralization and osteomalacia
- 25% of patients may become resistant to etidronate
- Not recommended in patients with lytic disease in weight-bearing bones
- Only use if patient is intolerant of more potent bisphosphonates

Dose
Adult oral dose: 5mg/kg/day (400mg/day, or 200mg/day for smaller patients) for 6 months, followed by 6 months of rest; repeated as necessary.

Efficacy
- The least effective FDA-approved bisphosphonate for the treatment of osteitis deformans
- Equivalent activity to calcitonin

Risks/Benefits
Risks:
- Use caution in renal disease, enterocolitis
- Use caution in pregnancy and nursing mothers
- Safety and efficacy have not been established in children

Benefit: may be of some use in patients who are intolerant to more potent bisphosphonates

Side-effects and adverse reactions
- Gastrointestinal: nausea, diarrhea, metallic taste, abdominal pain

- Musculoskeletal: hypocalcemia, bone pain and fractures in Paget's disease
- Genitourinary: abnormalities in renal function
- Hematologic: blood disorders

Interactions (other drugs)
- Aminoglycosides ⬛ Antacids ⬛ Calcium salts ⬛ Iron ⬛ Warfarin

Contraindications
- Severe renal disease ⬛ Overt osteomalacia ⬛ Hypersensitivity to the drug ⬛ Pregnancy and nursing mothers

Acceptability to patient
The instructions for oral administration are complicated, which may hinder compliance.

Follow up plan
- Monitor serum alkaline phosphatase at 3- to 6-month intervals
- Retreatment is suggested when levels rise above normal or 25% above the previous nadir

Patient and caregiver information
- Must be taken correctly to avoid gastrointestinal side-effects
- Patient/caregiver must be aware of side-effects and to report them if necessary

CALCITONIN
- Injectable salmon and human calcitonin are both FDA-approved treatments
- Intranasal salmon calcitonin is also available, but is not FDA-approved for this indication
- Useful in patients with expanding lytic lesions, lytic lesions of weight-bearing bones, treatment of fractures, or for preoperative therapy before elective surgery
- Has marked analgesic effects

Dose
Salmon calcitonin 50–100 IU daily or three times weekly, intramuscularly or subcutaneously, tapered to a lower dose when an adequate response has been attained (1–6 months).

Efficacy
- Serum alkaline phosphatase levels fall by 50%; activity equivalent to etidronate
- Some patients display therapeutic resistance; may be reversed by switching from salmon calcitonin to human calcitonin

Risks/Benefits
Risks:
- Use caution in hypocalcemia and heart failure
- Skin test is recommended in salmon calcitonin
- Use caution in pregnancy and breast-feeding
- In osteoporosis adequate intake of calcium salts and vitamin D is required

Benefits:
- Analgesic effects reduce bone pain
- Osteolytic lesions healing
- Decreases cardiac output
- Improvement in neurologic disease
- Stabilizes or improves hearing loss
- Reduces blood flow to affected regions

Side-effects and adverse reactions
- Gastrointestinal: nausea, vomiting, diarrhea, abdominal pain
- Central nervous system: headache, dizziness, chills
- Skin: rashes, edema of feet, flushing
- Ears, eyes, nose, and throat: rhinitis, irritation and bleeding of nose
- Musculoskeletal: tingling of hands
- Hypersensitivity: rare serious allergic reactions have been reported, including anaphylaxis

Interactions (other drugs)
None listed.

Contraindications
- Children ▪ Hypersensitivity to the drug ▪ Pregnancy category C

Acceptability to patient
- Medium
- Subcutaneous calcitonin imposes compliance problems, but the drug has few side-effects
- Compliance is likely to be higher if an intranasal formulation is used (off-label indication)

Follow up plan
Assess serum alkaline phosphatase levels after 3-6 months, and periodically thereafter.

Patient and caregiver information
Treatment must be taken indefinitely; disease activity recurs if treatment is stopped.

Surgical therapy
Preoperative treatment for at least 6 weeks (bisphosphonate or calcitonin) is advisable to suppress bone activity and vascularization before elective surgery.

SURGICAL INTERVENTION
Indications for surgery include:
- Intractable pain and/or significant functional impairment in joints (total joint replacement)
- Non-union of fractures
- Progressive deformity (e.g. bowing of long bones or malalignment of knees)
- Surgery also needed if neurologic complications are present or threatened

Efficacy
High.

Risks/Benefits
- Risk: often associated with copious blood loss due to heavy vascularization of lesions
- Benefit: interventions are often successful

Acceptability to patient
High.

Follow up plan
Monitor patient periodically for complications of surgery and signs of disease.

Patient and caregiver information
Patient should be made aware of the full benefits of treatment.

LIFESTYLE
Exercise and gaining/maintaining optimum bodyweight.

RISKS/BENEFITS
Risk: exercise program should be monitored to avoid placing undue stress on lesions

Benefits:
- Exercise program maintains health of skeleton and protects joints
- Weight loss reduces stress on existing lesions and protects joints
- High general health benefits

ACCEPTABILITY TO PATIENT
Exercise and weight-loss programs have a notoriously poor compliance record.

FOLLOW UP PLAN
Regular follow up visits may be required to raise compliance.

PATIENT AND CAREGIVER INFORMATION
- The potential benefits of compliance should be explained
- The condition is not curable and needs constant attention

EFFICACY OF THERAPIES
- Long-term treatment resumes lamellar bone formation and may elicit more normal radiographic appearances
- Long-term treatment may also reduce incidence of pathologic fracture
- Long-term treatment with bisphosphonates decreases bone enlargement and deformity
- Effective medical management improves slowly progressive spinal neurologic syndromes

Review period
- Check serum alkaline phosphatase levels 4–6 months after every course of bisphosphonate treatment
- Retreatment is suggested when levels rise above normal or 25% above the previous nadir

PROGNOSIS
- Monostotic lesions often remain asymptomatic
- Usually no spread to unaffected bones
- Slow progression is common in affected bones
- Fissure fractures unaffected by medical treatment
- Pathological fractures in long bones heal more slowly and with less success than normal
- Osteosarcoma occurs in <1% of patients and carries a grave prognosis

Clinical pearls
Sarcomatous degeneration is a rare occurrence, but when it does occur it does so most frequently in the pelvis, femur, and humerus.

Therapeutic failure
- Patients refractory to a particular bisphosphonate may be prescribed another
- Patients refractory to bisphosphonates may be prescribed calcitonin
- Patients refractory to bisphosphonates or calcitonin may be prescribed plicamycin or gallium nitrate
- Pharmacologic failure to arrest deformity and/or complications should prompt referral to the relevant department; surgical intervention may also be necessary

Deterioration
- Resistance may occur to a particular bisphosphonate after more than one course of treatment; another bisphosphonate can then be prescribed
- Bisphosphonate resistance may be countered with calcitonin
- Resistance may develop to either salmon or human calcitonin; the other type of calcitonin may be used as a replacement
- Patients refractory to bisphosphonates or calcitonin may be prescribed plicamycin or gallium nitrate. These are potentially toxic treatments and are reserved for specialist use in severe cases
- Pharmacologic failure to arrest deformity and/or complications should prompt referral to the relevant department; surgical intervention may also be necessary

Terminal illness
Osteosarcoma (<1% of patients) has a grave prognosis and cases should be immediately referred to oncology.

COMPLICATIONS
- Osteoarthritis: very common secondary condition due to bone deformation; hips and knees especially affected

- Pathologic fractures: occur due to weakening of bone; may cause extensive blood loss because of the heavy vascularization of Pagetic bone
- Hearing loss: due to cranial nerve compression from skull involvement; other manifestations, such as loss of vision, also occur but are less common
- Spinal cord compression from involvement of the spine
- Osteosarcoma occurs in <1% of patients; may be heralded by sudden onset or worsening of pain not caused by a fracture, a sudden increase in serum alkaline phosphatase levels and/or a large, soft-tissue mass; poor prognosis (6 months), and generally unresponsive to therapy or amputation
- High-output congestive heart failure due to chest and spine deformity and/or blood shunting to pagetic bone (rare)

CONSIDER CONSULT

- Refer to rheumatology if serum alkaline phosphatase levels remain high despite therapy
- Refer to rheumatology if functional deterioration affects quality of life
- Refer to rheumatology if either chronic pain or fractures emerge
- Refer to neurosurgery if symptoms of neural compression develop

PREVENTION

This condition can never be prevented, but early detection may aid management.

RISK FACTORS
Family history: follows a dominant inheritance pattern in families.

MODIFY RISK FACTORS
Lifestyle and wellness
FAMILY HISTORY
After the age of 40, siblings and children of patients with osteitis deformans should have a serum alkaline phosphatase test every 2–3 years.

SCREENING
Individuals over the age of 40 who have an immediate family member with the disease may be screened every 2–3 years.

SERUM ALKALINE PHOSPHATASE
This is a convenient test.

Cost/efficacy
Low cost and high rate of detection.

RESOURCES

ASSOCIATIONS

The Arthritis Foundation
PO Box 7669
Atlanta, GA 30357-0669
Tel: (800) 283 7800
www.arthritis.org

National Institutes of Health
Osteoporosis and Related Bone Diseases – National Resource Center
1232 22nd Street, NW
Washington DC 20037-1292
Tel: (202) 223 0344
Toll-free: (800) 624 BONE
Fax: (202) 293 2356
E-mail: orbdnrc@nof.org
www.osteo.org

The Paget Foundation
120 Wall Street, Suite 1602
New York, NY 10005
Tel: (212) 509 5335
Toll-free: (800) 23 PAGET
Fax: (212) 509 8492
E-mail: pagetrc@aol.com
www.paget.org

KEY REFERENCES

- Ankrom MA, Shapiro JR. Paget's disease of bone (osteitis deformans). Prog Geriat 1998;46:1025–33
- American College of Rheumatology. Guidelines for rheumatology referral.
  http://www.rheumatology.org/research/guidelines/refer/refer.html
- Paget's disease of bone. In: Beers MH, Berkow R, eds. The Merck manual of diagnosis and therapy. 17th edn.
  New Jersey: Merck & Co., 1999
- Coukell AJ. Pamidronate. A review of its use in the management of osteolytic bone metastases, tumour-induced
  hypercalcaemia and Paget's disease of bone. Drugs Aging 1998;12:149–68
- Gatti D. New bisphosphonates in the treatment of bone diseases. Drugs Aging 1999;15:285–96
- Hosking KJ, Eusabio RA, Cjines AA. Paget's disease of bone: reduction of disease activity with oral risedronate.
  Bone 1998;22:51–5
- Kaplan FS. Surgical management of Paget's disease. J Bone Miner Res 1999;14(Suppl 2):34–8
- Medline plus. Medical Encyclopedia. Paget's disease
  http://www.nlm.nih.gov/medlineplus/ency/article/000414.htm
- Morales-Piga A. Tiludronate. A new treatment for an old ailment: Paget's disease of bone. Expert Opin
  Pharmacother 1999;1:157–70
- National Institutes of Health Consensus Statement 1994;12:1–31
  http://odp.od.nih.gov/consensus/cons/098/098_intro.htm
- Singer FR. Clinical efficacy of salmon calcitonin in Paget's disease of bone. Calcif Tissue Int 1991;49(Suppl 2):S7–S8
- Siris ES. Goals of treatment for Paget's disease of bone. J Bone Miner Res 1999;14:49–52

FAQS

Question 1

Is osteitis deformans always progressive?

ANSWER 1

Yes, if untreated. Slow progression is common among the affected bones, but spread to unaffected bones is unusual.

Question 2

When should total hip replacement be considered in the treatment of osteitis deformans?

ANSWER 2

Joint replacement is an important consideration when medical and nonpharmacologic treatments have been maximized, and the patient remains dissatisfied with limitations on activity and quality of life.

Question 3

Can any treatment prevent the progression of osteitis deformans?

ANSWER 3

Remissions of disease activity can be induced by some newer bisphosphonate drugs in some patients, but it is unclear whether remissions can be made to last indefinitely.

CONTRIBUTORS

Randolph L Pearson, MD
Maria-Louise Barilla-LaBarca, MD
Elizabeth C Hsia, MD

OSTEOARTHRITIS

SUMMARY INFORMATION

DESCRIPTION

- A painful arthritis in which degeneration and loss of articular cartilage occur together with new bone formation at the joint surfaces and margins, leading to pain and deformity
- The cause of osteoarthritis is unknown. The disease process results in a reduction in proteoglycan content in cartilage, leading to reduced resiliency and deterioration
- Underlying bone responds by remodeling and formation of bone spurs (osteophytes), as the body is unable to repair articular cartilage
- Progression is unpredictable

URGENT ACTION

If joints are hot, swollen and inflamed, refer immediately for joint aspiration to rule out crystalline arthritis or infection

ICD9 CODE
715.0 Osteoarthritis and allied disorders.

SYNONYMS
Degenerative joint disease (DJD) is a misnomer, as degeneration is not the precise pathology of this disease.

CARDINAL FEATURES
- Most common joint disorder, affecting most people to some degree by age 70 years
- Slowly evolving, characterized by deterioration of articular cartilage and by formation of bony outgrowths or spurs (osteophytes)
- Two recognized forms, primary (idiopathic) which may be localized or generalized, and secondary
- Joints most often affected are knees, hips, distal interphalangeal (DIP) joints of the hands, carpometacarpal joints of thumb, and cervical and lumbrosacral spine
- Often benign, but severe changes may cause serious disability
- Initial pain may be alleviated with rest and simple analgesics, such as or nonsteroidal anti-inflammatory agents (NSAIDs)

CAUSES
Common causes
Primary osteoarthritis is of unknown cause.

Secondary osteoarthritis may result from a number of disorders:
- Acute trauma or injury: injury is followed by redness, swelling, and pain over the involved joint; with time these are replaced by a hard, painless enlargement
- Chronic trauma: an increased prevalence of has been associated with chronic trauma related to certain occupations such as professional athletics
- Obesity: excessive pressure on weight-bearing joints, especially the knees
- Rheumatoid arthritis or other inflammatory arthropathies
- Calcium pyrophosphate deposition disease (CPPD)
- Gout

Rare causes
- Hyperparathyroidism: degenerative changes may result from damage to cartilage, related either to excessive calcium pyrophosphate dihydrate crystal deposition or to subchondral bony erosion from the resorptive properties of parathyroid hormone
- Acromegaly: oversecretion of growth hormone in adults results in slowly progressive overgrowth of soft-tissue, cartilage and bone. Peripheral and spinal osteoarthritis is common, with peripheral joint symptoms in about 60% of patients
- Hypothyroidism
- Neuropathic arthropathy: such as Charcot's joints in which the loss of pain sensation may relax the normal protective mechanisms of the joint, leading to articular instability and exaggerated responses
- Congenital abnormalities of the joints/bones: localized osteoarthritis of the hip may be a result of congenital dysplasia of the hip, slipped capital epiphysis or Legg-Calve-Perthes disease
- Alkaptonuria (ochronosis): excessive deposition of homogentisic acid which binds to the connective tissues
- Wilson's disease: premature osteoarthritis has been described as one component of associated articular manifestations of this disorder. In some patients, copper is present in cartilage
- Hemochromatosis: excessive deposition of iron and fibrosis. Osteoarthritis changes occur in about 20–50% of patients, with hands, knees, and hips most commonly involved

- Gaucher's disease
- Kashin-Beck disease: abnormalities in bone growth and maturation may lead to dystrophic changes in epiphyseal and metaphyseal areas. Severe secondary osteoarthritis involves peripheral joints and spine

Contributory or predisposing factors
- Obesity
- Increasing age
- Repetitive joint overuse
- Joint trauma immobilization
- Joint instability

EPIDEMIOLOGY
Incidence and prevalence
FREQUENCY
- 2–6% of the general population affected at any one time
- About 33–90% of people aged over 65 years show radiographic evidence of osteoarthritis (OA), which may or may not cause symptoms

Demographics
AGE
- By age 40 years, 90% of people have osteoarthritic changes by radiographs in weight-bearing joints, although they are asymptomatic
- Under age 45 years, prevalence greater among men; prevalence greater in women than in men after age 55 years

GENDER
- Men and women equally affected when all ages considered together
- Pattern of joint involvement similar in men and women under age 55 years
- In older persons, distal interphalangeal, proximal interphalangeal, and first carpometacarpal joints more frequently affected in women; hips more commonly affected in men

RACE
- Higher rates of knee OA in African-American women than in Caucasian American women
- Southern Chinese, South African blacks and East Indians have a lower incidence of OA of the hip than European or American Caucasians

GENETICS
- Often there is a family history of Heberden's nodes, particularly in the female side of the family (mothers, daughters, and sisters)
- Primary generalized OA may due to mutations in type II collagen gene

GEOGRAPHY
- OA less frequent further north from equator
- Prevalence may be lower in Alaskan Eskimos
- Symptoms may be less severe in a warmer climate

SOCIOECONOMIC STATUS
- Mechanical stress related to occupation or sporting activity possibly implicated in the induction of OA
- Heavy manual labor involving gripping motions may lead to OA of the metacarpophalangeal joints, shoulder, and elbow (which are otherwise not affected by primary OA)

DIFFERENTIAL DIAGNOSIS
Infective arthritis
FEATURES
- Rapid onset
- Swollen, painful joint
- Limited range of motion
- Single joint affected in 80–90% of cases
- Febrile at presentation
- Most commonly affected joints are knee and hip

Rheumatoid arthritis
FEATURES
- Multiple joint involvement, most often in the hands and feet
- Joint effusions, tenderness, and restricted movement usually present in early stages
- Prolonged morning stiffness (over 1 h)
- Chronic, inflamed joints
- Systemic symptoms often present – possible mild anemia or mild leukocytosis
- Elevated ESR and C-reactive protein, positive rheumatoid factor

Bursitis and tendinitis
FEATURES
- Swelling
- Local tenderness with pain over affected area
- Inflammation in affected area
- Pain with joint movement
- Referred pain

Psoriatic arthritis
FEATURES
- Gradual onset
- Asymmetric involvement of scattered joints
- Selective involvement of the DIP joints, but only in 5% of cases
- Symmetric arthritis which is similar to rheumatoid arthritis in about 15% of patients
- Advanced form of hand involvement in some patients
- Pitting and ridging of the nails in patients with DIP joint involvement

Polymyalgia rheumatica
FEATURES
- Symptoms frequently of sudden onset, but often present before the diagnosis is made
- Most commonly neck, shoulder, low back, and thigh pain
- Morning stiffness lasts up to 2–3 h; patients have difficulty getting out of bed
- Mild, soft-tissue tenderness often present
- Synovitis may be present in peripheral joints
- Knee, wrist and metacarpophalangeal joints affected in 25–45% of patients
- Systemic symptoms include weight loss, malaise, depression, and low-grade fever

SIGNS & SYMPTOMS
Signs
- Crepitus: a creaking sound as the joint is moved
- Heberden's nodes: nodular swellings in the DIP joints of the hand
- Bouchard's nodes: nodular swellings in the proximal interphalangeal joints of the hand

Symptoms

- Aching pain at affected joints occurring after joint use and initially relieved by rest. As disease progresses, pain occurs even at rest or at night
- Stiffness on awakening and after periods of inactivity of less than 15 min duration
- Pain with range of motion
- Joint enlargement
- Referred pain away from the affected joint (for example, hip OA may present as knee pain)

INVESTIGATION OF THE PATIENT
Direct questions to patient

Q Has there been a trauma to the joint? Eliminate trauma as a cause of swelling and pain

Q Is there pain at rest? Patients with OA generally do not have pain at rest until late in the disease

Q Are symptoms worse after sustained activity?

Q Do you suffer from morning stiffness? One of the clinical features of arthritic conditions is stiffness of the joints first thing in the morning or after prolonged periods of inactivity

Q How long does the stiffness last? Stiffness associated with OA is of short duration, usually less than 15 min

Q Are you overweight? Obesity is a risk factor for OA

Q Do you have any systemic symptoms or signs, such a fever or rash? OA does not manifest any systemic signs or symptoms

Contributory or predisposing factors

Q Is there a history of repetitive joint overuse with regard to your occupation, sports activity? May have caused OA in specific joints

Q Is there history of a previous trauma involving joint immobilization? Such damage may eventually lead to OA of the affected joint

Q Is there a history of obesity, hyperparathyroidism, hypothyroidism, diabetes mellitus type 2?

Family history

Q Is there a family history of similar problems? Often there is a history of Heberden's nodes, particularly on the female side

Q Is there a family history of Wilson's disease, ochronosis, hemochromatosis, congenital anatomical abnormalities?

Examination

- Is the patient well/unwell? If systemically unwell, this suggests an inflammatory arthropathy such as rheumatoid arthritis, or other systemic disease
- The presence of infection is suggested by clinically evident inflammation of the joint, fever
- Obesity: define by BMI
- Is there inflammation at the joint? If yes, this suggests rheumatoid or other inflammatory arthritis
- Check range of motion at the affected joint
- Inspect joints and look for manifestations of new bone formation
- Inspect affected joints and detect warmth over a joint, tender effusion and pain on joint motion

Summary of investigative tests

- Synovial fluid analysis: generally not necessary. Useful for eliminating other forms of arthritis, including rheumatoid arthritis, especially if there is a significant effusion in a joint such as the knee
- Radiography: confirms a diagnosis of OA. Significant findings of OA are joint-space narrowing, subchondral sclerosis, and osteophyte formation

DIAGNOSTIC DECISION

- Radiography may confirm the diagnosis of OA and assess its severity; however, normal findings on radiographs do not rule out OA, as articular cartilage disease can be present without joint-space narrowing
- Suspect OA if the pain improves by resting the joint and is exacerbated by moving the joint or weight-bearing. Morning stiffness will be of short duration
- Previous traumas, injuries, fractures, or surgical procedures of the symptomatic joint should be documented
- Physical examination will help to distinguish between noninflammatory and inflammatory conditions. Osteoarthritic joints seldom display significant inflammation or swelling

Guidelines

- Guidelines for the Initial Evaluation of the Adult Patient with Acute Musculoskeletal Symptoms have been published by the American College of Rheumatology [1]
- American Academy of Orthopedic Surgeons Task Force on Clinical Algorithms; AAOS Committee on Clinical Policies. Clinical guideline on hip pain. Available online at the National Guidelines Clearinghouse [2]
- American Academy of Orthopedic Surgeons Task Force on Clinical Algorithms. Clinical guideline on knee pain. Available online at the National Guidelines Clearinghouse [3]

CLINICAL PEARLS

Laboratory evaluation in OA is generally noncontributory – normal ESR, complete blood count (CBC), negative antinuclear antibody (ANA), absent rheumatoid factor (RF) – and is not routinely indicated.

THE TESTS
Body fluids
SYNOVIAL FLUID ANALYSIS
Description
Joint aspiration.

Advantages/Disadvantages
Advantage: may help to distinguish between OA and inflammatory arthritis

Normal
White blood cell count in noninflammatory synovial fluid is less than 2000/mm^2.

Abnormal
- Slight increase in white blood cells of the mononuclear type
- Calcium pyrophosphate crystals may be present, especially in OA which appears to 'flare'
- Viscosity is decreased, protein level is >2.5g/dL, and mucin clot is friable in inflammatory conditions
- Keep in mind the possibility of a false-positive result

Cause of abnormal result
Increased mononuclear white blood cell count.

Imaging
RADIOGRAPHY
Advantages/Disadvantages
- Advantage: radiographs may confirm the diagnosis of OA and assess its severity
- Disadvantage: normal findings on radiographs do not rule out the presence of OA; conversely, the presence of OA on a radiograph does not necessarily indicate the cause of symptoms

Abnormal
- Joint-space narrowing
- Presence of osteophytes
- Subchondral sclerosis
- Presence of bone cysts
- Keep in mind the possibility of a false-positive result

Cause of abnormal result
- Deterioration and thinning of articular cartilage
- New bone formation (osteophytes)
- Increasing bone density

CONSIDER CONSULT
- Refer to physical and occupational therapists for design and implementation of exercise and activity programs, and ensure proper use of assistive devices
- Refer to a nutritionist to help the obese patient in a program of weight reduction
- Surgical consultation may be necessary for patients not responding to medical treatment, especially if pain at rest and at night is present

IMMEDIATE ACTION
If affected joint is hot, swollen and inflamed, refer immediately for joint aspiration and culture for suspected septic arthritis or crystalline arthritis.

PATIENT AND CAREGIVER ISSUES
Patient or caregiver request
Should I take an over-the-counter pain killer? Patients may consider taking an over-the-counter (OTC) nonsteroidal anti-inflammatory drug but be concerned about the risk of gastrointestinal (GI) side-effects

Health-seeking behavior
- **Has the patient been self-medicating?** Self-medication with acetaminophen or OTC NSAIDs likely to eliminate pain, so patients often do not consult in early stages
- **Has the patient undergone long periods of rest or physical inactivity?** Rest alleviates pain initially, but prolonged periods of inactivity and joint immobility are detrimental

MANAGEMENT ISSUES
Goals
- To reduce and control pain
- To minimize disability
- To educate the patient and his/her family about the disease and its treatment

Management in special circumstances
COEXISTING MEDICATION
Patients may be taking OTC medications such as NSAIDs or acetaminophen. Whereas acetaminophen may be continued with prescription doses of NSAIDs, the OTC NSAIDs should be discontinued.

SPECIAL PATIENT GROUPS
The elderly:
- Acetaminophen (maximum 4000mg/day) should be considered for the management of pain in elderly patients, as it lacks the potential GI and renal toxicity of NSAIDs
- Opioid analgesics should not be routinely used. They may be helpful for relieving moderate to severe pain, especially in patients who are unable to take NSAIDs or whom are not candidates for surgery
- NSAIDs should be used with caution and should be avoided in patients with abnormal renal function, in patients with a history of peptic ulcer disease and in patients with a bleeding diathesis
- They should be used with caution in any diabetic patients. The use of more than one type of NSAID at a time should be avoided

PATIENT SATISFACTION/LIFESTYLE PRIORITIES
- Pain is significant and can prevent patient from carrying out normal daily activities and from working

- Patient must address lifestyle issues such as weight, physical activity, and activities that result in repetitive joint injury
- Disability prevents patient from working, reduces quality of life and may result in psychosocial factors such as depression

SUMMARY OF THERAPEUTIC OPTIONS
Choices

- OA is relatively easy to manage in primary care. Independently of the pharmacologic or surgical therapy chosen, most patients will benefit from nonsurgical, nonpharmacologic therapies
- Rest and restricted use of weight-bearing joints
- Weight loss, if necessary
- Heat therapy and other modalities provided by physical therapists are of value
- Exercises including range of motion exercises, strengthening exercises, and aerobic aquatic exercises. Regular performance of quadriceps-strengthening exercise has been shown to reduce the pain associated with OA of the knee
- An evaluation by an occupational therapist of the patient's ability to perform daily activities and the provision of assistive devices for ambulation such as crutches, canes, and other walking aids are often helpful for weight-bearing joints
- Patient education programs improve clinical outcome
- Acetaminophen is the recommended first drug of choice for the treatment of the pain of OA, in view of its absence of GI toxicity. However, excessive doses may cause hepatic toxicity. It should be used with caution in patients with significant renal disease
- Judicious use of opioid analgesics, such as propoxyphene, codeine, and oxycodone may be appropriate in some patients, but long-term use should be reserved for patients who are not candidates for treatment with NSAIDs or surgery
- Tramadol is an opiate-like analgesic that has been shown to be of some benefit in OA, and it usually lacks the side-effects of constipation and sedation seen with narcotics. It is, however, expensive and may cause dizziness and somnolence
- Selective cyclo-oxygenase-2 (COX-2) inhibitors such as celecoxib and rofecoxib have been demonstrated to be as effective as traditional NSAIDs in the management of OA, but with a reduced GI risk. They are much more expensive than generic NSAIDs
- Topically applied capsaicin cream relieves local pain but may cause local burning and irritation
- Traditional NSAIDs (such as ibuprofen, naproxen and sulindac) and aspirin are useful in patients who fail to respond to acetaminophen and conservative treatment, and who have no contraindications to their use (e.g. gastritis, peptic ulcer disease, bleeding disorders, renal insufficiency)
- In patients with OA of the knee, judicious use of intra-articular corticosteroid injections (such as triamcinolone) is an effective short-term method of decreasing pain. In general, a given joint should not be injected more often than every once every 3 months
- Glucosamine and chondroitin supplementation may reduce pain, improving mobility and improving exercise tolerance in OA of the knee
- Acupuncture may be useful as an adjunctive therapy, or as an acceptable alternative therapy
- Vitamin D supplementation can be of benefit. People with lower bone density are at higher risk for incidence and progression of OA
- The injectable hyaluronate preparations Hyalgan and Synvisc have been shown to have comparable efficacy to NSAIDs for relief of OA of the knee. Benefit may last for 6–9 months. Weekly injections are required, and are technically difficult because osteoarthritic knees seldom have significant effusions

Guidelines

- The American College of Rheumatology Subcommittee on Osteoarthritis Guidelines. Recommendations for the medical management of osteoarthritis of the hip and knee. Also available online at the National Guidelines Clearinghouse [4]

- American Academy of Orthopedic Surgeons Task Force on Clinical Algorithms; AAOS Committee on Clinical Policies. Clinical guideline on hip pain. Available online at the National Guidelines Clearinghouse [2]
- American Academy of Orthopedic Surgeons Task Force on Clinical Algorithms. Clinical guideline on knee pain. Available online at the National Guidelines Clearinghouse [3]

Clinical pearls
Patients with severe hip or knee involvement should be referred for surgical consultation.

Never
There is NEVER a role for prednisone or methotrexate in the treatment of OA.

FOLLOW UP
Plan for review
- Follow range of motion and functional status at regular intervals
- Monitor for GI blood loss and follow cardiac, renal, and mental status in elderly patients on NSAIDs and/or aspirin
- Periodic blood counts, renal function tests, hepatic enzymes should be considered in patients on long-term NSAID therapy. Testing stool for occult blood is of uncertain value. A NSAID may cause occult blood in the stool, without causing clinically significant GI bleeding

Information for patient or caregiver
Progression is not always inevitable and prognosis is variable depending on the site and extent of disease.

DRUGS AND OTHER THERAPIES: DETAILS
Drugs
ACETAMINOPHEN (OTC)
Dose
Up to a maximum of 4000mg/day, orally.

Efficacy
Superior to placebo and comparable to naproxen and ibuprofen in OA of the knee.

Risks/Benefits
Risks:
- Caution in hepatic and renal impairment
- Overdosage results in hepatic and renal damage unless treated promptly
- Overdose may lead to multiorgan failure and may be fatal

Benefit: reduces fever and malaise

Side-effects and adverse reactions
- Acetaminophen rarely causes side-effects when used intermittently.
- Rare: nausea, vomiting, rashes, blood disorders, acute pancreatitis, acute hepatic, and renal failure

Interactions (other drugs)
- Alcohol ▪ Anticoagulants ▪ Anticonvulsants ▪ Isoniazid ▪ Cholestyramine ▪ Colestipol ▪ Domperidone ▪ Metoclopromide

Contraindications
Avoid in patients with known liver dysfunction (e.g. alcoholic liver disease, chronic hepatitis, etc)

Evidence
Acetaminophen is an effective first-line treatment choice for OA of the hip or knee.

- Two systematic reviews have shown that acetaminophen is an effective analgesic in the short-term management of osteoarthritis of the hip and knee [5] *Level M*
- Initial treatment of OA of the hip is symptomatic, with acetaminophen or low dose aspirin [3] *Level C*

Acceptability to patient
High.

Patient and caregiver information
Patient can self-medicate when pain symptoms occur, but must not exceed maximum stated dosage of 4000mg/day.

PROPOXYPHENE
Dose
Adult oral: 65mg every 4 h to a maximum of 390mg/day.

Risks/Benefits
Risks:

- Caution in renal and hepatic impairment
- Caution in children
- Caution in patients with a history of drug abuse
- Cautions in patients with a history of suicide attempts or at risk of suicide

Side-effects and adverse reactions

- Central nervous system: dizziness, dysphoria, headache, addiction, sedation
- Gastrointestinal: nausea, vomiting, abdominal pain, constipation
- Respiratory: respiratory depression
- Skin: rashes

Interactions (other drugs)

- Anticoagulants ▪ Antidepressants ▪ Antihistamines ▪ Barbiturates ▪ Beta-blockers
- Carbamazepine ▪ Ethanol ▪ Protease inhibitors ▪ Warfarin

Contraindications
Hypersensitivity to propoxyphene.

Acceptability to patient
High.

Follow up plan
Long-term therapy in selected cases, especially if NSAIDs or surgery contraindicated.

Patient and caregiver information
Long-term therapy in selected cases.

CODEINE
Dose
Adult oral: 15–60mg every 4 h.

Efficacy
Superior to placebo in clinical trials of OA pain.

Risks/Benefits

Risks:

- Use caution in the elderly
- Use caution in renal and hepatic disease
- Use caution in Addison's disease and hypothyroidism
- Use caution in recent head injury
- Use caution in patients with a history of drug abuse
- Use caution in GI disease
- Use caution in cardiac disease
- Use caution in pregnancy and breast-feeding

Side-effects and adverse reactions

- Cardiovascular system: bradycardia, tachcardia, palpitations, hypotension
- Central nervous system: headache, drowsiness, dizziness, dysphoria, addiction
- Gastrointestinal: nausea and vomiting, constipation, diarrhea, paralytic ileus, abdominal cramps
- Respiratory: respiratory depression
- Skin: rashes, urticaria

Interactions (other drugs)

- Alcohol ▪ Antidepressants (tricylcics and MAOIs) ▪ Antipsychotics ▪ Anxiolytics and hypnotics ▪ Cimetidine ▪ Ciprofloxacin ▪ Domperidone ▪ Metoclopramide ▪ Moclobemide ▪ Ritonavir

Contraindications

- Colitis ▪ Liver failure ▪ Diarrhea secondary to poisoning or infectious diarrhea ▪ Severe pulmonary disease or respiratory failure ▪ Children

Acceptability to patient

Low to moderate due to excessive sedation, constipation and abuse potential.

Follow up plan

Long-term therapy generally not indicated.

Patient and caregiver information

Long-term therapy is appropriate in selected cases only.

IBUPROFEN

Dose

Ibuprofen: analgesic dose 200mg 4 times/day up to a maximum of 3200mg/day (usually no more than 2400mg/day for osteoarthritis).

Efficacy

Excellent.

Risks/Benefits

Risks:

- Use caution in elderly
- Use caution in hepatic, renal and cardiac failure
- Use caution in bleeding disorders

Benefits:

- Faster onset of action than colchicines
- Inexpensive

Side-effects and adverse reactions
- Cardiovascular system: hypertension, peripheral edema
- Central nervous system: headache, dizziness, tinnitus
- Gastrointestinal: anorexia, nausea, dyspepsia, peptic ulceration, bleeding
- Genitourinary: nephrotoxicity
- Hematologic: blood cell disorders
- Hypersensitivity: rashes, bronchospasm, angioedema

Interactions (other drugs)
- Aminoglycosides   Anticoagulants   Antihypertensives   Baclofen   Corticosteroids
- Cyclosporine, tacrolimus   Digoxin   Diuretics   Lithium   Methotrexate
- Phenylpropanolamine   Warfarin

Contraindications
- Peptic ulceration   Hypersensitivity to NSAIDs   Coagulation defects
- Severe renal or hepatic disease

Evidence
NSAIDs are effective as first-line analgesics in the management of OA.
- Pain secondary to OA of the hip and knee may be effectively managed in the short term with NSAIDs, as found in three systematic reviews [5] *Level M*
- Joint damage in OA may be accelerated by indomethacin and other NSAIDs. Also NSAID use in older people may cause GI or renal damage [5]
- NSAIDs, along with acetaminophen should be one of the first-line treatment options in OA of the knee [3] *Level C*

Acceptability to patient
Generally good.

Follow up plan
It is useful to obtain liver function tests, serum hemoglobin, creatinine and potassium measurements before initiation of therapy and periodically to monitor for toxicity in patients on long-term NSAIDs.

Patient and caregiver information
Patients should be instructed about potential side-effects such as GI toxicity and advised to take the medication with food.

NAPROXEN
Dose
250–500mg twice daily by mouth.

Efficacy
Excellent.

Risks/Benefits
Risks:
- Use caution in hepatic, renal and cardiac disorders
- Use caution in elderly
- Use caution in bleeding disorders
- Use caution in porphyria
- Use caution in hepatic, renal, and cardiac failure

Benefit: faster onset of action than colchicines

Side-effects and adverse reactions
- Cardiovascular system: congestive heart failure, dysrhythmias, edema, palpitations, dyspnea
- Central nervous system: headache, dizziness, drowsiness, vertigo
- Gastrointestinal: constipation, heartburn, diarrhea, vomiting, nausea, dyspepsia, peptic ulceration, stomatitis
- Genitourinary: acute renal failure
- Hematolgic: thrombocytopenia
- Hypersensitivity: rashes, bronchospasm, angioedema
- Skin: pruritis, ecchymoses, sweating, purpura

Interactions (other drugs)
- Aminoglycosides
- Anticoagulants
- Antihypertensives
- Corticosteroids
- Cyclosporine
- Digoxin
- Diuretics
- Lithium
- Methotrexate
- Phenylpropanolamine
- Probenecid
- Triamterene

Contraindications
- Peptic ulceration
- Hypersensitivity to NSAIDs
- Coagulation defects
- Do not use naproxen and naproxen sodium concomitantly

Evidence
NSAIDs are effective as first-line analgesics in the management of OA.
- Pain secondary to OA of the hip and knee may be effectively managed in the short term with NSAIDs, as found in three systematic reviews [5] *Level M*
- Joint damage in OA may be accelerated by indomethacin and other NSAIDs. Also NSAID use in older people may cause GI or renal damage [5]
- NSAIDs, along with acetaminophen should be one of the first-line treatment options in osteoarthritis of the knee [3] *Level C*

Acceptability to patient
Generally good.

Follow up plan
It is useful to obtain liver function tests, serum hemoglobin, creatinine, and potassium measurements before initiation of therapy and periodically to monitor for toxicity in patients on long-term NSAIDs.

Patient and caregiver information
Patients should be instructed about potential side-effects such as GI toxicity and advised to take the medication with food.

SULINDAC
Dose
200 mg twice daily by mouth.

Efficacy
Excellent.

Risks/Benefits
Risks:
- Use caution in hepatic, renal and cardiac failure, renal calculi
- Use caution in GI bleeding
- Discontinue if pancreatitis is suspected

Benefit: faster onset of action than colchicines

Side-effects and adverse reactions
- Central nervous system: headache, dizziness, tinnitus
- Gastrointestinal: anorexia, constipation, diarrhea, nausea, dyspepsia, peptic ulceration, gastrointestinal pain
- Genitourinary: urine discoloration occasionally reported
- Hypersensitivity: rashes, bronchospasm, angioedema
- Hemetalogic: thrombocytopenia
- Skin: rash

Interactions (other drugs)
- Aminoglycosides ▪ Antihypertensives ▪ Corticosteroids ▪ Cyclosporin ▪ Digoxin
- Lithium ▪ Methotrexate ▪ NSAIDs ▪ Phenylpropanolamine ▪ Diuretics ▪ Warfarin

Contraindications
- Hypersensitivity to NSAIDs ▪ Bronchospasm ▪ Peptic ulceration ▪ Coagulation defects

Acceptability to patient
Generally good.

Follow up plan
It is useful to obtain liver function tests, serum hemoglobin, creatinine, and potassium measurements before initiation of therapy and periodically to monitor for toxicity in patients on long-term NSAIDs.

Patient and caregiver information
Patients should be instructed about potential side-effects such as GI toxicity and advised to take the medication with food.

ASPIRIN
Dose
2.6–5.2g/day in divided doses every 4–6 h, orally, for arthritis. 325–650mg every 4 h, as needed. Not to exceed 4000mg/day.

Efficacy
Excellent

Risks/Benefits
Risks:
- Use caution in anemia, Hodgkin's disease, bleeding disorders
- Use caution with gout, hepatic, and renal disease
- Use caution with asthma, nasal polyps, nasal allergies
- Use caution with children and teenagers (Reye's syndrome)

Benefit: simple dosing regimen allows for better patient compliance

Side-effects and adverse reactions
- Central nervous system: dizziness, headache
- Gastrointestinal: abdominal pain, nausea, dyspepsia, hepatotoxicity, gastrointestinal bleeding
- Eyes, ears, nose, and throat: hearing loss, tinnitus
- Hematologial: bleeding disorders, thrombocytopenia
- Respiratory: hyperpnea, asthma
- Skin: angioedema, bruising, rash, urticaria

Interactions (other drugs)
- ACE inhibitors ▪ Acetazolamide ▪ Antacids ▪ Corticosteroids ▪ Diltiazem ▪ Ethanol
- Griseofulvin ▪ Methotrexate ▪ Oral anticoagulants ▪ Anti-gout medicines ▪ Warfarin
(enhanced hypoprothrombinemic effect of warfarin

Contraindications
- Gastrointestinal bleeding ▪ Bleeding disorders ▪ Bone marrow suppression
- Hypersensitivity to salicylates, NSAIDS or tartrazine

Evidence
Initial treatment of OA of the hip is symptomatic, with acetaminophen or low-dose aspirin [3]
Level C

Acceptability to patient
High.

Follow up plan
It is useful to perform liver function tests, serum hemoglobin, creatinine, and potassium measurements before initiation of therapy and periodically in patients receiving long-term therapy.

Patient and caregiver information
Patients should be instructed about potential side-effects such as GI toxicity and easy bruising.

CELECOXIB
Dose
200mg/day in a single dose.

Efficacy
Excellent.

Risks/Benefits
Risk: use caution with patients with pre-existing asthma.

Side-effects and adverse reactions
- Central nervous system: dizziness, headache
- Gastrointestinal: abdominal pain, diarrhea, dyspepsia, flatulence, nausea
- Respiratory: respiratory tract infections
- Skin: rash

Interactions (other drugs)
- ACE inhibitors ▪ Furosemide ▪ Aspirin ▪ Fluconazole ▪ Lithium ▪ Warfarin

Contraindications
- Allergic reactions to sulfonamide ▪ Allergic reactions to NSAIDs ▪ Inflammatory bowel disease ▪ Severe congestive heart failure ▪ Renal impairment

Evidence
Some evidence exists that celecoxib achieves analgesic efficacy in OA comparable to that of traditional NSAIDs, and is well tolerated with no effect on platelet aggregation. Serious GI toxicity, such as GI ulceration may be reduced [6] *Level P*

Acceptability to patient
High.

Patient and caregiver information
Instruct patients to report signs and symptoms of GI ulceration or bleeding (may occur without warning), edema, or skin rash.

ROFECOXIB
Dose
12.5–50mg/day, orally; highest recommended for OA is 25mg/day.

Efficacy
- Similar to ibuprofen and naproxen, but with less GI toxicity
- Causes a 50% reduction in serious GI toxicity such as bleeding compared to naproxen, although GI intolerance (nausea, dyspepsia, diarrhea, etc.) may occur
- Improves physical functioning in OA patients compared with placebo

Risks/Benefits
Risks:
- Use caution with patients with pre-existing asthma
- Use caution in GI disease, perforation or history of bleeding, or peptic ulcer disease
- Use caution in the elderly or children
- Use caution in renal disease
- Use caution in fluid retention, hypertension or heart failure
- Use caution in breast-feeding or pregnancy
- Ensure patient is not dehydrated before commencing therapy

Side-effects and adverse reactions
- Cardiovascular system: edema, hypertension, congestive heart failure
- Central nervous system: dizziness, headache, fever
- Gastrointestinal: abdominal pain, diarrhea, nausea, vomiting, dyspepsia, gastritis, anorexia, cholecystitis, flatulence, esophagitis, constipation, gastrointestinal bleeding, pancreatitis, peptic ulcer, stomatitis, elevated hepatic enzymes
- Hematologic: anemia
- Musculoskeletal: back pain, fatigue
- Respiratory: sinusitis, bronchitis
- Skin: maculopapular rash, urticaria, dermatitis

Interactions (other drugs)
- ACE inhibitors ▪ Alendronate ▪ Antineoplastic agents ▪ Aspirin ▪ Corticosteroids
▪ Cyclosporine ▪ Diuretics ▪ Ethanol ▪ Lithium ▪ Methotrexate ▪ Rifampin ▪ Warfarin

Contraindications
▪ Salicylate hypersensitivity ▪ Severe hepatic impairment ▪ Advanced renal disease

Evidence
Rofecoxib is effective in the management of pain associated with OA, and is less likely to cause gastric ulceration than NSAIDs.
- A RCT compared rofecoxib with placebo in the management of patients with OA of the knee over a 6-week period. Analgesic benefit was noted in the treatment group. Rofecoxib was well tolerated in high and low doses [7] *Level P*
- A RCT compared rofecoxib (25mg and 50mg), ibuprofen (800mg three times a day) and placebo in patients with osteoarthritis. Patients were assessed for the development of gastroduodenal ulceration at 6, 12 and 24 weeks with endoscopy. Ulcers were significantly less common in the rofecoxib group at 12 and 24 weeks. The lower dose of rofecoxib was similar to placebo for ulcer incidence at 12 weeks [8] *Level P*

Acceptability to patient
High.

Patient and caregiver information
Instruct patients to report any signs of GI toxicity (bleeding may occur without warning) and pedal edema.

CAPSAICIN (OTC)
Dose
Topical cream: 0.025% and 0.075% applied 4 times/day; 0.25% applied twice daily.

Efficacy
A beneficial effect may require 1–2 weeks of therapy.

Risks/Benefits
Risks:
- Do not use on eyes
- Do not take a bath or shower either before or after applying capsaicin

Side-effects and adverse reactions
Burning or itching of skin where applied.

Interactions (other drugs)
None reported.

Contraindications
Broken or damaged skin.

Evidence
Capsaicin cream may be an effective and safe treatment of OA.
- A RCT compared capsaicin with placebo in the management of OA over a 4-week period. Capsaicin is superior to placebo in relieving the pain of OA. Mean reduction in pain was 33% [9] *Level P*
- A nonsystematic meta-analysis found that capsaicin was a more effective analgesic than placebo [5] *Level M*
- Capsaicin is an acceptable alternative, either as an adjunct or as monotherapy, for OA patients who do not desire systemic treatment [4] *Level C*

Acceptability to patient
Medium.

Patient and caregiver information
- Patients should be advised to apply cream wearing a glove or to wash hands immediately after application to avoid dispersal of cream to the eyes or mucous membranes
- Care should be taken to avoid getting the affected area wet after application, as that would increase the risk of a burning sensation

TRIAMCINOLONE
Dose
Intra-articular administration; 20–40 mg for large joints such as the knee.

Efficacy
Reduced pain within one week.

Risks/Benefits
Risks:

- Does not provide quick response; may take several hours for relief
- Risk of infection with intra-articular injection
- Use caution with glomerulonephritis, ulcerative colitis, renal disease
- Use caution with AIDS, tuberculosis, ocular herpes simplex, live vaccines, viral, and bacterial infections
- Use caution in diabetes mellitus, glaucoma, osteoporosis, hypertension
- Use caution in children and the elderly
- Use caution in recent myocardial infarction
- Use caution in psychosis
- Do not withdraw abruptly

Side-effects and adverse reactions

- Side-effects are minimized by short duration of therapy
- Cardiovascular system: hypertension, thromboembolism
- Central nervous system: insomnia, euphoria, depression, psychosis, seizures
- Endocrine: adrenal suppression, impaired glucose tolerance, growth suppression in children
- Eyes, ears, nose, and throat: cataract, glaucoma, blurred vision
- Gastrointestinal: dyspepsia, peptic ulceration, oesophagitis, oral candidiasis, nausea, vomiting
- Musculoskeletal: proximal myopathy, osteoporosis
- Skin: delayed healing, acne, striae

Interactions (other drugs)

- Aminoglutehamide ■ Antidiabetics ■ Barbiturates ■ Carbamazepine ■ Cholestyramine
- Cholinesterase inhibitors ■ Cyclosporine ■ Diuretics ■ Estrogens ■ Isoniazid
- Isoproterenal ■ NSAIDs ■ Phenytoin ■ Rifampin ■ Salicylates

Contraindications

- Local or systemic infection ■ Peptic ulcer ■ Pregnancy and breast-feeding

Evidence

Intra-articular steroid injections may produce a small and temporary analgesic effect for patients with OA.

- Two small prospective trials compared intra-articular corticosteroid injections with placebo in the management of knee OA. There was a greater reduction in pain and tenderness in the steroid-treated group; however the effects were temporary [10,11] *Level P*
- A systematic review of intra-articular steroid injections in OA of the knee found little analgesic benefit from steroids compared with placebo. Pain reduction lasted from one week to one month [5] *Level M*

Acceptability to patient
Low.

Physical therapy
EXERCISE
Efficacy

- Good with effects being seen within 8 weeks
- Quadriceps strengthening has been shown to reduce symptoms of pain in osteoarthritis of the knee
- Adherence to some programs low
- Long-term adherence to walking is critical to maintenance of initial gains in functional outcomes
- Exercise is integral in reducing impairment, improving function, and preventing disability

Risks/Benefits
- Risk: may worsen pre-existing symptoms.
- Benefit: improved flexibility, cardiovascular fitness, weight loss and improvement in wellbeing.

Evidence
Exercise may be effective in improving functioning in patients with OA of the hip and knee. Exercise must be continued for the benefit to be ongoing.
- A RCT assessed the efficacy of a program of supervised fitness, walking and education in patients with OA of the knee. Compared to standard medical therapy, fitness and education improved functional status without exacerbating pain or other symptoms [12] *Level P*
- A one-year follow up study of the above trial found that the failure of intervention patients to maintain regular walking resulted in loss of functional benefits [13]
- A RCT compared aerobic exercise with placebo (nonaerobic exercise) in the management of patients with OA. The treatment group showed significant improvement in physical activity, as well as in anxiety and depression over 12 weeks [14] *Level P*
- Three systematic reviews of people with knee and hip OA found that some evidence that exercise was beneficial, but more evidence is required [5] *Level M*

Acceptability to patient
Medium: adherence to exercise program can be problematic.

Patient and caregiver information
Long-term adherence to exercise is critical to maintenance of initial gains in functional outcomes.

Occupational therapy
EVALUATE ABILITY TO PERFORM DAILY ACTIVITIES AND PROVIDE ASSISTIVE DEVICES
Efficacy
An appropriately selected cane can reduce hip loading by 20–30%.

Risks/Benefits
- Risk: evaluating the patient's ability to perform daily activities and providing assistive devices as needed will help reduce further joint damage and assist in activities of daily life
- Benefit: reduction in joint loading allows increased periods of activity with reduced pain. Use of cushioned shoes helps lower extremity joint symptoms. Back pain can be reduced by a well-fitted brace

Acceptability to patient
High. The main reason for discarding aids is that patients have improved enough to manage without them.

Follow up plan
Monitor use of assistive device to assess efficacy.

Patient and caregiver information
The patient may be taught principles of joint protection and energy conservation.

Surgical therapy
JOINT REPLACEMENT SURGERY
Efficacy
- Pain relief achieved in over 90% of patients undergoing total joint replacement of the knee or hip
- Total joint replacement has an excellent outcome and dramatically improves quality of life

Risks/Benefits
- Risk: about 2% of patients undergo revisional surgery; operative mortality rates 0.5–1.9%; surgical complications such as loosening of the prosthesis, infection, and dislocation may occur
- Benefit: elimination of severe pain and end-stage structural disease markedly improved quality of life

Evidence
There is some evidence that joint replacement is effective in the management of OA.
- A systematic review was conducted on patients who underwent total hip replacement for the treatment of OA. 70% of patients without prosthetic failure rated functioning and pain control as good-excellent at 10-year follow up [5] *Level M*
- Many observational studies have found that hip replacement is beneficial and effective [5] *Level S*
- Evidence suggests that knee replacement is comparable to hip replacement in terms of benefits and harms [5]
- Two observational studies found that quality of life was superior in patients who underwent knee replacement for the treatment of OA [5] *Level S*

Acceptability to patient
Medium: patients concerned about complications of surgery, which increase with age.

Follow up plan
- Frequent postoperative monitoring to eliminate any postoperative complications
- Period of rehabilitation

OSTEOTOMY
Efficacy
Provides pain relief and may prevent progression of disease in patients not considered for total joint replacement.

Risks/Benefits
Risks:
- Operative mortality rates 0.5–1.9%
- Surgical complications such as loosening of the prosthesis, infection, and dislocation
- Long-term follow up results often disappointing. May only be a temporary measure, delaying total joint replacement

Benefits: provides short-term benefits

Evidence
- Osteotomy may be recommended for young, active patients with OA and loss of joint space in only one compartment [3] *Level C*
- Analgesia and the prevention of disease progression may be achieved with osteotomy in patients who are not suitable for total joint arthroplasty [4] *Level C*

Acceptability to patient
Medium: patients concerned about complications of surgery, which increase with age.

Follow up plan
Frequent postoperative monitoring to eliminate any postoperative complications.

Patient and caregiver information
Patients need to be aware that this may only provide temporary relief and that full joint replacement may be necessary at a later date.

Complementary therapy
GLUCOSAMINE & CHONDROITIN
Efficacy
Doses of chondroitin in the range of 400mg three times per day and glucosamine 500mg three times per day have shown efficacy in reducing pain, improving mobility, and improving exercise tolerance in osteoarthritis of the knee.

Risks/Benefits
Risks:
- Mild gastrointestinal complaints have been reported, but generally well tolerated
- Expense can be an issue for some patients

Interactions (other drugs)
- Insulin (glucosamine may increase insulin resistance) ■ Warfarin (chondroitin has antithrombotic activity)

Evidence
- A meta-analysis and systematic assessment of glucosamine and chondroitin preparations in patients with OA of the hip and knee found that some degree of efficacy is probable [15] *Level M*
- A systematic review found 16 RCTs that collectively provided evidence that glucosamine is effective and safe for the management of OA. The reviewers concluded that further research is required to determine the long-term effectiveness and safety of glucosamine [16] *Level M*

Acceptability to patient
Other than cost, quite acceptable. Occasional GI upset reported.

Follow up plan
Monitor response to treatment: pain, mobility, side-effects.

Patient and caregiver information
Safety has not been assessed in children or pregnant women.

ACUPUNCTURE
Efficacy
Determined by NIH Consensus Conference on Acupuncture to be an effective modality for managing the pain of OA.

Risks/Benefits
Risk: little risk associated with acupuncture; occasional hematoma at needle insertion site.

Evidence
Acupuncture may be useful as an adjunctive therapy, or as an acceptable alternative therapy [17] *Level C*

Acceptability to patient
Variable, depending upon patient acceptance of needle insertion. Acupuncture frequently not paid for by insurance, which is also a disincentive.

Follow up plan
Usual care.

NUTRITION

Efficacy

Data on the association of vitamin D deficiency and cartilage loss and OA progression in the knee and hip has been impressive. People with lower bone density are at higher risk for OA incidence and progression.

Risks/Benefits

Benefit: vitamin D supplementation of 400–800 IU daily appears to be quite safe. Serum 25-hydroxy-vitamin D (25-OH-vitamin D) levels can be monitored.

Evidence

A prospective observational study of 556 patients found that a low intake and low serum level of vitamin D are associated with an increased risk for progression of knee OA [18] *This study does not meet the criteria for level P*

Acceptability to patient

Well tolerated, inexpensive.

Follow up plan

Monitor serum 25-OH-vitamin D levels to assess effectiveness, toxicity.

Other therapies

PATIENT INFORMATION PROGRAMS

Efficacy

Patient education improves medication adherence and decreases utilization and cost.

Risks/Benefits

Benfits:

- Provide additional benefits that are 20–30% as great as the effects of NSAID treatment for pain relief in OA
- Improves knowledge, increase self-efficacy, maintain realistic expectation
- Facilitates adherence, resulting in more beneficial clinical outcomes

Evidence

Patient information programs may improve outcomes for OA patients.

- A double-blind RCT compared education on arthritis medication with general information for patients with OA of the knee or hip. The group receiving education were more involved in their management, and had better outcomes, in terms of improved stiffness [19] *Level P*
- A RCT found self-care education to be cost effective in the **primary care** management of OA of the knee [20] *Level P*
- A meta-analysis found that patient education programs may be more effective than NSAIDs in the treatment of pain in patients with OA. These results were not, however, statistically significant [21] *Level M*

Acceptability to patient

High.

Follow up plan

Programs are follow up in nature.

LIFESTYLE

- Obesity: weight reduction
- Fitness: exercise will improve physical symptoms of OA

RISKS/BENEFITS

Risk: excess or the wrong type of exercise can aggravate symptoms

Benefits:
- Exercise: improved flexibility, physical activity, cardiovascular fitness and wellbeing
- Weight loss: less impact on weight-bearing joints, improved wellbeing, possibly reduced progression of OA of the knee

ACCEPTABILITY TO PATIENT

- **Exercise:** adherence to an exercise program often low
- **Weight reduction:** adherence to a weight reduction diet may be difficult

FOLLOW UP PLAN

- After first symptoms, devise an exercise program
- Monitor adherence to exercise program – make changes as necessary to program to ensure compliance
- Monitor weight and set realistic, achievable goals for a weight loss program
- After weight loss, maintenance diet recommended

PATIENT AND CAREGIVER INFORMATION

- Adjustment of lifestyle issues (obesity, physical fitness) can improve outcome of OA
- A PDxMD Patient Information leaflet is available

EFFICACY OF THERAPIES

Osteoarthritis is relatively easy to manage in primary care. Remember that a combination of patient education and exercise with medical treatments such as NSAIDs improves outcomes significantly compared to NSAID therapy alone.

Evidence

- Acetaminophen and NSAIDs are effective analgesics in the short term management of osteoarthritis of the hip and knee [5] *Level M*
- Some evidence exists that celecoxib achieves analgesic efficacy in osteoarthritis [6] *Level P*
- Rofecoxib may be effective in the management of pain associated with osteoarthritis, and is less likely to cause gastric ulceration than NSAIDs [7,8] *Level P*
- Capsaicin is an effective topical analgesic [9] *Level P*
- Evidence shows little analgesic benefit from intra-articular steroid injections [5] *Level M*
- Exercise may be beneficial in improving functioning in patients with osteoarthritis of the hip and knee [5] *Level M*
- Joint replacement appears to be effective in the treatment of OA of the hip and knee [5] *Level M*
- Self-care education is cost effective in the **primary care** management of OA of the knee [20] *Level P*

Review period

Follow range of motion and joint function at regular intervals.

PROGNOSIS

- Disease may be progressive in some patients
- Initially, pain is relieved by rest; as condition progresses, pain may occur at rest and at night
- Joint effusions may occur, particularly in the knees
- Joint enlargement occurs later as a result of formation of bony enlargement
- Advanced stage with full loss of cartilage down to bone

Clinical pearls

Judicious exercise to maintain joint motion and muscle power will delay onset of significant disability in most patients.

Therapeutic failure

- If patients fail to respond to initial recommended drug of choice (acetaminophen), the use of a NSAID is indicated
- In the setting of an acute disabling exacerbation, short-term treatment with codeine or oxycodone may be given
- Consider a single intra-articular injection of corticosteroid for a temporary exacerbation of OA in the knee, or to prepare a patient for a special event such as a wedding. The benefit from corticosteroid injections usually lasts only a few weeks to perhaps 2–3 months, and should not be repeated more often than every 3 months

Deterioration

Refer for surgical consultation if there is incapacitating disease of a major weight-bearing joint that fails to respond to therapy.

CONSIDER CONSULT

Refer for surgical consultation if there is incapacitating disease of a major weight-bearing joint that fails to respond to therapy.

RISK FACTORS

- **Obesity:** excess weight increases impact on weight-bearing joints
- **Physical activity:** lack of physical exercise predisposes to musculoskeletal problems
- **Repetitive joint overuse:** manual labor may predispose to OA

MODIFY RISK FACTORS
Lifestyle and wellness
Obesity should be tackled as it is a risk factor for OA.

PHYSICAL ACTIVITY
A program of physical exercise should be initiated as it improves physical activity, flexibility, and function of the musculoskeletal system.

ENVIRONMENT
Ensure a variety in the tasks performed in the workplace, to avoid repetitive joint overuse.

SCREENING
General screening for OA is not necessary as asymptomatic OA should generally not be treated.

PREVENT RECURRENCE
- Advise a short period of rest if there is a flare up of severe hip or knee pain
- Advise continuation of isometric and nonweight-bearing exercises
- Advise avoidance of more prolonged inactivity and measures to limit joint stresses
- Prescribe use of a cane and other assistive devices
- Prescribe acetaminophen as first-line therapy for control of pain
- Consider NSAIDs for patients in whom acetaminophen is not effective
- Consider a single intra-articular injection of corticosteroid only if there is an inflammatory component to the arthritis and a single joint is involved. Repeat injections are to be avoided
- Refer for surgical consultation if the patient is unresponsive to all treatment and shows incapacitating disease of a major weight-bearing joint

RESOURCES

ASSOCIATIONS

American College of Rheumatology
1800 Century Place, Suite 250
Atlanta, GA 30345
Tel: (404) 633 3777
Fax: (404) 633 1870
www.rheumatology.org

American Geriatrics Society
The Empire State Building
350 Fifth Avenue, Suite 801
New York, NY 10118
Tel: (212) 308 1414
Fax: (212) 832 8646
www.americangeriatrics.org

Information is also available from:
Arthritis Foundation
1330 West Peachtree Street
Atlanta, GA 30309
Tel: (404) 872 7100
www.arthritis.org

KEY REFERENCES

- American College Of Rheumatology Ad Hoc Committee on Clinical Guidelines. Guidelines for the initial evaluation of the adult patient with acute musculoskeletal symptoms. Arthritis Rheum 1996;39:(1):1–8
- Edworthy SM, Devins GM. Improving medication adherence through patient education distinguishing between appropriate and inappropriate utilization. Patient Education Study Group. J Rheumatol 1999;26:1793–801
- Ehrich EW, Schnitzer TJ, McIlwain H, et al. Effect of specific COX-2 inhibition in osteoarthritis of the knee: a 6 week double blind, placebo controlled pilot study of Rofecoxib. Rofecoxib Osteoarthritis Pilot Study Group. J Rheumatol 1999;26:(11):2438–47
- Hawkey C, Laine L, Simon T, et al. Comparison of the effect of Rofecoxib (a cyclooxygenase 2 inhibitor), ibuprofen, and placebo on the gastroduodenal mucosa of patients with osteoarthritis: a randomized, double-blind, placebo-controlled trial. The Rofecoxib Osteoarthritis Endoscopy Multinational Study Group. Arthritis Rheum 2000;43:(2):370–77
- Kraus VB. Pathogenesis and treatment of osteoarthritis. Med Clin N Amer 1997;81:(1):85–112
- Manek NJ, Lane NE. Osteoarthritis: current concepts in diagnosis and management. Am Fam Physician 2000;61:(6):1795–804
- Mazzuca SA, Brandt KD, Katz BP, et al. Reduced utilization and cost of primary care clinic visits resulting from self-care education for patients with osteoarthritis of the knee. Arthritis Rheum 1999;42:1267–73
- Minor MA. Exercise in the treatment of osteoarthritis. Rheum Dis Clin N Am 1999;25:(2):397–415,viii
- Minor MA, Sanford MK. The role of physical therapy and physical modalities in pain management. Rheum Dis Clin N Am 1999;25:(1):233–48, viii
- Peloso PM, Bellamy N, Bensen W, et al. Double blind randomized placebo controlled trial of controlled release codeine in the treatment of osteoarthritis of the hip or knee. J Rheumatol 2000;27:(3):764–71
- Pincus T, Swearingen C, Cummins P, Callahan LF. Preference for nonsteroidal antiinflammatory drugs versus acetaminophen and concomitant use of both types of drugs in patients with osteoarthritis. J Rheumatol 2000;27:(4):1020–7
- Sullivan T, Allegrante JP, Peterson MG, et al. One-year follow-up of patients with osteoarthritis of the knee who participated in a program of supervised fitness walking and supportive patient education. Arthritis Care Res 1998;11:(4):228–33
- Superio-Cabuslay E, Ward MM, Lorig KR.. Patient education interventions in osteoarthritis and rheumatoid arthritis: a meta-analytic comparison with nonsteroidal antiinflammatory drug treatment. Arthritis Care Res 1996;9:(4):292–301

Evidence references and guidelines

1 Guidelines for the Initial Evaluation of the Adult Patient with Acute Musculoskeletal Symptoms have been published by the American College of Rheumatology

2 American Academy of Orthopedic Surgeons Task Force on Clinical Algorithms; AAOS Committee on Clinical Policies. Clinical guideline on hip pain. Available online at the National Guidelines Clearinghouse.

3 American Academy of Orthopedic Surgeons Task Force on Clinical Algorithms. Clinical guideline on knee pain. Available online at the National Guidelines Clearinghouse.

4 The American College of Rheumatology Subcommittee on Osteoarthritis Guidelines. Recommendations for the medical management of osteoarthritis of the hip and knee. Arthritis and rheumatism 2000; 43:1905–1915.Also available online at the National Guidelines Clearinghouse

5 Dieppe P, Chard J, Faulkner A, Lohmander S. Osteoarthritis: Musculoskeletal disorders. In Clinical Evidence 2001;5:808–822. BMJ Publishing Group, London.

6 Simon LS, Lanza FL, Lipsky PE, et al. Preliminary study of the safety and efficacy of SC-58635, a novel cyclo-oxygenase 2 inhibitor: efficacy and safety in two placebo-controlled trials in osteoarthritis and rheumatoid arthritis, and studies of gastrointestinal and platelet effects. Arthritis Rheum 1998; 41:1591–602. Medline

7 Ehrich EW, Schnitzer TJ, McIlwain H, et al. Effect of specific COX-2 inhibition in osteoarthritis of the knee: a 6 week double blind, placebo controlled pilot study of rofecoxib. Rofecoxib Osteoarthritis Pilot Study Group. J Rheumatol 1999; 26:2438–47. Medline

8 Hawkey C, Laine L, Simon T, et al. Comparison of the effect of rofecoxib (a cyclo-oxygenase 2 inhibitor), ibuprofen, and placebo on the gastroduodenal mucosa of patients with osteoarthritis: a randomized, double-blind, placebo-controlled trial. The Rofecoxib Osteoarthritis Endoscopy Multinational Study Group. Arthritis Rheum 2000; 43:370–77. Medline

9 Deal CL, Schnitzer TJ, Lipstein E, et al. Treatment of arthritis with topical capsaicin: a double-blind trial. Clin Ther 1991; 13:383–95. Medline

10 Dieppe PA, Sathapatayavongs B, Jones HE, et al. Intra-articular steroids in osteoarthritis. Rheumatol Rehabil 1980; 19:212–17. Medline

11 Friedman DM, Moore ME. The efficacy of intra-articular steroids in osteoarthritis: a double-blind study. J Rheumatol 1980; 7:850–6. Medline

12 Kovar PA, Allegrante JP, MacKenzie CR, et al. Supervised fitness walking in patients with osteoarthritis of the knee. A randomized, controlled trial. Ann Intern Med 1992; 116:529–34. Medline

13 Sullivan T, Allegrante JP, Peterson MG, et al. One-year follow-up of patients with osteoarthritis of the knee who participated in a program of supervised fitness walking and supportive patient education. Arthritis Care Res 1998; 11:228–33. Medline

14 Minor MA, Hewett JE, Webel RR, et al. Efficacy of physical conditioning exercise in patients with rheumatoid arthritis and osteoarthritis. Arthritis Rheum 1989; 32:1396–405. Medline

15 McAlindon TE, LaValley MP, Gulin JP, Felson DT. Glucosamine and chondroitin for treatment of osteoarthritis: a systematic quality assessment and meta-analysis. JAMA 2000;283:1469–75. Medline

16 Towheed TE, Anastassiaes TP, Shea B, et al. Glucosamine therapy for treating osteoarthritis (Cochrane Review). In: The Cochrane Library, 4, 2001. Oxford: Update Software.

17 NIH Consensus Development Panel on Acupuncture. Acupuncture. JAMA 1998;280:1518–24. Medline

18 McAlindon TE, Felson DT, Zhang Y, et al. Relation of dietary intake and serum levels of vitamin D levels to progression of osteoarthritis of the knee among participants in the Framingham study. Ann Intern Med 1996;125:353–9. Medline

19 Edworthy SM, Devins GM. Improving medication adherence through patient education distinguishing between appropriate and inappropriate utilization. Patient Education Study Group. J Rheumatol 1999; 26:1793–801. Medline

20 Mazzuca SA, Brandt KD, Katz BP, et al. Reduced utilization and cost of primary care clinic visits resulting from self-care education for patients with osteoarthritis of the knee. Arthritis Rheum 1999; 42:1267–73. Medline

21 Superio-Cabuslay E, Ward MM, Lorig KR. Patient education interventions in osteoarthritis and rheumatoid arthritis: a meta-analytic comparison with non-steroidal anti-inflammatory drug treatment. Arthritis Care Res 1996; 9:292–301. Medline

FAQS
Question 1
Is osteoarthritis always progressive?

ANSWER 1
No. The rate of radiographic or symptomatic progression is unpredictable, and many patients will not have progressive disease.

Question 2
When should total joint replacement be considered in the treatment of osteoarthritis?

ANSWER 2
Joint replacement is an important consideration when medical and non-pharmacologic treatments have been maximized, and the patient remains dissatisfied with limitations on activity and quality of life.

Question 3
Can any treatment prevent the progression of osteoarthritis?

ANSWER 3
Not at present, but promising treatments are under study.

CONTRIBUTORS
Fred F Ferri, MD, FACP
Jane L Murray, MD
Richard Brasington Jr, MD, FACP
Christine M Capio, MD

OSTEOMYELITIS

DESCRIPTION

- Acute or chronic infection of bone, usually bacterial
- Results from direct inoculation or hematogenous spread of infection
- Causes progressive inflammatory destruction of bone
- Requires prolonged course of antibiotic therapy for cure
- Surgery often needed to treat chronic disease

URGENT ACTION

- Suspected cases of osteomyelitis should be referred for diagnostic evaluation immediately
- Do not start empirical antibiotics
- Assess affected area for bony instability – immobilize if present

KEY! DON'T MISS!

- Osteomyelitis should be considered in any patient with constitutional symptoms and fever of unknown origin, especially children
- Reduction in limb movement may be an early sign
- Patients with persisting symptoms following orthopedic surgery, especially after insertion of a prosthetic device, should be suspected of having osteomyelitis
- Open fracture is a major risk factor for osteomyelitis. Persisting pain, systemic symptoms, or poor wound healing should prompt suspicion of osteomyelitis
- Suspect in nonhealing or recurrent cellulitis, particularly in immunosuppressed patients or those with diabetes mellitus

ICD9 CODE

- 730.0 Acute osteomyelitis
- 730.1 Chronic osteomyelitis
- 730.2 Acute or subacute osteomyelitis
- 526.4 Jaw osteomyelitis
- 3760.03 Orbital osteomyelitis

SYNONYMS

Bone infection.

CARDINAL FEATURES

- Acute or chronic infection of bone and related structures
- Affects children and older adults predominantly
- Hematogenous infection largely affects long bones of children and vertebrae in adults
- Direct infection usually associated with local vascular insufficiency, open fractures, or following orthopedic surgery
- Acute presentation is of local pain and redness, with systemic toxemia. Chronic presentation is more indolent and nonspecific
- Poorly treated acute infections often progress to chronic infection
- Preliminary diagnosis is radiologic
- Requires accurate microbiologic sampling and sensitivity testing
- Prolonged antibiotic therapy is necessary
- Chronic osteomyelitis often requires surgery
- Suspect diagnosis in patients with nonhealing or recurrent cellulitis

CAUSES

Common causes

- Acute hematogenous osteomyelitis is usually caused by infection with *Staphylococcus aureus* (60%)
- *Staph. aureus* (including methicillin-resistant *S. aureus*) – most frequent micro-organism in any type of osteomyelitis
- Osteomyelitis caused by direct spread of organisms (contiguous focus) is caused by *Staph. epidermidis* (30%) or mixed aerobic or anaerobic bacteria
- Osteomyelitis associated with prosthetic devices is usually caused by coagulase-negative Streptococci and *Staph. aureus*

Rare causes

- Coagulase-negative Staphylococci, *Hemophilus influenzae*, Gram-negative bacteria, and, very rarely, brucellosis, histoplasmosis, and fungi may cause acute hematogenous osteomyelitis
- Diptheroids and Gram-negative bacteria may cause contiguous focal osteomyelitis
- *Salmonella* species (predominantly in patients with sickle cell disease)
- *Mycobacterium tuberculosis* (usually as a result of hematogenous spread, occasionally directly from a lymph node); thoracic vertebrae are the most common site in adults
- Fungi (usually in immunosuppressed patients and intravenous drug abusers), most commonly *Candida albicans*, but also coccidiomycosis and blastomycosis; the most common presentation is a cold abscess overlying a lytic lesion; joints may be involved

Contributory or predisposing factors

- Open fractures – 70% contaminated; 2–9% get osteomyelitis. Open fractures are the most common predisposing factor for osteomyelitis despite careful wound cleansing and antibiotics

- Diabetes mellitus type 1 or type 2 – especially a risk factor for directly inoculated osteomyelitis from infected foot ulcers. 30–60% of diabetics with foot ulcers get osteomyelitis
- Intravenous drug abuse – bacteremia common, usually affects vertebrae, pubis, and clavicles. *Staph. aureus, Staph. epidermidis*, Gram-negative rods, and *Candida* species are the most commonly isolated pathogens
- Local bone trauma – often predisposes to hematogenous infection
- Prosthetic orthopedic implant – reduces numbers of bacteria necessary to cause osteomyelitis. Allows pathogens to persist on surface of foreign material. Causes painful unstable area. Staphylococci are the causative organisms in 75% of cases
- Peripheral vascular disease – similar to diabetes as a predisposing factor
- Peripheral neuropathy – common in diabetic patients. Responsible for late presentation as the condition is often pain-free
- Sickle cell disease – osteomyelitis common, especially Salmonella species. Difficult to differentiate from thrombotic marrow crisis
- Hemodialysis – cannulae are portals for bacterial entry. Usually 12–72 months after starting hemodialysis. Often ribs or vertebrae
- Following transient bacteremia occurring in major organ (e.g. kidney, lung) sepsis
- Long-term indwelling venous lines, especially nutritional lines in chronically malnourished patients. Associated with fungal osteomyelitis
- Bites (human or animal) or hand trauma after punching the mouth – Streptococci or anaerobic bacteria – associated with human or animal bites
- *M. tuberculosis* – osteomyelitis can occur in tuberculosis patients
- Predisposition in patients with liver or renal failure, malignancy, or tobacco use

EPIDEMIOLOGY
Incidence and prevalence
FREQUENCY
1 in 5000 children suffer osteomyelitis.

Demographics
AGE
Hematogenous infection (i.e. spread in the bloodstream) usually affects children (including neonates and infants), as well as elderly patients.

GENDER
Males affected more commonly than females.

RACE
No racial predisposition has been established.

GENETICS
No genetic predisposition has been established.

GEOGRAPHY
- Increased incidence in warm and humid climates
- Osteomyelitis associated with prosthetic devices is more common in developed countries

SOCIOECONOMIC STATUS
Patients with lower socioeconomic status are more prone to present with acute and chronic osteomyelitis.

DIFFERENTIAL DIAGNOSIS
Fracture
Fracture may mimic osteomyelitis by presenting with localized bone pain and immobility.

FEATURES
- History of trauma is usually present. May not be in young children or the cognitively impaired
- Systemic features are not found in fracture unless coexistent infection present. This may have predisposed to injury in elderly

Acute gout
The main features of acute gout are as follows.

FEATURES
- Joints affected
- History of previous gout common
- Gout rarely affects children
- Red, hot, tender joint
- Typically metatarsophalangeal joint of the big toe
- Negatively birefringent crystals in joint aspirate diagnostic

Soft-tissue infection
FEATURES
- May present with red, hot, tender tissue overlying bone
- Commonly associated with diabetic ulcers
- Radiologic studies are normal in the presence of infection that overlies bone
- Systemic features of infection common in both cellulitis and osteomyelitis

Systemic infection with bone-related symptoms
- Any source of infection may have coincident bony symptoms
- Focus of infection often obvious (e.g. chest, urinary tract)

FEATURES
- Specific radiologic abnormalities of osteomyelitis absent
- Difficult differential diagnosis in sickle cell crisis with infection as bone infarcts may mimic symptoms of osteomyelitis
- Bacterial endocarditis often presents with prominent musculoskeletal symptoms and systemic toxemia

Aseptic bone infarction
Often seen in sickle cell disease.

FEATURES
- May mimic osteomyelitis
- Evidence of systemic toxicity is absent
- Radiologic studies usually normal
- Areas of infarcted bone may develop osteomyelitis – ongoing pain with overlying redness and heat together with features of systemic toxemia

Bone tumors

- Primary bone tumors
- Bony secondaries associated with known primary cancers with tendency to metastasize to bone (bronchus, breast, thyroid, kidney, prostate)

FEATURES

- Usually more indolent course
- Absence of systemic toxemia
- Characteristic radiologic changes usual and easily differentiated from those of osteomyelitis
- Weight loss common
- Pathologic fracture much more common in bone tumors than osteomyelitis

Septic arthritis

- Septic arthritis affects joints
- Systemic symptoms usual
- Osteomyelitis may be associated with local joint effusions with pus and organisms found in joint aspirate in septic arthritis
- Occasionally, osteomyelitis infection can spread from the long bone to the joint, especially the hip, causing coexistent septic arthritis

FEATURES

- Red, hot, tender joint with decreased movement
- Joint effusions usual
- Microscopic examination of joint aspirate diagnostic

Gaucher's disease

Gaucher's disease is a lipid storage disease characterized by the deposition of glucocerebroside in cells of the macrophage-monocyte system, particularly in the bone marrow.

FEATURES

- Bone pain common, radiologically difficult to differentiate for osteomyelitis
- Splenomegaly and easy bruising (thrombocytopenia) common
- Systemic toxemia usually absent
- Usually found in Ashkenazi Jews

Brodie's abscess

Chronic localized bone abscess.

FEATURES

- Acute metaphyseal osteomyelitis contained locally by host defenses
- Infection becomes surrounded by scar tissue and rim of reactive bone
- Resulting cavity or cyst is filled with pus, which may ultimately become sterile – Brodie's abscess
- Subacute cases of Brodie's abscess may present with fever, pain, and periosteal elevation
- Chronic cases are often afebrile and present with long-standing dull pain
- Distal part of the tibia is the most common site
- 75% of patients less than 25 years of age
- Surgical debridement and culture – directed antibiotics are often curative

Charcot's joint

The main features of Charcot's joint are as follows.

FEATURES
- Joint may be unstable
- Crepitus
- Bony deformity may be present

SIGNS & SYMPTOMS
Signs
- Hematogenous long bone infection (usually in children) – fever, malaise, reduced movement of affected area, redness, heat, and swelling over affected bone common. Adjacent joint effusions sometimes seen
- Hematogenous infection of the vertebra in adults – usually insidious over 1–3 months. Fever in 50%, neurologic abnormalities in 10%. Lumbar spine 45%, thoracic spine 35%, cervical spine 20%. Systemic symptoms not marked
- Osteomyelitis affecting a long bone may be associated with local muscle spasm
- Contiguous osteomyelitis – history of trauma, surgery, or chronic soft-tissue infection. Local redness and inflammation, draining sinus, may present with loss of bone stability. Postsurgical wounds may be slow to heal or drain continually. Low-grade fever
- Osteomyelitis associated with vascular insufficiency (usually in patients with diabetes type 1 or type 2); affects small bones of feet following infected ulcers. Nonhealing ulcer and/or draining sinus. Associated cellulitis common. Bone often exposed in ulcer base. More common in large ulcers. Fever often absent
- Vertebral osteomyelitis occasionally causes neurologic signs such as paresis, sensory deficit, and bowel or bladder dysfunction
- Very occasionally, extension of infection from a vertebra affected by osteomyelitis causes retropharyngeal, iliopsoas, or subdiaphragmatic abcesses
- Chronic osteomyelitis may cause sinus formation and associated abscesses
- Suspect in nonhealing or recurrent cellulitis, particularly in immunosuppressed patients or those with diabetes mellitus

Symptoms
- Hematogenous long-bone infection (usually in children) with localized pain, irritability, malaise, general systemic symptoms. 50% present with vague symptoms
- Involuntary immobilization or guarding of affected area
- Hematogenous infection of the vertebra in adults – localized pain in 90%, patient may present with neurologic sequelae of spinal cord involvement
- Contiguous osteomyelitis – local pain. Loss of bone stability common. Slow resolution of pain and persisting wound drainage seen in osteomyelitis following surgery
- Osteomyelitis associated with vascular insufficiency – pain often absent due to associated peripheral neuropathy, especially in patients with diabetes
- Neurologic symptoms such as weakness, sensory deficits or bladder/bowel dysfuntion sometimes seen in vertebral osteomyelitis

ASSOCIATED DISORDERS
- More frequent in patients with diabetes mellitus, vascular insufficiency, or who are immunosuppressed
- Recent history of procedure or trauma to joint or bone

KEY! DON'T MISS!
- Osteomyelitis should be considered in any patient with constitutional symptoms and fever of unknown origin, especially children
- Reduction in limb movement may be an early sign
- Patients with persisting symptoms following orthopedic surgery, especially after insertion of a prosthetic device, should be suspected of having osteomyelitis

- Open fracture is a major risk factor for osteomyelitis. Persisting pain, systemic symptoms, or poor wound healing should prompt suspicion of osteomyelitis
- Suspect in nonhealing or recurrent cellulitis, particularly in immunosuppressed patients or those with diabetes mellitus

INVESTIGATION OF THE PATIENT
Direct questions to patient

Q **What is the duration of the symptoms?** Half of children with hematogenous osteomyelitis present within 3 weeks of onset of symptoms; the remainder between one and 3 months. Adults usually present with vague symptoms 1–3 months in duration

Q **Where is the pain?** Pain is the most common symptom of acute hematogenous osteomyelits. It is usually maximal over the affected area of bone. Children may be unable to locate pain and may present with irritability. Directly spread osteomyelitis in the feet of diabetics is often painless

Q **Have you been unable to move the affected area?** Characteristic in hematogenous osteomyelitis but not specific

Q **Is there a recent history of bony injury, procedure, or surgery?** Contiguous or directly spread osteomyelitis usually follows bony injury, especially open fracture, or surgery. Fracture is a major differential diagnosis

Q **Is there a recent history of a bacteremic episode?** A history of an infective illness that produced bacteremia is obtained in some patients with hematogenous osteomyelitis

Q **Do you have diabetes mellitus and/or peripheral vascular disease?** 30–70% of diabetics with chronic foot ulcers develop osteomyelitis. Systemic symptoms and pain are often absent or subtle

Q **Do you have sickle cell disease?** This is a risk factor for osteomyelitis due to bone infarcts. Presentation is usually with localized pain and swelling

Q **Do you have a history of repeated infections or HIV?** Patients may have an undiagnosed inherited or acquired immunodeficiency such as combined variable immunodeficiency or HIV and thus lead to a broader differential diagnosis of the responsible organism

Q **What medications are you taking?** Certain medications may lead to immunosuppression or, if taking antibiotics, select for certain organisms

Contributory or predisposing factors

- **Diabetes mellitus (type 1 or type 2):** especially a risk factor for directly inoculated osteomyelitis from infected foot ulcers. 30–70% of diabetics with foot ulcers get osteomyelitis
- **Open fractures:** 2–9% get osteomyelitis despite rigorous aseptic treatment and antibiotics
- **Local bone trauma:** allows seeding of bacteria when damage to periostium
- **Prosthetic orthopedic implant:** reduces numbers of bacteria necessary to cause osteomyelitis. Allows pathogens to persist on surface of foreign material
- **Vascular insuffiency:** similar in mechanism to diabetes as a risk factor. Inadequate blood supply and chronic ulcers predispose to osteomyelitis
- **Peripheral neuropathy:** predisposes to chronic infection as lack of perception of pain delays presentation
- **Sickle cell disease:** causes bony infarcts within which osteomyelitis can occur
- **Intravenous drug abuse:** bacteremia common
- **Transient bacteremia occurring in major organ (e.g. kidney, lung) sepsis:** hematogenous osteomyelitis may occur, particularly in the vertebrae of adults or long bones of children. These sites of predeliction due to circulatory factors
- **Hemodialysis:** cannulae are portals for bacterial entry. Usually 12–72 months after starrting hemodialysis. Often ribs or vertebrae
- Immunosuppression
- Joint deformity or previous joint surgery including prosthetic device

Examination

- Are there signs of systemic toxemia (e.g. fever, tachycardia, sweating, hypotension)? Systemic features common in acute hematogenous osteomyelitis which usually affects a long bone in a child or a vertebra in an adult. Chronic infection or directly spread osteomyelitis following trauma or surgery may present with less systemic toxemia
- Examine the painful area for redness, heat, and swelling. This may be a sign of underlying bone involvement with osteomyelitis or of associated cellulitis
- Is there reduced movement of the affected area? Seen particularly in children with osteomyelitis involving the long bones of the limbs. Reduced movement of the limb is suggestive of osteomyelitis
- Examine foot ulcers. Particularly in patients with diabetes or peripheral vascular disease. Pain and systemic symptoms may be absent if such patients develop osteomyelitis. Associated cellulitis and an ulcer base where bone is visible suggestive of osteomyelitis
- If there has been a recent open fracture or orthopedic surgery, is the operative site healing well? Delayed wound healing or chronically discharging wound sites suggestive of osteomyelitis
- Examine for neurologic abnormalities in adults with vertebral osteomyelitis. Paresis, sensory deficits, or bladder/bowel dysfunction possible
- Are there draining sinuses present? Suggestive of chronic osteomyelitis
- Is the area stable? Instability possible, especially in chronic osteomyelitis

Summary of investigative tests

- Any suspicion of osteomyelitis should prompt immediate referral for diagnostic evaluation
- X-ray of affected area – radiographic changes begin to develop 2 weeks after infection begins. Early signs are osteopenic or lytic lesions. Periostial elevation and thickening, new bone formation, and sclerosis and sequestra formation are late changes. Vertebral osteomyelitis causes disc-space narrowing and cortical destruction
- Inflammatory markers – erythrocyte sedimentation rate, C-reactive protein, and white cell count usually elevated in acute osteomyelitis but nonspecific. White cell count may be normal in chronic osteomyelitis. Inflammatory markers useful as markers of effectiveness of therapy
- A definitive microbiologic diagnosis vital to determine treatment. Blood cultures, sinus drainage site cultures, wound site cultures (if post surgical) should be sent
- If noninvasive techniques for obtaining microbiologic samples are negative, needle aspiration of the bone or bone biopsy should be done. Normally performed by a specialist
- Samples for culture should be obtained at surgical debridement. Normally performed by a specialist
- Cultures should be set up for bacteria, mycobacteria, and fungi. Normally performed by a specialist
- Bone scan – using technetium disphosphonate (radiopharmaceutical of choice), gallium citrate and indium-labeled leukocytes. Show increased tracer uptake, even early in infection (from 48h). More sensitive than X-ray but low specificity (fractures, neoplasms, and recent surgery also cause abnormal bone scans). Normally performed by a specialist
- Computed axial tomography – shows increased marrow density and possibly intramedullary (within bone) gas in affected area. Useful for identifying soft-tissue involvement and establishing surgical approach in chronic infection. Unsuitable if metal prostheses are present locally due to artifact. Normally performed by a specialist in this disorder
- Magnetic resonance imaging is useful for differentiating between bone and soft-tissue infection. Osteomyelitis shows abnormal marrow with changed signal intensity. Does not differentiate between osteomyelitis and neoplasms. Unsuitable if locally situated metallic bone implants, Normally performed by a specialist in this disorder

DIAGNOSTIC DECISION

Pain and reduced movement commonly present in all musculoskeletal conditions:

- Careful evaluation is necessary to differentiate benign conditions from potentially serious musculoskeletal disease
- 'Red flag' features that should prompt further investigation or referral in suspected osteomyelitis include constitutional symptoms (e.g. fever, malaise, weight loss) and heat and/or swelling at the site of pain
- Suspected infection in any bony structure should prompt immediate referral for diagnostic evaluation
- Clinician should have a high index of suspicion
- Bony instability is an indication for emergency referral – this is a late complication of osteomyelitis

Guidelines

Guidelines for the initial evaluation of the adult patient with acute musculoskeletal symptoms: American College of Rheumatology 1995. Also available online at the National Guideline Clearinghouse [1].

The American Academy of Family Physicians has published information on osteomyelitis: Carek, PJ et al. Diagnosis and Management of Osteomyelitis [2].

CLINICAL PEARLS

- Any unexplained musculoskeletal symptom in a diabetic patient should raise the question of infection, including osteomyelitis
- Osteomyelitis occurs almost always in patients with predisposing risk factors (e.g. diabetes, trauma, surgery)

THE TESTS
Body fluids
C-REACTIVE PROTEIN
Description

- Blood sent for C-reactive protein is a useful screening method for patients with bone symptoms
- Elevation of C-reactive protein in a patient with bony symptoms should raise the possibility of infection and prompt urgent referral to the hospital

Advantages/Disadvantages

Advantages:

- Relatively inexpensive, noninvasive screening test for patients with musculoskeletal symptoms
- Safe
- Can be used in conjunction with ESR for both diagnosis and monitoring of treatment of osteomyelitis

Disadvantages:

- Nonspecific: may be elevated in a range of other conditions
- In patients with hematogenous osteomyelitis, C-reactive protein increases and decreases significantly faster than ESR, reflecting the effectiveness of the therapy given and predicting recovery more sensitively than ESR or white cell count

Normal

C-reactive protein normally less than 10mg per liter (but normal values vary from laboratory to laboratory).

Abnormal
- Rise in C-reactive protein is approximately proportional to the degree of inflammation
- Elevation of C-reactive protein occurs in other infective and inflammatory conditions
- Elevation of C-reactive protein does not confirm the diagnosis of osteomyelitis but can serve to alert the primary care physician (PCP) of the need for urgent referral in a suspected case
- Keep in mind the possibility of a falsely abnormal result

Cause of abnormal result
Any etiology of systemic inflammation including connective tissue diseases, malignancy, and infectious causes.

Drugs, disorders and other factors that may alter results
- Systemic infection (e.g. sepsis in the respiratory or urinary tract, skin or soft-tissue infection) may cause elevation of the C-reactive protein
- Inflammatory conditions (e.g. connective tissue disease, arteritis) may cause elevation of the C-reactive protein

BLOOD CULTURES
Description
- Blood drawn into specific bottles under scrupulous aseptic technique and set up for cultures
- Usually performed in laboratory but may involve the PCP, especially in a rural setting

Advantages/Disadvantages
Advantages:
- Can act as an effective guide to therapy
- Noninvasive

Disadvantages:
- Requires sterile practice
- Nonspecific in that positive results in a range of infective conditions
- Contamination during the taking of the samples frequently gives rise to abnormal results
- Keep in mind the possibility of a falsely abnormal result

Normal
No growth on culture.

Abnormal
Growth of organisms is abnormal but may suggest contamination. Requires microbiologic expertise in the interpretation of the results.

Cause of abnormal result
- Bacteremia underlies positive blood cultures
- Most other bacterial infections give rise to bacteremia
- Drawing blood for culture when the patient has a fever increases the chance of bacteremia being present and a positive result

Drugs, disorders and other factors that may alter results
- Most other bacterial infections give rise to bacteremia
- The recent or ongoing use of antibiotics by the patient may substantially reduce the sensitivity of blood cultures

ERYTHROCYTE SEDIMENTATION RATE

Description

- Blood is drawn for measurement of ESR
- It is a measure of how rapidly red cells settle in a tube of blood, suggesting inflammation if the time to settle is prolonged
- ESR is a useful screening method for differentiating mechanical from infective or inflammatory bone symptoms

Advantages/Disadvantages

Advanatages:

- Can be used in conjunction with C-reactive protein for both diagnosis and monitoring treatment of osteomyelitis
- Relatively inexpensive, noninvasive screening test for patients with vague musculoskeletal symptoms

Disadvantages:

- Nonspecific: may be elevated in a range of other conditions
- Less specific and of less predictive value than C-reactive protein

Abnormal

- Rise in ESR is approximately proportional to the degree of inflammation
- Elevation of ESR occurs in other infective and inflammatory conditions
- Elevation of ESR does not confirm the diagnosis of osteomyelitis but can serve to alert the primary care physician of the need for urgent referral in a suspected case
- Keep in mind the possibility of a falsely abnormal result

Cause of abnormal result

- Infective nature of osteomyelitis responsible for elevations in markers of systemic infection such as ESR
- Rate may be 'falsely low' in conditions in which red blood cells do not undergo rouleaux formation, i.e. sickle cell anemia and hereditary spherocytosis

Drugs, disorders and other factors that may alter results

- Cancers may cause elevation of the ESR, particularly hematologic cancers such as multiple myeloma
- Systemic infection (e.g. sepsis in the respiratory or urinary tract, skin, or soft-tissue infection) may cause elevation of the ESR
- Inflammatory conditions (e.g. connective tissue disease, arteritis) may cause elevation of the ESR

WHITE BLOOD CELL (LEUKOCYTE) COUNT

Description

- Blood is drawn and the total and differential white blood cell count is measured
- Neutrophils are the most discriminatory subfraction of the white cell count in bacterial infection (the usual type of infecting organism osteomyelitis)

Advantages/Disadvantages

Advantages: relatively inexpensive, noninvasive screening test for patients with musculoskeletal symptoms

Disadvantges:

- Nonspecific: maybe elevated in a range of other conditions
- Less specific and of less predictive value than C-reactive protein or ESR

- Should be used in conjunction with C-reactive protein and ESR for diagnosis of suspected osteomyelitis. Not widely used for monitoring of treatment of osteomyelitis
- Sensitivity – white cell count may be normal in chronic or directly spread osteomyelitis

Normal
- Total leukocyte count in adults: 4.3–10.8x10^9/L
- Differential count (as a percentage of total count): neutrophils 45–74%; lymphocytes 16–45%; monocytes 4–10%; eosinophils 0–7%; basophils 0–2%

Abnormal
- Differential white cell count should be examined
- Total white cell count may be raised but the element of the total cell count responsible for this rise may not be suggestive of osteomyelitis. For example, eosinophilia suggests helminthic infection while lymphophilia suggests viral infection
- Keep in mind the possibility of a falsely abnormal result

Cause of abnormal result
Infective nature of osteomyelitis responsible for elevations in markers of systemic infection such as white cell count.

Drugs, disorders and other factors that may alter results
Other infections, inflammatory conditions, and hematologic malignancies can all increase white cell count.

SINUS DRAINAGE CULTURE
Description
- Bacteriologic swabs should be taken of any drainage from sinuses associated with the site of osteomyelitis
- Sinus formation occurs in chronic osteomyelitis
- Usually performed in laboratory but may involve the primary care physician, especially in a rural setting

Advantages/Disadvantages
Advantages:
- Inexpensive, noninvasive
- Can act as an effective guide to therapy

Disadvantage: test is subject to contamination and therefore false results

Normal
- Drainage from sinuses following osteomyelitis is abnormal and suggests treatment failure and chronic disease
- In this instance, referral should not be delayed in order to await results of swabs

Abnormal
- Growth of organisms is abnormal but may suggest contamination. Requires microbiologic expertise in the interpretation of the results
- Keep in mind the possibility of a falsely abnormal result

Cause of abnormal result
The organisms responsible for the infection in osteomyelitis will be discharged in sinus drainage and will be responsible for the abnormal result.

Drugs, disorders and other factors that may alter results
The recent or ongoing use of antibiotics by the patient may substantially reduce the sensitivity of sinus drainage cultures.

ORTHOPEDIC WOUND-SITE CULTURE
Description
- Drainage from wounds following discharge from hospital after any orthopedic surgery, especially prosthetic device or open fracture, is abnormal
- Wound-site drainage should raise the suspicion of osteomyelitis, especially if associated with pain, systemic toxemia, or bony instability
- Referral to the hospital should be made and if possible material from the wound site sampled with bacteriologic swabs
- Usually performed in the hospital but may involve the primary care physician, especially in a rural setting

Advantages/Disadvantages
Advantages:
- Inexpensive, noninvasive
- Can act as an effective guide to therapy

Disadvantage: test is subject to contamination and therefore false results

Normal
- Drainage from wounds following orthopedic surgery is abnormal and if cultures are sterile this should not dissuade from referral
- In this instance, referral should not be delayed in order to await results of swabs

Abnormal
- Growth of organisms is abnormal but may suggest contamination. Requires microbiologic expertise in the interpretation of the results
- Keep in mind the possibility of a falsely abnormal result

Cause of abnormal result
The organisms responsible for the infection in osteomyelitis will be discharged in wound site drainage and will be responsible for the abnormal result.

Drugs, disorders and other factors that may alter results
The recent or ongoing use of antibiotics by the patient may substantially reduce the sensitivity of wound site drainage cultures.

Imaging
X-RAY
Advantages/Disadvantages
Advantages:
- Plain radiography of affected area is a useful screening test
- Relatively inexpensive, noninvasive. Dose of radiation varies according to location (lumbar spine X-ray equivalent to over 12 months' background radiation)
- Sensitive for the diagnosis of fracture, a major differential diagnosis

Disadvantages:
- Nonspecific – in cases of eventually proven osteomyelitis, <5% of radiographs are initially abnormal and less than one-third are positive at one week; about 90% are positive by 3–4 weeks

- May be normal, especially in first 2 weeks of symptoms
- Requires expert evaluation of films as abnormalities are subtle

Abnormal
- Early X-ray changes of osteomyelitis are osteopenic or lytic lesions
- Periosteal elevation and thickening, new bone formation, and sclerosis and sequestra formation are late changes
- Vertebral osteomyelitis causes disc-space narrowing and cortical destruction
- A normal X-ray does not exclude the diagnosis of osteomyelitis, especially in the first 2-4 weeks after the onset of symptoms
- Keep in mind the possibility of a falsely abnormal result

Cause of abnormal result
- Normal bone tissue destruction causes radiographic changes
- X-ray changes tend to lag behind clinical condition by approximately 2 weeks

Drugs, disorders and other factors that may alter results
Malignant invasion of bone may cause similar X-ray changes.

TREATMENT

CONSIDER CONSULT

- Refer to an orthopedic surgeon if bone biopsy or surgical debridement is necessary. Infectious disease consultation is also advisable
- Prompt diagnostic evaluation should be made as soon as osteomyelitis is suspected. If the suspicion is strong, hospital referral should be made before awaiting the results of investigations
- Any patient with continuing pain and/or systemic symptoms (e.g. fever, malaise, anorexia) following open fracture or orthopedic surgery should be referred to the hospital immediately
- A patient with a history of musculoskeletal symptoms and systemic symptoms (e.g. fever, malaise, anorexia) should be referred immediately for diagnostic evaluation
- Patients with vague symptoms should have C-reactive protein, ESR, and white cell count measured and an X-ray of any area of bony pain. Any abnormalities suggestive of osteomyelitis should prompt referral. These investigations may be normal, especially soon after the onset of symptoms. Normal blood tests and X-rays do not rule out the diagnosis of osteomyelitis
- A patient with bony pain and loss of bone stability should be referred to the hospital immediately

IMMEDIATE ACTION

- Empirical antibiotic therapy should not be started in the primary care setting for suspected osteomyelitis
- Accurate antibiotic therapy, guided by microbiologic samples, is necessary for effective treatment of osteomyelitis
- Early referral to the hospital is necessary in suspected osteomyelitis as delayed diagnosis and treatment may materially affect outcome, necessitating surgery and/or causing permanent disability
- Any areas of bony instability should be immobilized
- Provide analgesia if necessary

PATIENT AND CAREGIVER ISSUES
Health-seeking behavior
Self-medication with simple analgesia may have delayed definitive presentation.

MANAGEMENT ISSUES
Goals

- Identify osteomyelitis and differentiate it from other less serious musculoskeletal diseases
- Facilitate prompt referral to appropriate hospital specialist (orthopedic surgeon) if osteomyelitis suspected
- Provide analgesia as necessary
- Assess bony stability and immobilize affected area pending further evaluation if signs of bony instability

Management in special circumstances
COEXISTING DISEASE

- Diabetes mellitus (type 1 or type 2) or peripheral vascular disease tends to give rise to contiguously spread osteomyelitis of the foot. Different organisms are responsible for the infection in these circumstances (compared to hematogenously spread infection) so treatment is different
- Any infection may worsen diabetic control, and blood sugars should be carefully monitored in a patient with osteomyelitis. It may be necessary to increase doses of insulin

COEXISTING MEDICATION
- Certain antibiotics interact with various medications, particularly warfarin
- A patient on warfarin should have their clotting profile monitored closely during treatment for osteomyelitis

SPECIAL PATIENT GROUPS
- Osteomyelitis is primarily managed medically in children with prolonged antibiotic therapy
- Adults with osteomyelitis often require surgery
- Allergies to specific antibiotics should be carefully documented and should guide antibiotic therapy
- A rheumatology consult should be obtained in patients with an underlying connective tissue disease requiring immunosuppression

PATIENT SATISFACTION/LIFESTYLE PRIORITIES
- Relief of pain and systemic toxemia are likely to be the patient's immediate priorities
- Maintenance of bony integrity and stability are long-term goals of therapy

SUMMARY OF THERAPEUTIC OPTIONS
Choices
General supportive measures include rest and immobilization of the affected area, fluids, analgesia, antipyretics, and physical therapy when initial acute phase over.

First choice – medical therapy with antibiotics:
- Appropriate antibiotic treatment will be effective in producing a cure in the majority of patients if given before the formation of pus
- Following culture of samples, a parenteral antimicrobial regimen should be initiated for suspected organisms
- Once pathogen identified, the antibiotic regimen should be tailored to particular organism and sensitivities
- Choice of agent(s) guided by infection type, infecting organism, sensitivity results, and antibiotic characteristics
- Penicillin is active against Streptococci
- Fluoroquinolones such as ciprofloxacin are active against enterococci, *Pseudomonas* species, Staphylococci, and Streptococci
- Clindamycin has variable activity against anaerobes (including clostridia), *Bacteroides* species, Staphylococci, and Streptococci
- Rifampin is used for infection with *M. tuberculosis* along with a range of other antituberculous therapy. Rifampin is used in conjunction with other antibiotic treatments for *Staphylococcus* species
- Amphotericin B is the most commonly used agent in the treatment of fungal osteomyelitis
- Fewer than 5% of patients with acute hematogenous osteomyelitis develop chronic disease with adequate antibiotic therapy
- Medical therapy includes improving any host deficiencies (e.g. malnutrition, immunosuppression and coexisting conditions)
- Empirical antibiotics are given for 24–48h; if the patient does not appear to be responding, these can be changed

Antituberculous and antifungal therapies are given in appropriate circumstances
- Antibiotic levels should be measured whenever possible
- Initial treatment usually with intravenous antibiotics, usually for 2 weeks
- Antibiotic therapy should be given for 4–6 weeks in acute infection, longer in chronic infection
- Oral antibiotics can be used in the following circumstances: resolving clinical course; adequate surgical debridement; adequate serum level of the antibiotic (verified); reliable parents; no vomiting or diarrhea with the antibiotic; identification of the organism (relative indication)

Second choice – surgery:

- Necessary in chronic infection or when pus has formed or when necrotic tissue present
- Surgical treatment involves debridement of necrotic bone and tissue, obtaining appropriate cultures, managing dead space and, when necessary, obtaining bone stability
- Necrotic tissue and purulent material must be removed surgically
- Antibiotics need to be given after surgery

Third choice – hyperbaric oxygen:

- This controversial therapy may be used in addition to antibiotic therapy and surgery
- Tends to be used in patients with severe and/or prolonged infections
- Given once per day for 90–120 min at 2–3 atmospheres at 100% oxygen

Guidelines

The American Academy of Family Physicians has provided information on osteomyelitis [2].

Practice guidelines for community-based parenteral anti-infective therapy are available from Infectious Diseases Society of America [3].

Clinical pearls

- Successful treatment of osteomyelitis depends on adequate sampling for cultures; this often requires a bone biopsy
- Anaerobic infection is common in diabetics, and should be strongly suspected

Never

- Never attempt to manage osteomyelitis in the community without close supervision by the specialists (an orthopedic surgeon, usually in conjunction with an infectious disease specialist)
- Never delay referral in cases of suspected osteomyelitis

FOLLOW UP

- Follow up should be for at least 6 months after 'cure'
- Serum C-reactive protein and ESR should be monitored during and after treatment
- Post-treatment plain radiography should be done to assess healing
- If after 6 weeks of antibiotics there are signs that the osteomyelitis has been inadequately treated (e.g. persisting radiographic abnormalities, elevations of serum inflammatory markers, sinus formation), surgery should be considered
- At least 6 weeks of appropriate antibiotic therapy should be given following surgical treatment

Plan for review

- Physical examination and history
- ESR and C-reactive protein level

Information for patient or caregiver

- Osteomyelitis is an infection of bone
- It is important to rest the affected area
- All antibiotic treatment must be taken to avoid severe long-term problems that may require surgery

DRUGS AND OTHER THERAPIES: DETAILS
Drugs
PENICILLIN
Given to treat infections with streptococcus species.

Dose
- Initial therapy: 2–4mU 4- to 6-hourly intravenously
- Can be continued orally after 2 weeks of intravenous therapy as guided by an infectious diseases consultant
- Usual oral dosage: 500mg every 6h in adults

Efficacy
Treatment of choice only for penicillin-sensitive *Staph. aureus.*

Risks/Benefits
Risks:
- Use caution in patients allergic to cephalosporins
- Use caution in severe renal failure

Side-effects and adverse reactions
- Gastrointestinal: diarrhea, nausea, vomiting
- Respiratory: anaphylaxis
- Skin: erythema multiforme, rash, urticaria
- Hematologic: bone marrow suppression, coagulation disorder
- Renal: interstitial nephritis
- Central nervous system: anxiety, coma, seizures
- Hypersensitivity reactions

Interactions (other drugs)
- Chloramphenicol ▪ Glucocorticoids ▪ Macrolide and tetracyclines antibiotics
- Methotrexate ▪ Oral contraceptives ▪ Phenindione ▪ Probenecid ▪ Warfarin

Contraindications
Penicillin hypersensitivity.

Acceptability to patient
- Antibiotic therapy is usually acceptable to patients
- Outpatient parenteral therapy may necessitate the use of indwelling intravenous catheters

Follow up plan
- Follow up should be by infectious diseases consultant and PCP
- Serum C-reactive protein and/or ESRs should be monitored
- Post-treatment plain radiography should be done to assess healing
- If after 6 weeks of antibiotic therapy there are signs that the osteomyelitis has been inadequately treated (e.g. persisting radiographic abnormalities, elevations of serum inflammatory markers, sinus formation), surgery should be considered
- At least 6 weeks of appropriate antibiotic therapy should be given following surgical treatment

Patient and caregiver information
Compliance with therapy is vital. Adverse outcomes of incompletely treated osteomyelitis include need for surgery and amputation.

CIPROFLOXACIN
- Various flouroquinolones have been used in the treatment of osteomyelitis including ciprofloxacin
- Variable activity against Enterococci, *Pseudomonas* species, Staphylococci, Streptococci

Dose
- Dose is based on microbiologic diagnosis and patient characteristics
- Usual adult oral dosage range is 500–750mg every 12h

Efficacy
- Ciprofloxacin is extremely effective when used for susceptible organisms
- Ciprofloxacin and ofloxacin have reported 70–80% cure rates in patients with osteomyelitis due to susceptible Gram-negative bacilli

Risks/Benefits
Risks:
- Not suitable for children or growing adolescents
- Caution in adolescents, pregnancy, epilepsy, glucose-6-phosphate dehydrogenase deficiency
- Use caution in renal disease

Benefit: is curative against sensitive organisms

Side-effects and adverse reactions
- Gastrointestinal: abdominal pain, altered liver function, anorexia, diarrhea, heartburn, vomiting
- Central nervous system: anxiety, depression, dizziness, headache, seizures
- Eyes, ears, nose, and throat: visual disturbances
- Skin: photosensitivity, pruritus, rash

Interactions (other drugs)
- Antacids ■ Beta-blockers ■ Cyclosporine ■ Caffeine ■ Didanosine ■ Diazepam
- Mineral supplements (zinc, magnesium, calcium, aluminium, iron) ■ NSAIDs ■ Opiates
- Oral anticoagulants ■ Phenytoin ■ Theophylline ■ Warfarin

Contraindications
Use is not recommended in children because arthropathy has developed in weight-bearing joints in young animals.

Evidence
Use of ciprofloxacin is comparable to conventional intravenous antibiotics for osteomyelitis caused by susceptible organisms.
- A RCT compared oral ciprofloxacin with a broad-spectrum cephalosporin or a nafcillin-aminoglycoside combination intravenously in osteomyelitis patients. Clinical success rates were 24 of 31 (77%) for the ciprofloxacin group and 22 of 28 (79%) for the intravenous group [4] Level P

Acceptability to patient
Ciproflaxacin is active orally in osteomyelitis. This is likely to be acceptable to patients.

Follow up plan
- Follow up should be by infectious diseases specialist and PCP
- Serum C-reactive protein and/or ESR should be monitored
- Post-treatment plain radiography should be done to assess healing
- If after 6 weeks of antibiotic therapy there are signs that the osteomyelitis has been inadequately treated (e.g. persisting radiographic abnormalities, elevations of serum inflammatory markers, sinus formation), surgery should be considered
- At least 6 weeks of appropriate antibiotic therapy should be given following surgical treatment

Patient and caregiver information
Compliance with therapy is vital. Adverse outcomes of incompletely treated osteomyelitis include need for surgery and amputation.

CLINDAMYCIN
- Variable activity against anaerobes (including clostridia), *Bacteroides* species, Staphylococci, Streptococci
- Useful in the treatment of diabetics with osteomyelitis in the bases of ulcers

Dose
- Dose guided by infecting agent and patient characteristics
- Usual adult intravenous dosage range is 1.2–1.8g/day in 2–4 divided doses. The oral dosage range is 150–450mg every 6–8h

Efficacy
Useful for:
- Outpatient oral dosing. Initiated intravenously
- Susceptible organisms, especially those affecting diabetics

Risks/Benefits
Risks:
- Not suitable for children or growing adolescents
- Use caution in adolescents, pregnancy, epilepsy, glucose-6-phosphate dehydrogenase deficiency, renal disease
- Risk of inadequately treated osteomyelitis is chronic infection and need for surgery

Side-effects and adverse reactions
- Gastrointestinal: abdominal pain, altered liver function, anorexia, diarrhea, heartburn, vomiting
- Central nervous system: anxiety, depression, dizziness, headache, seizures
- Eyes, ears, nose, and throat: visual disturbances
- Skin: photosensitivity, pruritus, rash

Interactions (other drugs)
- Antacids ▪ Beta-blockers ▪ Cyclosporine ▪ Caffeine ▪ Didanosine ▪ Diazepam
- Mineral supplements (zinc, magnesium, calcium, aluminium, iron) ▪ NSAIDs ▪ Opiates
- Oral anticoagulants ▪ Phenytoin ▪ Theophylline ▪ Warfarin

Contraindications
- Use is not recommended in children because arthropathy has developed in weight-bearing joints in young animals ▪ Pregnancy category B. Compatible with breast-feeding

Evidence
Clindamycin was the most commonly used antibiotic in a series of diabetic patients with osteomyelitis, and resolution with antibiotic therapy was achieved in 77% of cases [5] *Level S*

Acceptability to patient
Can be used orally in osteomyelitis. This is likely to be acceptable to patients.

Follow up plan
- Follow up should be by infectious diseases specialist and PCP
- Follow up should be for at least 6 months after 'cure'
- Serum C-reactive protein and ESR should be monitored during and after treatment
- Diabetic control should be carefully monitored

- After treatment, plain radiography should be done to assess healing
- If after 6 weeks of antibiotics there are signs that the osteomyelitis has been inadequately treated (e.g. persisting radiographic abnormalities, elevations of serum inflammatory markers, sinus formation), surgery should be considered
- At least 6 weeks of appropriate antibiotic therapy should be given following surgical treatment

Patient and caregiver information
Importance of compliance should be stressed.

RIFAMPIN

- Efficacy in osteomyelitis due to mycobacteria including tuberculosis. Used with a range of other antituberculous regimes
- Also activity against *Staph. aureus* and can act synergistically when co-administered with a penicillin-class antibiotic

Dose

- Dose guided by careful microbacterial input, especially when treating drug-resistant organisms
- Given in combination with at least one other antituberculous drug in the treatment of tuberculosis
- Usual adult dose: 600mg once daily

Efficacy

- Rifampin is used for infection with *M. tuberculosis* along with a range of other antituberculous therapy
- Rifampin is used in the treatment of methicillin-resistant and other drug-resistant strains of *Staph. aureus*

Risks/Benefits
Risks:

- Rifampin resistance coupled with resistance to isoniazid and other antituberculosis agents is common in many multidrug-resistant isolates in the US
- Use caution in pregnancy, hepatic impairment, renal impairment

Benefits:

- Suitable for use in children
- Benefits of rifampin relate to efficacious antibiotic activity. There are rarely effective alternatives to its use in infections with tuberculosis and drug-resistant *Staph. aureus*

Side-effects and adverse reactions

- Gastrointestinal: nausea, vomiting, diarrhea
- Central nervous system: fever, headache, dizziness, behavioral changes, confusion
- Genitourinary: acute renal failure, nephritis, hematuria, orange discoloration of urine and secretions
- Respiratory: shortness of breath, collapse, and shock
- Skin: rashes, urticaria, pemphigoid reaction
- Hematologic: blood cell disorders

Interactions (other drugs)

Acetaminophen ▪ Aminosalicylic acid ▪ Anticoagulants ▪ Antimalarials ▪ Azole antifungals ▪ Beta-blockers ▪ Calcium channel blockers ▪ Chloramphenicol ▪ Clofibrate ▪ CNS depressants ▪ Corticosteroids ▪ Dapsone ▪ Disopyramide ▪ Hypoglycemic agents ▪ Isoniazid ▪ Oral contraceptives ▪ Phenytoin ▪ Protease inhibitors ▪ Theophyllines ▪ Thyroid hormone ▪ Tricyclic antidepressants ▪ Zidovudine

Contraindications
■ Hypersensitivity to rifamycins ■ Rifampin should not be used if drug susceptibility tests show a high degree of resistance

Acceptability to patient
■ Serious side-effects are rare
■ Patients should be warned that rifampin discolors bodily secretions such as urine orange/red

Patient and caregiver information
Compliance with therapy is essential to avoid relapse or development of drug resistance.

AMPHOTERICIN B
Dose
Initial test dose of 1mg over 20–30min then 250mcg/kg daily, gradually increased if tolerated to 1mg/kg daily. Do not exceed 1.5mg/kg daily or on alternate days.

Efficacy
Used for fungal osteomyelitis. Affects drug abusers and immunosuppressed patients.

Risks/Benefits
Risks:
■ Reduced renal function is common
■ Other toxicities include anemia, anorexia, nausea, fever, hypokalemia, thrombophlebitis
■ Extremely toxic drug. Given under careful monitoring in the hospital
■ Intravanous form should not be used to treat noninvasive fungal infections (such as oral thrush and vaginal cadidiasis)
■ Renal disease
■ Rapid intravenous infusion
■ Prior total body irradiation
■ Leukocyte infusion
■ Avoid eye contact
■ Relapse of blastomycosis after treatment with amphotericin B is uncommon
■ Pregnancy category B

Side-effects and adverse reactions
■ Cardiovascular system: cardiac failure, pulmonary edema, shock, myocardial infarction, hemoptysis, tachypnea, thrombophlebitis, pulmonary embolus, cardiomyopathy, pleural effusion, arrhythmias
■ Central nervous system: cerebral vascular accident, convulsions, encephalopathy, tinnitus, visual impairment, hearing loss, peripheral neuropathy, vertigo, diplopia
■ Gastrointestinal: acute liver failure, anorexia, cholecystitis, diarrhea, dyspepsia, epigastric pain, hepatitis, hepatomegaly, jaundice, melena, veno-occlusive liver disease
■ Genitourinary: anuria, dysuria, decreased renal function, impotence, oliguria
■ Hematologic: blood dyscrasias, eosinophilia, coagulation defects, leukocytosis
■ Metabolic: hypomagnesemia, hyperkalemia, hypocalcemia, hypercalcemia, hyperglycemia, hyperuricemia, hypophosphatemia, acidosis
■ Musculoskeletal: myasthenia
■ Skin: exfoliative dermatitis, erythema multiforme, maculopapular rash, pruritus

Interactions (other drugs)
■ Antineoplastic agents ■ Corticosteroids and corticotrophin ■ Cyclosporin A ■ Digitalis glycosides ■ Flucytosine ■ Imidazoles ■ Leukocyte transfusions ■ Nephrotoxic agents ■ Skeletal muscle relaxants ■ Zidovudine

Contraindications
Hypersensitivity to amphotericin.

Acceptability to patient
- Amphotericin B is usually given intravenously as it is erratically absorbed orally
- This is less acceptable to patients than oral therapy

Follow up plan
Careful monitoring of renal and liver function as well as hematologic parameters is necessary when using amphotericin B.

Patient and caregiver information
Toxicity should be explained. The fact that the drug is justified for the treatment of fungal osteomyelitis should be emphasized.

Physical therapy
EXERCISES TO IMPROVE MOBILITY OF AFFECTED AREA
- Wide range of strength and mobility excercises can be used
- Specific techniques depend on patient characteristics and site of osteomyelitis
- Should not be done in the acute phase of the disease
- Careful expert supervision is required for a physiotherapy program following osteomyelitis
- Patients can practice set exercises at home

Efficacy
- Physiotherapy is useful to return affected areas to full functioning
- Especially used after prolonged immobilization or after surgery
- Associated joint stiffness and muscle atrophy can be improved by physical therapy
- Physiotherapists can advise on the use of mobility or functional aids if necessary

Risks/Benefits
Risk: injury minimized by careful supervision.

Acceptability to patient
- Some patients may require encouragement to maintain an exercise program
- Resulting return of strength and function of a limb affected by osteomyelitis should ensure compliance with exercise regimen

Follow up plan
- Physiotherapy is usually done on an outpatient basis
- Frequent visits for assessment and progression of exercises are necessary

Patient and caregiver information
Importance of practice of exercises outside the physiotherapy department should be stressed.

Surgical therapy
- The goal of surgical treatment is to convert an infection with dead bone to a situation with well-vascularized tissues that are readily penetrated by blood-borne antibiotics, making prolonged drug treatment unnecessary
- Necessary in chronic infection, when pus has formed or when necrotic tissue present. Occasionally necessary in acute osteomyelitis when a tense collection of intraosseous pus is causing continuing pain

SURGICAL DEBRIDEMENT

- A number of techniques are used in the surgical management of osteomyelitis
- Surgical treatment involves debridement of necrotic bone and tissue, obtaining appropriate cultures, managing dead space (usually with bone graft) and, when necessary, obtaining bone stability
- Necrotic tissue and purulent material must be removed surgically
- Usually necessary to cover the wound with a tissue graft after surgical treatment
- Postoperatively the area is splinted and/or rested
- Popular surgical approach is the Ilarazov technique – remove affected bone and bridge gap by bone grafts, bone distraction using an external fixator and osteogenesis
- Requires average of 8.5 months treatment

Efficacy
Results of the Ilarazov technique evaluated in 28 patients in one series showed good results in 72%, complications in 2.5%, and amputation in one patient.

Risks/Benefits
- Risk: poor outcomes in surgery include nonunion, persisting infection, deformity
- Benefit: appropriate surgery may preserve function and prevent the need for amputation

Follow up plan
- Careful postoperative follow up by the surgical team is necessary
- Antibiotics need to be given for at least 6 weeks after surgery
- Amputation is occasionally required in cases where failure to achieve bone union occurs or in the rare condition of an osteosarcoma forming in the affected area

OUTCOMES

EFFICACY OF THERAPIES

- Majority of adults will need surgical debridement
- Following culture of samples, a parenteral antimicrobial regimen should be initiated for suspected organisms
- Once pathogen is identified, the antibiotic regimen should be tailored to particular organism and sensitivities
- Parenteral therapy should be continued for 4–6 weeks
- Majority of childhood osteomyelitis may be managed with 2 weeks parenteral antibiotic therapy then changed to an oral antibiotic
- Chronic osteomyelitis requires surgical debridement of all nonviable tissue and then 6 weeks of appropriate parenteral antibiotic therapy
- Studies are currently under way to investigate the utility of oral antibiotics alone and in combination with parenteral antibiotics

Evidence

- Treatment of pediatric cases of acute staphylococcal osteomyelitis may be simplified by keeping surgery at a minimum and shortening the course of intravenous antimicrobials by switching to oral medication early
- A RCT of 50 children with acute staphylococcal osteomyelitis were treated with cephradine or clindamycin (intravenous followed by oral treatment). No treatment failure occurred, and no long-term (one year) sequelae were observed [6] *Level P*
- PDxMD are unable to cite evidence which meets out criteria for all therapies used in the management of osteomyelitis

Review period

Review should be by the orthopedic team with appropriate input from infectious disease physician as necessary. Follow up should be for at least 6 months from the resolution of the osteomyelitis.

PROGNOSIS

Clinical pearls

Effective management of the patient with osteomyelitis requires co-operation with specialists from orthopedics and infectious disease.

Therapeutic failure

Failure of antibiotics requires surgical treatment.

Recurrence

- Failure of medical therapy with antibiotics occurs if there is pus formation within the bone
- Surgical therapy is necessary in this instance

Deterioration

- Hyperbaric oxygen can be used in severe infections
- In an area affected by osteomyelitis that is not successfully treated by surgery, amputation is the only option

COMPLICATIONS

- Loss of bony stability
- Pathologic fracture of bone affected by osteomyelitis
- Systemic septicemic complications
- Amyloidosis
- Squamous cell metaplasia of sinus tract leading to squamous cell carcinoma or fibrosarcoma

MODIFY RISK FACTORS
Lifestyle and wellnes
TOBACCO

Tobacco should be discouraged in diabetic patients or those with established peripheral vascular disease. These are risk factors for osteomyelitis in foot ulcer bases.

ALCOHOL AND DRUGS

Intravenous drug abuse is a risk factor for hematogenously spread osteomyelitis.

PREVENT RECURRENCE
In diabetes, scrupulous care of the feet is necessary, especially if there is coexistent neuropathy.

RESOURCES

ASSOCIATIONS

American Academy of Orthopedic Surgeons
6300 North River Road
Rosemont, IL 60018-4262
Tel: (847) 823-7186, (800) 346-AAOS
Fax: (847) 823-8125
www.aaos.org

American Academy of Family Physicians
11400 Tomahawk Creek Parkway
Leawood, KS 66211-2672
Tel: (913) 906-6000
www.aafp.org

Infectious Diseases Society of America
99 Canal Center Plaza, Suite 210
Alexandria, VA 22314
Tel: (703) 299-0200
Fax: (703) 299-0204
www.idsociety.org

KEY REFERENCES

- Lew DP, Waldvogel FA. Osteomyelitis. N Engl J Med 1997;336(14):999–1007
- Peltola H, Unkila-Kallio L, Kallio MJ. Simplified treatment of acute staphylococcal osteomyelitis of childhood. The Finnish Study Group. Pediatrics 1997;99(6):846–50
- Leet AI, Skaggs DL. Evaluation of the acutely limping child. Am Fam Physician 2000;61:1011–8
- Mader JT, Shirtliff ME, Bergquist SC, Calhoun J. Antimicrobial treatment of chronic osteomyelitis. Clin Orthop 1999;(360):47–65
- Karwowska A, Davies HD, Jadavji T. Epidemiology and outcome of osteomyelitis in the era of sequential intravenous-oral therapy. Pediatr Infect Dis J 1998;7(11):1021–6
- Armstrong EP, Rush DR. Treatment of osteomyelitis. Clin Pharm 1983;2(3):213–24
- Calhoun JH, Cobos JA, Mader JT. Does hyperbaric oxygen have a place in the treatment of osteomyelitis? Orthop Clin North Am 1991;22(3):467–71
- Dendrinos GK, Kontos S, Lyritsis E. Use of the Ilizarov technique for treatment of nonunion of the tibia associated with infection. J Bone Joint Surg Am 1995;77(6):835–46
- Unkila-Kallio L, Kallio MJ, Eskola J, Peltola H. Serum C-reactive protein, erythrocyte sedimentation rate, and white blood cell count in acute hematogenous osteomyelitis of children. Pediatrics 1994;93(1):59–62
- Gentry LO, Rodriguez GG. Oral ciprofloxacin compared with parenteral antibiotics in the treatment of osteomyelitis. Antimicrob Agents Chemother 1990;34(1):40–3
- Wheeler's textbook of Orthopedics online: http://www.medmedia.com/ortho1/981.html

Evidence references and guidelines

1 Guidelines for the initial evaluation of the adult patient with acute musculoskeletal symptoms: American College of Rheumatology, 1995. Also available online at the National Guideline Clearinghouse
2 The American Academy of Family Physicians has provided the following guidelines: Carek PJ, Dickerson LM, Sack JL. Diagnosis and management of osteomyelitis. Am Fam Phycisian 2001;63(12):2413–20
3 Practice guidelines for community-based parenteral anti-infective therapy. Clin Infect Dis 1997;25(4):787–801. Available at Infectious Diseases Society of America (IDSA) – Medical Specialty Society, 1999, and at the National Guideline Clearinghouse
4 Gentry LO, Rodriguez GG. Oral ciprofloxacin compared with parenteral antibiotics in the treatment of osteomyelitis. Antimicrob Agents Chemother 1990;34(1):40–3. Medline

5   Venkatesan P, Lawn S, Macfarlane RM, et al. Conservative management of osteomyelitis in the feet of diabetic patients. Diabet Med 1997;14(6):487–90. Medline

6   Peltula H, Urkila-Kallio L, Kallio MJ. Simplified treatment of acute staphyloccocal osteomyelitis of childhood. The Finnish Study Group. Pediatrics 1997;99:846–50. Medline

FAQS
Question 1
When should osteomyelitis be suspected?

ANSWER 1
Unexplained musculoskeletal problems in diabetics; recurring joint and soft-tissue infections, especially in the setting of trauma and surgery.

Question 2
What is the appropriate antibiotic for the treatment of osteomyelitis?

ANSWER 2
This must be determined by appropriate tissue sampling, often including a surgical biopsy of bone.

Question 3
What are the indications for Doppler studies in patients with osteomyelitis?

ANSWER 3
Doppler studies should be considered in patients with peripheral vascular disease to determine vascular adequacy.

CONTRIBUTORS
Fred F Ferri, MD, FACP
Shane Clarke, MD
Keith M Hull, MD, PhD

POLYARTERITIS NODOSA

DESCRIPTION

- A vasculitis disorder that presents as a necrotizing inflammation of the media of small and medium-sized arteries, inflammatory cell infiltration, and development of lesions
- Common features include peripheral neuropathy, mononeuritis multiplex, and skin lesions (palpable purpura, livedo reticularis, necrotic ulcers, digital infarcts)
- Vascular lesions occur in all stages of development and healing, are segmental, and tend to involve bifurcations and branchings of arteries
- Disease progression results in a compromised lumen, partial occlusion of arteries, thrombosis, infarction of the tissues supplied by the involved vessel, and, in some cases, palpable or visible aneurysms with occasional rupture

URGENT ACTION

- Toxic patients should be referred to the emergency department
- Referral to the emergency department will be required for patients with life-threatening presentations, such as ischemic bowel, or other rapidly progressing major organ disease

ICD9 CODE
446.0 Polyarteritis nodosa.

SYNONYMS
- PAN
- Periarteritis noditis
- Periarteritis
- Necrotizing arteritis
- Panarteritis
- Polyarteritis

CARDINAL FEATURES
- A vasculitis disorder that presents as a necrotizing inflammation of the media of small and medium-sized arteries, inflammatory cell infiltration, and development of lesions
- Constitutional symptoms are common and >50% of patients present with fever, malaise, anorexia, and weight loss
- Common features include peripheral neuropathy, mononeuritis multiplex, and skin lesions (palpable purpura, livedo reticularis, necrotic ulcers, digital infarcts)
- Skin lesions are present in about one-third of patients
- Dominant feature is organ infarction; cardiac, peripheral nerve, skin, and gastrointestinal involvement are most frequent
- Lesions occur in all stages of development and healing, are segmental, and tend to involve bifurcations and branchings of arteries
- The infiltration of polymorphonuclear neutrophils and mononuclear cells in the vessel wall and perivascular area leads to fibrinoid necrosis
- Microaneurysm formation occurs
- As lesions heal, collagen deposits may further occlude arteries
- Disease progression results in a compromised lumen, partial occlusion of arteries, thrombosis, infarction of the tissues supplied by the involved vessel, and, in some cases, palpable or visible aneurysms with occasional rupture
- Hypertension, which can be severe, can occur in about one-third of patients due to renal artery involvement. It is usually accompanied by mild azotemia

CAUSES
Common causes
- Cause is unknown, but immune mechanisms appear to be involved
- Hepatitis B antigenemia is seen in 30% of cases, and polyarteritis nodosa may be due to an abnormal immune response to the virus
- The wide range of clinical and pathologic features of polyarteritis nodosa suggests that more than one pathogenic mechanism is involved

Contributory or predisposing factors
Hepatitis B virus has been implicated in the development of polyarteritis nodosa in some patients. It appears that hepatitis B antigen triggers the immune complex response that leads to polyarteritis nodosa.

EPIDEMIOLOGY
Incidence and prevalence
Polyarteritis nodosa is extremely rare. In addition, overlapping diagnostic criteria with other vasculitis syndromes makes determining epidemiology of this disorder difficult.

INCIDENCE
0.007/1000.

PREVALENCE
0.063/1000.

Demographics

AGE
Occurs in all age groups, with predominance between 40 and 60 years.

GENDER
2.5:1 to 3:1 male:female ratio.

RACE
Observed in all racial groups.

DIFFERENTIAL DIAGNOSIS

- Accurate diagnosis is important because treatment and prognosis vary for different vasculitic disorders
- The main differential diagnoses include other vasculitides and autoimmune diseases, infections, and malignancies

Cryoglobulinemia

Essential mixed cryoglobulinemia may present as cutaneous vasculitis.

FEATURES
- Palpable purpura
- Digital vessel occlusion
- Glomerulonephritis
- Chronic infection with hepatitis C is common

Systemic lupus erythematosus

Systemic lupus erythematosus is a systemic disease that is not organ-specific.

FEATURES
- Erythematous rash
- Alopecia
- Leg, nasal, or oropharyngeal ulcerations
- Livedo reticularis
- Pallor
- Petechiae
- Joint tenderness, swelling, or effusion
- Pericardial rub (in patients with pericarditis) and heart murmurs (if endocarditis or valvular thickening or dysfunction is present)
- Fever

Henoch-Schoenlein purpura

Henoch–Schoenlein purpura is a systemic vasculitic disorder resulting from immune complex deposition.

FEATURES
- Purpuric rash, commonly on buttocks or extensor surfaces
- Nephritis may occur in one-third of patients
- Abdominal pain
- Arthralgias
- Usually lasts only weeks or months

Wegener's granulomatosis

Wegener's granulomatosis is a necrotizing vasculitis affecting mainly small arteries in the respiratory tract.

FEATURES
- Respiratory symptoms are common
- Skin lesions include papules, vesicles, and palpable purpura
- Necrotizing glomerulonephritis may occur
- Associated with presence of antineutrophil cytoplasmic autoantibodies

Churg-Strauss syndrome

Churg-Strauss syndrome is characterized by necrotizing granulomas of mainly small arteries.

FEATURES

- Fever, malaise, anorexia, and weight loss occur
- Lung involvement is the predominant clinical feature
- Patients have significant history of asthma
- Associated with presence of antineutrophil cytoplasmic autoantibodies

Microscopic polyangiitis

Microscopic polyangiitis is a necrotizing arteritis of mainly small arteries (capillaries, venules, arterioles).

FEATURES

- Few or no immune deposits
- Necrotizing glomerulonephritis
- Pulmonary capillaritis
- Associated with presence of antineutrophil cytoplasmic autoantibodies

Giant cell (temporal) arteritis

Giant cell arteritis is an inflammation of medium and large arteries, with frequent involvement of the temporal artery.

FEATURES

- Headache, tenderness over the temporal artery and scalp, and visual disturbances are common and may progress rapidly to complete blindness
- Malaise, anorexia, weight loss, fever, and arthralgias may also be seen
- Occurs most frequently in patients >50 years
- Often associated with polymyalgia rheumatica

Takayasu's arteritis

Takayasu's arteritis is characterized by granulomatous inflammation of the aorta and major branches.

FEATURES

- Malaise, fever, weight loss, and anorexia are common systemic symptoms
- Pain secondary to vessel inflammation and organ infarction may occur
- Occurs most frequently in patients <50 years

Kawasaki disease

Kawasaki disease is an acute multisystem disease.

FEATURES

- Arteritis of large, medium, and small arteries
- Mucocutaneous lymph node syndrome
- Frequently involves coronary arteries
- Fever is common
- Generally occurs in children

Hypersensitivity vasculitis

Hypersensitivity vasculitis is also known as predominantly cutaneous vasculitis and cutaneous leukocytoclastic vasculitis.

FEATURES
- Vasculitis of the small vessels of the skin
- Presumed to be triggered by a drug, infection, or other allergen
- Palpable purpura is the typical feature
- Macules, papules, and vesicles may occur
- Systemic signs of fever, malaise, anorexia, and arthralgia may be present

Rheumatoid arthritis
Rheumatoid arthritis affects 3% of the population.

FEATURES
- A deforming peripheral arthropathy with extra-articular manifestations
- Weight loss and fever
- Arthritis, which is usually symmetrical and deforming
- Can have associated polyarthritis similar to polyarteritis nodosa

Trichinosis infection
Trichinosis occurs after ingestion of meat containing cysts of *Trichinella*.

FEATURES
- Abdominal pain
- Nausea and vomiting
- Mild, transient diarrhea
- Malaise
- Low-grade fever
- Myalgias
- Headache
- Rash

Rickettsial infection
Vector-borne bacterial infection caused by *Rickettsia* sp.

FEATURES
- Triad of fever, rash, and headache
- Macular rash which becomes purpuric and slightly papular and is variable depending on infectious agent
- Malaise

Lyme disease
Lyme disease is caused by *Borrelia burgdorferi* infection, which is tick-borne.

FEATURES
- Erythema chronicum migrans
- Malaise, arthralgia, and lymphadenopathy may be associated
- Peripheral neuropathy may also be seen

Infective endocarditis
Fever and a changing heart murmur should be assumed to be infective endocarditis until proven otherwise.

FEATURES
- Fever, malaise, and weight loss
- Heart murmur

- Vasculitis may occur, causing splinter hemorrhages, Janeway lesions, Osler's nodes, Roth's spots, and hematuria
- Splenomegaly is common

Lymphoma

Lymphoma often presents with vague constitutional symptoms.

FEATURES
- Pruritus
- Fever
- Weight loss
- Night sweats
- Hepatomegaly
- Splenomegaly

Hairy cell leukemia

Hairy cell leukemia is rare, and commonly occurs in older males.

FEATURES
- Splenomegaly and pancytopenia are common presenting features
- Vasculitis may be associated

Other disorders

Cholesterol embolization, left atrial myxoma, and ergot poisoning are rare disorders that may present with similar features to polyarteritis nodosa.

FEATURES
- Purpura and skin ulcers may occur with cholesterol emboli
- Left atrial myxoma may present with constitutional symptoms and signs such as anorexia, weight loss, fever, malaise, arthralgia, and skin rash
- Ergot poisoning can cause vessel constriction, leading to numbness or gangrene in the extremities

SIGNS & SYMPTOMS
Signs

General signs include fever, weight loss, and livedo reticularis. Other signs tend to reflect the particular organ system being affected.

Cardiac involvement:
- Pericarditis: friction rub
- Congestive heart failure: jugular venous distention, hepatic enlargement, orthopnea, dyspnea on exertion, peripheral edema, signs of pleural fluid
- Arrhythmias: abnormal pulse
- Myocardial infarction: signs of its complications

Gastrointestinal involvement:
- Hepatomegaly
- Mucosal ischemia, with or without perforation: abdominal tenderness and guarding with abnormal bowel sounds
- Appendicitis, cholecystitis, or hemorrhagic pancreatitis: abdominal tenderness and guarding
- Liver involvement can cause hepatomegaly, with or without jaundice, to signs of extensive hepatic necrosis

Renal involvement:
- Hypertension – may be severe
- Mild azotemia, hematuria, proteinuria

Skin involvement:
- Subcutaneous hemorrhages
- Polymorphic rashes

Musculoskeletal involvement:
- Reduced muscle power
- Features of synovitis

Eye involvement:
- Retinal hemorrhages or detachment may be seen during ophthalmoscopy

Other manifestations:
- Digital infarcts
- Subcutaneous nodules (uncommon but characteristic)
- Raynaud's phenomenon (rare)

Symptoms
General symptoms:
- Fever
- Weakness
- Weight loss
- Malaise
- Myalgia
- Headache

Other symptoms tend to reflect the particular organ system in which the arterial supply is impaired.
Cardiac involvement:
- Chest pain
- Dyspnea

Gastrointestinal involvement:
- Recurrent and severe abdominal pain
- Vague abdominal discomfort
- Anorexia
- Nausea (less prominent)
- Vomiting (less prominent)
- Bloody diarrhea

Musculoskeletal involvement:
- Myalgias
- Muscle weakness
- Migratory arthralgias
- Arthritis symptoms

Neurologic involvement:
- Paresthesia
- Limb weakness
- Seizures

Skin involvement:
- Urticaria

Genitourinary involvement:
- Usually asymptomatic
- May have testicular pain

Eye involvement:
- Flashing lights, floaters, or a scotoma in the peripheral visual field are symptoms of detachment

ASSOCIATED DISORDERS
- Hepatitis B antigen is detected in 20–30% of patients with systemic vasculitis, and is especially associated with polyarteritis nodosa
- Hepatitis C has been associated, and is present in 5% of patients with polyarteritis nodosa
- Hairy cell leukemia may be linked to polyarteritis nodosa

CONSIDER CONSULT
- Patients with suspected polyarteritis nodosa should be evaluated by a rheumatologist
- Patients should be referred for biopsy in cases of diagnostic uncertainty
- Patients proven to have polyarteritis nodosa should be followed by a rheumatologist

INVESTIGATION OF THE PATIENT
Direct questions to patient
Q **Do you feel sick or tired overall?** General feelings of malaise are characteristic of polyarteritis nodosa; malaise may also occur with cardiac or renal involvement

Q **Have you lost weight recently without trying?** Weight loss >4kg is a symptom of polyarteritis nodosa

Q **Have you been running a fever lately?** Unexplained fever is a characteristic symptom of polyarteritis nodosa

Q **Have you experienced any unexplained muscle pain or weakness?** Although not diagnostic, muscle pain and weakness occur frequently with polyarteritis nodosa

Q **Are you experiencing any abdominal pain?** Although not diagnostic, severe abdominal pain may indicate that the arteries that feed the gastrointestinal (GI) system are involved. It is critical to determine this, as complications can include perforation of the gastrointestinal structures and subsequent death

Q **Have you noticed a lack of desire to eat?** Although not diagnostic, anorexia may be associated with polyarteritis nodosa with GI involvement

Q **Have you experienced any bloody diarrhea?** Although not diagnostic, bloody diarrhea may be associated with polyarteritis nodosa with GI involvement

Q **Have you noticed any odd marks or lesions on your skin?** Livedo reticularis is a common finding in patients with polyarteritis nodosa

Q **Have you noticed any numbness in your extremities or elsewhere?** Peripheral neuropathy is a common manifestation

Q **Have you experienced pain in your joints?** Arthritis will cause joint pain and swelling

Q **Have you experienced unexplained headaches recently?** Headaches are a symptom of polyarteritis nodosa

Q **Have you experienced any chest pain, shortness of breath, or unexplained swelling?** Although not diagnostic, these symptoms could indicate polyarteritis nodosa with cardiac involvement

Q **Have you experienced any testicular pain?** The patient may be embarrassed to mention this, and so should be asked directly to ascertain if there is possible genital involvement

Q **Have you noticed any changes in your vision?** Retinal hemorrhages and detachment are rare features

Contributory or predisposing factors

Have you been diagnosed with or exposed to hepatitis B virus? Hepatitis B virus has been implicated in the pathogenesis of polyarteritis nodosa in some patients.

Examination

- **Check for fever**: fever is associated with the occurrence of polyarteritis nodosa
- **Check the pulse**: an abnormal pulse rate may appear in patients with cardiac involvement
- **Check the blood pressure**: patients with renal involvement may experience hypertension
- **Check patient for weight loss**: weight loss may occur with polyarteritis nodosa or as a consequence of anorexia, one of the symptoms of the disorder
- **Examine the skin**: livedo reticularis, (cyanotic discoloration surrounding pale central areas of skin) is a common finding in patients with polyarteritis nodosa. In addition, subcutaneous hemorrhages, polymorphic rashes, and subcutaneous nodules are characteristic findings. The digits should be inspected for infarcts and ulcers
- **Palpate the abdomen**: hepatomegaly may be present in patients with cardiac involvement. In addition, abdominal tenderness and guarding with abnormal bowel sounds may be seen in patients with GI involvement
- **Auscultate the lungs**: pleural fluid can form in patients with cardiac involvement
- **Perform a neurologic examination**: look especially for paresthesia and muscle weakness
- **Perform ophthalmoscopy**: look for retinal hemorrhages or detachment (rare findings)

Summary of investigative tests

Investigations are directed at diagnosing the condition and assessing the degree of organ involvement:

- Blood tests: a sample of venous blood is required to check for leukocytosis, erythrocyte sedimentation rate, renal function tests (blood urea nitrogen and creatinine levels), liver function tests, and viral hepatitis serology
- Urine test: urine dipstick test is required to detect hematuria and proteinuria. Microscopy should also be performed
- Electrocardiogram: an ECG is needed for patients with suspected cardiac involvement to check for arrhythmias
- Biopsy: a biopsy is the preferred test to diagnose the presence of polyarteritis nodosa. Biopsies are usually performed by a specialist, except, perhaps, for skin biopsy
- Arteriogram: is needed for a conclusive diagnosis of polyarteritis nodosa if a biopsy specimen cannot be obtained (e.g. if biopsy would be difficult or dangerous). Arteriograms are also useful for diagnosis if involvement of medium or large arteries is suspected, and if there is no obvious symptomatic site to biopsy. Arteriograms are usually performed by a specialist
- Electromyography (EMG): is performed if the patient has symptoms of neuropathy – usually performed by a specialist

DIAGNOSTIC DECISION

The American College of Rheumatology states that patients must have three of the following 10 criteria for a diagnosis of polyarteritis nodosa:

- Weight loss >4kg
- Livedo reticularis
- Testicular pain or tenderness
- Myalgias, weakness, or leg tenderness
- Mononeuropathy or polyneuropathy
- Diastolic blood pressure >90mmHg
- Elevated blood urea nitrogen or creatinine
- Hepatitis B virus
- Arteriographic abnormality
- Biopsy of small or medium artery containing polyarteritis nodosa

CLINICAL PEARLS

- The presenting symptoms of polyarteritis nodosa can be protean and nonspecific, such as fever, weight loss, and abdominal pain, so this diagnosis is often overlooked
- Mononeuropathy, such as wrist drop or foot drop, should always raise the question of vasculitis even without skin lesions
- When palpable purpura appears on the skin, the critical differential is whether the disease is limited to the skin or whether it is systemic

THE TESTS
Body fluids
COMPLETE BLOOD COUNT
Description
Venous blood sample.

Advantages/Disadvantages
Advantages:
- Inexpensive
- Easy to perform

Disadvantage: not specific for polyarteritis nodosa

Normal
- Leukocytes: 3200–9800/mm^3 (3.2–9.8x10^9/L)
- Hemoglobin: male 13.5–18.0g/dL; female 11.5–16.0g/dL
- Platelets 150–400x10^9/L

Abnormal
- Leukocytes above normal reference range, mainly polymorphonuclear neutrophils
- Hemoglobin below normal reference range
- Platelets outside normal reference range
- Keep in mind the possibility of a false-positive result

Cause of abnormal result
- Leukocytes: inflammatory response within arteries
- Anemia of chronic disease
- Thrombocytosis is associated with inflammation

Drugs, disorders and other factors that may alter results
Leukocytes are raised with coexistent infection.

ERYTHROCYTE SEDIMENTATION RATE
Description
Venous blood sample.

Advantages/Disadvantages
Advantages:
- Inexpensive
- Easy to perform

Disadvantage: not specific for polyarteritis nodosa

Normal
- Men <50 years: 0–15mm/h

- Men >50 years: 0–20mm/h
- Women <50 years: 0–20mm/h
- Women >50 years: 0–30mm/h

Abnormal
- ESR >50mm/h
- Keep in mind the possibility of a false-positive result

Cause of abnormal result
- Inflammatory response within arteries
- Other inflammatory process

Drugs, disorders and other factors that may alter results
- May be elevated in the presence of collagen-vascular disease, infections, myocardial infarction, hyperthyroidism or hypothyroidism
- May be decreased with use of corticosteroids and in presence of sickle cell disease, polycythemia, liver disease, or some cancers

RENAL FUNCTION TESTS
Description
Venous blood sample.

Advantages/Disadvantages
Advantages:
- Inexpensive
- Easy to perform

Disadvantage: not specific for polyarteritis nodosa

Normal
- Blood urea nitrogen: 8–18mg/dL (3–6.5mmol/L)
- Creatinine: 0.6–1.2mg/dL (50–110mmol/L)

Abnormal
- Blood urea nitrogen: >40mg/dL (14.3mmol/L)
- Creatinine: >1.5mg/dL (132mmol/L)
- Keep in mind the possibility of a false-positive result

Cause of abnormal result
- Inflammatory response within renal arteries
- Other causes of azotemia

Drugs, disorders and other factors that may alter results
Blood urea nitrogen:
- May be elevated with use of aminoglycosides, antibiotics, diuretics, lithium, or corticosteroids; or the presence of dehydration, GI bleeding, decreased renal blood flow, renal disease, or urinary tract obstruction
- May be decreased with liver disease, malnutrition, overhydration, acromegaly, and celiac disease

Creatinine:
- May be elevated with use of aminoglycosides, cephalosporins, hydantoin, diuretics, or methyldopa; or the presence of renal insufficiency, dehydration, congestive heart failure, or urinary tract infections

459

▨ May be decreased in persons who are amputees, older people, or individuals with prolonged debilitation

LIVER FUNCTION TESTS
Description
Venous blood sample.

Advantages/Disadvantages
Advantages:
▨ Inexpensive
▨ Easy to perform

Disadvantage: not specific for polyarteritis nodosa

Normal
▨ AST (aspartate aminotransferase; SGOT): 5–35 IU/L
▨ ALT (alanine aminotransferase; SGPT) : 5–35 IU/L
▨ ALP (alkaline phosphatase): 30–300 IU/L
▨ Albumin: 35–50g/L
▨ Bilirubin: 3–17mcmol/L (0.25–1.5mg/100mL)

Abnormal
▨ Results outside normal reference range (increased enzymes and bilirubin; decreased albumin)
▨ Keep in mind the possibility of a false-positive result

Cause of abnormal result
▨ Inflammatory response affecting the liver may cause transaminitis, increased ALP, and decreased albumin
▨ Hepatomegaly secondary to cardiac failure may cause deranged liver function

Drugs, disorders and other factors that may alter results
Wide variety of drugs may alter liver functions tests, including:
▨ Acitretin
▨ Aminoglutethimide
▨ Ampicillin
▨ Angiotensin II receptor antagonists
▨ Bentiromide
▨ Captopril
▨ Clonazepam
▨ Enoxaparin
▨ Gentamicin
▨ Ivermectin
▨ Leflunomide
▨ Mycophenolate mofetil
▨ Nandrolone
▨ Niacin
▨ Norfloxacin
▨ Pentamidine isetionate
▨ Pioglitazone
▨ Pyridoxine
▨ Sildenafil
▨ Statins

- Tibolone
- Vitamin B6

URINE TEST
Description
Urine dipstick test and microscopy.

Advantages/Disadvantages
Advantages:
- Easy to perform
- Inexpensive
- Pain-free

Disadvantages:
- Not diagnostic of polyarteritis nodosa
- False-positive results may occur

Normal
- Negative for microscopic hematuria
- Negative for protein
- No casts or sediment

Abnormal
- Presence of hematuria
- Proteinuria
- Presence of urinary sediment

Cause of abnormal result
- Renal involvement
- Keep in mind the possibility of a false-positive result

Drugs, disorders and other factors that may alter results
- Hematuria may be due to trauma to the urinary tract, renal disease, bladder lesions, or prostate cancer
- Urine protein may be elevated with use of anticoagulants or aspirin, and in the presence of renal disease, congestive heart failure, hypertension, or cancer of the renal pelvis or bladder

VIRAL HEPATITIS SEROLOGY
Description
Venous blood sample.

Advantages/Disadvantages
Advantages:
- Easy to perform
- May identify a potentially causative factor

Normal
Hepatitis B:
- Hepatitis B surface antigen negative
- HBeAg negative
- Hepatitis anti-core antibody negative or positive (if positive, indicates past infection if other two markers are negative)

461

Hepatitis C:

- Anti-hepatitis C virus antibody negative

Abnormal
Hepatitis B (acute infection):

- Hepatitis B surface antigen positive
- HBeAg positive (indicates active viral replication)
- Hepatitis B anti-core antibody positive

Hepatitis B (chronic infection):

- Hepatitis B surface antigen positive
- HBeAg positive or negative
- Hepatitis B anti-core antibody positive

Hepatitis C :

- Antihepatitis C virus antibody positive

Cause of abnormal result
Active or chronic hepatitis B or C virus infection.

Drugs, disorders and other factors that may alter results

- Patients who are immunocompromised may give false-negative results, especially in the detection of hepatitis C virus
- Viral levels below the limits of detection

Tests of function
ELECTROMYOGRAPHY
Description
Electrical patterns of the muscle are recorded using a needle electrode inserted into the muscle.

Advantages/Disadvantages
Advantage: may help confirm the diagnosis of peripheral nerve disorders

Disadvantages:

- Discomfort at the site of needle insertion
- Results may require specialist interpretation

Abnormal

- The pattern of muscles affected may localize the disorder to a particular peripheral nerve
- Keep in mind the possibility of a false-positive result

Cause of abnormal result
Peripheral neuropathy.

Drugs, disorders and other factors that may alter results

- NSAIDs should be avoided for one week before testing
- Position of electrodes and skin temperature may affect results
- Anticholinergic and muscle-relaxing medications affect results

Biopsy
BIOPSY OF AFFECTED AREA
Description

- Biopsy should target skin, subcutaneous tissue, or sural nerve or muscle at clinical sites of disease

- A deep, open surgical biopsy sample, including subcutaneous tissue and underlying muscle should be taken whenever possible from skeletal muscle that exhibits pain and tenderness
- Nerve and muscle are most frequent sites for biopsy
- Electromyography can help to direct biopsy of muscle or sural nerve

Advantages/Disadvantages
Advantages: can confirm diagnosis of polyarteritis nodosa

Disadvantages:
- Diagnosis by nerve biopsy has difficulties linked to sampling
- Some nerve biopsies, such as the sural nerve, may not show diagnostic features
- Expensive
- Painful for patient
- In some cases (e.g. testicular biopsy), general anesthesia is required
- Other vasculitides may show similar inflammatory changes

Abnormal
- Histologic changes demonstrate all levels of progression and healing
- Lesions of small and medium-sized arteries are focal, panmural, and necrotizing
- Fibrinoid necrosis, disruption of the vessel wall architecture, pleomorphic cellular infiltration (predominantly polymorphonucleocytes) are features of inflammation
- There may be thrombosis, aneurysmal dilatation, and fibrous tissue causing vessel occlusion

Cause of abnormal result
Inflammatory response within the arterial wall.

Drugs, disorders and other factors that may alter results
Glucocorticoid and immunosuppressive treatment can decrease the yield of biopsy.

Imaging
ARTERIOGRAM
Advantages/Disadvantages
Advantages:
- May help detect aneurysms of medium-sized arteries in renal, hepatic, or intestinal sites
- Can be used to help confirm diagnosis of polyarteritis nodosa
- Acceptable alternative to biopsy

Disadvantages:
- Expensive
- Uncomfortable and sometimes painful for the patient
- Contrast dye is contraindicated for individuals with contrast allergy, and patients with significant renal insufficiency
- Findings are nonspecific

Abnormal
- Aneurysms or occlusions of the visceral arteries, not due to arteriosclerosis, fibromuscular dysplasia, or noninflammatory causes
- Narrowing and tapering of blood vessels in combination with the presence of aneurysms leads to the classical 'string of beads' appearance

Cause of abnormal result
Inflammatory response within the arteries.

Drugs, disorders and other factors that may alter results
Arteriosclerosis, fibromuscular dysplasia, or noninflammatory disease states could cause an abnormal result.

Other tests
ELECTROCARDIOGRAM
Advantages/Disadvantages
Advantages:
- Easy to perform
- Cheap

Disadvantage: not diagnostic of polyarteritis nodosa; can only be used to show damage caused by the disease

Abnormal
Abnormalities consistent with conduction defects, ischemia, or pericarditis may be seen.

Cause of abnormal result
- Involvement of small to medium-sized arteries that supply the heart
- Heart failure

Drugs, disorders and other factors that may alter results
- Certain drugs, including digitalis and quinidine, can cause ECG abnormalities
- Electrolyte disorders, including hypokalemia and hypocalcemia, can cause changes in the ECG
- A pulmonary embolus can produce ECG abnormalities

TREATMENT

CONSIDER CONSULT
- Referral to a rheumatologist is required for treatment of major organ involvement

IMMEDIATE ACTION
- Toxic patients should be transferred to the emergency department
- If the disease is rapidly progressing, referral to hospital should be immediate, with rapid consultation by a rheumatologist

PATIENT AND CAREGIVER ISSUES
Patient or caregiver request
- **What are the short- and long-term implications of steroid treatment?** High-dose steroid therapy can cause emotional instability and even psychosis in the short term. Long-term use has many adverse effects, including cushingoid appearance, osteoporosis, hypertension, decreased glucose tolerance, and acne
- **Is there a cure for this disease?** There are effective treatments to induce remission

MANAGEMENT ISSUES
Goals
- Treat the patient's symptoms
- Reduce pain
- Prevent disease progression

Management in special circumstances
Five factors are associated with excess mortality with polyarteritis nodosa: renal insufficiency (serum creatinine concentration of 1.58mg/dL (140mcmol/L) or higher), proteinuria (>1g/day), and visceral involvement of the GI system, central nervous system, or cardiac function:

- Presence of one factor = 5-year mortality of 25%
- Presence of two factors = 5-year mortality of 46%
- Presence of no factors = expected 5-year mortality of 12% or less

Assess for these five factors and treat accordingly.

Surgery is necessary in the case of bowel perforation, hemorrhage, digestive tract infarction, pancreatitis, appendicitis or cholecystitis.

COEXISTING DISEASE
- Hypertension is common in patients with polyarteritis nodosa. Close attention to treatment of hypertension can lessen morbidity and mortality associated with renal, cardiac, and central nervous system complications of polyarteritis nodosa. Treatment with angiotensin-converting enzyme (ACE) inhibitors or angiotensin II receptor blockers can control severe or malignant hypertension
- Patients with polyarteritis nodosa associated with hepatitis B virus infections have been shown to respond to treatment regimens that include interferon-alpha 2b and plasma exchange. When this approach was combined with short-term steroid therapy, a significant number of patients had long-term remission and seroconversion in terms of hepatitis

PATIENT SATISFACTION/LIFESTYLE PRIORITIES
The risk of not treating the disease is greater than the side-effects of treatment.

SUMMARY OF THERAPEUTIC OPTIONS
Choices

Nonhepatitis-associated polyarteritis nodosa:

- Prednisone is the first-choice treatment
- Second-choice treatment is prednisone in combination with cyclophosphamide

Hepatitis-associated polyarteritis nodosa:

- Excessive immunosuppression worsens hepatitis B viremia and outcomes. Prednisone is therefore quickly tapered after approx. 2 weeks, and an antiviral should be used
- The antiviral drug of choice is interferon-alpha
- Plasma exchange with interferon-alpha is a second-line option. This would be performed by a specialist in the hospital setting
- Lifestyle measures such as smoking, diet, and exercise should be addressed, as these factors may contribute to vascular complications

Clinical pearls

- Virtually all patients with polyarteritis nodosa will require treatment with high-dose prednisone
- Some patients with severe disease will require treatment with cyclophosphamide
- Other immunosuppressive agents, such as methotrexate, may have a role, but evidence of support is lacking

Never

Never prescribe long-term prednisone for polyarteritis nodosa associated with active hepatitis.

FOLLOW UP
Plan for review

- Carefully monitor the patient for infection
- Measure ESR periodically
- Watch for delayed appearance of neoplasms in patients who have received cyclophosphamide

Information for patient or caregiver

- Patient should be informed of the expected duration of treatment
- The effects of corticosteroid use should be communicated
- The potential risks of cyclophosphamide with regard to infertility, infection, and malignancy, must be conveyed to the patient

DRUGS AND OTHER THERAPIES: DETAILS
Drugs
PREDNISONE

Prednisone is the first-line treatment for patients with polyarteritis nodosa not associated with hepatitis.

Dose

- 5–60mg/day in single or divided doses
- May be increased if disease is not controlled at this dose
- Dosing must be individualized for each patient
- Treatment is usually given for one year, but low-dose prednisone treatment may sometimes be required indefinitely

Efficacy

- Provides symptomatic relief
- May or may not improve one-year survival rate

- The acceptance of glucocorticoids to treat polyarteritis nodosa was based on uncontrolled data from retrospective studies, showing that patients with polyarteritis nodosa who were treated had better survival rates of approx. 70% at one year and 50% at 5 years vs 35% and 10%, respectively, if left untreated

Risks/Benefits

Risks:
- Use caution with peptic ulcer
- Use caution in patients with congestive heart failure, diabetes mellitus, renal disease, ulcerative colitis
- Use caution in patients with glaucoma, osteoporosis
- Use caution in the elderly

Benefits:
- Provides symptomatic relief
- Can help control swelling of arteries

Side-effects and adverse reactions
- Side-effects are minimized by short duration of therapy
- Cardiovascular system: hypertension, thromboembolism
- Central nervous system: insomnia, euphoria, depression, psychosis, seizures
- Endocrine: adrenal suppression, impaired glucose tolerance, growth suppression in children
- Eyes, ears, nose, and throat: cataract, glaucoma, blurred vision
- Gastrointestinal: dyspepsia, peptic ulceration, esophagitis, oral candidiasis
- Musculoskeletal: proximal myopathy, osteoporosis
- Skin: delayed healing, acne, striae, fragile skin

Interactions (other drugs)
- Aminoglutethamide (increased clearance of prednisone) ■ Antidiabetics (hypoglycemic effect inhibited) ■ Antihypertensives (effects inhibited) ■ Barbiturates (increased clearance of prednisone) ■ Cardiac glycosides (toxicity increased) ■ Cholestyramine, colestipol (may reduce absorption of corticosteroids) ■ Clarithromycin, erythromycin, troleandomycin (may enhance steroid effect) ■ Cyclosporine (may increase levels of both drugs; may cause seizures) ■ Diuretics (effects inhibited) ■ Isoniazid (reduced plasma levels of isoniazid) ■ Ketoconazole ■ Nonsteroidal antiinflammatory drugs (increased risks of bleeeding) ■ Oral contraceptives (enhanced effects of corticosteroids) ■ Rifampin (may inhibit hepatic clearance of prednisone) ■ Salicylates (increased clearance of salicylates) ■ Warfarin (alters clotting time)

Contraindications
- Systemic infection ■ Avoid live virus vaccines in patients receiving immunosuppressive doses ■ History of tuberculosis ■ Cushing's syndrome ■ Recent myocardial infarction

Acceptability to patient
- Patients may complain of weight gain with prednisone and may be noncompliant with therapy
- Hyperexcitability and irritability may make it less acceptable

Follow up plan
- Decrease daily dose of prednisone in patients with reduced fever, decreased ESR, improved cardiac and renal function, disappearance of cutaneous lesions, and diminished pain
- Monitor blood pressure regularly
- Perform glucose and electrolytes regularly
- Watch for signs of masked infection, including oral *Candida* infection

- Watch for changes in mood and behavior, emotional stability, sleep patterns, and psychomotor activity
- If long-term steroids are required at a dose >7.5mg daily, alendronate or risedronate should be commenced for the prevention of glucocorticoid-induced osteoporosis

Patient and caregiver information
- Therapy should be taken as prescribed
- The patient should not stop therapy without informing the physician; withdrawal symptoms may occur
- Any side-effects should be reported to the physician immediately

CYCLOPHOSPHAMIDE

- Cyclophosphamide may be given to patients who do not respond to corticosteroids during the first few weeks of treatment, or for whom prohibitively high doses of corticosteroids are needed to control disease
- Cyclophosphamide and prednisone are used in combination for patients without active hepatitis
- The drug dose should be adjusted to maintain a peripheral leukocyte count of 2000–3500/cm^3, and more importantly an absolute neutrophil count of >1000/cm^3

Dose
1–2mg/kg per day orally.

Efficacy
- Provides symptomatic relief
- Combination therapy with prednisone has been reported to result in remission

Risks/Benefits
Risk: bone marrow supression and hepatotoxicity

Benefits:
- Provides symptomatic relief
- Can help control swelling of arteries
- Can help stop progression of disease

Side-effects and adverse reactions
- Cardiovascular system: cardiotoxicity (at high doses)
- Central nervous system: dizziness, headache
- Gastrointestinal: nausea, vomiting, diarrhea
- Genitourinary: amenorrhea, azoospermia, ovarian fibrosis, sterility, hematuria, hemorrhagic cystitis, neoplasms
- Hematologic: leukopenia, myelosuppression, pancytopenia, thrombocytopenia
- Metabolic: bone marrow suppression
- Respiratory: fibrosis
- Skin: alopecia, dermatitis

Interactions (other drugs)
- Allopurinol (increased cyclophosphamide toxicity) - Clozapine (may cause agranulocytosis) - Digoxin (decreased digoxin absorption from tablet form) - Pentostatin (increased toxicity with high dose cyclophosphamide) - Phenytoin (reduced absorption of phenytoin) - Succinylcholine (prolonged neuromuscular blockade) - Suxamethonium (enhanced effect of suxamethonium) - Warfarin (inhibits hypoprothrombinemic response to warfarin)

Contraindications
- Serious infections, including chickenpox and herpes zoster ▪ Myelosuppression

Evidence

Cyclophosphamide may be effective in inducing and maintaining remission for patients with polyarteritis nodosa.
- A randomized controlled trial compared treatment with prednisone plus plasma exchange vs prednisone, plasma exchange, and cyclophosphamide in patients with polyarteritis nodosa and Churg-Strauss angiitis. The two groups had comparable survival but the patients who had received cyclophosphamide had fewer relapses [1] *Level P*
- One small, uncontrolled trial, in which patients with severe necrotizing vasculitis were treated with 2mg/kg per day of oral cyclophosphamide, resulted in a high rate of remission. Patients who had been previously treated with glucocorticoids were able to reduce the steroid dose, and thus decrease corticosteroid-related adverse effects [2] *This study does not meet the criteria for level P*

Acceptability to patient
- Cyclophosphamide is associated with alopecia in 33% of patients; this side-effect may cause noncompliance with therapy
- Other side-effects, including nausea and vomiting, are severe in some patients and may lead to discontinuation of therapy

Follow up plan
- Watch for hematuria or dysuria
- Complete blood count and urinalysis should be performed periodically to monitor for myelosuppression and cystitis
- Urine cytology is recommended yearly, even after treatment is completed

Patient and caregiver information
- Therapy should be taken as prescribed
- The cyclophosphamide should be taken in the morning
- Copious quantities of liquid should be consumed throughout the day to maintain high urine output
- The patient should not stop therapy without discussing with the physician
- Any side-effects should be reported to the physician immediately
- Treatment may result in amenorrhea, which can last up to one year after therapy is stopped
- Patients should use some form of birth control while on cyclophosphamide

INTERFERON-ALPHA

Good results have been achieved with interferon-alpha and plasma exchange in polyarteritis nodosa related to hepatitis B.

Dose
- The recommended dose of interferon-alpha for chronic hepatitis B is 5 million units a day; however, in patients with HBV-related polyarteritis nodosa, interferon-alpha has only been used at doses of 3–5 million units, three times weekly
- Chronic active hepatitis C dose is 3 million units, three times weekly, either by intramuscular or subcutaneous injection

Efficacy
- The antiviral drug of choice is interferon-alpha
- Favorable results may be achieved for patients with hepatitis B antigenemia when used in combination with plasma exchange

Risks/Benefits

Risks:

- Use caution in patients with cardiac disease, pulmonary disease, diabetes mellitus, and renal or hepatic disease
- Use caution in patients with dental disease, thyroid disease, seizure disorders, psoriasis
- Use with caution during pregnancy, breast-feeding, and in the elderly
- Adverse effects are generally dose-related
- Flu-like symptoms are common

Benefit: useful in the treatment of viral hepatitis

Side-effects and adverse reactions

- Cardiovascular system: chest pain, hypertension, edema, arrhythmias, myocardial infarction, cardiomyopathy
- Central nervous system: depression, suicidal ideation, dizziness, anxiety, confusion, paresthesias, insomnia, seizures, coma, flu-like symptoms
- Eyes, ears, nose, and throat: retinal hemorrhage, visual impairment
- Gastrointestinal: nausea, vomiting, diarrhea, weight loss, abdominal pain, taste disturbances, raised liver enzymes, gastrointestinal bleeding
- Hematologic: blood dyscrasias
- Metabolic: hyperthyroidism, hypothyroidism, hyperglycemia
- Skin: injection site reaction, rash, alopecia, pruritus, exacerbation of psoriasis, dry skin
- Respiratory: cough, dyspnea, sinusitis

Interactions (other drugs)

- Aldesleukin ▪ Aminophylline, theophylline ▪ Antineoplastic agents ▪ Zidovudine

Contraindications

▪ Benzyl alcohol hypersensitivity ▪ *Escherichia coli* protein hypersensitivity ▪ Neonates, children under one year ▪ History of depression or severe psychiatric disorders ▪ History of hepatitis, autoimmune disease ▪ Immunosuppression ▪ Visceral AIDS-related Kaposi's sarcoma associated with rapidly progressive disease ▪ Intramuscular injections ▪ Women of childbearing age (unless undertaking contraceptive measures)

Evidence

A small prospective trial involving six patients with HBV-related polyarteritis nodosa showed that treatment with interferon-alpha and plasma exchange controlled disease manifestations [3] *This study does not meet the criteria for level P*

Acceptability to patient

- Generally acceptable
- GI symptoms may make this medication more difficult to tolerate

Follow up plan

- Patients will need to be followed closely when on this medication
- Complete blood count should be monitored periodically

Patient and caregiver information

- Patients should be instructed to drink plenty of fluids
- If fever and headache occur secondary to treatment, acetaminophen may be given

LIFESTYLE

- Smokers should be advised to quit, as the nicotine-induced vasospasm may worsen ischemia
- Risk factors for stroke and heart disease should be addressed, as patients with polyarteriitis nodosa are already at increased risk for these conditions
- Diet should be addressed, and a low-fat, low-cholesterol diet recommended
- An appropriate level of exercise should be determined

RISKS/BENEFITS
Benefits:

- Improvement of overall health
- Risk reduction for vascular diseases

ACCEPTABILITY TO PATIENT
Smoking is extremely addictive, and patients may not be able to comply with this advice.

PATIENT AND CAREGIVER INFORMATION
Consultation with a dietitian may be helpful.

EFFICACY OF THERAPIES

- Prednisone with or without the addition of cyclophosphamide is effective as first-line treatment when there is no association with hepatitis
- Many patients will require the addition of cyclophosphamide
- Interferon-alpha and plasma exchange improve the outcome in patients with hepatitis-associated polyarteritis nodosa
- After remission is achieved, patients should be monitored closely throughout their lifetime, because relapses occur in about one-third of patients. Relapse risk continues to decrease the longer the patient remains in remission without active treatment

Evidence

- Treatment with prednisone plus plasma exchange was compared with prednisone, plasma exchange, and cyclophosphamide in patients with polyarteritis nodosa and Churg-Strauss angiitis in a small randomized controlled trial. The two groups had comparable survival but the patients who had received cyclophosphamide had fewer relapses [1] *Level P*
- Because polyarteritis nodosa is such a rare disease, few definitive studies have been performed that compare treatment options. Therefore, in the absence of such evidence, clinical experience and longitudinal studies will provide the basis for treatment

Review period

Patients should be monitored closely for at least one year, but will require lifelong follow up, as relapse is seen in about one-third of patients.

PROGNOSIS

- The course of untreated polyarteritis nodosa is progressive, with destruction of vital organs
- Expected course of untreated polyarteritis nodosa is poor, with a 5-year survival rate of 10–13%
- Death in the first year usually results from renal failure, GI complications (bowel infarcts or perforation), or cardiovascular events secondary to uncontrolled vasculitis. Infectious complications of treatment are the other major cause of mortality
- After the first year, death usually results from complications of treatment (infection) and vascular disease such as acute myocardial infarction and stroke
- Although survival rates are poor, the extent of the progression of the illness is variable among patients, with some having only limited disease
- Steroid treatment may increase survival rate to 50–60%
- Renal and GI signs are associated with the most serious prognosis

Clinical pearls

- Once patients are treated intensively for approx. one year, it is often possible to withdraw treatment and follow the patient clinically for disease activity. Many patients enjoy long disease-free remissions
- For younger patients, the risk of sterility and ovarian failure from cyclophosphamide treatment must be weighed against the life-threatening nature of this disease

Recurrence

- About one-third of patients who are in remission may relapse
- The patient should be followed lifelong for assessment and need for further treatment

COMPLICATIONS

- Cardiac involvement: pericarditis, heart failure, arrhythmias, and myocardial infarction
- Hypertension

- Gastrointestinal involvement: liver involvement, mucosal perforation, appendicitis, cholecystitis, pancreatitis
- Peripheral neuropathy and mononeuropathy, such as wrist drop and foot drop
- Skin involvement
- Migratory arthralgia and arthritis

CONSIDER CONSULT

Patients who have relapsed or who develop complications after treatment should be referred to a specialist.

RISK FACTORS

- Hepatitis B virus infection: may be a risk factor
- Hepatitis C virus infection: may be a risk factor
- Smoking: smokers should be advised to quit smoking, as the nicotine-induced vasospasm may worsen ischemia
- Risk factors for stroke and heart disease: should be addressed, as patients with polyarteritis nodosa are already at increased risk for these conditions
- Diet: should be addressed, and a low-fat, low-cholesterol diet recommended
- Exercise: an appropriate level should be determined

MODIFY RISK FACTORS
Lifestyle and wellness
IMMUNIZATION

Immunization against hepatitis B has been recommended as part of routine childhood vaccinations.

Cost/efficacy

Vaccination is effective for at least 5 years in 80–90% of people who are immunocompetent.

RESOURCES

ASSOCIATIONS
American College of Rheumatology
1800 Century Place, Suite 250
Atlanta, GA 30345
Tel: (404) 633 3777
Fax: (404) 633 1870
www.rheumatology.org

KEY REFERENCES
- Gay RM Jr, Ball GV. Vasculitis. In: Koopman WJ. Arthritis and Allied Conditions. A Textbook of Rheumatology. Baltimore: Williams and Wilkins, 1997, p1491–524
- Jennette JC, Falk RJ. Small-vessel vasculitis. N Engl J Med 1997;337:1512–23
- Watts RA, Scott DGI. Classification and epidemiology of the vasculitides. Bailliere's Clin Rheumatol 1997;11(2):191–217
- Guillevin L. Treatment of classic polyarteritis nodosa in 1999. Nephrol Dial Transplant 1999;14:2077–9
- Guillevin L, Lhote F, Gherardi R. Polyarteritis nodosa, microscopic polyangiitis, and Churg-Strauss syndrome: clinical aspects, neurologic manifestations, and treatment. Neurol Clin 1997;15(4):865–86
- Lightfoot RW Jr, Michel BA, Bloch DA, et al. The American College of Rheumatology. 1990 criteria for the classification of polyarteritis nodosa. Arthritis Rheum 1990;33:1088–93

Evidence references
1 Guillevin L, Jarrousse B, Lok C, et al. Long-term follow-up after treatment of polyarteritis nodosa and Churg-Strauss angiitis with comparison of steroids, plasma exchange and cyclophosphamide to steroids and plasma exchange: A prospective randomized trail of 71 patients. The Cooperative Study Group for Polyarteritis Nodosa. J Rheumatol 1991;18:567–74. Medline
2 Fauci AS, Katz P, Haynes BF, Wolff SM. Cyclophosphamide therapy of severe systemic necrotizing vasculitis. N Engl J Med 1979; 301: 235–8. Medline
3 Guillevin L, Lhote F, Sauvaget F, et al. Treatment of polyarteritis nodosa related to hepatitis B virus with interferon-alpha and plasma exchanges. Ann Rheum Dis 1994; 53: 334–7. Medline

FAQS
Question 1
How does polyarteritis nodosa usually present?

ANSWER 1
Patients will present with three of the following 10 signs or symptoms:
- Weight loss >4kg
- Livedo reticularis
- Testicular pain or tenderness
- Myalgias, weakness, or leg tenderness
- Mononeuropathy or polyneuropathy
- Diastolic blood pressure >90mmHg
- Elevated blood urea nitrogen or creatinine
- Hepatitis B virus
- Arteriographic abnormality
- Biopsy of small or medium artery contain polyarteritis nodosa

Question 2
How is polyarteritis nodosa differentiated from other vasculitis disorders?

ANSWER 2
The key differences between polyarteritis nodosa and other necrotizing vasculitides are:

- Lack of granuloma formation
- Sparing of veins, except by contiguous spread
- Sparing of pulmonary arteries
- Predilection for medium-sized arteries
- Absence of renal involvement

Question 3
What causes polyarteritis nodosa?

ANSWER 3
The cause of polyarteritis nodosa is not known, but it is believed to involve immune mechanisms. Because of the wide range of clinical and pathologic features of polyarteritis nodosa, it is believed that more than one pathogenic mechanism is responsible for the disease.

Question 4
What is the prognosis for patients with polyarteritis nodosa?

ANSWER 4
The course of polyarteritis nodosa may be progressive, with destruction of vital organs. The expected course of untreated polyarteritis nodosa is poor, with a 5-year survival rate of 10–13%. Steroid treatment may increase survival rates to 50–60%. However, it should be noted that the extent and progression of the disease can be quite variable among patients, with some having only limited and nonprogressive disease.

Question 5
What is the best treatment for patients with polyarteritis nodosa?

ANSWER 5
Patients should be treated with prednisone or a combination of prednisone and cyclophosphamide as first choices.

CONTRIBUTORS
Russel C Jones, MD, MPH
Richard, Brasington Jr, MD, FACP
Elizabeth C Hsia, MD

POLYMYALGIA RHEUMATICA

DESCRIPTION

- Polymyalgia rheumatica is characterized by muscle stiffness and pain predominately in neck, shoulder, and pelvic girdle muscles
- Stiffness and pain are typically worse in the morning, improving during the day, and are exacerbated by rest
- Symptoms are usually bilateral and symmetrical. There are no definitive diagnostic signs, symptoms, or laboratory tests
- Most patients are over 50 years old
- Steroid therapy is the mainstay of management. Patients can expect a dramatic response within 2–4 days at a starting prednisolone dose of 10–20mg daily
- Patients with polymyalgia rheumatica often develop giant cell arteritis (temporal arteritis) and vice versa

URGENT ACTION

- Commence corticosteroids immediately if giant cell arteritis (temporal arteritis) is suspected – classic presentation is unilateral headache with scalp tenderness (but symptoms may be vague)
- The patient with giant cell arteritis is at risk of blindness or stroke. Delaying treatment to confirm diagnosis carries significant risk and should be avoided

KEY! DON'T MISS!

Giant cell arteritis – needs urgent treatment and higher dose of steroids.

ICD9 CODE

725 Polymyalgia rheumatica.

CARDINAL FEATURES

- Polymyalgia rheumatica is a syndrome that may contain a complex of disease processes and whose pathophysiology is poorly understood
- Most frequently occurs after the age of 50; incidence increases with age
- Pain and stiffness in neck, shoulder, and pelvic girdle
- Dramatic response to steroids. In the absence of a rapid and dramatic response to steroids, the diagnosis must be reconsidered

There are no absolute diagnostic criteria. However, the following clinical features suggest the diagnosis:

- Pain in two of three areas (neck, shoulder, and pelvic girdle)
- Morning stiffness
- Duration of symptoms for one month or longer
- Age over 50 years
- Elevated erythrocyte sedimentation rate (ESR) usually over 50mm/h
- Absence of another diagnosis, such as rheumatoid arthritis, malignancy, or chronic infection

CAUSES

Common causes

- Cause is unknown and the precise nature of the inflammation is unclear
- Muscle biopsy shows nonspecific findings, without myositis or vasculitis
- An infectious cause has long been suspected, but never proven
- Polymyalgia rheumatica is more common in individuals of northern European ancestry, and very uncommon in blacks and Asians, suggesting a genetic predisposition

Contributory or predisposing factors

- More common over the age of 50 years
- Females twice as likely to be affected
- Genetic factors may play a part. Polymyalgia rheumatica is more common in individuals of northern European ancestry, and very uncommon in blacks and Asians
- Patients with polymyalgia rheumatica may develop giant cell arteritis (and vice versa). The precise incidence has not been established, but is probably in excess of 30%

EPIDEMIOLOGY

Incidence and prevalence

Data are limited, and cannot be generalized from one location to another. There are fewer studies specifically for polymyalgia rheumatica than for giant cell arteritis.

INCIDENCE

Approximately 0.5 per 1000 in Sweden and in Minnesota for the population 50 years and older.

PREVALENCE

6 per 1000 age 50 years and older in Minnesota.

FREQUENCY

Up to 2% of the population over 70 years.

Demographics

AGE
Rare under the age of 50 years. Incidence rises with increasing age.

GENDER
Female:male 2:1.

RACE
More frequent in patients with northern European ancestry, and rare in blacks and Asians.

GENETICS
Some studies show incidence of HLA-DR4 allele is twice as high in patients with polymyalgia rheumatica and giant cell arteritis compared with controls. Cases of familial aggregation have been described.

DIFFERENTIAL DIAGNOSIS
Rheumatoid arthritis
Rheumatoid arthritis may be difficult to distinguish from polymyalgia rheumatica, especially in the elderly. Both polymyalgia rheumatica and giant cell arteritis respond dramatically to low doses of corticosteroids.

FEATURES
- 80% of patients with rheumatoid arthritis are seropositive for rheumatoid factor
- Synovitis (inflammation localized to the joint) is much more common in rheumatoid arthritis than polymyalgia rheumatica
- Small peripheral joints in the hand are almost always involved in rheumatoid arthritis
- Onset of rheumatoid arthritis is often more gradual than polymyalgia rheumatica
- Morning stiffness in rheumatoid arthritis is more localized to the joints, rather than the proximal muscles as in polymyalgia rheumatica

Relapsing seronegative symmetric synovitis with peripheral edema (RS3PE)
FEATURES
- Abrupt onset of synovial inflammation in the hands and feet with pitting edema in the hands
- Rheumatoid factor is negative
- ESR is elevated
- Responds dramatically to corticosteroids
- Usually resolves within a few months of onset

Fibromyalgia
FEATURES
- Pain is diffuse, and not limited to a proximal muscle distribution
- Patients usually have nonrefreshing sleep
- Headaches and irritable bowel syndrome often accompany fibromyalgia
- Examination shows tenderness at specific locations
- Laboratory tests, including complete blood count and ESR should be normal
- May respond to low-dose corticosteroids, but not dramatically

Hypothyroidism
FEATURES
- Weight gain, dry skin, constipation, and voice change may occur
- Not associated with elevated ESR
- Thyroid-stimulating hormone is elevated (should be normal in polymyalgia rheumatica)
- Does not respond to corticosteroid treatment

Malignant disease
FEATURES
A number of malignancies can present with nonspecific symptoms such as myalgia, fatigue, anemia, and elevated ESR. Although any malignancy can present in this way, lymphoma, leukemia, and multiple myeloma should be especially considered.

Inflammatory myopathies
Polymyopathy and dermatomyositis may present with muscle pain.

FEATURES
- Muscle weakness is present, and is more pronounced than muscle pain and stiffness. Patients with polymyalgia rheumatica may appear to be weak because muscle effort during testing is

limited by pain
- Morning stiffness is unusual in inflammatory myopathies
- Elevated creatine kinase, electromyogram abnormalities, and specific muscle biopsy findings are present
- Dermatomyositis is associated with a distinctive rash

Osteoarthritis
Osteoarthritis may coexist in the elderly.

FEATURES
- X-rays confirm the presence of osteoarthritis
- Chronic onset
- ESR normal

Joint capsulitis
Bilateral adhesive capsulitis can give similar features.

FEATURES
Limitation of passive movement of the shoulders.

Myalgia due to infectious disease
Infectious diseases can cause myalgias. Viral etiologies are the most common, but septicemia and endocarditis must always be considered.

FEATURES
- Associated with fever
- Heart murmur often present with endocarditis
- White cell count often elevated

Drug-induced myalgia
The statins used for hypercholesterolemia are particularly prone to cause myalgias, sometimes with elevated creatine kinase. Other medications to consider include colchicine, hydroxychloroquine, and quinine.

FEATURES
Introduction of a new drug prior to the onset of symptoms should always be suspicious.

SIGNS & SYMPTOMS
Signs
- Limited active abduction and elevation of the shoulders
- Temporal artery tenderness and reduced pulse if associated with giant cell arteritis
- Usually minimal or no joint swelling (synovitis)

Symptoms
- Onset usually insidious, but may be acute
- Duration of symptoms over one month
- Involvement of proximal neck, shoulder, and pelvic girdle muscles
- Morning stiffness and nocturnal pain (trouble getting out of bed and trouble rolling over in bed during the night)
- Nonspecific constitutional symptoms including weight loss, anorexia, general malaise, and depression
- Occasionally have low-grade fever
- Inflammation of joints can occasionally occur

- Anemia: normocytic normochromic
- Sometimes associated with giant cell arteritis. Most common presentations include headache, visual disturbance, tongue or jaw claudication, and scalp tenderness

ASSOCIATED DISORDERS
Giant cell arteritis. Most common presentations are:
- Visual disturbance
- Jaw or tongue claudication
- Headache
- Scalp tenderness

KEY! DON'T MISS!
Giant cell arteritis – needs urgent treatment and higher dose of steroids.

CONSIDER CONSULT
- Uncertainty over diagnosis
- Urgent ophthalmologic referral is indicated in the presence of symptoms of visual loss

INVESTIGATION OF THE PATIENT
Direct questions to patient
Q How quickly did your pain come on? Onset usually gradual, but may be sudden
Q What is the distribution of pain and stiffness? Predominantly limb girdle
Q Have you experienced headache, tongue or jaw claudication, visual disturbance, or scalp tenderness? Be alert for other manifestations of giant cell arteritis
Q Do you have other symptoms, particularly morning stiffness, anorexia, weight loss, general malaise, depression? Be aware of other presentations of muscle pain

Contributory or predisposing factors
Q What is the patient's age? More common over the age of 50 years, and increasingly common with advancing age
Q What is the patient's sex? Females twice as likely to be effected
Q Does the patient have giant cell arteritis? Over one-third of patients with giant cell arteritis will develop polymyalgia rheumatica

Examination
Q Is the patient systemically ill? Be alert for malignancy or infection
Q Is muscle strength reduced? More likely to be a myopathy
Q Is joint movement limited? Limitation of shoulder movement is almost universal with this diagnosis
Q Is synovitis present? May be present, but less prominent than in rheumatoid arthritis
Q Is the patient febrile? Low-grade fever may occur
Q Is a heart murmur present? Consider endocarditis
Q Is there scalp tenderness, or tenderness or reduced pulse of either temporal artery? These findings suggest giant cell arteritis
Q Are multiple tender points present? This suggests fibromyalgia
Q Is the thyroid gland enlarged? Rule out hypothyroidism

Summary of investigative tests
Although laboratory tests are useful, they are not definitive. The main characteristic is acute-phase reaction.

- The ESR is almost always elevated
- C-reactive protein is raised and may be elevated when the ESR is normal

- Full blood count may reveal a mild normochromic normocytic anemia
- Liver function tests may be mildly abnormal in some patients

DIAGNOSTIC DECISION
There are no absolute diagnostic criteria. Diagnosis is based on clinical presentation and rapid response to steroids.

Polymyalgia rheumatica should be considered in the presence of one or more of the following symptoms:
- Neck, or bilateral shoulder or pelvic pain and stiffness
- Morning stiffness
- ESR greater than 40mm/h
- Aged 50 years or more
- Unexplained fever

Diagnostic guidelines:
The American College of Rheumatology has prepared diagnostic guidelines for evaluating patients with acute musculoskeletal symptoms:
- American College Of Rheumatology Ad Hoc Committee on Clinical Guidelines. Guidelines for the initial evaluation of the adult patient with acute musculoskeletal symptoms. Arthritis Rhematism 1996; 39:1–8; also available on-line from the National Guideline Clearinghouse

CLINICAL PEARLS
- Patients often complain of devastating symptoms, which severely interfere with quality of life and activities of daily living
- Frequent complaints are difficulty rolling over in bed at night or getting out of bed
- Substantial limitation of shoulder abduction and elevation (putting the arms together above the head) is almost always present

THE TESTS
Body fluids
ERYTHROCYTE SEDIMENTATION RATE
Description
ESR is a measure of acute-phase proteins.

Advantages/Disadvantages
Disadvantages:
- Can be normal in polymyalgia rheumatica
- Can be raised in other conditions that give a similar picture such as infection or malignancy

Normal
- Females: 0–20mm/h
- Males: 1–15mm/h

Abnormal
- Usually above 50mm/h in polymyalgia rheumatica, but rarely may be normal
- Raised ESR is helpful but not diagnostic. May be elevated in other conditions that give similar picture such as infection or malignancy
- Keep in mind the possibility of a falsely abnormal result

Cause of abnormal result
Increased fibrinogen levels in response to inflammation.

Drugs, disorders and other factors that may alter results
- Anemia due to any cause tends to increase ESR
- Many inflammatory and autoimmune conditions cause a raised ESR
- Corticosteroid therapy will typically lower ESR

C-REACTIVE PROTEIN
Description
C-reactive protein may be raised if ESR is normal.

Advantages/Disadvantages
Advantages:
- The C-reactive protein is unaffected by anemia
- Rises and falls more rapidly than the ESR

Disadvantage: may be raised in other conditions that give a similar picture, such as infection or malignancy

Normal
<1.0mg/dL (depending upon each laboratory's range).

Abnormal
- May be raised in other conditions that give a similar picture such as infection or malignancy
- Keep in mind the possibility of a falsely abnormal result

COMPLETE BLOOD COUNT
Description
Venous blood sample.

Advantages/Disadvantages
- Adavantage: simple, universally available test
- Disadvantage: nonspecific

Normal
Hemoglobin:
- Males: 13.6–17.7g/dL
- Females: 12–15g/dL

White blood cells:
- 3200–9800 cells/mm^3

Platelet count:
130,000–400,000 platelets/mm^3

Abnormal
- Values outside the normal ranges
- Keep in mind the possibility of a falsely abnormal result

Cause of abnormal result
Polymyalgia rheumatica is often associated with a mild, normochromic or hypochromic, normocytic anemia, hemoglobin 10g/dL or above.

TREATMENT

CONSIDER CONSULT

- When symptoms of headache, tongue and jaw claudication, scalp tenderness, or visual loss suggest the possibility of giant cell arteritis, a temporal artery biopsy should be performed without delay
- When symptoms do not respond dramatically to low-dose steroids

IMMEDIATE ACTION

If there is clinical evidence of giant cell arteritis (headache, visual disturbance, tongue or jaw claudication, or scalp tenderness), commence high-dose corticosteroids (40–60mg/day) immediately, then refer for a temporal artery biopsy.

PATIENT AND CAREGIVER ISSUES
Health-seeking behavior

- Patients may be reluctant to take steroids
- The importance of continuing with this medication should be emphasized, and patients should be warned that they will have to be on steroids for as long as 1–2 years.

MANAGEMENT ISSUES
Goals

- To resolve patient symptoms and improve quality of life
- To monitor for the associated condition of giant cell arteritis
- To monitor for exacerbations of polymyalgia rheumatica
- To minimize the side-effects of steroids

Management in special circumstances
COEXISTING DISEASE

- Be aware of the potential coexistence of giant cell arteritis. This condition will require a much higher dose of steroids and performance of a temporal artery biopsy
- Specialist opinion should be considered if there is a possibility that steroids might exacerbate a coexisting problem, such as diabetes, osteoporosis, or chronic infection
- Coexisting fibromyalgia, osteoarthritis, or rheumatoid arthritis may cloud the diagnosis

COEXISTING MEDICATION
Nonsteroidal anti-inflammatories (NSAIDs) may be useful in relieving symptoms, but in combination with steroids increase the risk of upper gastrointestinal toxicity. A selective cyclo-oxygenase-2 (COX-2) inhibitor (-coxib) such as celecoxib or rofecoxib may be a safer choice in an elderly patient on steroids (although neither agent has been specifically studied in polymyalgia rheumatica).

PATIENT SATISFACTION/LIFESTYLE PRIORITIES

- Patient may be unhappy with the thought of steroid medication for a median duration of 2 years
- Warn of possible adverse affects
- Emphasize importance of continuing with medication

SUMMARY OF THERAPEUTIC OPTIONS
Choices

- First and only real choice is prednisolone at a dose of 10–20mg a day (although there remains some controversy regarding the optimum dosage)
- No immunosuppressive or 'steroid-sparing' agent has been proven effective, although methotrexate and hydroxychloroquine are sometimes used
- Rapid response to prednisone supports the diagnosis

- There is no evidence that physical therapy addresses the cause, although it may help the patient recover range of motion of neck, shoulders, and hips, and may temporarily relieve discomfort
- Lifestyle changes may help reduce risk of osteoporosis secondary to steroid therapy; but prophylactic treatment is recommended

Guidelines:

The American Academy of Family Physicians have published guidelines:

- Meskimen S, Cook TD, Blake RL. Management of giant cell arteritis and polymyalgia rheumatica. Am Fam Phys 2000;61:2061–8.

Clinical pearls

- All patients on corticosteroids should receive prophylactic treatment to prevent osteoporosis: supplemental calcium, vitamin D, and a bisphosphonate such as alendronate 5mg/day or risedronate 5 mg/day. In women, hormone (estrogen) treatment may be considered. A baseline bone density study (DEXA) may be performed
- Because steroid-related osteoporosis occurs rapidly during the first 6 months of steroid treatment, prophylaxis should be implemented immediately to be effective
- If prednisolone cannot be tapered to an acceptable dose, refer to a rheumatologist for consideration of an additional agent, such as methotrexate or hydroxychloroquine
- Significant corticosteroid toxicity is very common in older patients on chronic corticosteroids: osteoporosis with fracture, avascular necrosis, formation or progression of cataract, development or worsening of diabetes, and elevated blood pressure

Never

Never use low doses of steroids if there is evidence of giant cell arteritis, in which case the recommended dose is 40–60mg prednisone (or 1mg/kg body weight).

FOLLOW UP

- Average treatment with steroids is 1–2 years
- The aim of monitoring is to identify toxicity of steroid treatment, exacerbations of polymyalgia rheumatica, and onset of giant cell arteritis (which can occur at any time during the disease and is not prevented by low-dose steroids used for polymyalgia rheumatica)
- Review in one week to assess clinical response, which should be rapid. In the absence of dramatic improvement, the diagnosis must be re-evaluated
- Remain at 10–20mg a day for the first month before reducing the dose
- Time course of steroid reduction must be individualized for each patient. In general, doses of 10–20mg a day can be reduced by 2.5 mg every month. Below 10mg a day, the dose should be reduced by 1mg per month
- Maintenance dose is that which is necessary to control the symptoms
- Acute phase reactants can be useful to monitor disease activity but are less important than clinical symptoms for two reasons: ESR or C-reactive protein can remain elevated in some patients who are clinically well; a rise in ESR or C-reactive protein can have many other causes (such as infection or malignancy) other than polymyalgia rheumatica

Plan for review

Review after one week to assess acute clinical response, monthly until stable, then every 3 months until treatment is discontinued.

Information for patient or caregiver

- Explain nature of the disease and its association with giant cell arteritis
- Emphasize the need for long-term steroids and the importance of regular review
- Emphasize the likelihood of toxicity related to corticosteroids and the importance of measures to prevent osteoporosis

DRUGS AND OTHER THERAPIES: DETAILS
Drugs
PREDNISOLONE

Prednisolone is the drug of choice prescribed as a single morning dose.

Dose
- Starting dose of 10–20mg a day for at least one month
- Average duration of treatment with steroids is 1–2 years
- 30–50% of patients need continuous management for more than 2 years
- The aim of monitoring is to identify steroid-related toxicity, exacerbations of polymyalgia rheumatica, and onset of giant cell arteritis, which can occur at any time during the disease
- Review in one week to assess clinical response, which should be rapid and dramatic
- Remain at 10–20mg a day for the first month
- The time course of steroid reduction must be individualized for each patient. In general, doses of 10–20mg a day can be reduced by 2.5 mg every month. Below 10mg a day, the dose should be reduced by 1mg per month
- The maintenance dose is that which is necessary to control the symptoms
- Acute-phase reactants can be useful to monitor disease activity but are less important than clinical symptoms for two reasons. First, ESR or C-reactive protein can remain elevated in some patients who are clinically well. Second, a rise in ESR or C-reactive protein can have many other causes (such as infection or malignancy) other than polymyalgia rheumatica

Efficacy
A rapid response with complete relief of symptoms should occur if the diagnosis of polymyalgia rheumatica is correct.

Risks/Benefits
Risks:
- Overwhelming septicemia if patient has an infection
- Loss of control of blood glucose in those with diabetes
- Prolonged use causes adrenal suppression

Benefit: the benefits are worthwhile given the severity of symptoms in polymyalgia rheumatica, but it must be recognized that medication-related toxicity is very likely to occur

Side-effects and adverse reactions
- Side-effects are minimized by short duration of therapy
- Gastrointestinal: dyspepsia, peptic ulceration, esophagitis, oral candidiasis
- Cardiovascular system: hypertension, thromboembolism
- Central nervous system: insomnia, euphoria, depression, psychosis
- Endocrine: adrenal suppression, impaired glucose tolerance, growth suppression in children
- Musculoskeletal: proximal myopathy, osteoporosis
- Skin: delayed healing, acne, striae
- Eyes, ears, nose and throat: cataract, glaucoma, blurred vision

Interactions (other drugs)
- Aminoglutethamide
- Barbiturates
- Cholestyramine
- Clarithromycin, erythromycin
- Colestipol
- Isoniazid
- Ketoconazole
- NSAIDs
- Oral contraceptives
- Rifampin
- Salicylates
- Troleandomycin

Contraindications
- Systemic infection
- Avoid live virus vaccines in those receiving immunosuppressive doses

Acceptability to patient
Patients may be reluctant to adhere to long-term steroids. Compliance with regular follow up and compliance with medication cannot be over-emphasized.

Follow up plan
- Follow blood pressure, blood glucose, cholesterol, and bone density
- Advise patients about increased risk from infectious contacts, including chicken pox if nonimmune
- Recommend preventive measures for osteoporosis in all patients

Patient and caregiver information
- Emphasize importance of compliance
- Average duration of medication treatment is 1–2 years
- Self-monitor for exacerbation of condition and need for increased steroid dose
- Giant cell arteritis can occur even if on steroids. Review immediately if headache, visual disturbance, temporal headache, or jaw or tongue claudication occur

LIFESTYLE

The lifestyle changes that will have a beneficial effect are those that prevent the side-effects of long-term corticosteroid therapy. These include weight control and prevention of osteoporosis:
- Daily intake of elemental calcium (males 1000mg, females 1500mg), and 400–800IU of vitamin D
- Stop smoking
- Avoid excessive alcohol consumption
- At least 30 min each day of weight-bearing activity (walking or running)

EFFICACY OF THERAPIES
Treatment with corticosteroids usually leads to rapid and dramatic resolution of symptoms.

Evidence
PDxMD are unable to cite evidence which meets our criteria for evidence.

PROGNOSIS
If adequately treated, the prognosis of polymyalgia rheumatica is good provided that the clinician is alert for the development of steroid-related toxicity, or the development of giant cell arteritis. The major problems arise from the side-effects of long-term steroid medication.

Clinical pearls
- Toxicity from steroid treatment is common in these patients, especially osteoporosis. All patients should be treated prophylactically for this
- A surprising number of patients require long-term steroid therapy at doses that cause complications or are not tolerated. These patients should be evaluated by a rheumatologist for a 'steroid-sparing' agent

Therapeutic failure
- If steroid therapy does not produce rapid and dramatic improvement, the diagnosis should be re-evaluated
- Secondary treatment failure may occur in a patient whose prednisolone dose cannot be reduced to an acceptable level, in which case a 'steroid-sparing' agent should be considered

Recurrence
For recurrences that do not respond to an increase in steroid dosage, specialist referral is indicated.

Deterioration
Further options include methotrexate, hydroxychloroquine, and possibly other immunosuppressive agents. Referral to a rheumatologist is indicated for these drugs.

COMPLICATIONS
- Patients with polymyalgia rheumatica are at increased risk of giant cell arteritis, the complications of which are stroke and blindness. Early intervention in giant cell arteritis is important to minimize the risk
- The complications of this disorder accompany its functional limitation and, in treatment, are associated with adverse effects of steroid use

PREVENTION

There are no known preventative factors for polymyalgia rheumatica.

RISK FACTORS
Northern European ancestry.

MODIFY RISK FACTORS
Lifestyle and wellness
TOBACCO
Stop smoking.

ALCOHOL AND DRUGS
Alcohol and drugs should be reduced.

DIET
At least 1.5g calcium/day.

PHYSICAL ACTIVITY
At least 30 min of weight-bearing activity each day.

PREVENT RECURRENCE
- There may be recurrence at any time during the treatment of polymyalgia rheumatica and occasionally after medication has been stopped
- The patient should be closely monitored during the early stages of the disease, while the dose is being reduced, and for several months following the withdrawal of treatment

RESOURCES

ASSOCIATIONS

American College of Rheumatology
1800 Century Place
Suite 205
Atlanta, GA30345-4300
Tel: (404) 633 3777
Fax: (404) 633 1870
www.rheumatology.org

National Inststute of Arthritis and Musculoskeletal Diseases
National Institute for Health
Bethesda, MD 20892-2350
www.nih.gov/niams

Canadian Arthritis Network
600 University Avenue, Suite 600
Toronto, Ontario M5G 1X5
Canada
Tel: (416) 586 4770
Fax: (416) 586 8628
www.arthritis.ca

KEY REFERENCES

- American College Of Rheumatology Ad Hoc Committee on Clinical Guidelines. Guidelines for the initial evaluation of the adult patient with acute musculoskeletal symptoms. Arthritis Rhematism 1996;39:1–8; also available on-line from the National Guideline Clearinghouse
- Jones JG, Hazelman B. Prognosis and management of polymyalgia rheumatica. Ann Rheum Dis 1981;40:1–5
- Kyle V, Hazleman BL. The Clinical Cause of Polymyalgia Rheumatica – giant cell arteritis. Br J Rheumatol 1988;27(Suppl 1):7
- Meskimen S, Cook TD, Blake RL. Management of giant cell arteritis and polymyalgia rheumatica. Am Fam Phys 2000;61:2061–8.
- Pountaing, Hazleman BL. Polymyalgia rheumatica and giant cell arteritis. BMJ 1995;310:1057–9

CONTRIBUTORS

Eric F Pollak, MD, MPH
Richard Brasington Jr, MD, FACP
Deborah L Shapiro, MD

PROLAPSED INTERVERTEBRAL DISC

SUMMARY INFORMATION

DESCRIPTION

- Frequently asymptomatic
- Common degenerative change of aging
- Symptomatic disc prolapse causes radiculopathy in distribution of compressed nerve root
- May be difficult to distinguish from other causes of back and neck pain

URGENT ACTION

Immediate surgical referral for symptoms indicative of possible cauda equina syndrome:

- Difficult urination
- Incontinence
- Impotence
- Saddle anesthesia

Surgical consultation should be sought if the patient has a history of progressive motor weakness.

KEY! DON'T MISS!

Do not miss signs/symptoms of potential cauda equina syndrome, or high or midline lumbar disc herniation, including:

- Unilateral or bilateral leg weakness
- Rectal pain
- Perineal numbness
- Sphincter paralysis, with concomitant loss of bowel and/or bladder control

BACKGROUND

ICD9 CODE

- 722.0 Herniated disc: cervical
- 722.10 Herniated disc: lumbar
- 722.11 Herniated disc: thoracic
- 722.2 Herniated disc: site unspecified
- 722.3 Degeneration of intervertebral disc: cervical
- 722.4 Degeneration of intervertebral disc: thoracic
- 722.5 Degeneration of intervertebral disc: lumbar
- 722.6 Degenerative disc disease
- 722.7 Herniated disc with myelopathy
- 722.8 Other and unspecified disc disorder

SYNONYMS

- Herniated disc
- Slipped disc
- Herniated nucleus pulposus

CARDINAL FEATURES

- Protrusion of the nucleus pulposus of the intervertebral disc partially or completely through the outer annulus fibrosus
- May impinge on spinal nerve roots
- Prolapsed intervertebral discs may be asymptomatic; a significant number are found incidentally on studies
- Nerve root compression may lead to radiculopathy
- Prolapsed intervertebral discs most commonly present at the L4–L5 and L5–S1 levels, although cervical and thoracic discs may also prolapse

CAUSES
Common causes

- Degenerative changes due to aging, including: decreased height, dehydration of the nucleus pulposus, tears and fissures in the annulus fibrosus
- Disc becomes subject to repeated microtrauma
- Natural progression leads to nucleus pulposus prolapse
- Trauma, injuries

Contributory or predisposing factors

- Family tendency
- History of repeated heavy lifting, twisting, vibration, bending in occupation or recreation
- Cigarette smoking
- Poor nutrition
- Frequent diving from a diving board
- Tall stature
- Overweight, obesity
- Pregnancy and childbirth
- Sedentary lifestyle
- Pre-existing spinal disorders, including: fused vertebrae, vertebral malformations, lumbar spinal stenosis secondary to short pedicles, ankylosing spondylitis, degenerative arthritis

EPIDEMIOLOGY
Incidence and prevalence

The true incidence and prevalence of prolapsed intervertebral discs in the population is not known. Some statistics are available for generalized low back pain.

INCIDENCE

- Thoracic intervertebral disc prolapse: 0.025–0.05 per 1000 cases of intervertebral disc rupture
- Among patients with acute back pain, 1% have nerve root symptoms

PREVALENCE

- Life-time prevalence of low back pain is 60–90%
- 95% of diseased discs are localized to L4–L5 and L5–S1

Demographics

AGE

Peak incidence: 30–50 years.

GENDER

- Cervical – male:female 1.4:1
- Lumbar – male:female 1:1

GENETICS

Family tendency noted.

DIFFERENTIAL DIAGNOSIS
Trauma (sprains and strains, fracture)
Mechanical lower back pain and fractures are examples of trauma that may be encountered.

FEATURES
Mechanical lower back pain:
- Onset usually related to new or unusually intense exertion
- Patient usually lacks history of major trauma, systemic infection, or malignancy
- Pain may be quite severe
- Pain improves when supine
- Physical examination may reveal paravertebral tenderness and/or spasm, scoliosis, loss of lumbar lordosis, or absence of focal neurologic signs

Fracture:
- History of major trauma
- Elderly or known osteoporotic patient may have virtually no known mechanism of injury

Osteoarthritis/cervical spondylosis
Osteoarthritis may occur at the apophyseal and Luschka joints, and/or the intervertebral disc in the cervical or lumbosacral spine. 'Cervical spondylosis' is the term used for degenerative changes in cervical vertebra and/or disc, with spur formation and subsequent impingement of neural elements in a narrow cervical canal.

FEATURES
- Pain in the posterior neck often associated with radiation into the arms
- Radicular pain into the arms or scapular area may be present without neck pain
- Scapular pain
- Weakness of upper and/or lower extremities
- If osteophyte develops and extends laterally on neurocentral joint, then this can encroach on the vertebral artery and may cause dizziness, vertigo, tinnitus, or interorbital blurring of vision. Symptoms are exacerbated by extremes of movement and even minor neck trauma
- Commonly, loss of neck extension
- Lateral flexion of the cervical spine is limited in the erect position but greatly increases on lying down
- Spondylolisthesis (forward motion of one vertebral body over the one below it) usually occurs at L4–L5 or L5–S1, and may contribute to pain

Rheumatoid arthritis
Rheumatoid arthritis, usually advanced cases, may cause atlantoaxial subluxation. The thoracic and lumbar spine are spared.

FEATURES
- Chronic, insidious, autoimmune disorder characterized by a symmetric polyarthritis affecting mainly small joints in the hands and feet
- Symptoms of atlantoaxial subluxation include pain radiating to the occiput and sensation of head falling forward during flexion; less commonly there may be spastic quadriparesis, parasthesias during neck motion, altered consciousness, difficulty speaking or swallowing
- X-ray reveals >3mm between odontoid and axis

Thoracic outlet syndrome
Thoracic outlet syndrome is a differential diagnosis of cervical symptoms.

FEATURES

- Neurovascular compression of the subclavian vessels or the brachial plexus in the thoracic outlet
- More common in women
- Age 35–55 years
- Symptoms may be vascular or neurologic, depending on whether the subclavian vessels or the brachial plexus, respectively, are compromised. Neurologic symptoms may include pain and paresthesias over shoulders, supraclavicular area, medial arms, and/or anterior chest wall, and motor and sensor changes over the palmer fourth and fifth digits
- A specialist can determine whether surgery or conservative treatment is warranted

Referred pain from visceral or vascular origin
FEATURES

- Pain may be colicky, episodic in nature
- No positional relief; patient may present writhing in an attempt to find a comfortable position
- Positive finding on abdominal examination
- Patient may present with fever, evolving shock state
- The visceral organ involved may refer pain: from the innervating spinal segment (i.e. pelvic sources, such as endometriosis, uterine cancer, chronic prostatitis, and cancer) to the sacral area; from lower abdominal disease (colitis, diverticulitis) to the lower lumbar region; and from upper abdominal disease (retroperitoneal extension of peptic ulcer or tumor, pancreatitis, abdominal aortic aneurysm) to the lower thoracic or upper lumbar area
- No local signs of spasm or pain on movement during examination

Metastatic disease (including multiple myeloma)
Multiple myeloma is a malignancy of plasma cells.

FEATURES

- Positive past history or current suspicion of malignancy
- Pain not relieved by rest
- Positive systemic symptoms may include weight loss, anorexia, fever, night sweats
- May present with neurologic signs, including weakness, bowel and/or bladder dysfunction
- Physical examination may note tenderness to palpation of spinous process, or neurologic findings specified by level of involvement (may progress to full paraplegia)

Infection, including epidural abscess, vertebral osteomyelitis, septic discitis
The key features of infection, including epidural abscess, vertebral osteomyelitis, and septic discitis, are as follows.

FEATURES

- Pain not relieved by rest
- Patient may present with fever, signs of shock
- Past history or current suspicion of active infection
- History of pelvic or genitourinary surgery
- Known diabetes mellitus, intravenous drug abuse, immunosuppressive medications or illness
- May present with neurologic signs, including weakness, bowel and/or bladder dysfunction
- Physical examination may identify tenderness to palpation of spinous process, neurologic findings specified by level of involvement (may progress to full paraplegia), and signs of specific systemic infection
- Elevated erythrocyte sedimentation rate (ESR)
- White blood cell count indicative of infection
- May have positive blood cultures
- Abscess suggested by radionuclide scan

Ankylosing spondylitis

Ankylosing spondylitis is a chronic inflammatory condition involving the sacroiliac joints and axial skeleton.

FEATURES
- Onset slowly progressive, insidious
- Back pain (lower) most severe in morning
- Back pain relieved with exercise
- Patient's age <40 years at onset of symptoms
- Sacroiliac joints ankylosed
- Decreased spinal mobility
- Decreased expansion of chest wall
- X-rays reveal ankylosed sacroiliac joints and lumbosacral spine
- Elevated ESR
- Positive human leukocyte antigen (HLA)-B27
- Anterior uveitis revealed on ophthalmologic examination

Reactive spondyloarthropathies
FEATURES
- May have noted prodromal urethritis, rash, colitis
- Onset slowly progressive, insidious
- Back pain most severe in morning
- Back pain relieved with exercise
- Patient's age <40 years at onset of symptoms
- Sacroiliac joints ankylosed
- Decreased spinal mobility
- Decreased expansion of chest wall
- X-rays reveal ankylosed sacroiliac joints and lumbosacral spine
- Elevated ESR
- Positive HLA-B27
- Anterior uveitis revealed on ophthalmologic examination
- Gastrointestinal radiographic studies may reveal inflammatory or infectious bowel disease
- Genitourinary cultures may reveal infectious urethritis

Spinal stenosis
FEATURES
- Variable intensity of back pain (absent to severe)
- May note pseudoclaudication (neurogenic claudication) of anterior thigh due to constriction of spinal cord when spine is in extension
- Pain increases throughout the day
- Pain exacerbated by standing and walking, and improves with sitting
- May present with neurologic signs, including weakness, bowel and/or bladder dysfunction
- Physical examination may suggest osteoarthritis
- Neurologic examination may reveal radiculopathy at more than one spinal level
- X-ray examination reveals vertebral osteophytes, degenerative disc disease

SIGNS & SYMPTOMS
Signs
Cervical disc prolapse:
- If nerve root compression is present, signs follow predictable dermatomal distribution
- Pain elicited or improved with particular maneuvers
- Distraction or compression may increase or decrease cervical disc pain
- Cervical paraspinal spasm

- Decreased neck mobility
- Motor weakness evident when testing grip strength, resistance maneuvers
- Reproduction of paresthesias numbness via limb or neck positioning
- Fasciculations in hand muscles
- Muscle atrophy
- Hypo-, hyper-, or areflexia

Thoracic disc prolapse:
- If root compression is present, signs follow predictable dermatomal distribution
- Unilateral or bilateral weakness in both leg and abdominal muscles
- Gait disorders
- Spinal deformity
- Kyphosis demonstrated rarely
- Rarely, complete paraplegia
- Rarely, acute-onset Brown-Séquard's syndrome (unilateral motor paralysis with contralateral sensory loss)
- Deep tendon reflex usually hyper-reflexic
- Extensor plantar reflex
- Clonus

Lumbar disc prolapse:
- If root compression is present, signs follow predictable dermatomal distribution
- Straight leg raise increases pain (lumbar disc)
- Motor weakness evident when testing limb strength, resistance maneuvers
- Reproduction of paresthesias numbness via limb positioning
- Hypo-, hyper-, or areflexia
- Clonus
- Muscle atrophy
- Gait disorders

Symptoms
Cervical discogenic pain:
- Pain in neck, medial scapula, shoulder
- Headache
- Vertigo, dizziness
- Tinnitus
- Visual disturbances

Cervical nerve root compression:
- Radiating pain, running down arm and/or into chest; may appear cardiogenic
- Paresthesias, numbness in hands, fingers
- Motor weakness in arm, hands, fingers
- Neck and shoulder pain
- Predictable dermatomal distribution

Cervical myelopathy:
- Paresthesias, numbness, pain secondary to neck extension
- Motor weakness, sensory deficit specific to compressed nerve root
- Predictable dermatomal distribution

Thoracic intervertebral disc prolapse:
- Pain in thoracic area
- May note lower back, abdominal, or leg pain

- May note unilateral or bilateral numbness, paresthesias, hyperesthesias, difficulty walking
- If root compression is present, symptoms follow predictable dermatomal distribution

Lumbar intervertebral disc prolapse:
- Back pain (sometimes for months or years before other initiation of other symptoms)
- Back pain may improve with rest
- Pain usually increases with sitting, may improve when standing, lying
- Back pain exacerbated by increased exertion, particularly bending and/or twisting motions
- Pain radiates into sacroiliac region, buttocks, posterior thigh
- Radicular pain will continue to radiate below the knee
- Any movement involving the Valsalva maneuver increases pain, including coughing, sneezing, straining to urinate or defecate
- Groin, testicular, rectal pain of concern
- Perineal numbness
- Bowel or bladder incontinence
- If nerve root compression is present, symptoms follow predictable dermatomal distribution

KEY! DON'T MISS!
Do not miss signs/symptoms of potential cauda equina syndrome, or high or midline lumbar disc herniation, including:
- Unilateral or bilateral leg weakness
- Rectal pain
- Perineal numbness
- Sphincter paralysis, with concomitant loss of bowel and/or bladder control

CONSIDER CONSULT
- Patients with possible cauda equina syndrome or high/midline lumbar disc herniation should be referred immediately for urgent surgical consult
- Patients with hyper-reflexia in upper or lower limbs, or other upper motor signs should also receive urgent surgical referral
- Surgical consultation should be sought with a history of progressive motor weakness, recurrent incapacitating pain with conservative nonoperative methods, or incapacitating pain despite conservative nonoperative methods

INVESTIGATION OF THE PATIENT
Direct questions to patient
Q When did your pain begin?
Q How long has it been since you first began noticing symptoms?
Q Do you recall any injury that may have led to your symptoms? The patient may volunteer information that will indicate the cause of the problem
Q What is the exact location and radiation of the pain you're experiencing? Radicular pain generally follows a predictable dermatomal pattern
Q What is the quality of the pain you're experiencing? Radicular pain may be described as sharp, burning, and stabbing
Q Have you noticed any weakness? Where? Nerve root compression may lead to weakness in hands or legs, which may be unilateral or bilateral
Q Have you noticed any tingling sensations or numbness? Where? Nerve root irritation may result in paresthesias, hyperesthesias, or numbness
Q What makes your symptoms worse? Twisting, bending, and lifting may exacerbate pain, as may sitting for a long time
Q What makes your symptoms better? Standing or lying down may improve pain, whereas symptoms may be exacerbated by sitting

Q **Have you experienced any loss of bladder or bowel control?** Loss of sphincter control may indicate a serious problem (e.g. cauda equina syndrome) that requires immediate aggressive intervention

Q **Are you having any trouble walking?** Gait disturbances are common in lumbar disc prolapse

Q **Do you have any other symptoms, such as fever or weight loss?** Systemic symptomatology may suggest the presence of infection or malignancy

Q **Do you do a lot of heavy lifting, twisting, or bending, or are you exposed to vibration in your job or during recreational activities?** All of these impose increased stress on the spine, and may predispose to prolapsed intervertebral disc

Contributory or predisposing factors

Q **Do you smoke?** Cigarette smoking has been associated with increased risk for prolapsed intervertebral disc

Q **Do you have any known spinal deformities or conditions?** Congenital spinal defects (fused vertebrae, vertebral malformations, lumbar spinal stenosis secondary to short pedicles) and acquired spinal defects (ankylosing spondylitis, degenerative arthritis) are all associated with a higher risk for prolapsed intervertebral disc

Q **What is your occupation? Do you need to perform physical labor or lifting? Do you have young children that need to be carried? In what kinds of recreational activities do you participate?** Jobs, childcare tasks, recreation that requires lifting, physical exertion, bending, twisting, or exposure to vibration may predispose to prolapsed intervertebral disc

Family history

Do other family members have a history of prolapsed intervertebral disc? Family history of prolapsed intervertebral disc may be a risk factor.

Examination

- Observe patient's posture while sitting. In particular, look for 'sciatic list'
- Observe patient's gait. In particular, look for 'sciatic list'
- Survey patient's back for visual suggestion of paraspinal spasm
- Observe relevant muscle groups for suggestion of atrophy
- Palpate spinous processes and interspinous ligaments for presence of tenderness
- Assess range of motion of back, neck, arms, and legs
- Assess motor function bilaterally. Assess using active and passive methods, and applying resistance
- Assess sensory function (pain, light touch, vibration) bilaterally
- Assess reflexes bilaterally
- Observe for muscle fasciculations, clonus
- To identify potential cervical disc prolapse, assess whether pain: is exacerbated during neck extension and rotation, or during Spurling maneuver (extend, bend laterally, and hold down patient's neck); is exacerbated or relieved via neck flexion; or is exacerbated or relieved when symptomatic arm is held over the top of the head
- To identify lumbar disc prolapse, assess exacerbation or relief of pain during: seated straight leg raise, supine straight leg raise, Braggart test, or prone hip extension test

Summary of investigative tests

- Complete blood count (CBC) can help to determine the presence of infection. May also suggest the presence of metastatic disease
- Erythrocyte sedimentation rate (ESR) will help to differentiate between inflammatory/metastatic and other disorders
- Plain spine films give minimal information but are always appropriate as an initial step in the evaluation

- Computed tomography (CT) scan is helpful for better delineating bony anatomy and pathology
- Magnetic resonance imaging (MRI) scan is excellent for soft-tissue imaging, revealing narrowing and compression of spinal structures
- Nerve conduction studies and electromyogram (EMG): these are not routinely performed for back pain, but may be of benefit when investigating some patients who present with a neurologic deficit in the lower limbs. Several weeks of symptoms are necessary before studies will show any abnormality
- Discography: although controversial, proponents believe discography can evaluate whether visualized disc disease is truly the source of patient's pain. This is normally performed by a specialist
- Myelography has been largely replaced by MRI, although some spine surgeons prefer a myelogram/CT combination

CLINICAL PEARLS

- A critical distinction is between pain from disc disease and paresthesias caused by nerve root compression
- Motor deficits from cervical nerve root compression are unusual unless several nerve roots are compromised
- Aggravation by cough and sneeze is typical of discogenic pain
- Cervical spine stenosis presents indolently with upper and lower extremity motor signs, rather than symptoms of paresthesias

THE TESTS
Body fluids
COMPLETE BLOOD COUNT
Description
Venous blood sample.

Advantages/Disadvantages
Advantages:
- Simple, standard test
- Relatively inexpensive
- Results rapidly available

Disadvantage: nonspecific – indicates presence of infection/inflammation but not source

Normal
Hemoglobin:
- Males – 13.6–17.7g/dL (136–177g/L)
- Females – 12.0–15.0g/dL (170–150g/L)

Leukocyte profile:
- Total – 3.9–9.8x10^3/mcL
- Lymphocytes – 1.2–3.3x10^3/mcL
- Mononuclear cells – 0.2–0.7x10^3/mcL
- Granulocytes – 1.8–6.6x10^3/mcL

Platelet count:
- 130–400x10^3/mm^3 (130–400x10^9/L)

Abnormal
- White blood cells may be increased in infection

- Low hemoglobin or pancytopenia may suggest presence of malignant disease
- Keep in mind the possibility of a false-positive result

Cause of abnormal result
May be abnormal in infection, inflammation, or because of a blood disorder.

Drugs, disorders and other factors that may alter results
Steroid medications, lithium, and NSAIDs may falsely elevate leukocyte count.

ERYTHROCYTE SEDIMENTATION RATE
Description
Blood sample.

Advantages/Disadvantages
- Advantage: simple, safe to obtain
- Disadvantage: not definitive for a specific disease but may help to sort out differential. May be positive with infection (including epidural abscess, vertebral osteomyelitis, septic discitis), ankylosing spondylitis, reactive spondyloarthropathies, malignancy

Normal
- Males: 0–15mm/h
- Females: 0–20mm/h

Abnormal
- Values outside the normal range
- Keep in mind the possibility of a false-positive result

Cause of abnormal result
- Marked elevation suggests inflammatory or malignant process
- Keep in mind the possibility of a false-positive or false-negative result

Drugs, disorders and other factors that may alter results
Abnormal test result may reflect another inflammatory disorder.

Imaging
PLAIN BACK FILMS
Advantages/Disadvantages
Advantages:
- Noninvasive
- Inexpensive
- Readily obtained at most hospitals

Disadvantages:
- May reveal abnormalities that are not responsible for symptomatology
- Not terribly specific or sensitive
- May be falsely negative

Abnormal
- May note loss of disc height
- May visualize vertebral fracture

Cause of abnormal result
- Loss of disc height may occur as a normal part of aging, or may be indicative of a pathologic process

- Bone destruction may signal metastatic process
- Vertebral fracture could indicate metastasis or sequelae of severe osteoporotic disease

Drugs, disorders and other factors that may alter results
A full bowel may prevent adequate visualization of lumbar spine.

COMPUTED TOMOGRAPHY SCAN
Advantages/Disadvantages
Advantages:
- Provides detailed information regarding vertebral anatomy and pathology
- Compared with plain back films, CT studies have higher sensitivity and specificity for most conditions of the spine

Disadvantages:
- Compared with MRI, CT studies have lower sensitivity and specificity for most conditions of the spine
- Generally, will require use of contrast, and intrathecal contrast is necessary to show detail of spinal cord and nerve roots

Abnormal
- Bony destruction
- Collapse of vertebral body
- Vertebral fracture
- Spinal stenosis
- Filling defect suggests compression of spinal nerve roots
- Keep in mind the possibility of a false-positive result

Cause of abnormal result
- Bony destruction may signal metastatic process
- Vertebral collapse or fracture may be due to metastatic disease, trauma, or severe osteoporosis
- Spinal stenosis may be secondary to facet joint hypertrophy
- Compressed spinal root may be secondary to prolapsed intervertebral disc

MAGNETIC RESONANCE IMAGING
Advantages/Disadvantages
Advantage: provides detailed images for diagnosis of soft-tissue disease

Disadvantages:
- Requires specialized, expensive equipment
- Cannot be performed on individuals with significant metal prostheses or pacemakers
- May be difficult to keep patient comfortable for lengthy imaging time (40–60min)

Abnormal
- May note cord or cauda equina compression
- May note compression of nerve roots

Various classifications exist for evaluating MRI results, including the following terms:
- Normal – disc does not extend beyond intervertebral space
- Bulge – symmetric, circumferential extension of disc past intervertebral space
- Protrusion – asymmetric extension of disc past intervertebral space (more extensive than bulge). The protruding disc is on a narrowed pedicle of disc material. May also be called a contained herniation

- Extrusion – very extensive extension of disc past intervertebral spasm, with separation of extruded disc from original disc. May also be called a sequestered or free fragment herniation
- High-intensity zone – a high-intensity signal believed by some to indicate a painful area

Cause of abnormal result
Cord, cauda equina, or nerve root compression may be secondary to prolapsed intervertebral disc, spinal stenosis, or tumor.

ELECTROMYOGRAM
Description
Using a needle electrode inserted into muscle, the pattern of electrical activity of that muscle may be determined.

Normal
Relaxed muscle is electrically silent.

Abnormal
- Spontaneous activity during rest
- Fibrillation
- Positive sharp waves

Cause of abnormal result
- Denervation muscle
- Inflammatory muscle disease

Special tests
NERVE CONDUCTION STUDIES
Description
- Not routinely performed for back or neck pain
- May be of benefit when investigating patients who present with a neurologic deficit in the limbs

Advantages/Disadvantages
Advantage: can help to differentiate between a neurologic deficit due to nerve root compression and other conditions such as a diabetic peripheral neuropathy

Disadvantages:
- Time-consuming, invasive, and expensive
- Not always very helpful
- Symptoms must have been present for several weeks for study to be positive

Normal
Motor and sensory latencies unaffected.

Abnormal
- Delayed conduction in the affected nerves
- Keep in mind the possibility of a false-positive result

Cause of abnormal result
- Nerve root compression
- Peripheral neuropathy
- Any other neurologic condition that affects nerve conduction

Drugs, disorders and other factors that may alter results
The results of nerve conduction studies can be very difficult to interpret in patients with nerve root compression superimposed on an underlying peripheral neuropathy or any other chronic neurologic condition.

TREATMENT

CONSIDER CONSULT
If imaging studies reveal significant impingement on spinal cord or nerve roots, or cauda equina syndrome, then immediate surgical referral is justified.

IMMEDIATE ACTION
Assess serious risk factors (i.e. history of cancer, trauma, or infection).

PATIENT AND CAREGIVER ISSUES
Forensic and legal issues
Legal issues may complicate a patient's care if injury is occupational and workman's compensation issues are involved.

Impact on career, dependants, family, friends
Symptomatic prolapsed intervertebral discs may interfere with a patient's job, childcare tasks, or recreational pursuits.

MANAGEMENT ISSUES
Goals
- To ascertain whether serious complications of prolapsed intervertebral disc (cauda equina syndrome, spinal cord, or nerve root impingement/entrapment) are present
- To help patient make appropriate lifestyle choices to aid in recovery from symptoms of prolapsed intervertebral disc
- To provide appropriate pain management techniques to improve patient's comfort

Management in special circumstances
SPECIAL PATIENT GROUPS
Sciatica is often a maternal complication of pregnancy.

PATIENT SATISFACTION/LIFESTYLE PRIORITIES
Lifestyle changes may be significant, and may cause significant hardship for patients whose occupations, family (childcare) obligations, or recreational pursuits involve activities that may exacerbate the symptoms of prolapsed intervertebral disc.

SUMMARY OF THERAPEUTIC OPTIONS
Choices
Conservative treatment for cervical prolapsed intervertebral disc:
- Rest, for not more than 2 days
- Anti-inflammatory analgesia
- Physical therapy – these optional measures include neck and shoulder exercises, massage, and ice (note that proof of its efficacy is lacking and use is controversial)
- A cervical collar may be used. This measure is normally instituted by an orthopedic specialist

Thoracic prolapsed discs are generally not amenable to conservative measures.

Conservative treatment for lumbar prolapsed intervertebral disc (note that 95% of patients with lumbar prolapsed intervertebral disc will improve with conservative treatment):
- Rest, for not more than 2 days
- Anti-inflammatory analgesia and selective cyclo-oxygenase 2 (COX-2) inhibitors
- Muscle relaxants
- Narcotic analgesia (rarely)

- Acetaminophen
- Physical therapy – optional; may include application of heat or ice, ultrasound treatment to muscles, massage, transcutaneous electrical nerve stimulation (TENS) therapy, and posture education. Note that proof of its efficacy is lacking and its use is controversial
- Back braces or corsets
- Epidural steroid injections

Surgical treatment:
- Patients who have continued to have severe symptomatology despite conservative treatment, those with significant radiculopathy, and those with thoracic prolapsed intervertebral discs will most likely be referred to a specialist and offered surgery
- Surgical treatments for prolapsed intervertebral disc include open disc surgery, percutaneous lumbar discectomy, chemonucleolysis

Lifestyle:
Modifications to lifestyle may have beneficial effects on both prolapsed intervertebral disc and other aspects of health.

Clinical pearls
- Conservative, nonoperative treatment is always appropriate, and may be successful even in the setting of radiculopathy
- Surgical treatment is reserved for symptoms caused by spinal cord or nerve root compression that do not resolve with conservative measures
- Spinal fusion is performed to compensate for any spinal instability that might result from laminectomy, and not to relieve pain from disc disease
- Surgery is more likely to benefit neuropathic symptoms, rather than neck or back pain

FOLLOW UP
Most patients will be able to return to normal activities at the 2-week follow up visit.

DRUGS AND OTHER THERAPIES: DETAILS
Drugs
NSAIDS
- Ibuprofen
- Indomethacin
- Naproxen
- Diclofenac
- Sulindac

Dose
- Ibuprofen:1200–3200mg daily (300mg four times daily; 400, 600 or 800mg three to four times daily). Individual patients may show a better response to 3200mg daily, as compared with 2400mg daily
- Indomethacin regular strength capsules: 25mg two to three times daily. If this is well tolerated, increase the daily dosage by 25mg or 50mg, if required by continuing symptoms, at weekly intervals until a satisfactory response is obtained or until a total daily dose of 150–200mg is reached
- Indomethacin extended-release capsules: initiate with 75mg once daily. For patients who require 150mg indomethacin per day and have demonstrated acceptable tolerance, indomethacin extended-release may be prescribed as one 75mg capsule twice daily
- Naproxen: initiate with 500mg (20mL), followed by 250mg (10mL) every 6–8h as required. The total daily dose should not exceed 1250mg (50mL)
- Diclofenac: the recommended starting dose of diclofenac potassium immediate-release

tablets is 50mg three times daily. Some patients may benefit from an initial dose of 100mg diclofenac potassium immediate-release tablets, followed by 50mg doses. After the first day, when the maximum recommended dose may be 200mg, the total daily dose should generally not exceed 150mg

- Sulindac: 150mg orally twice per day with food; maximum dosage is 400mg/day. May increase to maximum dosage on the basis of patient response to lower dosage

Efficacy
Considered good for acute and chronic back pain.

Risks/Benefits
Risks:
- Use caution in the elderly, pregnancy, and breast-feeding
- Use caution in renal, cardiac, gastrointestinal, and hepatic disease
- Use caution in Addison's disease, recent head injury, and hypothyroidism
- Use caution in patients with a history of drug abuse
- Small risk of dependency

Benefits:
- Decreased inflammation
- Analgesia

Side-effects and adverse reactions
- Cardiovascular system: hypertension, peripheral edema, congestive heart failure
- Central nervous system: headache, dizziness, tinnitus, fever
- Gastrointestinal: anorexia, nausea, dyspepsia, peptic ulceration, bleeding
- Genitourinary: nephrotoxicity
- Hematologic: blood cell disorders
- Hypersensitivity: rashes, bronchospasm, angioedema
- Skin: pruritus, rash

Interactions (other drugs)
- ACE inhibitors - Acetazolamide - Alcohol - Antacids - Antihypertensives, beta-blockers - Antineoplastic agents - Aminoglycosides - Baclofen - Corticosteroids - Cyclosporine, tacrolimus - Diltiazem - Digoxin - Diuretics - Ethanol - Griseofulvin - Lithium - Methotrexate - NSAIDs (other concurrent) - Phenylpropanolamine - Platelet inhibitors, salycitlates, thrombolytic agents - Oral anticoagulants

Contraindications
- Peptic ulcer - Gastrointestinal bleeding - Bleeding disorders - Bone marrow suppression (aspirin) - Hypersensitivity to salicylates, NSAIDs, or tartrazine - Severe renal or hepatic disease - Dehydration

Acceptability to patient
Usually acceptable, although some patients have gastrointestinal discomfort that makes NSAID treatment difficult.

Follow up plan
Schedule return visits to verify that patient is receiving pain relief, and to ascertain that no new neurologic signs have presented.

Patient and caregiver information
Recommend that all doses of NSAIDs should be taken with food.

SELECTIVE CYCLO-OXYGENASE-2 INHIBITORS

- Celecoxib
- Rofecoxib

Dose

- Celecoxib: initiate with 400mg orally, followed by an additional 200mg dose if needed on the first day. On subsequent days, the recommended dose is 200mg twice daily as needed
- Rofecoxib: initial with 50mg once daily, followed by 50mg once daily as needed. Use of rofecoxib for >5 days in management of pain has not been studied

Efficacy

Considered good for acute and chronic back pain.

Risks/Benefits

Risk (celecoxib): use caution with patients with pre-existing asthma

Risks (rofecoxib):

- Use caution with patients with pre-existing asthma
- Use caution in gastrointestinal disease, perforation or history of bleeding, or peptic ulcer disease
- Use caution in the elderly, children, pregnancy, and breast-feeding
- Use caution in renal disease
- Use caution in fluid retention, hypertension, or heart failure
- Ensure patient is not dehydrated before commencing therapy

Benefits:

- Decreased inflammation
- Analgesia

Side-effects and adverse reactions

Celecoxib:

- Central nervous system: dizziness, headache
- Gastrointestinal: abdominal pain, diarrhea, dyspepsia, flatulence, nausea
- Respiratory: respiratory tract infections
- Skin: rash

Rofecoxib:

- Cardiovascular system: edema, hypertension, congestive heart failure
- Central nervous system: dizziness, headache, fever
- Gastrointestinal: abdominal pain, diarrhea, nausea, vomiting, dyspepsia, gastritis, anorexia, cholecystitis, flatulence, esophagitis, constipation, gastrointestinal bleeding, pancreatitis, peptic ulcer, stomatitis, elevated hepatic enzymes
- Hematologic: anemia
- Musculoskeletal: back pain, fatigue
- Respiratory: sinusitis, bronchitis
- Skin: maculopapular rash, urticaria, dermatitis

Interactions (other drugs)

Celecoxib:

- ACE inhibitors ■ Furosemide ■ Aspirin ■ Fluconazole ■ Lithium ■ Warfarin

Rofecoxib:

- ACE inhibitors ■ Alendronate ■ Antineoplastic agents ■ Aspirin ■ Corticosteroids
- Cyclosporine ■ Diuretics ■ Ethanol ■ Lithium ■ Methotrexate ■ Rifampin ■ Warfarin

Contraindications
Celecoxib:

▪ Allergic reactions to sulfonamide ▪ Allergic reactions to NSAIDs ▪ Inflammatory bowel disease ▪ Severe congestive heart failure ▪ Renal impairment

Rofecoxib:

▪ Salicylate hypersensitivity ▪ Severe hepatic impairment ▪ Advanced renal disease

MUSCLE RELAXANTS
▫ Cyclobenzaprine
▫ Carisoprodol

Dose
▫ Cyclobenzaprine: 10mg three times a day, with a range of 20–40mg a day in divided doses. Dosage should not exceed 60mg a day. Use for periods longer than 2 or 3 weeks is not recommended
▫ Carisoprodol: one 350mg tablet, three times daily and at bedtime. Usage in patients under age 12 is not recommended

Efficacy
May be helpful if prolapsed intervertebral disc is causing significant muscle spasm.

Risks/Benefits
Risk (cyclobenzaprine): use caution in glaucoma, urinary retention, epilepsy, and the elderly

Risks (carisoprodol):
▫ Requires high doses for efficacy in masticatory muscles
▫ No direct efficacy on skeletal muscles; should be used as an adjunct to physical therapy

Benefits:
▫ May provide palliation in patients with significant muscle spasm
▫ May help potentiate effectiveness of NSAIDs

Side-effects and adverse reactions
Cyclobenzaprine:
▫ Gastrointestinal: constipation, nausea, dry mouth
▫ Cardiovascular: palpitations, arrythmias, hypotension, dizziness, drowsiness
▫ Genitourinary: hesitancy, frequency, retention
▫ Central nervous system: headache, insomnia, confusion, weakness
▫ Eye: visual disturbance

Carisoprodol:
▫ Dizziness, drowsiness, and weakness
▫ Nausea common

Interactions (other drugs)
Cyclobenzaprine:
▪ Antidepressants (SSRIs and MAOIs) ▪ Droperidol

Carisoprodol:
Use with caution with alcohol.

Contraindications
Cyclobenzaprine:
- Recent myocardial infarction ■ Arrhythmias ■ Child <12 years of age ■ Porphyria
- Hypothyroidism, hyperthyroidism

Carisoprodol:
- Should not be used in patients with sensitivity to related compounds ■ Should not be used in children ■ Acute intermittent porphyria ■ Hypersensitivity to this medication and other meprobamate derivatives

Acceptability to patient
Usually acceptable, although elderly patients may experience confusion with these medications. Sedation is common with cyclobenzaprine.

Follow up plan
Schedule return visits to verify that patient is receiving pain relief, and to ascertain that no new neurologic signs have presented.

Patient and caregiver information
- Notify caregiver of elderly patient of potential for initiating confusion
- Be wary of prescribing to patient known to have history of substance abuse, due to addictive/abuse potential

ACETAMINOPHEN
Dose
325–1000mg orally every 4h as necessary, not to exceed 4g/day.

Efficacy
Effective pain relief.

Risks/Benefits
Risks:
- Use caution in hepatic and renal impairment
- Overdosage results in hepatic and renal damage unless treated promptly
- Overdose may lead to multiorgan failure and may be fatal
- Accidental overdosage can occur if over-the-counter preparations containing acetaminophen are taken with prescribed drugs that contain acetaminophen

Side-effects and adverse reactions
- Acetaminophen rarely causes side-effects when used intermittently
- Gastrointestinal: nausea, vomiting
- Hematologic: blood disorders
- Metabolic: acute hepatic and renal failure
- Skin: rashes
- Other: acute pancreatitis

Interactions (other drugs)
- Alcohol ■ Anticoagulants ■ Anticonvulsants ■ Isoniazid ■ Cholestyramine ■ Colestipol
- Domperidone ■ Metoclopromide

Contraindications
- Hypersensitivity to acetaminophen ■ Known liver dysfunction

Physical therapy
PHYSICAL THERAPY
May include application of heat or ice, ultrasound treatment to muscles, transcutaneous electrical nerve stimulation (TENS) therapy, and posture education.

Efficacy
- Many of these physical therapy modalities have no proven efficacy
- Use of some modalities is controversial
- Although there is little specific evidence that these treatments are efficacious, the conventional wisdom is that they help reduce symptoms

Acceptability to patient
- Some patients may be aware of and ask for these treatment modalities
- Others may consider these modalities to be 'alternative' and may feel skeptical about their benefits

Follow up plan
Schedule return visits to assess whether symptoms are resolving, and to evaluate to see whether new neurologic signs have presented.

Surgical therapy
- Patients who have continued to have severe symptomatology despite conservative treatment, those with significant radiculopathy, and those with thoracic prolapsed intervertebral discs will most likely be referred to a specialist and offered surgery
- Surgical treatments for prolapsed intervertebral disc include: open disc surgery, percutaneous lumbar discectomy, and chemonucleolysis

Other therapies
EPIDURAL STEROID INJECTIONS
May be combined with local anesthetic for injection into epidural space or into trigger points.

Efficacy
Thought to be efficacious by some, although good evidence is lacking.

Risks/Benefits
Risks:
- Risk of inadvertent intrathecal injection small, but can be catastrophic
- Symptoms may not improve, or may intensify

Benefit: may decrease radicular symptomatology

Follow up plan
Schedule return visits to assess whether symptoms are resolving, and to evaluate to see whether new neurologic signs have presented.

Patient and caregiver information
Make sure patient is aware that repeated injections may be necessary after effects wear off.

LIFESTYLE
Lifestyle aspects that may predispose to or exacerbate prolapsed intervertebral disc include:
- Heavy lifting
- Bending, twisting
- Exposure to vibration

- Occupations, childcare tasks, recreational pursuits that involve heavy lifting, bending, twisting, exposure to vibration, repeated diving from board
- Cigarette smoking
- Poor nutrition
- Obesity

RISKS/BENEFITS

- Risk: modification of activities may be most difficult, especially if lifting or certain movements are necessary for employment or childcare
- Benefit: modifications of risk factors may have beneficial effects on other areas of health

ACCEPTABILITY TO PATIENT

- Compliance may be difficult for patients who have to inform employer of curtailed physical activity
- Lifestyle modifications involving cigarette smoking or diet are notoriously difficult for patients

FOLLOW UP PLAN

Reasonable frequency of follow up appointments is necessary to:

- Re-evaluate to see whether symptoms are improving
- Reassess for the development of new or more severe symptoms
- Support patient in lifestyle changes

PATIENT AND CAREGIVER INFORMATION

Carefully explain to patient and caregiver the rationale for lifestyle changes, particularly those that may be difficult to maintain.

Prolapsed intervertebral disc – OUTCOMES

EFFICACY OF THERAPIES

More studies are needed to compare conservative vs surgical therapies, and to help determine the best surgical candidates.

PROGNOSIS

- Back injuries have a high likelihood of recurrence, and of conversion from acute to chronic
- Most instances of acute back pain, however, will respond to conservative therapy in 2 weeks

Clinical pearls

- For back pain that has been present for months, the likelihood of significant relief is low; patients should be counseled so that they do not expect dramatic results from any therapeutic intervention. A chronic pain management approach will be appropriate for many such individuals
- Elderly patients with discogenic pain are likely to have multiple risk factors for NSAID-induced gastrointestinal toxicity; caution must be exercised in prescribing such medications for this group
- 'Muscle relaxants', such as cyclobenzaprine, are often beneficial, but may be associated with sedation
- Exercise is especially important in the management of chronic pain from these disorders

CONSIDER CONSULT

- Urgent referral is necessary for progressive neurologic disability, especially disability suggestive of cauda equina syndrome (saddle anesthesia, loss of sphincter control, evidence of upper motor neuron disease)
- Refer if conservative therapy fails to relieve symptoms

RISK FACTORS

- Heavy lifting
- Bending, twisting
- Exposure to vibration
- Occupations, childcare tasks, recreational pursuits that involve heavy lifting, bending, twisting, exposure to vibration, repeated diving from board
- Cigarette smoking
- Poor nutrition
- Obesity

MODIFY RISK FACTORS
Lifestyle and wellness
TOBACCO

Cigarette smoking (but not, interestingly, cigar or pipe smoking) has been associated with the development of prolapsed intervertebral disc.

DIET
- Both obesity and malnutrition have been implicated as risk factors for the development of prolapsed intervertebral disc
- Encourage patient to achieve and then maintain a healthy weight
- Encourage nutritious diet

PHYSICAL ACTIVITY

Sedentary lifestyle may contribute to predisposition to prolapsed intervertebral disc.

FAMILY HISTORY
- Tendency to develop prolapsed intervertebral disc may run in families
- Patients with a positive family history may wish to attend a healthy back class to learn more about, for example, safe lifting

PREVENT RECURRENCE

- Advise patient on safe lifting practices
- Give advice regarding positions to be avoided (i.e. twisting, bending, heavy lifting, lifting from waist instead of knees)
- Recommend that patient avoids diving from boards
- Recommend that patient avoids vibration
- Give advice regarding modifiable risk factors, including cigarette smoking, obesity, and malnutrition

RESOURCES

ASSOCIATIONS

American Academy of Neurology
1080 Montreal Avenue
St Paul, MN 55116
Tel: (651) 695 1940
Fax: (651) 695 2791
www.aan.com

American Academy of Orthopaedic Surgeons
6300 North River Road
Rosemont, IL 60018-4262
Tel: (847) 823 7186 or (800) 346 AAOS
Fax: (847) 823 8125
www.aaos.org

American Academy of Physical Medicine and Rehabilitation
One IBM Plaza, Suite 2500
Chicago, IL 60611-3604
Tel: (312) 464 9700
Fax: (312) 464 0227
E-mail: info@aapmr.org
www.aapmr.org/

American College of Rheumatology/Association of Rheumatology Health Professionals
1800 Century Place, Suite 250
Atlanta, GA 30345
Tel: (404) 633 3777
Fax: (404) 633 1870
E-mail: acr@rheumatology.org
www.rheumatology.org

Arthritis Foundation
PO Box 7669
Atlanta, GA 30357-0669
Tel: (800) 283 7800
www.arthritis.org

KEY REFERENCES

- Gibson JNA, Grant IC, Waddell G. Surgery for lumbar disc prolapse. In: The Cochrane Library, 2001, 4. Oxford: Update Software
- Humphreys SC, Eck JC. Clinical evaluation and treatment options for herniated lumbar disc. Am Fam Physician 1999;59:575–82
- McCall IW. Imaging of low back pain, I: lumbar herniated disks. Radiol Clin North Am 2000;38:1293–309
- Tierney LM, McPhee SJ, Papadakis MA. Current medical diagnosis and treatment. New York: Lange Medical Books/McGraw-Hill, 2001

FAQS
Question 1
What symptoms should suggest the presence of disc disease?

ANSWER 1
Pain in the neck or back that is aggravated by coughing and sneezing, or back pain aggravated by sitting should raise the suspicion of a discogenic cause.

Question 2
What is the role for decompressive laminectomy and spinal fusion?

ANSWER 2
Such surgery may be beneficial for the relief of symptoms of spinal cord or nerve root compromise, not for the relief of pain.

Question 3
What can patients with painful disc disease do to help themselves?

ANSWER 3
Smoking cessation, proper lifting techniques, and regular exercise can be beneficial.

CONTRIBUTORS
Fred F Ferri, MD, FACP
Richard Brasington Jr, MD, FACP
Maria-Louise Barilla-LaBarca, MD

PSEUDOGOUT

DESCRIPTION

- Rheumatic manifestation of calcium pyrophosphate dihydrate crystal deposition in articular cartilage (chondrocalcinosis), synovium, and periarticular ligaments and tendons
- Identification of crystals is the only means of positive diagnosis
- Usually affects the knee (50% of cases) but often also the wrist, elbow, shoulder, ankle, and hand

URGENT ACTION

Infectious arthritis should always be considered if the patient presents with inflammatory arthritis of a single joint. Refer for aspiration of synovial fluid for culture and Gram staining immediately.

KEY! DON'T MISS!

Infectious arthritis is always in the differential diagnosis of monoarticular inflammatory arthritis.

BACKGROUND

ICD9 CODE

275.4 Chondrocalcinosis
712.2 Chondrocalcinosis due to calcium phosphate crystals

SYNONYMS

- Calcium pyrophosphate deposition disease
- CPPD
- Calcium pyrophosphate dihydrate crystal deposition disease
- CPPD crystal deposition disease
- CPPD deposition disease
- Pyrophosphate arthropathy

CARDINAL FEATURES

- Rheumatic manifestation of calcium pyrophosphate dihydrate crystal deposition in articular cartilage (chondrocalcinosis), synovium, and periarticular ligaments and tendons
- Identification of crystals is the only means of positive diagnosis
- Usually affects the knee (50% of cases) but often also the wrist, elbow, shoulder, ankle, and hand joints

CAUSES
Common causes

- Crystal deposition may be secondary to degenerative or biochemical changes in the affected tissues
- Acute attacks are sometimes triggered by trauma, surgery, or systemic illness

Contributory or predisposing factors

- Aging (for acute and chronic disease)
- Previous trauma (for acute and chronic disease)
- Family history (<1% of cases; for acute and chronic disease)
- Certain metabolic diseases may underlie a small fraction of cases; should be suspected if the patient is under 55 years of age
- Hyperparathyroidism (for acute disease)
- Hemochromatosis (for acute and chronic disease)
- Hypophosphatasia (for acute disease)
- Hypomagnesemia (for acute disease)
- Hypothyroidism (chondrocalcinosis)

EPIDEMIOLOGY
Incidence and prevalence

Uncertain. Most data reflect the presence of chondrocalcinosis, which is asymptomatic in the majority of cases.

PREVALENCE
Approximately 3/1000 persons in the total population.

FREQUENCY
Chondrocalcinosis has a prevalence of 81/1000 in the age range 63–93 years.

Demographics

AGE

- Increasing age is a predisposing factor; more than 80% of patients are over 60 years old
- Peak age 65–75 years

GENDER
Female/male 2:1.

RACE
Hereditary patterns (<1% of cases) have been observed in Slovakian-Hungarian, Chilean-Spanish, French, Swedish, Dutch, Canadian, Mexican-American, Italian-American, German-American, Japanese, Tunisian, Jewish, and English families.

GENETICS
Genetic defects on chromosomes 5p and 8q have been found in hereditary cases.

DIFFERENTIAL DIAGNOSIS

Infectious arthritis is the most important differential diagnosis; it requires urgent attention to avoid severe and irreversible joint destruction. The following disorders may also coexist with pseudogout.

Osteoarthritis

Osteoarthritis, especially inflammatory osteoarthritis, may closely mimic chronic pseudogout. Pseudogout should always be suspected in cases of apparent osteoarthritis in which inflammatory flares occur.

FEATURES

- Affects one or a few joints; typically those that are weight bearing or have suffered previous injury
- Only rarely involves the wrist, hand, elbow, or shoulder
- Slowly progressive with occasional exacerbations, which are usually not associated with effusion, warmth, and redness
- No rest pain (unless disease is end stage); symptoms worse with or after sustained activity
- Joints show bony swelling, crepitus, and restricted movement
- Osteophytes may be palpable
- No systemic illness
- Synovial fluid noninflammatory (fewer than 2000 white blood cells/mL)
- X-rays display typical joint space narrowing, subchondral sclerosis, and osteophytic spurring

Rheumatoid arthritis

May be mimicked by chronic polyarticular pseudogout.

FEATURES

- Chronic, gradually progressive arthritic disease, often with acute exacerbations
- Symmetric, polyarticular joint pain with swelling, warmth, effusion, and synovial thickening
- Almost always involves hands and feet symmetrically
- Prolonged morning stiffness; restricted movement early in the disease
- Systemic features: weakness, fatigue, weight loss
- Eventually leads to characteristic deformities: subluxations, dislocations, and joint contractures
- Rheumatoid nodules over bony prominences
- Tenosynovitis and possible tendon rupture
- X-rays display typical marginal erosions and periarticular osteopenia in established disease
- Synovial fluid has 2000–50,000 white blood cells/mm^3
- Elevated serum rheumatoid factor levels in 80% of cases
- Rarely associated with splenomegaly, pericarditis, or vasculitis

Gout

Acute gout may closely mimic acute attacks of pseudogout, and chronic gout may resemble chronic pseudogout.

FEATURES

- Recurrent acute gout and chronic gout may also strongly resemble rheumatoid arthritis
- Most common in middle-aged men
- Typically affects first metatarsophalangeal joint, ankles, and midfoot
- Joints hot, red, swollen, and extremely tender or painful
- Attacks may be precipitated by illness, surgery, exercise, dietary indiscretions, or stress
- Associated with history of diuretic use, hypertension, and alcohol consumption

- Soft tissue tophi are common around joints, in bursae, in Achilles' tendons, and at the extensor surface of the forearm
- In long-standing disease, X-rays may show typical cystic erosions with thin, overhanging edges of bone resulting from reparative changes ('punched-out erosions with overhanging osteophytes')
- Synovial fluid contains 3000–white blood cells/mm^3
- Positively diagnosed by deposition of monosodium urate crystals, visible under polarized light microscopy
- In transplant patients, cyclosporine may cause a particularly rapidly progressing form of the condition
- Renal stones may occur as a complication of hyperuricosuria

Infectious arthritis

This condition is highly destructive and should always be considered in the differential diagnosis of monoarticular inflammatory arthritis.

FEATURES

- Usually one joint is affected (acute monoarthritis)
- Usually affects knee or hip
- Affected joint(s) are hot, painful, and swollen, with restricted range of movement
- Fever is often present
- Suspect in a febrile patient with established arthritis who displays an acute flare in a single joint
- Often caused by hematogenous spread of infection from a distant site, direct puncture of the joint, or spread from adjacent osteomyelitis
- Often associated with history of previously abnormal joint, rheumatoid arthritis, old age, immunocompromised status, or intravenous drug use
- Synovial fluid contains >50,000 white blood cells/mm^3
- Synovial fluid is positive for culture and Gram stain
- Causes rapidly progressing radiographic abnormality
- If untreated, can lead to irreversible joint damage

Calcium hydroxyapatite deposition disease

Similar to pseudogout, except that the rheumatologic manifestation is due to calcium apatite deposition.

FEATURES

- Associated with articular and periarticular deposition of calcium hydroxyapatite crystals, identified in a wet preparation of synovial fluid stained with Alizarin red S. Unlike gout and pseudogout, these crystals are not detectable with polarized microscopy
- Short history with rapid and destructive progression
- Typically involves knees and shoulders ('Milwaukee shoulder') but also hips and fingers
- Acute and chronic forms may occur
- Pain is the most common symptom, but joints may show erythema and swelling
- Bursitis and periarthritis may occur in addition to arthritis
- X-rays show marked destructive changes, osteophytes, and soft-tissue calcification (nummular calcification of tendon inserts is typical)
- Synovial fluid is usually noninflammatory
- Treated in the same manner as pseudogout

Calcium oxalate deposition disease

Similar to pseudogout, except the rheumatologic manifestation is due to calcium oxalate deposition.

FEATURES

- Associated with articular deposition of calcium oxalate crystals
- X-rays reveal chondrocalcinosis and soft-tissue calcification
- Acute or chronic joint effusions
- May affect any joint
- Oxalate deposits in blood vessels may mimic vasculitis
- Vertebral deposition may cause spinal cord compression
- Primary disease is a rare hereditary disorder
- Associated with patients with renal failure maintained on chronic hemodialysis or peritoneal dialysis
- May be potentiated by vitamin C supplements
- Synovial fluid is usually noninflammatory
- Treated in the same manner as pseudogout

SIGNS & SYMPTOMS
Signs

- Variable presentation: usually presents as acute arthritis involving a single joint (mimicking gout), but can present acutely involving multiple joints (mimicking osteoarthritis, rheumatoid arthritis or polyarticular gout)
- Most common cause of acute inflammatory monoarthritis in the elderly
- Most typically observed in the knee (50% of cases) but also often in the wrist, elbow, shoulder, ankle, and hand
- Acute attacks associated with swelling, restricted movement and increased heat in the affected joints, and fever. The intensity of the periarticular inflammation may suggest cellulitis
- Joints in chronic disease may show bony swelling, crepitus, and restricted movement, with varying levels of synovitis
- Severe joint disease may ultimately result (usually observed in elderly women)
- X-rays display calcification of articular cartilage and tendon inserts and often hypertrophic appearance of bone, with exuberant formation of cysts and osteophytes
- A severe destructive arthropathy resembling neuropathic joint disease can rarely occur

Symptoms

- Most typically experienced in the knee (50% of cases) but also often in the wrist, elbow, shoulder, ankle, and hand
- Acute attacks may be incapacitating
- Acute attacks are associated with swelling, effusion, redness, severe pain, and stiffness in the affected joints and fever
- Patients are usually symptom-free between acute attacks, or low-grade symptoms may persist
- Chronic disease may be associated with morning or inactivity stiffness, and joints may show bony swelling, crepitus, restricted movement, and inflammation
- Severe joint damage may be associated with severe night or rest pain

ASSOCIATED DISORDERS

- Osteoarthritis
- Gout
- Hypothyroidism
- Amyloidosis
- Ochronosis
- Hemochromatosis

KEY! DON'T MISS!
Infectious arthritis is always in the differential diagnosis of monoarticular inflammatory arthritis.

CONSIDER CONSULT

- Suspected or confirmed infectious arthritis
- For arthrocentesis and X-ray of affected joint(s)

INVESTIGATION OF THE PATIENT
Direct questions to patient

Q **Has there been trauma to the joint?** Eliminate trauma as a cause of joint swelling and pain (usually obvious from the patient's history, but alcohol intoxication may impair the memory of trauma)

Q **How long have you had this problem, and has it happened before?** The answer will provide information about the pattern of the disease

Q **Which joint(s) are affected?** Pseudogout typically affects the knee but also occurs often in the wrist, elbow, shoulder, ankle, and hand, in any number of joints - the answer is important for early differential diagnosis

Q **Are your affected joint(s) stiff in the morning, or after extended inactivity?** A positive answer is consistent with any form of inflammatory arthritis

Q **Do you have severe night or rest pain?** A positive answer is consistent with severe joint damage

Q **What is hard for you to do now that you could do before, and does this affect your daily life?** The answer to this question will help assess functional ability

Contributory or predisposing factors

Q **How old is the patient?** Pseudogout is typically found in patients over 60 years of age (if pseudogout is suspected in a patient under the age of 50 years, an underlying metabolic disease should be suspected)

Q **Is there a history of other predisposing factors?** Hyperparathyroidism, hemochromatosis, hypophosphatasia, or hypomagnesemia

Family history

Does anyone in the near family suffer from a similar condition? Pseudogout is rarely (<1% of cases) hereditary.

Examination

- **Inspect affected joints.** Record skin color, tender effusion, signs of tracking infection, other signs of arthropathy (including gouty tophi)
- **Check pain and movement in joints.** Record the level and quality of pain in joints and the range of movement
- **Check temperature.** Pyrexia may reflect pseudogout, gout, or infectious arthritis
- **Look for other signs of systemic illness.** Rheumatoid arthritis is associated with weakness, fatigue, and anorexia

Summary of investigative tests

- Arthrocentesis is essential for diagnosis of pseudogout and for differential diagnosis. Culture and Gram staining of synovial fluid should be performed if an effusive joint is present to diagnose or exclude infectious arthritis
- X-ray imaging may show chondrocalcinosis, which supports, but does not prove, the diagnosis. It will also provide an indication of the progress of the condition
- Serum test: a rheumatoid factor assay should be performed if rheumatoid arthritis is suspected. Underlying metabolic disease may be screened for if a confirmed pseudogout sufferer is under 55 years of age

DIAGNOSTIC DECISION

- Pseudogout can be positively diagnosed only by polarized microscopy, showing calcium pyrophosphate crystals, which have been phagocytosed by neutrophils

- Note, however, that the confirmed presence of calcium pyrophosphate dihydrate crystals does not exclude the presence of other arthropathies, including infectious arthritis

Guidelines:
- The American College of Rheumatology has produced guidelines that cover the diagnosis of pseudogout [1]
- The American Academy of Family Physicians has published a paper that covers the diagnosis of pseudogout in the knee [2]
- The American Academy of Orthopaedic Surgeons has produced guidelines that cover the diagnosis of knee pain [3]

CLINICAL PEARLS
- Calcium pyrophosphate dihydrate crystals in synovial fluid are diagnostic of pseudogout arthritis only if the crystals are contained within neutrophils
- Chronic pseudogout arthritis should be suspected if a patient who apparently has osteoarthritis experiences periodic inflammatory 'flares' of disease
- The periarticular soft-tissue inflammation with acute pseudogout arthritis may be so intense as to resemble cellulitis

THE TESTS
Body fluids
SERUM TEST
Description
Serum: rheumatoid factor, calcium, albumin, alkaline phosphatase, magnesium, alanine aminotransferase, transferrin saturation, and ferritin levels.

Advantages/Disadvantages
Advantage: may be useful to identify a predisposing metabolic disease in patients under 55 years of age

Disadvantages:
- Rheumatoid arthritis may be difficult to distinguish from polyarticular pseudogout with a symmetric distribution
- The rheumatoid factor may be positive in many conditions other than rheumatoid arthritis

Normal
- Rheumatoid factor: negative
- Calcium: 8.8–10.3mg/dL (2.2–2.58mmol/L)
- Alkaline phosphatase: 30–120U/L (0.5–2.0mckat/L)
- Magnesium: 1.8–3.0mg/dL (0.80–1.20mmol/L)
- Albumin:4–6g/dL (40–60g/L)
- Alanine aminotransferase: 0–35U/L (0.058mckat/L)

Abnormal
- Rheumatoid factor: present
- Calcium: >10.3mg/dL (2.58mmol/L)
- Alkaline phosphatase: <30U/L (2.0mckat/L)
- Magnesium: <1.8mg/dL (0.80mmol/L)
- Albumin: <4g/dL (40g/L)
- Alanine aminotransferase: >35U/L (0.058mckat/L)
- Keep in mind the possibility of a false-positive result

Cause of abnormal result
- Rheumatoid factor present: rheumatoid arthritis, lupus, hepatitis, tuberculosis and other chronic infections, sarcoidosis, cryoglobulinemia
- High calcium: hyperparathyroidism, sarcoidosis, multiple myeloma, diuretic therapy, malignancy
- Low alkaline phosphatase: possible hypophosphatasia
- Low magnesium: hypomagnesemia
- Abnormal alanine aminotransferase, elevated transferrin saturation: possible hemochromatosis
- Low albumin: hypoalbuminemia will result in a falsely low or normal calcium level because of a decrease in protein-bound calcium (decreased total serum calcium but normal free (ionized) calcium)

Drugs, disorders and other factors that may alter results
- Rheumatoid factor present: chronic inflammatory processes, old age, infections, liver disease
- High calcium: thiazide diuretics, neoplasia, hyperparathyroidism
- Low alkaline phosphatase: hypothyroidism, pernicious anemia
- Low magnesium: alcoholism, congestive heart failure, severe diarrhea, loop and thiazide diuretics
- Low albumin: malnutrition, malabsorption

Biopsy
ARTHROCENTESIS
Description
Synovial fluid:
- Inspection of fresh fluid
- Crystal identification (calcium pyrophosphate, monosodium urate)
- Total and differential white blood cell counts
- Culture with Gram stain

Advantages/Disadvantages
Advantages:
- Identification of calcium pyrophosphate dihydrate crystals in synovial fluid is necessary for a positive diagnosis of pseudogout or a differential diagnosis of gout (gout, acute; gout, chronic tophaceous) and other arthritides
- Elevated white blood cell count indicates inflammation, and possibly infection if extremely elevated
- Gram stain will be positive in most cases of nongonococcal bacterial arthritis
- Identification of crystals can be performed only with a polarized microscope

Normal
- Synovial fluid is clear and viscous
- Absence of calcium pyrophosphate dihydrate or monosodium urate crystals under polarized microscopy
- White blood cell count under $2000/mm^3$ and less than 75% polymorphonuclear leukocytes
- Gram stain negative

Abnormal
- Synovial fluid is turbid or blood-stained, and viscosity is reduced
- Presence of calcium pyrophosphate dihydrate or monosodium urate crystals under polarized microscopy
- White blood cell count over $2000/mm^3$ and more than 75% polymorphonuclear leukocytes (a count over $50,000/mm^3$ is consistent with infectious arthritis)
- Gram stain positive
- Keep in mind the possibility of a false-positive result

Cause of abnormal result

- Presence of calcium pyrophosphate dihydrate crystals: pseudogout
- Presence of monosodium urate crystals: gout, acute; gout, chronic tophaceous
- Elevated white blood cell count: inflammatory reaction consistent with pseudogout, gout, rheumatoid arthritis, or infectious arthritis
- Gram stain positive: infectious arthritis

Imaging
X-RAY OF AFFECTED JOINTS
Advantages/Disadvantages
Disadvantage: the presence of chondrocalcinosis on an X-ray does not establish the diagnosis of pseudogout arthritis.

Abnormal

- Punctate and linear calcification of hyaline and articular cartilage (chondrocalcinosis)
- If chondrocalcinosis is not present in the knee, wrist, or symphysis pubis, it is unlikely to exist elsewhere
- Arthropathy similar to that of osteoarthritis plus patellofemoral osteoarthritis ('three-compartment osteoarthritis')
- Keep in mind the possibility of a false-positive result

Cause of abnormal result
Chondrocalcinosis is associated with a variety of disorders other than pseudogout arthritis.

TREATMENT

CONSIDER CONSULT

- Incapacitating pain
- Severe polyarticular disease
- Intractable symptoms
- Pregnant women requiring systemic treatment
- Destructive joint changes necessitating surgery
- The presence of more than 50,000 white blood cells/mm^3 in synovial fluid

IMMEDIATE ACTION

If infectious arthritis is suspected, refer immediately to rheumatologist or orthopedist.

PATIENT AND CAREGIVER ISSUES
Patient or caregiver request

- **Can the condition be cured?** No, the symptoms can only be managed
- **Will joint replacement be necessary?** Sometimes, if destructive joint changes occur
- **Will nonsteroidal anti-inflammatory drugs (NSAIDs) induce side-effects?** Mild 'nuisance' gastrointestinal side-effects such as nausea and diarrhea are common. Ulcer complications develop in approximately 2–4% per year of patients taking NSAIDs. The risk of such complications is increased in the elderly
- **Is steroid treatment dangerous?** Not usually, because the steroids prescribed are different from anabolic steroids (those abused by athletes) – moreover, the steroids are injected directly into the affected joints, which will limit systemic side-effects

Health-seeking behavior

- **How long has the patient waited before consulting a physician?** The answer given may indicate the pattern of the disease: if a long time has elapsed, the patient is more likely to have the chronic form of the disease
- **Has the patient tried to treat the condition with NSAIDs or analgesics, and have they been effective?** The answer given may indicate the intensity of the pain and which drugs are effective in that patient. The extent of the pain or inflammation may have been affected, and the medication taken may affect immediate treatment
- **Has the patient visited the emergency room?** If so, acute trauma or a serious complaint is unlikely
- **Have the patient visited any other physicians for this disorder?** The condition may already be diagnosed, previous treatments may affect future choices, and information about compliance may be available

MANAGEMENT ISSUES
Goals

- To reduce pain and swelling
- To identify and treat any possible triggering illness
- To mobilize the affected joints in chronic disease or between acute attacks

Management in special circumstances

Pseudogout primarily affects the elderly, who are more susceptible to drug side-effects and are more likely to be taking other medications.

COEXISTING DISEASE
Patients with gastrointestinal, renal, cardiovascular, or hepatic problems should be prescribed NSAIDs only with great caution. Use of selective cyclo-oxygenase-2 (Cox-2) inhibitors (celocoxib, rofecoxib) will lessen the risk of gastrointestinal toxicity.

COEXISTING MEDICATION
NSAIDs have a wide range of interactions with other drugs. In the elderly, interactions with antihypertensive agents and sulfonylurea antidiabetic compounds may be especially relevant.

SPECIAL PATIENT GROUPS
Pregnancy is unlikely in this patient group, but NSAIDs should be used with caution in such patients.

PATIENT SATISFACTION/LIFESTYLE PRIORITIES
- Therapy should be chosen to maximize mobility
- The side-effects associated with NSAIDs are a major disadvantages to their use
- Intra-articular corticosteroids induce relatively few side-effects but necessitate regular appointments for the injections to be administered
- Alcohol consumption should be limited when NSAIDs are prescribed

SUMMARY OF THERAPEUTIC OPTIONS
Choices
Acute attacks:
- Immobilize and elevate the affected joints
- Aspiration of joint may provide immediate relief
- NSAIDs, intra-articular corticosteroid injection, and oral colchicine are suitable approaches, depending on the patient

Chronic disease:
- Reduction in obesity (if necessary), use of a walking aid, and education in appropriate joint usage
- Exercise therapy
- NSAIDs are more likely to be useful than intra-articular steroids or colchicine
- Joint replacement may be considered if structural joint damage occurs

Guidelines:
The American Academy of Orthopaedic Surgeons has produced guidelines that cover the management of knee pain, including pseudogout [3].

Clinical pearls
- Joint aspiration and corticosteroid injection are often the best treatment for acute pseudogout involving the knee
- Acute pseudogout, like acute gout, may respond to colchicine

Never
- Never treat acute inflammatory monoarticular arthritis without adequately assessing the possibility of infectious arthritis
- Never administer colchicine intravenously without consulting a rheumatologist (the role for intravenous colchicine in this disease will be limited, and this treatment can be dangerous if given incorrectly)

FOLLOW UP
Regular follow up consultations are necessary to determine the most effective treatment for the patient, to monitor the development of side-effects, and to monitor the progress of the disease.

Plan for review
- Re-evaluate response to therapy after 48–72 h and then after one week. For acute pseudogout arthritis, no additional follow up is necessary once the attack has resolved
- NSAIDs should be assessed for effectiveness and potential gastrointestinal toxicity

Information for patient or caregiver

- Side-effects of NSAIDs or colchicine should be reported immediately
- Patients should be educated concerning exercise therapy and appropriate joint use
- Weight reduction and the use of a walking aid, if necessary, should be encouraged

DRUGS AND OTHER THERAPIES: DETAILS
Drugs
NSAIDS

Any drug in this class is suitable, but attention should be paid to the side effect profiles. Selective COX-2 inhibitors (refecoxib, celecoxib) are preferred for patients who have had gastrointestinal side-effects to other NSAIDs.

Dose

- Normal anti-inflammatory doses
- Ibuprofen: 400–800mg four times a day by mouth not to exceed 3200mg/day
- Indomethacin: 100mg by mouth initially, then 50mg three times a day until pain relieved
- Celecoxib: 100–200mg twice a day

Efficacy

Effective at reducing pain and inflammation.

Risks/Benefits

Risks:

- All currently available NSAIDs have unwanted effects, especially in the elderly
- Substantial individual variation in clinical response to NSAIDs
- Have a range of actions: anti-inflammatory, analgesic, antipyretic
- Use caution in renal, cardiac, and hepatic impairment

Benefit: may improve the patient's symptoms

Side-effects and adverse reactions

- Gastrointestinal: diarrhea, dyspepsia, nausea, vomiting, gastric bleeding and perforation
- Skin: rashes, urticaria, photosensitivity
- Genitourinary: reversible renal insufficiency, renal disease (high doses over long periods)
- Respiratory: worsening of asthma
- Eyes, ear, nose, and throat: tinnitus, decreased hearing
- Central nervous system: headache, dizziness

Interactions (other drugs)

- Antihypertensives ■ Antidysrhythmics ■ Antiplatelet agents ■ Baclofen ■ Cyclosporine ■ Corticosteroids ■ Heparins ■ Lithium ■ Methotrexate ■ Moclobemide ■ Nitrates ■ Pentoxifylline ■ Phenytoin ■ Quinolones ■ Ritonavir ■ Sulfonylureas ■ Tacrolimus ■ Warfarin ■ Zidovudine

Contraindications

- Patients with active peptic ulceration ■ Patients with allergic disorders, including asthma, that have been precipitated by aspirin or other NSAIDs ■ Pregnancy and breast-feeding ■ Coagulation defects

Acceptability to patient

Some patients are unable to tolerate NSAIDs.

Patient and caregiver information
Patients should be advised to take the medication after meals to minimize gastrointestinal side-effects.

CORTICOSTEROIDS
- These may be prescribed if NSAIDs are ineffective or contraindicated, or as an alternative to them
- To be administered intra-articularly

Dose
- Standard intra-articular doses
- Hydrocortisone injection: large joints, 25mg; small joints, 10–25mg

Efficacy
Usually effective in reducing symptoms in acute disease.

Risks/Benefits
Benefits:
- The side-effects are limited because corticosteroids are administered locally, but limited systemic absorption occurs
- May present less risk than NSAIDs, especially in elderly patients

Side-effects and adverse reactions
- Side-effects are minimized by short duration of therapy
- Gastrointestinal: dyspepsia, peptic ulceration, esophagitis, oral candidiasis, nausea, diarrhea
- Cardiovascular system: hypertension, thromboembolism
- Central nervous system: insomnia, euphoria, depression, psychosis
- Endocrine: adrenal suppression, impaired glucose tolerance, growth suppression in children, Cushing syndrome
- Musculoskeletal: proximal myopathy, osteoporosis
- Skin: delayed healing, acne, striae
- Eyes, ear, nose, and throat: cataract, glaucoma, blurred vision

Interactions (other drugs)
- Adrenergic neuron blockers, alpha-blockers, beta-blockers, beta$_2$-agonists
- Aminoglutethimide ■ Anticonvulsants (carbemazepine, phenytoin, barbiturates)
- Antidiabetics ■ Antidysrhythmics (calcium channel blockers, cardiac glycosides)
- Antifungals (amphotericin, ketoconazole) ■ Antihypertensives ■ Cyclosporine
- Erythromycin ■ Methotrexate ■ Nitrates ■ Nitroprusside ■ NSAIDs ■ Oral contraceptives ■ Rifampin ■ Ritonavir ■ Somatropin ■ Vaccines

Contraindications
- Systemic infection ■ Avoid live virus vaccines in those receiving immunosuppressive doses

Acceptability to patient
This treatment requires repeated meetings with a healthcare professional, which may be inconvenient.

Follow up plan
The effectiveness of this treatment should be monitored at regular intervals.

Patient and caregiver information
Any side-effects, worsening of symptoms, or signs of infection should be immediately reported.

COLCHICINE
May be prescribed to prevent repeated acute attacks or if first-line treatment fails.

Dose
- For prophylactic purposes: 0.6mg orally twice daily
- For treatment of an attack: 0.6mg orally every hour until pain is controlled (up to a maximum of 4–6g) or side-effects intervene

Efficacy
Effective in treating acute attacks and in preventing repeated acute attacks.

Risks/Benefits
Risk: colchicine must be given with caution to elderly patients, who may be at particular risk of cumulative toxicity

Benefits:
- May be effective in controlling an acute attack if previous options have failed, but its relative efficacy is low
- May be used in patients who cannot tolerate NSAIDs

Side-effects and adverse reactions
- Neuropathy or myopathy may arise if the patient has hepatic or renal disease
- Gastrointestinal: diarrhea, nausea, vomiting, abdominal pain
- Central nervous system: peripheral neuritis, myopathy
- Skin: alopecia
- Hematologic: blood cell disorders

Interactions (other drugs)
- Cyclosporine, tacrolimus   Macrolide antibiotics: clarithromycin, erythromycin, troleandomycin

Contraindications
- Pregnancy and nursing   Significant renal, hepatic, or cardiac impairment
- Blood dyscrasias

Acceptability to patient
Side-effects may introduce compliance problems.

Follow up plan
Regular follow up consultations are necessary to prevent cumulative toxicity and monitor effectiveness of treatment.

Patient and caregiver information
- The prescribed doses should be adhered to under all circumstances
- Any side-effects should be reported immediately

Physical therapy
- Mobilization is important in chronic disease and between acute attacks
- Isometric exercises may be performed to maintain muscle strength during acute attacks

EXERCISE OF AFFECTED JOINT
Walking (with an aid, if needed) and exercises to improve strength.

Efficacy
The efficacy of physical therapy has not been published.

Risks/Benefits
Risks:
- Improved muscle tone may reduce mechanical stress and thus slow joint destruction
- General mobilization in the elderly is important because prolonged immobility may provoke complications
- Risk is minimal with correct instruction

Evidence
There is no evidence for benefits of this treatment, but it is recommended by most authorities.

Acceptability to patient
Compliance with exercise can be poor.

Follow up plan
Regular contact may be necessary to motivate or instruct the patient.

Patient and caregiver information
- Specific instructions on the prescribed exercises
- The importance of exercise should be emphasized

Surgical therapy
JOINT REPLACEMENT
To be considered if structural joint damage occurs.

Efficacy
Provides benefit equal to that in patients with uncomplicated osteoarthritis.

Risks/Benefits
The risk of surgery should be weighed against the benefit of improved mobility and decreased pain.

Acceptability to patient
Joint replacement is a major operation, which may discourage some patients.

Follow up plan
Regular exercise therapy sessions may be required.

Patient and caregiver information
The pros and cons of the treatment should be explained.

Other therapies
ELEVATION AND IMMOBILIZATION OF AFFECTED JOINT
Necessary during acute attacks.

Efficacy
Reduces symptoms during an attack.

Risks/Benefits
Risk: there is no risk attached to this treatment.

Evidence
There is no published evidence for benefits of this treatment, but it is recommended by most authorities.

Acceptability to patient
No acceptability problems are associated with this treatment.

Follow up plan
None necessary.

Patient and caregiver information
Patients should promptly report onset of any fever (may indicate infectious process).

WALKING AID
Aids mobility if a hip, leg, or foot joint is affected.

Efficacy
The efficacy of such aids is widely known.

Risks/Benefits
Risk: no risk is attached to the use of such aids.

ARTICULAR ASPIRATION
May be considered in cases of effusion, with or without concomitant intraarticular injection of corticosteroids.

Efficacy
Induces rapid relief of symptoms; fluid may reaccumulate unless corticosteroids are also administered.

Risks/Benefits
There is immediate benefit for the patient. The benefit/risk ratio is high; there is a very small risk of infection if strict aseptic technique is not used.

Acceptability to patient
This treatment requires repeated meetings with a healthcare professional, which may be inconvenient.

Follow up plan
The effectiveness of this treatment should be monitored at regular intervals.

Patient and caregiver information
Signs of infection should be reported immediately.

LIFESTYLE
Reduction in obesity and appropriate joint usage.

RISKS/BENEFITS
Benefits:
- Decreases stress on joints
- No risks are attached to such lifestyle changes

ACCEPTABILITY TO PATIENT
Changes in diet and body usage often present compliance problems.

FOLLOW UP PLAN
Regular contact may be required to ensure compliance.

PATIENT AND CAREGIVER INFORMATION
The importance of these measures should be emphasized.

EFFICACY OF THERAPIES
- An acute attack usually responds well to standard treatment
- The pain and inflammation can usually be controlled

Evidence
PDxMD are unable to cite evidence which meets our criteria for evidence.

Review period
- Re-evaluate response to therapy after 48–72 hours and then after one week
- NSAIDs should be assessed for effectiveness 3 weeks after prescription and changed if necessary

PROGNOSIS
- The prognosis for the resolution of an acute attack is very good
- Recurrent acute attacks may be prevented to some degree
- Some patients suffer progressive joint damage, with consequent loss of mobility

Clinical pearls
- Decompression of an acutely swollen knee joint provides immediate relief, even if corticosteroids are not injected
- Colchicine once or twice daily may prevent recurrent attacks

Therapeutic failure
Referral to a rheumatologist is advisable if a patient does not respond to the treatment listed above.

Deterioration
Joint replacement may be indicated if structural joint damage occurs.

COMPLICATIONS
Structural joint damage may result, mimicking neuropathic (Charcot) joints.

PREVENTION

- This condition can generally not be prevented
- Certain metabolic disorders thought to be predisposing factors should be controlled

RISK FACTORS

- Hyperparathyroidism: metabolic disease thought to underlie some cases
- Hemochromatosis: metabolic disease thought to underlie some cases
- Hypophosphatasia: metabolic disease thought to underlie some cases
- Hypomagnesemia: metabolic disease thought to underlie some cases

MODIFY RISK FACTORS

For each of the metabolic diseases in the above section, treat the condition. There is no significant evidence that treating any of these disorders affects the incidence of pseudogout.

PREVENT RECURRENCE

Recurrent acute attacks may be prevented by prescribing prophylactic colchicine.

RESOURCES

ASSOCIATIONS
American College of Rheumatology
1800 Century Place
Atlanta, GA 30345
Tel: (404) 633 3777
Fax: (404) 633 1870
www.rheumatology.org/index.asp

The Arthritis Foundation
1330 West Peachtree Street
Atlanta, GA 30309
www.arthritis.org

American Academy of Orthopaedic Surgeons
6300 North River Road
Rosemont, IL 60018-4262
Tel: (847) 823 7186
Fax: (847) 823 8125
www.aaos.org

KEY REFERENCES
- Doherty M. Calcium pyrophosphate dihydrate. In Klippel JH, Dieppe PA, eds. Rheumatology. London: Mosby; 1998: Section 8, Chapter 16, pp.1–12
- Lefkowith JB, Kahl LE. Crystal-induced synovitis. In Carey CF, Lee HH, Woeltje KF, eds. The Washington Manual of Medical Therapeutics, 29th Edn. Philadelphia: Lippincott - Williams & Wilkins; 1998: pp.464–6
- Pyrophosphate arthropathy. In Marshall KG. Mosby's Family Practice Sourcebook: Evidence-based Emphasis, 2nd Edn. St Louis: Mosby; 2000; p.207
- Schumacher HR. Crystal deposition arthropathies. In Goldman L, Bennett JC, eds. Cecil Textbook of Medicine, 21st Edn. Philadelphia: WB Saunders; 2000; Chapter 300

Guidelines
1 American American College of Rheumatology Ad Hoc Committee on Clinical Guidelines. Guidelines for the initial evaluation of the adult patient with acute musculoskeletal symptoms. Arthritis Rheum 1996;39:1–8
2 Johnson MW. Acute knee effusions: a systematic approach to diagnosis. Arm Fam Physician 2000;61:2391–400
3 Anonymous. Clinical guideline on knee pain. Rosemont, IL: American Academy of Orthopaedic Surgeons; 1999; summary available online at the National Guideline Clearinghouse

FAQS
Question 1
What are the different presentations of calcium pyrophosphate deposition disease?

ANSWER 1
- Acute synovitis (pseudogout)
- Chronic pyrophosphate arthropathy
- Asymptomatic chondrocalcinosis
- Pseudoneuropathic arthropathy

Question 2
Which metabolic diseases predispose to calcium pyrophosphate dihydrate crystal deposition?

ANSWER 2

Metabolic predisposition is rare and should be considered in:

- Early onset arthritis (under 55 years of age)
- Polyarticular presentation
- Recurrent acute attacks

The metabolic diseases that should be considered are hemochromatosis, hypophosphatemia, hypomagnesemia, gout, acromegaly, hyperparathroidism, and hypothyroidism.

Question 3

Is all chondrocalcinosis caused by calcium pyrophosphate dihydrate crystal deposition?

ANSWER 3

Calcium salts other than calcium pyrophosphate dihydrate, such as calcium hydroxyapatite and calcium oxalate, can appear as chondrocalcinosis on X-rays.

Question 4

Do any features suggest pseudo-osteoarthritis from calcium pyrophosphate dihydrate crystal deposition rather than typical osteoarthritis?

ANSWER 4

Pseudo-osteoarthritis is seen in about half of patients with the diagnosis of calcium pyrophosphate dihydrate crystal deposition. The pattern of joint involvement is different from that seen in osteoarthritis and includes severe degenerative changes in the metacarpophalangeal joints, wrists, elbows, shoulders, and the patellofemoral compartment of knees, which are atypical for osteoarthritis.

Question 5

Can recurrent attacks of pseudogout be prevented?

ANSWER 5

If patients are having recurrent acute attacks, colchicine 0.6mg orally twice daily can be used to prevent attacks.

CONTRIBUTORS

Fred F Ferri, MD, FACP
Richard Brasington Jr, MD, FACP
Dinesh Khanna, MD

PSORIATIC ARTHRITIS

SUMMARY INFORMATION

DESCRIPTION

- Psoriatic arthritis is a chronic, inflammatory spondyloarthritis, usually seronegative for rheumatoid factor, that develops in patients with psoriasis
- Develops in 5–10% of patients with psoriasis (lag time often two decades after the onset)
- Usually benign but a subset have severe (mutilating) disease
- There are five general patterns of psoriatic arthritis, but they are not absolutely discrete
- Psoriatic nail lesions are strongly associated with the development of psoriatic arthritis

URGENT ACTION

- Erythrodermic psoriasis is a dermatologic emergency requiring urgent specialist referral
- If acute iritis (uveitis), a severe inflammatory complication, is present, immediate referral to ophthalmologist is mandatory

KEY! DON'T MISS!

- Don't miss hidden psoriasis, for example on the scalp, perineum, natal cleft, umbilicus
- Flare-ups of psoriasis and psoriatic arthritis may indicate associated pathology such as viral infection, including HIV
- Don't miss concurrent common joint diseases such as osteoarthritis (when patient presents with distal interphalangeal joint disease) and rheumatoid arthritis in the patient with simple psoriasis

ICD9 CODE
696.0 Psoriatic arthritis.

SYNONYMS
Psoriasis, arthropathic.

CARDINAL FEATURES
- Psoriatic arthritis is a systemic inflammatory disease with articular and extra-articular features. It is usually seronegative for rheumatoid factor and develops in patients with psoriasis
- Develops in 5–10% of patients with psoriasis. Most patients with psoriatic arthritis have classical psoriasis vulgaris skin lesions, which may not always be apparent, although there is no direct correlation between severity of skin lesions and the degree of joint inflammation
- Usually benign but a minority (<5%) have severe (mutilating) disease – arthritis mutilans
- In contrast with rheumatoid arthritis, psoriatic arthritis is often asymmetric. Although there is pain and swelling in the joints, they are generally less tender than those of rheumatoid arthritis
- Nail lesions (pitting, ridging, and oncholysis) are the only clinical feature of psoriasis correlated with the development of psoriatic arthritis; 90% of patients with psoriatic arthritis show these nail lesions, as opposed to 40% of psoriatics without arthritis

CAUSES
Common causes
- Unknown etiology. Familial clustering suggests a genetic component
- Bacterial infection and trauma have been suggested as trigger factors for psoriatic arthritis

Contributory or predisposing factors
- Psoriasis
- Family history of psoriasis
- Disease may be exacerbated by infection with HIV

EPIDEMIOLOGY
Incidence and prevalence
INCIDENCE
Unknown.

PREVALENCE
0.75–1.5/1000.

FREQUENCY
Affects 5–10% of patients with psoriasis.

Demographics
AGE
- Psoriatic arthritis classically develops between the ages of 30 and 55 years
- In the majority of patients there is a lag time of some two decades between the onset of uncomplicated psoriasis and the development of psoriatic arthritis
- Psoriatic spondyloarthropathy develops in older patients, especially men

GENDER
- No gender bias, contrasting with 3:1 female preponderance in seropositive arthritis
- Psoriatic spondyloarthropathy affects males more than females
- Asymmetric arthritis occurs more frequently in women than in men

RACE
No association.

GENETICS
- A genetic predisposition to psoriatic arthritis is generally accepted, although the evidence suggests susceptibility may be heterogeneous, conferred by multiple genes with partial penetrance. Some studies have suggested a heavier emphasis on transmission of paternal predisposing genes
- HLA-B7 and HLA-B27 are markers for the development of psoriatic arthritis in patients with psoriasis. Patients with established psoriatic arthritis show a high frequency of HLA-DR7alpha

GEOGRAPHY
No association.

SOCIOECONOMIC STATUS
No association.

DIFFERENTIAL DIAGNOSIS
Rheumatoid arthritis
Rheumatoid arthritis is a chronic, multisystem inflammatory disease of unknown etiology.

FEATURES
- The characteristic feature of rheumatoid arthritis is persistent inflammatory synovitis, usually involving the peripheral joints in a symmetric distribution
- Early on in the disease, painful joint effusions restricting movement are common as is prolonged morning stiffness, while in late disease characteristic deformities can occur (subluxation, dislocation, and joint contractures)
- Systemic involvement may be marked with fevers, anorexia, splenomegaly, pericarditis, vasculitis, and uveitis
- In rheumatoid arthritis, a raised rheumatoid factor occurs in 80%, often with elevated erythrocyte sedimentation rate (ESR) and C-reactive protein level
- Radiographs usually reveal soft-tissue swelling and osteoporosis in early disease, while later showing joint-space narrowing, erosion, and deformity as the articular surface is destroyed

Osteoarthritis
Osteoarthritis is the most common form of arthritis, resulting from degenerative changes in the articular surface of any synovial joint.

FEATURES
- Affects 2–6% of the general population, may be primary (idiopathic) or secondary (to trauma or disease)
- Typically, pain is localized to the involved joint, exacerbated by joint use and relieved by rest
- Joint tenderness, bony hypertrophy (swelling), crepitus, and a decreased range of movement are features of osteoarthritis
- Involvement of distal interphalangeal joints with characteristic Herberden's nodes may occur
- No diagnostic test exists for this degenerative joint disease
- Characteristic radiologic features include joint-space narrowing as articular cartilage is lost, subchondral bone sclerosis, subchondral cysts, and marginal osteophytes

Gouty arthritis
Gout can cause an arthritis due to the deposition of urate crystals in the joints.

FEATURES
- An excruciatingly painful arthritis, principally affecting middle-aged men
- Typically but not exclusively monoarticular
- Classically the first metatarsophalangeal joint is involved (swelling, heat, and redness). Later, crystals may be deposited in subcutaneous tissues (tophi)
- Gout is caused by hyperuricemia, but a definitive diagnosis requires the demonstration of intracellular monosodium urate crystals in polymorphonuclear leukocytes or in tophaceous aggregates of synovial fluid aspirated from the involved joint or tissue
- Serum urate level is raised, ESR may be elevated, and mild leukocytosis may be present
- Radiographs show no abnormalities in acute disease, but later may demonstrate the characteristic punched-out lesions of joint destruction

Ankylosing spondylitis
Ankylosing spondylitis is a chronic condition in which inflammatory changes and new bone formation occur.

FEATURES

- Mainly involves the axial skeleton and sacroiliac joints; may also involve other large joints and occasionally peripheral joints
- Prevalence in men is approx. 10 times that in women, with onset occurring between 15 and 35 years
- Ankylosing spondylitis has extraskeletal manifestations, including cardiovascular, respiratory (loss of chest expansion), and ocular systems (uveitis)
- Symptoms are classically persistent low back pain (limited lumbar spine movement), improved by exercise, not relieved by rest, together with morning stiffness and other systemic features (fatigue, anorexia, weight loss)
- ESR may be elevated, absent rheumatoid factor and antinuclear factor; 90% of sufferers are positive for HLA-B27
- Radiographs may show sacroiliitis, the vertebral bodies may be demineralized and squared off, and later the typical 'bamboo spine' appearance occurs as calcification of the paravertebral ligaments and annulus fibrosus occurs

Reiter's syndrome/reactive arthritis

Reiter's syndrome, also referred to as reactive arthritis, is a seronegative spondylarthropathy producing an asymmetric polyarthritis mainly affecting the lower extremities, associated with one or more of the following: urethritis, cervicitis, dysentery, inflammatory eye disease, and mucocutaneous lesions.

FEATURES

- Predominantly occurs in men, aged 20–40 years; strongly associated with HLA-B27
- Asymmetrical polyarthiritis commonly affecting knee and ankle, often with large effusions
- Keratoderma blenorrhagicum is characteristic (hyperkeratosis lesions that occur on soles of feet, toes, hands, and penis) and closely resembles psoriasis
- Uveitis (can be severe and sight-threatening) or conjunctivitis occur
- Aortic regurgitation may occur
- Syndrome may develop following infection with certain pathogens in genetically susceptible individuals
- No specific laboratory tests to confirm diagnosis, but ESR may be elevated
- Radiographs may show erosions and joint-space narrowing in more advanced disease, plus features of sacroiliitis

SIGNS & SYMPTOMS
Signs

- Skin lesions of psoriasis (although these may be in hidden regions, for example, scalp, perineum, natal cleft, umbilicus)
- Heat and swelling of joints and the soft-tissue around them; pattern may be asymmetrical
- Restricted movement of joints
- Reduced spinal movements
- Sausage digits – enlarged digits caused by swelling and inflammation of the tendons
- Psoriatic nail changes (pitting, ridging, onchyolosis)
- Severe joint destruction of the hand ('opera glass' deformity) in arthritis mutilans
- Redness and pain in the eye (conjunctivitis or uveitis)
- Occasionally signs of dactylitis, tenosynovitis, and enthesitis
- Aortic regurgitation (uncommon)

Oligoarticular (asymmetric) arthritis:

- The most characteristic pattern of joint involvement in psoriasis (16–70%)
- Usually affects only one to three joints (commonly knee, hip, ankle, hands, feet, wrist)

- Hands and feet often involved, causing enlarged sausage digits (because of swelling and inflammation of the tendons and joint involvement (DIP/PIP))

Distal interphalangeal (DIP) predominant:
- The classic type, however, only affects 5–10% of people with psoriatic arthritis
- Involves the distal joints of fingers and toes
- Highly associated with psoriatic nail changes

Arthritis mutilans:
- Aggressive, destructive arthritis with severe deformity and bone dissolution
- Affects 5% of people with psoriatic arthropathy
- Particularly affects the small joints of the hands and feet
- Often associated with neck and lower back pain (sacroiliitis)
- Arthritic flares and remissions tend to coincide with skin flares and remissions

Symmetric polyarthropathy:
- Similar to rheumatoid arthritis but rheumatoid factor is negative
- Accounts for 25% of people with psoriatic arthritis
- Affecting multiple symmetrical pairs of joints and can be disabling
- Associated psoriasis is often severe
- Approx. 50% of people with this type will develop varying degrees of progressive destructive disease that can be disabling

Psoriatic spondylitis:
- Inflammation of the axial column is the predominant feature
- Accounts for 20–40% of people with psoriatic arthritis
- May occur in the absence of peripheral arthropathy
- There is a tendency for the sacroiliac involvement to be asymmetric (unlike ankylosing spondylitis)
- Tends to affect men and older patients and occurs later in the course of the disease

Symptoms
- Presence of rash, skin, or scalp lesions
- Morning stiffness and lethargy
- Pain, heat, and joint tenderness (often restricting hand dexterity)
- Back stiffness and pain
- Nail lesions
- May complain of hand or foot deformity
- Painful red eyes
- Clinical depression/anxiety

ASSOCIATED DISORDERS
There may be an association of severe disease with HIV infection.

KEY! DON'T MISS!
- Don't miss hidden psoriasis, for example on the scalp, perineum, natal cleft, umbilicus
- Flare-ups of psoriasis and psoriatic arthritis may indicate associated pathology such as viral infection, including HIV
- Don't miss concurrent common joint diseases such as osteoarthritis (when patient presents with DIP joint disease) and rheumatoid arthritis in the patient with simple psoriasis

CONSIDER CONSULT
Refer to rheumatologist if diagnosis is in doubt.

INVESTIGATION OF THE PATIENT
Direct questions to patient
General:

Q **Are you generally well?** Malaise and fevers may be present, but not mentioned by patients unless specifically sought

Q **Is there any family history of disease?** There is a genetic predisposition to psoriasis and psoriatic arthritis, as well as differential diagnoses such as rheumatoid arthritis

Q **Are you taking any medication, including skin preparations?** May indicate underlying disease, or suggest drug reaction etiology, and choice of future therapy

Q **Have you had any past illnesses?** For example pre-existing immunocompromising disease (HIV, lymphoma), previous streptococcal infection (guttate psoriasis), previous gastrointestinal infections (Reiter's syndrome)

Skin:

Q **Do you suffer from or have you ever had skin disease or psoriasis?** Psoriatic arthritis almost always accompanies skin lesions, but may appear to be separated in time or the rashes not recognized for what they are

Q **Do you have or have you ever had scalp disease?** Many patients will not have recognized scalp psoriasis as different from common dandruff, but often their hairdresser will comment, especially on patchy lesions

Q **Do you ever suffer from pitted, ridged, or brittle nails?** Psoriatic nail disease is strongly correlated with the development of psoriatic arthritis

Joints:

Q **Do you experience stiffness on waking (lasting >30min)?** This is a common complaint in patients with forms of inflammatory arthritis (as opposed to noninflammatory), including psoriatic arthritis

Q **Which joints are affected and what problem does this cause?** Pattern of joint involvement may narrow differential diagnosis; joints commonly affected by psoriatic arthritis are wrists, knees, ankles, lower back, and neck

Q **How have your joint problems behaved over time?** Typically, inflammatory arthritis is characterized by flare and remissions, unlike degenerative arthritis

Q **Have you noticed any deformity?** Unless there is the arthritis mutilans pattern of psoriatic arthritis, deformity tends to be less noticeable than in rheumatoid arthritis

Eyes:

Q **Have you had any problems with your eyes?** Inflammatory conjunctivitis and uveitis may be associated with any inflammatory arthritis

Contributory or predisposing factors

Q **Is there a history of psoriasis/rashes?** Psoriatic arthritis nearly almost always occurs with psoriatic skin lesions somewhere/sometime on the patient

Q **Is there a family history of psoriasis?** Genetic predisposition

Q **Is there a history of immunocompromising disease (HIV, lymphoma)?** May exacerbate arthritis and skin lesions

Family history

Q **Is there any family history of joint disease?** There is a genetic predisposition to psoriasis and psoriatic arthritis, as well as differential diagnoses such as rheumatoid arthritis

Q **Is there a family history of psoriasis?** Genetic predisposition

Examination

General examination:

◻ **What is the general state of the patient?** Look for anemia, signs of immunosuppression, lymphadenopathy, etc

◻ **What is the cardiovascular state of the patient?** Look for aortic incompetence (occurs late in psoriatic arthritis)

◻ **Is there any evidence of respiratory compromise?** Consider differential diagnosis of ankylosing spondylitis in young men with restricted chest and back movements

◻ **Is there any indication of eye disease?** If history or observation suggests pathology, then do a formal eye examination

◻ **Is there any nail disease?** A strong indicator of predisposition to arthritis if psoriatic nail present

◻ **Is there evidence for enthesitis?** Look for inflammation and pain at sites such as the Achilles tendon insertion into the calcaneus

◻ **Is there any skin disease present?** Don't miss hidden psoriasis, e.g. scalp, perineum, natal cleft, umbilicus

Joint examination:

◻ **Do the joints show signs of inflammation (redness, swelling, deformity, restricted movement)?** Joints commonly affected by psoriatic arthritis are wrists, knees, ankles, lower back, and neck; be sure to examine the specific joints indicated by the patient as symptomatic, and document the findings in detail including any deformities ('sausage-like' fingers, 'opera glass' hand)

Summary of investigative tests

There are no specific diagnostic laboratory tests for psoriatic arthritis. The tests suggested are largely to rule out differential diagnoses.

- ESR and C-reactive protein levels to determine whether inflammation is present
- Rheumatoid factor: positive rheumatoid factor suggests rheumatoid arthritis; negative indicates either noninflammatory or seronegative arthritis, including psoriatic
- Uric acid levels: high in gout, but levels are often high in psoriasis (reflecting the active turnover of skin), and therefore care must be taken in diagnosing monoarthritis in the presence of raised uric acid levels (crystals must be demonstrated in the joint to confirm gout)
- Radiology: several radiologic findings are suggestive of inflammatory arthritis, some of which are peculiar to psoriatic arthritis. Interpretation by specialist radiologist is necessary

Note that although HLA-B27 may be positive in up to 50% of psoriatic patients with arthritis and spondylitis, it is also positive in as many as 7% of the normal population. It should not be used unless there is 50% doubt as to the true diagnosis. That is, for ankylosis spondylititis where its prevalence is much higher, a negative HLA-B27 makes the diagnosis unlikely, but a positive one makes the diagnosis more likely. In psoriatic arthritis, where the positive predictive value of the test is much lower, it has little if any role and will, therefore, not be discussed further.

DIAGNOSTIC DECISION

To establish the diagnosis with certainty, psoriatic skin disease will be present, however, the arthritis may precede or occur at the same time as the skin disease in as many as one-third of patients.

Five different clinical patterns of psoriatic arthritis are recognized, but it is important to remember that these patterns are not permanent and that >60% change from their initial pattern. All peripheral joints can be affected in psoriatic arthropathy.

Oligoarticular (asymmetric) arthritis:

- The most characteristic pattern of joint involvement in psoriasis (16–70%)
- Usually affects only one to three joints (commonly knee, hip, ankle, hands, feet, wrist)
- Hands and feet often involved, causing enlarged sausage digits (because of swelling and inflammation of the tendons and joint involvement (DIP/PIP))

Distal interphalangeal (DIP) predominant:

- The classic type, however, only affects 5–10% of people with psoriatic arthritis
- Involves the distal joints of fingers and toes
- Highly associated with psoriatic nail changes

Arthritis mutilans:

- Aggressive, destructive arthritis with severe deformity and bone dissolution
- Affects 5% of people with psoriatic arthropathy
- Particularly affects the small joints of the hands and feet
- Often associated with neck and lower back pain (sacroiliitis)
- Arthritic flares and remissions tend to coincide with skin flares and remissions

Symmetric polyarthropathy:

- Similar to rheumatoid arthritis but rheumatoid factor is negative
- Accounts for 25% of people with psoriatic arthritis
- Affecting multiple symmetrical pairs of joints and can be disabling
- Associated psoriasis is often severe
- Approx. 50% of people with this type will develop varying degrees of progressive destructive disease that can be disabling

Psoriatic spondylitis:

- Inflammation of the axial column is the predominant feature
- Accounts for 20–40% of people with psoriatic arthritis
- May occur in the absence of peripheral arthropathy
- There is a tendency for the sacroiliac involvement to be asymmetric (unlike ankylosing spondylitis)
- Tends to affect men and older patients and occurs later in the course of the disease

These findings along with a negative RF and characteristic radiographic features will support a diagnosis of psoriatic arthritis.

CLINICAL PEARLS

- Arthritis may precede the skin disease in as many as one-third of patients
- There may be ocular findings (conjunctivitis, uveitis) in up to one-third of patients

THE TESTS
Body fluids
ERYTHROCYTE SEDIMENTATION RATE AND C-REACTIVE PROTEIN
Description

- Specimen: venous blood
- Testing for nonspecific inflammatory markers

Advantages/Disadvantages
Advantages:

- Easy to perform, rapid results
- Indicates if generalized inflammation is present

Disadvantage: tests are nonspecific

Normal
Erythrocyte sedimentation rate:
- Male: 0–15mm/h
- Female: 0–20mm/h

C-reactive protein:
- 6.8–820mcg/dL

Abnormal
- Raised ESR and C-reactive protein above normal levels
- Keep in mind the possibility of a false-positive result

Cause of abnormal result
- Many systemic causes of inflammation or chronic disease
- 40–60% of patients with psoriatic arthritis have a raised ESR

RHEUMATOID FACTOR
Description
Specimen: venous blood.

Advantages/Disadvantages
Advantages:
- Easy to perform, rapid results
- Negative rheumatoid factor makes a diagnosis of rheumatoid arthritis far less likely

Disadvantage: rheumatoid factor may be weakly positive in many other states, including symmetric psoriatic arthritis

Normal
Rheumatoid factor is normally absent.

Abnormal
- Rheumatoid factor is present in titers greater than one in 20
- Keep in mind the possibility of a false-positive result

Cause of abnormal result
- Rheumatoid factor is positive in 75% of patients with rheumatoid arthritis, and many other conditions
- Low titers of rheumatoid factor may be present in psoriatic arthritis (5–16% of patients)

URIC ACID
Description
Specimen: venous blood.

Advantages/Disadvantages
- Advantage: easy to perform, rapid results

Disadvantages:
- Can occur in any condition with increased tissue turnover, and many diseases
- Not specific

Normal
2–7mg/dL (120–420mcmol/L).

Abnormal
- Values outside the normal range
- Keep in mind the possibility of a false-positive result

Cause of abnormal result
- Elevated uric acid level reflects increased cell turnover
- Occurs in renal disease, myeloproliferative disease, hereditary enzyme deficiency, hypothyroidism, Addison's disease, active psoriasis, and gout (this list is not exhaustive)

Drugs, disorders and other factors that may alter results
Raised levels occur in lead poisoning, renal disease, myeloproliferative disease, hereditary enzyme deficiency, hypothyroidism, Addison's disease, active psoriasis, and gout (this list is not exhaustive).

Lowered levels occur in inappropriate ADH secretion, alcoholism, liver disease, renal tubular deficit (this list is not exhaustive).

Many drugs increase or reduce urate levels:
- Increase – diuretics, salicylates, ethambutol, nicotinic acid
- Reduce – allopurinol, high-dose salicylates, probenecid, warfarin, corticosteroids

Imaging
RADIOLOGY
Advantages/Disadvantages
Advantages:
- Relatively easy to perform
- Rapid results
- Noninvasive
- Some radiologic findings are characteristic of psoriatic arthritis
- Generally, levels of irradiation are small and acceptably safe

Disadvantages:
- Most radiologic findings indicating inflammatory arthritis are not specific for psoriatic arthritis
- Requires specialist interpretation
- Specific radiologic markers of psoriatic arthritis may require most complex radiologic techniques, including computed topography
- Safety concerns when X-raying lower spine/sacroiliacs in women who may be pregnant

Normal
Normal skeletal anatomy demonstrated and confirmed by radiologist.

Abnormal
General radiographic findings indicative of inflammatory arthritic disease include:
- Soft-tissue swelling
- Loss of cartilage space
- Erosions
- Bony ankylosis
- Subluxations
- Subchondral cysts

Signs suggestive of psoriatic arthritis include:

- Asymmetric oligoarticular distribution
- Erosions at distal interphalangeal joints
- Expansion of the base of the terminal phalanx
- Tapering of the proximal phalanx and cup-like erosions of and bony proliferation of the distal terminal phalanx ('pencil-in-cup' appearance)
- Proliferation of bone near osseous erosions (usually thick and fluffy)
- Terminal phalangeal osteolysis
- Bone proliferation and periostitis
- Telescoping of one bone onto its neighbor ('opera-glass' hand)
- Sacroiliitis and spondylitis (syndesmophytes are usually bulky asymmetric and nonmarginal)

Cause of abnormal result

- The presence of arthritis
- Certain features may distinguish one type of arthropathy from another (e.g. periarticular osteopenia is found in rheumatoid arthritis but not in psoriatic arthritis)

Drugs, disorders and other factors that may alter results

Trauma, previous disease affecting the skeletal system and congenital abnormalities may affect the appearance of radiographs.

TREATMENT

CONSIDER CONSULT
- Refer to rheumatologist if disease is severe or aggressive, and if simple measures such as NSAIDs are ineffective
- Many of the disease-modifying treatments are licensed for specialist use only

IMMEDIATE ACTION
Refer to hospital urgently if patient has erythrodermic psoriasis or is systemically unwell.

PATIENT AND CAREGIVER ISSUES
Patient or caregiver request
- **Am I going to be disabled by the arthritis?** Possibly in about 5% of cases, depending on the type of psoriatic arthritis
- **Will it affect my work?** This depends on the type of work, the type of psoriatic arthritis, and the joints affected
- **Can it be cured?** No, treatment is aimed at control of symptoms, although some disease-modifying agents may improve the condition
- **Is it inherited?** Not directly, but there is a familial susceptibility to both psoriasis and psoriatic arthritis

MANAGEMENT ISSUES
Goals
- There is no cure, and therefore treatment is directed at combating psoriasis, arthritis, or both
- Management is geared toward reducing joint pain, stiffness, and destruction
- Patients effectively have to cope with two chronic, incurable diseases – they will need information, a sympathetic ear, and may benefit from counseling to allow them to talk about their concerns and fears

Management in special circumstances
COEXISTING DISEASE

HIV carrier status is a poor prognostic feature in psoriatic arthritis. HIV infection not only enhances susceptibility to spondyloarthropathies, but also correlates strongly with aggressive and sustained disease. However, the incidence of psoriatic arthritis in HIV-infected patients has probably fallen with the use of more effective HIV treatments such as protease inhibitors.

COEXISTING MEDICATION
- Sulfa drugs, ketaconazole, and NSAIDs may interfere with renal function, increasing the risk of methotrexate toxicity when co-prescribed
- Systemic steroids may be useful in helping to control flares of disease, but there is a substantial risk of severe rebound flaring when the steroids are stopped

SPECIAL PATIENT GROUPS
- Psoriatic arthritis may improve or worsen during pregnancy
- Postpartum flare has been reported
- Several drugs including methotrexate are teratogenic and therefore contraindicated in pregnant women or those likely to get pregnant
- Women of childbearing age should use birth control while taking any drug with significant teratogenic potential
- Methotrexate is contraindicated in women who are breast-feeding

PATIENT SATISFACTION/LIFESTYLE PRIORITIES
- Control of skin symptoms (appearance)

- Control of joint symptoms and prevention of deformity
- Appropriate aids to overcome disability with activities of daily living
- Women contemplating pregnancy will need to consider treatment options very carefully to avoid risk to the fetus

SUMMARY OF THERAPEUTIC OPTIONS
Choices
In psoriatic arthritis it is important to tailor the treatment to the severity of the disease. Unfortunately it is often difficult to judge this at the onset, so regular review is necessary.

Nonpharmacologic therapies include:
- Occupational therapy for the hand problems and aids to daily living
- Physical therapy, including isometric exercises to maintain strength and flexibility and possibly hydrotherapy
- Lifestyle changes may also prove beneficial

Pharmacologic therapies include:
- NSAIDs: first-line treatment. Many patients with psoriatic arthritis respond well to NSAIDs alone. No evidence for superiority of any one NSAID in psoriatic arthritis
- Persistent monoarthritis is often improved by intra-articular corticosteroid injections. Triamcinolone hexacetonide is used due to minimization of systemic absorption leading to maximized local effect

Pharmacologic therapies that may be instituted by a specialist:
- Under specialist care, patients with severe articular disease commonly need combined treatment with NSAIDs and disease-modifying antirheumatic drugs (DMARDs). The DMARDs are numerous and largely overlap with those used in rheumatoid arthritis. Antimalarials such as hydroxychloroquine and gold (off label) are seldom used for fear that they will exacerbate cutaneous psoriasis. A subset of 'RA-like' patients may respond well to gold therapy. Methotrexate is the second-line treatment of choice, followed by sulfasalazine. Cyclosporine may be considered by specialists for those who have not responded to the other DMARDs. It is effective in the treatment of psoriasis and arthritis, but there are concerns over its renal toxicity. Combination therapies are used by rheumatologists in those who do not respond adequately to DMARD monotherapy. Most recently, intermittent therapy has also been studied
- Systemic corticosteroids are best avoided because severe flare-ups of disease can occur after ceasing the course. Specialists may use them in severe flares
- Photochemotherapy

Surgical options:
- Surgical intervention (synovectomy, arthroplasty) is indicated in those patients with severe deformity in progressive arthritis
- The heterogeneity of the disease combined with the lack of adequately sized randomized controlled trials stands in the way of evidence-based guidelines

Clinical pearls
HLA-B27 may be positive in up to 7% of the normal population, therefore diagnosis and treatment should not be made based on the haplotyping.

Never
Do not initiate systemic corticosteroid therapy without specialist advice.

FOLLOW UP

The type of follow up will depend on the condition of the patient and the monitoring requirement of the medication initiated.

Plan for review

Review plan is agreed on with the patient having regard to the need for monitoring the disease and medication, including specific tests for side-effects. If a DMARD was initiated by a specialist, regular follow-up appointments are essential for assessment of treatment and related side-effects (e.g. complete blood counts and LFTs at monthly intervals for patients on methotrexate). Patients with psoriatic arthritis, as opposed to rheumatoid arthritis, will also require a liver biopsy after a defined amount of methotrexate).

DRUGS AND OTHER THERAPIES: DETAILS
Drugs
NONSTEROIDAL ANTI-INFLAMMATORY DRUGS (NSAIDS)

- NSAIDs are the mainstay of therapy in psoriatic arthritis
- Indomethacin was originally studied in this disease, but more recent investigations have shown good success with other NSAIDs as well

Dose

Indomethacin:
- 25–50mg orally after food twice to three times a day (maximum 200mg/day)
- Sustained release formula – 75mg once a day after food, may increase to 75mg twice daily

Efficacy
- Effectively controls pain, may help stiffness and/or joint swelling
- Pain begins to ease within 2h

Risks/Benefits

Risks:
- Use caution in elderly
- Use caution in hepatic, renal, and cardiac failure
- Use caution in bleeding disorders
- There is no evidence that final outcome changed by NSAIDs

Benefits:
- The main benefit is relief of pain
- Targets the main symptoms of arthritis
- Easy to take and fairly well tolerated
- Flexible choice of different NSAIDs and dosage to treat a wide variety of patients

Side-effects and adverse reactions
- Cardiovascular system: hypertension, peripheral edema, congestive heart failure
- Central nervous system: headache, dizziness, tinnitus, fever
- Gastrointestinal: anorexia, nausea, dyspepsia, peptic ulceration, bleeding
- Genitourinary: nephrotoxicity
- Hematologic: blood cell disorders
- Hypersensitivity: rashes, bronchospasm, angioedema
- Skin: pruritus, rash

Interactions (other drugs)
- Aminoglycosides ▪ Anticoagulants ▪ Antihypertensives ▪ Baclofen ▪ Corticosteroids
- Cyclosporine, tacrolimus ▪ Digoxin ▪ Diuretics ▪ Lithium ▪ Methotrexate
- Phenylpropanolamine ▪ Warfarin

Contraindications
- Peptic ulceration
- Hypersensitivity to NSAIDs
- Coagulation defects
- Severe renal or hepatic disease

Acceptability to patient
- Usually very acceptable, depending on effectiveness in controlling symptoms
- Common gastrointestinal side-effects may limit acceptability

Follow up plan
Complete blood count yearly, LFTs, creatinine testing may be required.

Patient and caregiver information
Take after food.

TRIAMCINOLONE HEXACETONIDE
- The choice of corticosteroid for intra-articular injection is governed by the knowledge that a poorly absorbed preparation will lead to the least amount of systemic absorption
- All intra-articular injections must be performed using strict aseptic technique

Dose
- 2–20mg (0.1–1.0mL) given by injection into the affected joint space
- 2–6mg for small joints; 10–20mg for large joints

Efficacy
Usually produces good response in treated joint.

Risks/Benefits
Risks:
- Does not provide quick response; may take several hours for relief
- Risk of infection with intra-articular injection
- Use caution with glomerulonephritis, ulcerative colitis, renal disease, AIDS, tuberculosis, ocular herpes simplex, live vaccines, viral and bacterial infections, diabetes mellitus, glaucoma, osteoporosis, hypertension, recent myocardial infarction
- Use caution in children and the elderly
- Use caution in psychosis
- Do not withdraw abruptly

Benefits:
- Can provide localized symptomatic relief
- Avoids many adverse effects of steroids due to the lack of systemic absorption

Side-effects and adverse reactions
- Side-effects are minimized by short duration of therapy
- Cardiovascular system: hypertension, thromboembolism
- Central nervous system: insomnia, euphoria, depression, psychosis, seizures
- Endocrine: adrenal suppression, impaired glucose tolerance, growth suppression in children
- Eyes, ears, nose, and throat: cataract, glaucoma, blurred vision
- Gastrointestinal: dyspepsia, peptic ulceration, esophagitis, oral candidiasis, nausea, vomiting
- Musculoskeletal: proximal myopathy, osteoporosis
- Skin: delayed healing, acne, striae, transient atrophy at injection site

Interactions (other drugs)
- Aminoglutehamide
- Antidiabetics
- Barbiturates
- Carbamazepine
- Cholestyramine

- Cholinesterase inhibitors ▪ Cyclosporine ▪ Diuretics ▪ Estrogens ▪ Isoniazid
- Isoproterenal ▪ NSAIDs ▪ Phenytoin ▪ Rifampin ▪ Salicylates

Contraindications
- Local or systemic infection ▪ Peptic ulcer ▪ Pregnancy and breastfeeding

Acceptability to patient
Targeted relief for painful joint highly acceptable, but initial pain of injection procedure may restrict use in some individuals.

Follow up plan
Review in 7–10 days to reassess joint pain and mobility.

Patient and caregiver information
- Injected joint may feel more painful during initial 24h
- After this it is important to mobilize joint

Physical therapy
The aim of physical therapy is to maintain joint mobility, prevent contracturesm, and maintain muscle strength.

ISOMETRIC EXERCISE
Individual program designed by specialist physical therapist after careful assessment of the patient's problems.

Efficacy
Improves strength and flexibility of affected joints.

Risks/Benefits
Risks:
- May be exhausting and increase pain levels during and immediately after therapy session
- May encourage dependence on therapist

Benefits:
- Increases patient mobility and sense of well being
- One-to-one therapy has beneficial effect on patient motivation and self-esteem

Acceptability to patient
Variable: depends on individual motivation and levels of pain.

Follow up plan
Tailored to the individual and the prevailing level of disability.

Patient and caregiver information
- May take a while for benefits to become apparent
- Must be continued regularly for optimal benefit

HYDROTHERAPY
Part of the physical therapy program. Given by specialist physical therapist after careful assessment of the patient's problems.

Efficacy
Improves strength and flexibility of affected joints.

Risks/Benefits
Risks:
- May be tiring during and immediately after therapy session
- May encourage dependence on therapist

Benefits:
- Increases patient mobility and sense of well being
- One-to-one therapy has beneficial effect on patient motivation and self-esteem
- Generally pleasant for the patient

Acceptability to patient
Variable: depends on individual motivation and levels of pain.

Follow up plan
Depends on the individual.

Patient and caregiver information
May take a while for benefits to become apparent.

Occupational therapy
OCCUPATIONAL THERAPY
Occupational therapy is required:
- To provide a functional assessment
- To provide aids and assistive devices, including splints
- To provide education regarding modification of daily activities
- To advise regarding modifications to the workplace

Efficacy
- Enables individual patients to overcome specific disabilities and difficulties with activities of daily living
- Especially effective in patients with problems with dexterity

Acceptability to patient
Patients are usually very grateful for the help provided to live as independently as possible.

Follow up plan
This is a specialized therapy, and follow up must be tailored to the individual.

Patient and caregiver information
Therapy and adaptations are designed to aid independent living.

LIFESTYLE
- The physician can educate the arthritic patient in joint preservation techniques. In particular, not to use a painful joint or overuse a fatigued joint; in remissions keep joints as active as possible (physical therapist will advise)
- Adaptive equipment (provided by the occupational therapist) is helpful; e.g. enlarged handles for writing or eating utensils

ACCEPTABILITY TO PATIENT
Depends on individual severity of problems and motivation to overcome them.

OUTCOMES

EFFICACY OF THERAPIES

- No treatment for psoriatic arthritis is curative
- There is no evidence that one NSAID is superior to another

Review period

Depends on the pattern of the disease and the treatment given.

PROGNOSIS

- The course of psoriatic arthritis is usually characterized by flares and remissions
- Generally, psoriatic arthritis will follow a relatively benign course without serious systemic complications
- The course of the disease is mild in most people and affects only a few joints. (Note, this is not the case for patients with arthritis mutilans)
- Younger age of onset, female gender, and acute onset of arthritis are more common in patients with severe arthritis
- The course for any individual may be difficult to predict at presentation, because one pattern type can change unpredictably into another

Clinical pearls

- The course of arthritis is unrelated to the severity of skin disease
- Arthritis involving the DIP joints virtually never occurs without concomitant nail changes of psoriasis

Therapeutic failure

Therapeutic failures may require surgical management.

Deterioration

Refer to rheumatologist or possibly orthopedic surgeon for surgical intervention if necessary (7% of sufferers will require surgery, on average after 13 years of disease).

COMPLICATIONS

- Arthritis mutilans progresses to severe deforming and destructive arthritis
- Systemic complications, especially eye involvement (conjunctivitis/uveitis) and aortic incompetence

CONSIDER CONSULT

If patient has coexisting HIV infection, refer to infectious disease specialist.

PREVENTION

There are no known preventive measures that can be taken to avoid psoriatic arthritis.

MODIFY RISK FACTORS
Lifestyle and wellness
DIET
Polyunsaturated ethylester lipids (such as are commonly found in fish) have been reported to be a useful adjuvant to standard therapy.

PHYSICAL ACTIVITY
- Rest and exercise are indicated to increase mobility
- Useful information on exercise in psoriatic arthritis is available from the National Psoriasis Foundation

RESOURCES

ASSOCIATIONS

The National Psoriasis Foundation
6600 SW 92nd Avenue, Suite 300
Portland, OR 97223-7195
Tel: (503) 244 7404
Fax : (503) 245 0626
E-mail: getinfo@npfusa.org
www.psoriasis.org

Psoriatic Arthritis Support (Website support group for sufferers and families)
www.wpunj.edu

Arthritis Foundation
PO Box 7669
Atlanta, GA 30357-0669
Tel: (800) 283 7800
www.arthritis.org

The Road Back Foundation
PO Box 447
Orleans, MA 02653
Voice mail: (614) 227-1556
http://roadback.org

The Johns Hopkins University Division of Rheumatology
Johns Hopkins Hospital Outpatient Center
601 North Caroline Street
Baltimore, MD 21287
Tel: (410) 955 3052
Fax: (410) 614 0498
www.hopkins-arthritis.som.jhmi.edu

National Institute of Arthritis and Musculoskeletal
and Skin Diseases
National Institutes of Health
Bethesda, MD 20892
www.nih.gov

KEY REFERENCES

- Cohen MR, Reda DJ, Clegg DD. Department of Veterans Affairs Cooperative Study Group on Seronegative Spondyloarthropathies. Baseline relationships between psoriasis and arthritis: analysis of 221 patients with active psoriatic arthritis. J Rheumatol 1999;26:1752–6
- Scarpa R, Pucino A, Iocco M, et al. The managemnt of 138 psoriatic arthritis patients. Acta Derm Venereol 1989;146:199–200
- Clegg DO, Reda DJ, Abdellatif M. Comparison of sulfasalazine and placebo for the treatment of axial and peripheral articular manifestations of the seronegative spondyloarthropathies: A Department of Veterans Affairs cooperative study. Arthritis Rheum 1999;42:2325–9
- Pitzalis C, Pipitone N. Psoriatic arthritis. J Roy Soc Med 2000;93:412–15
- Gladman DD. Psoriatic arthritis. Rheum Dis Clin North Am 1998;24:829–44
- Rahman P, Gladman DD, Cook RJ, et al. The use of sulphasalazine in psoriatic arthritis: a clinic experience. J Rheumatol 1998;25:1957–61
- Cuellar ML, Espinoza LR. Rheumatic manifestations of HIV-AIDS. Baillieres Best Pract Res Clin Rheumatol 2000;14:579–93

- Spadarow A, Riccieri V, Sili-Scavalli A, et al. A comparison of cyclosporin A and methotrexate in the treatment of psoriatic arthritis: a one year prospective study. Clin Exp Rheumatol 1995;13:589–93
- Jones G, Crotty M, Brooks P. Interventions for treating psoriatic arthritis (Cochrane Review). In: The Cochrane Library, 1, 2002. Oxford: Update Software
- Gladman DD, Rahman P. Psoriatic arthritis. In: Ruddy S, Harris Jr ED, Sledge CB, eds. Kelley's Textbook of Rheumatology, 6th edn. Philadelphia: WB Saunders, 2001

FAQS
Question 1
Can the diagnosis of psoriatic arthritis be made without evidence of skin involvement?

ANSWER 1
In up to one-third of patients, skin involvement occurs concurrently or after the diagnosis of psoriatic arthritis is suspected. It is important to look for skin involvement in areas such as the scalp, navel, and intergluteal cleft.

Question 2
How likely is it that a patient with psoriasis will get psoriatic arthritis?

ANSWER 2
5% of psoriasis patients will develop the arthritis.

Question 3
How useful is haplotyping in the diagnosis of psoriatic arthritis?

ANSWER 3
Checking for HLA-B27 will likely only add confusion to the clinical picture. It occurs in only 50% of psoriatic arthritis patients and may be present in 7% of normal individuals.

Question 4
Can RF be present in psoriatic arthritis?

ANSWER 4
Psoriatic arthritis is classically thought of as a seronegative (RF negative) inflammatory arthritis. Hence, by definition, the rheumatoid factor should be negative. However, as RF may occur in a very small percentage of the population, it is possible that a low titer RF may be positive. However, caution must be exercised as early rheumatoid arthritis may present in a similar way as psoriatic arthritis.

CONTRIBUTORS
Mary Jo Groves, MD
Maria-Louise Barilla-LaBarca, MD
Deborah L Shapiro, MD

REITER'S SYNDROME

DESCRIPTION

- Arthritis
- Nongonococcal urethritis and cervicitis
- Conjunctivitis or iritis
- Mucocutaneous lesions

URGENT ACTION

Acute uveitis in Reiter's syndrome is most often characterized by unilateral ocular pain and requires urgent referral to an ophthalmologist to confirm diagnosis and initiate cycloplegic agents and topical corticosteroids.

KEY! DON'T MISS!

Severe eye pain, blurred vision, and photophobia suggest acute anterior uveitis (iridocyclitis), which should be referred to an ophthalmologist. Gonorrhea should always be considered in the differential diagnosis of genitourinary symptoms.

BACKGROUND

ICD9 CODE
099.3 Reiter's disease.

SYNONYMS
Reactive arthritis, seronegative spondyloarthropathy.

CARDINAL FEATURES
- Onset of symptomatology within 1–4 weeks of infections with a sexually transmitted urethritis or bacterial gastroenteritis in some cases. However, for most cases, an infectious etiology is not clinically apparent
- Classic triad of features include arthritis, urethritis, conjunctivitis
- Musculoskeletal manifestations, including axial arthritis (including sacroiliitis and spondylitis) and/or peripheral arthritis (usually asymmetrical and oligoarticular with a lower extremity predominance); enthesopathy; spondyloarthropathy
- Dermatological manifestations, including oral aphthous ulcers, keratoderma blennorrhagica, circinate balanitis, circinate ulcerative vulvitis
- Urogenital manifestations, including urethritis, prostatitis, cystitis, balanitis, cervicitis
- Ocular manifestations, including conjunctivitis, scleritis, keratitis, corneal ulcerations, uveitis, iritis
- Cardiovascular manifestations, including pericarditis, myocarditis, first-degree AV block, aortic regurgitation
- Systemic manifestations, including fever, malaise, fatigue, anorexia, weight loss

CAUSES
Common causes
- Nongonococcal urethritis secondary to sexually-transmitted organisms, including *Chlamydia trachomatis, C. psittaci, C. pneumoniae, Ureaplasma urealyticum*
- Enteric infection secondary to *Shigella flexneri, Salmonella typhimurium, S. enteritidis, S. paratyphi, S. heidelberg, Yersinia enterocolitica, Y. pseudotuberculosis, Campylobacter jejuni, C. fetus*

Contributory or predisposing factors
- HLA-B27 genotype
- Pre-existing HIV infection

EPIDEMIOLOGY
Incidence and prevalence
PREVALENCE
In USA, 3.5–4.0 cases per 1000 men per year

Demographics
AGE
- Peak onset in third decade
- Occasionally occurs in pediatric and geriatric patients

GENDER
- Post-venereal Reiter's syndrome is more common in men (20:1)
- Post-enteric Reiter's syndrome is equally common in men and women

GENETICS
- Reports show greatly increased risk of Reiter's syndrome in individuals with positive HLA-B27 genotype

- Some studies show that 60–80% of Reiter's syndrome patients possess HLA-B27; other studies show 90–96% of Reiter's syndrome patients possess this antigen
- However, only 20% of individuals infected with arthritogenic bacteria and possessing a positive HLA-B27 genotype will ultimately develop Reiter's syndrome
- There is no role for determining HLA B-27 status in the diagnosis of Reiter's in an individual patient

DIFFERENTIAL DIAGNOSIS
Rheumatoid arthritis
FEATURES

- Morning stiffness, generally over an hour prior to improving
- Arthritis involves three or more joints
- Frequent involvement of the hand (proximal interphalangeal joints, metacarpophalangeal joints, wrists)
- Usually symmetric
- Constitutional symptoms may include fever, weight loss, malaise
- Seropositive for rheumatoid factor
- May exhibit rheumatoid nodules
- X-rays are characteristic

Conjunctivitis
FEATURES

- Conjunctival erythema
- Itching, burning, gritty feeling to eyes
- May have watery or purulent discharge

Gout or pseudogout
FEATURES

- In gout, male:female ratio is 9:1; in pseudogout, male:female ratio is 1.5:1
- For gout, podagra is most common acute presentation
- Sites for gout include ankle, wrist, knee; sites for pseudogout include knee, wrist, shoulder, occasional carpal tunnel syndrome
- Usually monarticular
- May precipitate systemic symptoms, including fever, chills, malaise
- Other problems associated with crystal-induced arthritides include development of kidney stones and/or tophi

Psoriatic arthritis
FEATURES

- Asymmetric, oligoarticular inflammatory polyarthritis
- Onychodystrophy
- Rash sometimes on penis mimicking circinate balanitis

Rheumatic fever
FEATURES

- Tends to strike younger children
- Sequela of streptococcal pharyngitis
- Causes polyarticular, migratory arthritis of large joints (especially ankles, wrists, knees, and elbows)
- Carditis is serious complication, may be manifested as pericarditis, congestive heart failure, development of a new murmur, cardiomegaly
- Arthralgia and fever considered minor criteria for diagnosis
- May also result in Aschoff bodies, erythema marginatum, Sydenham's chorea

Sarcoidosis
FEATURES

- Affects females slightly more frequently than males
- Affects all body systems

- Constitutional symptoms include fever, night sweats, malaise, fatigue, weight loss
- Transient, migratory arthritis of large joints, often with a predilection for the ankles
- Dermatological manifestations include erythema nodosum, maculopapular eruption, development of subcutaneous nodules, and/or lupus pernio
- Interstitial lung disease, resulting in dyspnea, cough
- Anterior or posterior uveitis
- Radiologic evidence of bone cysts, punched-out bone lesions
- Left ventricular dysfunction, arrhythmias, conduction disturbances frequent

SIGNS & SYMPTOMS
Signs
- 'Sausage' digit
- Signs of sacroiliac inflammation, decreased spinal mobility
- Ocular inflammation
- Conduction disturbance picked up by ECG
- Aortic regurgitation, new murmur
- Prostatic tenderness
- Circinate balanitis

Symptoms
- Fever, malaise, anorexia, weight loss, fatigue
- Dysuria, urinary urgency, frequency
- Mucopurulent penile discharge, vaginal discharge
- Prostatitis, including fever, chills, dysuria, urinary frequency
- Arthritis, especially of the knees, ankles, feet, usually asymmetric
- Spondylitis, sacroiliitis with low back pain
- Enthesopathy, including Achilles tendinitis, plantar fasciitis, digital periostitis, calcaneal spurring, heel pain, dactylitis
- Conjuncitivitis, with redness, tearing, photophobia, pain, lid edema
- Uveitis
- Circinate balanitis
- Keratoderma blennorrhagica
- Mouth ulcers
- Onycholysis, nail pitting, subungual hyperkeratosis

KEY! DON'T MISS!
Severe eye pain, blurred vision, and photophobia suggest acute anterior uveitis (iridocyclitis), which should be referred to an ophthalmologist. Gonorrhea should always be considered in the differential diagnosis of genitourinary symptoms.

CONSIDER CONSULT
Patients with refractory arthritis that is not controlled with NSAIDs should be referred to a rheumatologist for consideration of treatment with agents such as methotrexate or sulfasalazine.

INVESTIGATION OF THE PATIENT
Direct questions to patient
Q Have you had an illness or infection any time over the last month? Seek information in particular about symptoms of urethritis or gastroenteritis; question about sexual activity, partners' illnesses/infections; question about any outbreaks of food poisoning or bacterial dysentery in patient's family/community

Q How has your energy level been? Any difficulty with your appetite, or unintended weight loss? Have you noted any fever?

Q Do you have any problems or pain urinating?

Q Have you noticed any discharge from your penis/any unusual vaginal discharge? Question also regarding unusual skin eruptions in the genital area

Q Have you had any joint pain, stiffness, redness? If arthritis is present, determine which joints

Q Have you noticed any rashes or changes to your nails?

Q Have you noticed any eye redness, burning, discharge, eyelid swelling? Be sure to ask the patient about any visual disturbances noted

Contributory or predisposing factors

Q Do you have any other illnesses? In particular, has patient been recently tested for HIV?

Family history

Q Do you have any family members with any arthritic conditions? This is an attempt to see if HLA-B27-associated diseases may run in the family

Examination

- Is patient well/unwell? If unwell, consider systemic diseases, including sarcoidosis, rheumatic fever, septic arthritis
- Take temperature
- Inspect joints, looking for redness, swelling, heat, stiffness, tenderness; assess for symmetry versus asymmetry of findings; evaluate spine for tenderness, decreased range of motion
- Inspect skin, looking for psoriatic-like skin eruptions, especially soles and palms for keratoderma blennorrhagicum; include skin in genital area for circinate balanitis, circinate or ulcerative vulvitis
- Inspect nails for onycholysis, pitting, subungual hyperkeratosis
- Examine eyes, looking for redness, discharge, lid edema, evaluate for pain, visual disturbances
- Examine genital area, looking for mucopurulent penile or vaginal discharge; in men, evaluate prostate for tenderness, hypertrophy; in women, evaluate for cervicitis
- Carefully auscultate heart, listening for new murmur

Summary of investigative tests

- Full blood count with differential should be performed
- ESR, if markedly elevated, indicates the presence of an inflammatory process
- C-reactive protein, if present, also indicates the presence of infection
- Rheumatoid factor
- Culture of penile or vaginal discharge can identify causative pathogens
- Stool cultures
- Arthrocentesis and synovial fluid analysis to exclude gout, pseudogout, and infection
- X-rays of affected joints, spine, and pelvis

DIAGNOSTIC DECISION

Reiter's syndrome can be diagnosed according to guidelines from the American College of Rheumatology [1]:

- Episode of arthritis of more than one month with urethritis and/or cervicitis
- Episode of arthritis of more than one month and *either* urethritis *or* cervicitis, or bilateral conjunctivitis
- Episode of arthritis, conjunctivitis, and urethritis
- Episode of arthritis of more than one month, conjunctivitis, and urethritis

CLINICAL PEARLS

- The clinical triad of urethritis, conjunctivitis, and arthritis is observed in <40 % of patients with Reiter's syndrome

- HIV infection can sometimes present as a mimic of Reiter's syndrome. Serologic testing should be considered.
- Post-dysenteric Reiter's syndrome affects both sexes equally

THE TESTS
Body fluids
FULL BLOOD COUNT WITH DIFFERENTIAL
Description
Blood.

Advantages/Disadvantages
Advantage: simple, safe to obtain.

Abnormal
- May note slight anemia, neutrophilic leukocytosis
- Keep in mind the possibility of a false-positive result

Cause of abnormal result
May be Reiter's syndrome, or some other inflammatory process.

Drugs, disorders and other factors that may alter results
If patient is on steroids, white cell demargination can skew results.

ERYTHROCYTE SEDIMENTATION RATE
Description
Blood sample.

Advantages/Disadvantages
- Advantage: simple, safe to obtain
- Disadvantage: not definitive for Reiter's syndrome

Normal
- Males: 0–15mm/h
- Females: 0–20mm/h

Abnormal
- Values outside the normal range
- Keep in mind the possibility of a false-positive result

Cause of abnormal result
- Marked elevation suggests inflammatory process
- Keep in mind possibility of a false-positive or false-negative result

Drugs, disorders and other factors that may alter results
Abnormal test result may reflect another inflammatory disorder.

C-REACTIVE PROTEIN
Description
Blood sample.

Advantages/Disadvantages
- Advantage: easy to procure
- Disadvantage: non-specific

Cause of abnormal result
- Abnormally high C-reactive protein level suggests presence of inflammation; not specific for Reiter's syndrome
- Keep in mind the possibility of a false-positive or false-negative result

Drugs, disorders and other factors that may alter results
Inflammatory disorders other than Reiter's syndrome may cause abnormal test result.

RHEUMATOID FACTOR
Description
Blood sample.

Advantages/Disadvantages
Advantage: relatively easy to obtain.

Normal
Rheumatoid factor is not normally present in blood.

Abnormal
- Presence of rheumatoid factor in blood specimen is generally considered abnormal
- Keep in mind the possibility of a false-positive result

Cause of abnormal result
Keep in mind the possibility of a false-positive or false-negative result.

Drugs, disorders and other factors that may alter results
Other inflammatory disorders may cause abnormal test result.

SEROLOGY FOR CHLAMYDIAL ANTIBODIES
Description
Blood specimen.

Advantages/Disadvantages
Advantages:
- Fairly simple to obtain
- Presence of chlamydial antibodies may indicate past chlamydial infection

Disadvantage: doesn't indicate when infection occurred

Normal
No chlamydial bodies present.

Abnormal
- Chlamydial bodies present
- Keep in mind the possibility of a false-positive result

CULTURE OF VAGINAL OR PENILE DISCHARGE
Description
Vaginal or penile discharge.

Advantages/Disadvantages
Advantage: relatively simple and safe to obtain.

Abnormal
- Any discharge is abnormal; culture may grow gonococcus or other micro-organisms
- Keep in mind the possibility of a false-positive result

Cause of abnormal result
Infection, which may be sexually transmitted.

Imaging
X-RAY OF AFFECTED JOINTS
Advantages/Disadvantages
Advantage: radiography can show distinctive changes to affected joints, spine.

Abnormal
- Periosteal reaction at inferior calcaneus
- Significant periosteal thickening, proliferation
- Erosive lesions with adjacent bony proliferation
- Tendinous and ligamentous calcification
- Sacroiliitis, spondylitis
- Keep in mind the possibility of a false-positive result

Cause of abnormal result
- While radiography may well be suggestive of Reiter's syndrome, appearance may not be definitive
- Abnormal radiography may suggest presence of arthropathic/spondylitic process, without necessarily confirming Reiter's syndrome as the specific entity

Drugs, disorders and other factors that may alter results
Other arthropathic or spondylitic processes may appear the same on radiograph.

Special tests
ARTHROCENTESIS/SYNOVIAL FLUID ANALYSIS
Description
Synovial fluid.

Advantages/Disadvantages
Advantage: can differentiate between some forms of arthritis, help rule out certain arthropathic processes, help support presumptive diagnosis of Reiter's syndrome

Disadvantages:
- Somewhat painful
- Care must be taken to avoid iatrogenic infection

Normal
Normal synovial fluid is clear and viscous, whereas inflammatory fluid is turbid with reduced viscosity.

Abnormal
- Synovial fluid that is turbid or purulent indicates inflammatory arthritis or infection
- Laboratory analysis can indicate other abnormalities, such as the presence of crystals, white blood cells bacteria
- Keep in mind the possibility of a false-positive result

Cause of abnormal result
Results may indicate a variety of arthropathic conditions, including crystal-induced arthritides (gout, pseudogout), other inflammatory conditions (rheumatoid arthritis), or septic arthritis.

Other tests

STOOL CULTURES

Description
Stool sample.

Advantages/Disadvantages
Advantage: stool sample is usually easily procured.

Normal
Red blood cells, white blood cells, micro-organisms should be absent from sample.

Abnormal
- Presence of micro-organisms may indicate Reiter's syndrome secondary to enteric infection, continued need for antibiotic treatment
- Inflammatory cells in absence of bacterial infection may indicate arthritis secondary to inflammatory bowel disease
- Keep in mind the possibility of a false-positive result

Cause of abnormal result
May be due to bacterial gastroenteritis, may be due to inflammatory bowel disease.

Drugs, disorders and other factors that may alter results
Recent ingestion of red meat, ingestion of fruits/vegetables containing high levels of peroxidase or vitamin C, imbibing alcohol, bleeding gums, taking certain medications (aspirin, ibuprofen, steroids), in days just prior to testing of stool sample may cause result to be falsely Hemoccult-positive.

CONSIDER CONSULT

Severe eye pain and redness should prompt an immediate referral to an ophthalmologist.

IMMEDIATE ACTION

A single inflamed joint should be aspirated to rule out infection.

PATIENT AND CAREGIVER ISSUES
Patient or caregiver request

- Patient may have concerns about the chronicity of the condition and about disability associated with it
- Patient may wonder if Reiter's syndrome is considered a sexually transmitted disease

Health-seeking behavior

Have you tried medications (such as over-the-counter ibuprofen, aspirin)? Have you tried other palliative techniques (resting, heat, ice)? Such measures may have delayed medical assessment.

MANAGEMENT ISSUES
Goals

- Reduce pain, swelling, and stiffness
- Maintain/restore optimal level of functioning

Management in special circumstances

Patient's HIV status should be determined before treatment with any potentially immunosuppressant medications is initiated.

PATIENT SATISFACTION/LIFESTYLE PRIORITIES

Patient may have significant limitation of activity during acute episodes of inflammation; this may significantly interfere with employment, care of family.

SUMMARY OF THERAPEUTIC OPTIONS
Choices

- First-line drugs are all nonsteroidal anti-inflammatory drugs (NSAIDs), replacing previous use of salicylates. Of the NSAIDs, indomethacin (particularly sustained-release formulation) is usually the first choice. This is an off-label indication
- Other NSAID choices include diclofenac, naproxen, Sulindac. Phenylbutazone is rarely chosen, owing to risk of aplastic anemia, although it may be used for patients who fail other types of NSAIDs
- Intra-articular injections of corticosteroids (e.g. triamcinolone) are sometimes used
- However, systemic corticosteroids are almost never used to treat Reiter's syndrome, except for the most refractory cases
- The use of antibiotic therapy is somewhat controversial, except for clearcut indications
- Slow-acting antirheumatics including sulfasalazine and methotrexate may be used for NSAID-unresponsive patients
- Physical therapy should be utilized to improve joint mobility and muscle tone, thus maintaining mobility, preventing disability, and optimizing the chance for a return to patient's previous level of functioning
- Occupational therapy can help teach the patient strategies for accomplishing the activities of daily living with minimum pain
- Rarely, surgical intervention in the form of arthroplasty is required in the event of joint deformity, destruction which permanently interferes with an individual's lifestyle
- Patients should be educated about the chance of recurrence and chronicity

Clinical pearls
Maximum doses of NSAIDs are usually required to treat this disorder (e.g. indomethacin 50mg four times a day, naproxen 500mg three times a day).

Never
If patient is at risk of positive HIV status, and testing has yet to be performed, do not give patient cytotoxic agents (high-dose corticosteroids, methotrexate, cyclosporine); these can complicate pre-existing immunosuppression.

FOLLOW UP
- The frequency and duration of follow up depends upon the severity and chronicity of the patient's disease
- Some patients will require only as-needed follow up when acute episodes of arthritis occurs
- Patients with more chronic arthritis, especially if treated with agents such as methotrexate or sulfasalazine, need to be seen on a regular schedule every 2–3 months

Information for patient or caregiver
- Practitioner should communicate effectively with patient to encourage appropriate rest during acute episodes of inflammation, but with quick return to monitored exercise/physical therapy, to improve strength, prevent permanent disability
- Patient should be educated about the chance of relapse
- Patient should be educated about complications for which immediate medical care should be sought in order to avoid potentially serious sequelae such as iritis

DRUGS AND OTHER THERAPIES: DETAILS
Drugs
NONSTEROIDAL ANTI-INFLAMMATORY DRUGS
Dose
Depends on specific agent.

Indomethacin:
- Sustained release formula more convenient, dosed at 75–150mg/day
- Regular formulation: 25mg by mouth four times a day; can be increased to 50mg four times a day as necessary

Naproxen:
250–500mg by mouth twice daily, adjusted according to response. May be increased to 500mg three times daily.

Diclofenac:
- 50–75mg by mouth twice daily
- Base any increase on patient responsiveness to lower dose

Sulindac:
- 150mg by mouth twice daily
- Maximum dosage is 400mg/day
- May increase to maximum dosage on the basis of patient response to lower dosage

Efficacy
Considered to be good.

Risks/Benefits
- Risk: caution required in elderly patients and in patients with allergic disorders or a history of peptic ulceration

Benefit: provides relief of arthritic symptoms of Reiter's syndrome

Side-effects and adverse reactions

- Gastrointestional: abdominal pain, nausea, diarrhea, bleeding, peptic ulceration, pancratitis
- Skin: rashes, Stevens-Johnson syndrome
- Pulmonary: bronchospasm, alveolitis, pulmonary eosinophilia
- Central nervous system: Headache, dizziness, tinnitus, photosensitivity, aseptic meningitis
- Cardiovascular: edema
- Renal: renal failure
- Allergic-like symptoms: angioedema, rhinitis
- Gastrointestinal: colitis

Interactions (other drugs)

Angiotensin-converting enzyme inhibitors Angiotensin II antagonists Antihypertensive drugs Baclofen Bisphosphonates Cimetidine Corticosteroids Cyclosporine Desmopressin Digoxin Diuretics Haloperidol Heparin Levothyroxine Lithium Methotrexate Mifepristone Moclobemide Pentoxifylline Pheynytoin Probenecid Quinolone antibiotics Ritonavir Tacrolimus Warfarin Zidovudine

Contraindications

History of hypersensitivity to aspirin or any NSAID Active gastrointestinal bleeding Pregnancy Lactation

Acceptability to patient
Good.

INTRA-ARTICULAR TRIAMCINOLONE
Dose
40mg injected intra-articularly into the knee.

Efficacy
Good.

Risks/Benefits
Risks:

- Full aseptic precautions are essential
- Second-line therapy
- Does not provide quick response; make take several hours for relief
- Risk of infection with intra-articular injection
- Risk of joint destruction and sepsis if septic arthritis is misdiagnosed as gout

Side-effects and adverse reactions

- Pain at injection site
- Flushing

Interactions (other drugs)

Antidiabetics Isoniazid Rifampicin Salicylates

Contraindications
Local or systemic infection.

Acceptability to patient
Moderate: involves invasive procedure but may provide good relief of symptoms.

Physical therapy
STRENGTH TRAINING, FLEXIBILITY, INCREASE IN MOBILITY
Efficacy
Physical therapy can help maintain joint and spine range of motion, and prevent atrophy around large joints such as the knee.

Acceptability to patient
Generally good.

LIFESTYLE
- Rest may be helpful initially, during acute episode
- It is important for the patient to return to mobility as soon as possible, to avoid muscle atrophy and loss of motion
- Physical therapy and monitored exercise help to improve mobility, strengthen muscles which support affected joints

ACCEPTABILITY TO PATIENT
Patient may have difficulty resting if it will interfere with employment or caring for family.

EFFICACY OF THERAPIES

Even with therapy, recurrence of Reiter's syndrome is common. Long-term problems include:
- Persistent arthritis and back pain
- Progressive iritis

PROGNOSIS

- Initial arthritic episode lasts a mean of 2–3 months, but may last up to one year
- Disease-free intervals may be interspersed with relapses (particularly likely in those patients who have the classic triad of urethritis, conjunctivitis, and arthritis)
- Patients who do not have the classic triad are at risk of chronicity
- Only about 15% of patients are at risk of severe disability
- Death is rare and usually secondary to cardiac complications or amyloidosis

Clinical pearls

Patients who do not have the classic triad of urethritis, conjunctivitis, and arthritis are at risk of developing chronic disease.

Therapeutic failure

- Slow-acting antirheumatic agents include sulfasalazine, methotrexate, cyclosporine
- Patients with joint deformity, severe interruption of lifestyle may benefit from arthroplasty

Recurrence

- Recurrence of Reiter's syndrome is common
- Disease-free intervals may be interspersed with relapses (particularly likely in those patients who have the classic triad of urethritis, conjunctivitis, and arthritis)

COMPLICATIONS

Severe complications are rare, but can include severe lower extremity arthritis, severe axial arthritis, blindness, cardiac complications, amyloidosis.

CONSIDER CONSULT

Referral to rheumatologist and ophthalmologist is recommended when diagnosis is suspected and when patients experience recurrent attacks after disease-free intervals.

MODIFY RISK FACTORS
Lifestyle and wellness
SEXUAL BEHAVIOR

For patients with documented sexually transmitted disease, condom use is advised.

SCREENING
Screening for Reiter's syndrome is not necessary.

PREVENT RECURRENCE
Some researchers recommend condom usage to avoid repeated exposure to potentially inductive micro-organisms.

RESOURCES

ASSOCIATIONS

American College of Rheumatology
1800 Century Place, Suite 250
Atlanta, GA 30345
tel: (404) 633 3777
Fax: (404) 633 1870
www.rheumatology.org

National Institute of Arthritis and Musculoskeletal and Skin Diseases
National Institutes of Health
Bethesda, MD 20892-2350
www.nih.gov/niams

KEY REFERENCES

■ Reiter's syndrome. In Beers MH, Berkow R, eds. The Merck Manual of Diagnosis and Therapy, 17th Edn. Whitehouse Station: Merck & Co, 1999

Guidelines

1 Wilkens RF, Arnett FC, Bitter T, et al. Reiter's syndrome: evaluation of preliminary criteria for definite disease. Arthritis Rheum 1981;24:844–9

FAQS

Question 1

Is Reiter's syndrome usually associated with a history of sexually transmitted disease?

ANSWER 1

No. Such a history is usually not present. However, it must always be considered.

Question 2

Is the triad of 'conjuctivitis, urethritis, and arthritis' necessary for the diagnosis of Reiter's syndrome?

ANSWER 2

No. Most patients will not have all three of these. Other features such as inflammatory back pain, stomatitis, dactylitis, and stomatitis are equally important to consider in making the diagnosis.

Question 3

What is the prognosis of Reiter's syndrome?

ANSWER 3

Fortunately, few patients develop chronic, severe disease. The majority have intermittent episodes, punctuated by symptom-free intervals. Occasionally, a patient will have a single episode of disease without recurrence.

CONTRIBUTORS

Fred F Ferri, MD, FACP
Richard Brasington Jr, MD, FACP
Dinesh Khanna, MD

RHEUMATOID ARTHRITIS

DESCRIPTION

- Chronic, insidious, autoimmune inflammatory disorder
- Symmetric polyarthritis affecting mainly small joints in the hands and feet, as well as larger joints such as the wrists and shoulders
- Characteristic deformities include subluxations, dislocations, rheumatoid nodules, and joint contractures
- Treated with a combination of disease-modifying antirheumatic drugs (DMARDs), nonsteroidal anti-inflammatory drugs (NSAIDs), analgesics, rest, exercise (including physical therapy), and surgery

URGENT ACTION

Refer immediately to rheumatology if septic arthritis is suspected.

Effective treatment should be started before a firm diagnosis, including:

- Patient education
- Pain control, especially NSAIDs
- Rest and exercise
- Physical therapy

KEY! DON'T MISS!

Refer to rheumatology immediately if septic arthritis is suspected.

ICD9 CODE
714.0 Rheumatoid arthritis.

CARDINAL FEATURES
- Chronic, insidious, autoimmune inflammatory disorder
- Symmetric polyarthritis affecting mainly small joints in the hands and feet, as well as larger joints such as the wrists and shoulders
- Characteristic deformities include subluxations, dislocations, rheumatoid nodules, and joint contractures
- May lead to progressive joint destruction, deformity, disability, and premature death
- Treated with a combination of disease-modifying antirheumatic drugs (DMARDs), nonsteroidal anti-inflammatory drugs (NSAIDs), analgesics, rest, exercise (including physical therapy), and surgery

CAUSES
Common causes
- The cause of rheumatoid arthritis (RA) is unknown
- People with a genetic predisposition to developing RA may experience an environmental event (such as infection) that triggers the development of the condition, after which an inappropriate self-directed immune response persists
- Infectious agents, immunoregulatory and hormonal irregularities, and autoimmunity are among the factors currently being considered

EPIDEMIOLOGY
Incidence and prevalence
INCIDENCE
- Women: 0.36/1000
- Men: 0.14/1000

PREVALENCE
0.05–0.15/1000 in developed nations.

Demographics
AGE
- Disease onset most common at 25–55 years of age
- Incidence rises with age

GENDER
Women: men 2.5:1.

RACE
There is a higher incidence (3–5%) in some native North American tribes (Pima, Yakima, Chippewa, and Inuit).

GENETICS
- Patients with HLA-DRB1 alleles may have a poorer prognosis
- The condition clusters in families
- A shared epitope among several HLA-DR1 and HLA-DR4 alleles appears to predispose to the disease
- HLA-DQw7 has been proposed as an important marker gene

GEOGRAPHY
Remarkably constant worldwide, but slightly lower (0.3%) in China.

SOCIOECONOMIC STATUS
Lack of formal education correlates with increased mortality in RA.

DIFFERENTIAL DIAGNOSIS

- Rheumatoid arthritis (RA) can be very difficult to diagnose, especially in early disease
- If there is any uncertainty over diagnosis, referral to a rheumatologist is strongly indicated
- Systemic lupus erythematosus, psoriatic arthritis, and spondyloarthropathies may mimic RA

Osteoarthritis

Erosive osteoarthritis may coexist with RA in the elderly. It affects the distal interphalangeal (DIP) joints, which are not affected by RA.

FEATURES

- X-rays display typical joint-space narrowing, subchondral sclerosis, and osteophytic spurring. More abnormality at the interfaces of the phalanges is seen compared with typical osteoarthritis
- Joints show soft-tissue inflammation, bony swelling, crepitus, and restricted movement
- Slowly progressive with occasional exacerbations, which may be associated with warmth and redness. Effusion may be present
- Affects one or a few joints, typically those that are weight-bearing or have suffered previous injury
- Only rarely affects the wrist
- Erythrocyte sedimentation rate (ESR) normal
- No systemic illness
- Synovial fluid noninflammatory (<2000 white blood cells (WBCs)/mL)

Fibromyalgia

Fibromyalgia is a chronic musculoskeletal disorder of poorly understood pathophysiology.

FEATURES

- Widespread, diffuse pain with distinct tender points
- No evidence of inflammatory cause
- Associated problems include sleep disorders, fatigue, headaches, and irritable bowel syndrome
- ESR and complete blood count tests are normal
- May respond to corticosteroids, but not dramatically

Gout

Gout (acute or chronic) is caused by crystals of monosodium urate becoming deposited in tissue as a result of hyperuricemia.

FEATURES

- Most common in middle-aged men
- Typically affects first metatarsophalangeal joint, ankles, and midfoot. It is rare for the initial presentation of gout to affect multiple joints; polyarticular involvement generally develops later in the disease
- Associated with history of diuretic use, hypertension, alcohol consumption, renal insufficiency
- Soft tissue tophi are common around joints, in bursae, in Achilles' tendons, and at the extensor surface of the forearm; however, these are usually absent in the early stages of disease
- X-rays may show typical cystic erosions with thin overhanging edges of bone resulting from reparative changes (punched out erosions with overhanging osteophytes – 'rat bite')
- Synovial fluid contains 3000–50,000 WBCs/mm^3
- Positively diagnosed by deposition of monosodium urate crystals, visible under polarized light microscopy

Polymyalgia rheumatica

Polymyalgia rheumatica is a syndrome which may contain a complex of disease processes and whose pathophysiology is poorly understood.

FEATURES

- A syndrome in the elderly characterized by morning stiffness, stiffness and aching of the neck, shoulders, and hips. Patients almost always have a very elevated ESR
- Muscle stiffness and pain predominantly in neck, shoulder, and pelvic girdle muscles
- Knee, wrist, and metacarpophalangeal joints may be affected in some patients, although the extent of synovitis in polymyalgia rheumatica is controversial
- Stiffness and pain typically worse in the morning, improving during the day, and exacerbated by rest
- Symptoms are usually bilateral and symmetrical
- Symptoms frequently of sudden onset
- Systemic symptoms include weight loss, malaise, depression, and low-grade fever. Frequent association with temporal arteritis (giant cell arteritis)

Reiter's syndrome

Reiter's syndrome is sometimes, but not always, associated with infection by sexually transmitted urethritis or bacterial gastroenteritis.

FEATURES

- Classic triad of arthritis, urethritis, and conjunctivitis or uveitis is rarely seen
- Musculoskeletal manifestations: axial arthritis and/or peripheral arthritis (usually asymmetrical and oligoarticular with a lower extremity predominance); enthesopathy; spondyloarthropathy 'sausage digits' (dactylitis) are seen in Reiter's, but not in RA
- Dermatologic manifestations: oral aphthous ulcers, keratoderma blenorrhagica, circinate balanitis, circinate ulcerative vulvitis
- Urogenital manifestations: urethritis, prostatitis, cystitis, balanitis, cervicitis
- Ocular manifestations: conjunctivitis, scleritis, keratitis, corneal ulcerations, uveitis, iritis
- Cardiovascular manifestations: pericarditis, myocarditis, first-degree arteriovenous block, aortic regurgitation
- Systemic manifestations: fever, malaise, fatigue, anorexia, weight loss

Pseudogout

Calcium hydroxyapatite and calcium oxalate deposition diseases, such as pseudogout, should also be considered.

FEATURES

- Caused by calcium pyrophosphate dihydrate crystal deposition in articular cartilage, synovium, and periarticular ligaments and tendons
- Usually affects the knee, but also the wrist, elbow, shoulder, ankle, and hand joints
- Usually monoarticular; most common cause of acute inflammatory monoarthritis in the elderly
- Acute attacks are associated with severe pain, swelling, restricted movement, increased heat in the affected joints, and fever
- Joints in chronic disease may show bony swelling, crepitus, and restricted movement, with varying levels of synovitis; morning stiffness may also occur
- X-rays may display calcification of articular cartilage (chondrocalcinosis) and tendon inserts, and often hypertrophic appearance of bone, with exuberant formation of cysts and osteophytes

Ankylosing spondylitis

Ankylosing spondylitis is a chronic inflammatory condition involving the sacroiliac joints and axial skeleton.

FEATURES

- Most frequently found in young men under 40 years of age
- The peripheral joint involvement in ankylosing spondylitis is usually asymmetric in the lower extremity large joints
- 'Sausage digits' (dactylitis) may be seen in ankylosing spondylitis, but not in RA
- Low back pain, with prominent morning stiffness, sometimes nocturnal
- Often insidious in onset
- Chronic and progressive inflammation of the axial skeleton and sacroiliac joints
- Loss of chest expansion
- Progressive, fixed spinal deformity, with characteristic X-ray findings
- Associated with peripheral arthritis, enthesitis, and extra-articular manifestations, such as iritis

Inflammatory bowel diseases

Divided into Crohn's disease and ulcerative colitis.

FEATURES

- Peak onset is at 15–35 years of age; also at 70–80 years
- Peripheral joint involvement is usually asymmetric and in large joints. A spondyloarthopathy pattern may also be seen. The activity of the arthritis will sometimes, but not always, parallel the activity of the bowel disease
- Diarrhea (with or without blood) and abdominal pain
- Fever
- Weight loss

Systemic lupus erythematosus

Systemic lupus erythematosus is a chronic multisystemic disease of autoimmune origin.

FEATURES

- Malar or discoid rash
- Photosensitivity
- Nasal or oropharyngeal ulcerations
- Anemia
- Thrombocytopenia
- Inflammatory peripheral joint arthritis, which is rarely deforming or erosive. Jaccoud's arthropathy due to joint laxity may produce reducible ulnar drift of the fingers that may resemble RA; however, in RA, the ulnar drift is often not reducible due to subluxation of the metacarpophalangeal joints
- Pericardial and pleural effusions
- Alopecia
- Fever
- Conjunctivitis, sicca syndrome
- Abdominal tenderness, abdominal serositis
- Raynaud's phenomenon

Lyme disease

Lyme disease is a multisystem infection primarily involving skin, joints, and nervous system.

FEATURES

- Joint pain, swelling, and fatigue are common
- Positive serology (enzyme-linked immunosorbent assay (ELISA) – Western blot)
- Characteristic erythema chronicum migrans rash, not always observed
- History of deer tick bite

- Geographic distribution with endemic areas
- Possible neurologic and cardiac abnormalities
- Fibromyalgia symptoms may appear after a bout of Lyme disease

Infective endocarditis

Infective endocarditis is a syndrome resulting from microbial infection of the cardiac valves, usually by bacteria, though fungi, rickettsiae, mycoplasmas, and chlamydiae may be the cause.

FEATURES

- Fever and/or chills
- Heart murmur
- WBC count is often elevated. High titer rheumatoid factor
- Embolic phenomenon with peripheral manifestations
- Skin manifestations: petechiae, Osler nodes, splinter hemorrhages, Janeway lesions
- Splenomegaly

Sarcoidosis

A multisystem granulomatous disorder of unclear etiology, sarcoidosis is characterized pathologically by the presence of noncaseating granulomas.

FEATURES

- Affects multiple systems
- Fever, night sweats, malaise, fatigue, weight loss
- Transient, migratory arthritis of large joints, often the ankles
- Dermatologic manifestations: erythema nodosum, maculopapular eruption, development of subcutaneous nodules, and/or lupus pernio
- Interstitial lung disease, resulting in dyspnea, cough
- Anterior or posterior uveitis
- Radiologic evidence of bone cysts, punched-out lesions
- Left ventricular dysfunction, arrhythmias, conduction disturbances

Septic arthritis

Septic arthritis is highly destructive; referral is essential if suspected.

FEATURES

- Usually affects one joint (monoarthritis) – most often knee or hip
- Affected joint(s) hot, painful and swollen, with restricted range of movement
- Fever often present
- Also suspect in patient with established RA who develops an acute flare, especially after local corticosteroid therapy
- Often caused by spread of infection from a distant site, direct puncture of the joint, or spread from adjacent osteomyelitis
- Often associated with history of previously abnormal joint, RA, old age, immunocompromised status, or intravenous drug use
- Synovial fluid contains >50,000 WBCs/mm^3
- Synovial fluid positive for culture and Gram stain
- Causes no early radiographic abnormality
- If untreated, can lead to irreversible joint damage

SIGNS & SYMPTOMS
Signs

- Typically affects small joints in hands (except DIP joints) and feet; these joints are usually the first joints affected

- Wrist, elbow, neck, shoulder, hip, and ankle joints may also be involved
- Lumbar or thoracic spine not affected
- Multiple, symmetric involvement is typical
- Initial articular manifestations: swelling/effusion, restricted motion, warmth
- Eventual characteristic deformities include subluxations, dislocations, and joint contractures
- Rheumatoid nodules: subcutaneous nodules over bony prominences (e.g. the elbow and shaft of the ulna) in 20–30% of patients
- Chronic inflammation of the tendon sheaths
- Possible tendon rupture
- Low-grade fever may be apparent
- Swollen lymph glands
- Anemia
- Leg ulcers
- Splenomegaly

Symptoms

- Symptoms usually have gradual onset and may last for years
- Constitutional symptoms may precede articular involvement: fatigue (especially early afternoon), malaise, loss of appetite, and weakness
- Low-grade fever may also be apparent
- Typically affects small joints in hands (except DIP joints) and feet; these joints are usually the first joints affected
- Wrist, elbow, neck, shoulder, hip, and ankle joints may also be involved
- Lumbar or thoracic spine not affected
- Multiple, symmetric involvement is typical
- Initial articular manifestations: swelling/effusion, restricted motion, warmth
- Stiffness, lasting more than one hour, especially after sleep or rest
- Eventual characteristic deformities include subluxations, dislocations, and joint contractures
- Rheumatoid nodules: painless, subcutaneous nodules over bony prominences (e.g. the elbow and shaft of the ulna)
- Chronic inflammation of the tendon sheaths
- Possible tendon rupture
- Swollen glands
- Burning or itching sensation in eyes; inflammation
- Pallor
- Numbness or tingling
- Leg ulcers
- Shortness of breath

ASSOCIATED DISORDERS

- Depression: living with arthritis can cause depression in some patients
- Interstitial lung disease
- Septic arthritis

KEY! DON'T MISS!

Refer to rheumatology immediately if septic arthritis is suspected.

CONSIDER CONSULT

- Refer to rheumatology to confirm or establish diagnosis (differential diagnosis may be difficult, and early treatment is essential). All patients with RA should be followed by a rheumatologist, possibly in conjunction with the primary care physician (PCP)
- Refer to rheumatology immediately if septic arthritis is suspected

INVESTIGATION OF THE PATIENT

Direct questions to patient

Q How long have you had the symptoms? Owing to the chronic nature of the disease, the patient may not seek a diagnosis immediately. Treatment is most successful within 1–2 years of onset

Q What were you doing when you first noticed the pain? Rules out trauma as source of pain

Q Have you had any illnesses or accidents that may have caused the pain? Rules out other causes of the symptoms

Q Is there a family history of arthritis/joint pain? Indicates presence or absence of familial connection

Q On a scale of 1–10, how bad is your joint pain? How much pain have you had in the last week? Indicates level of disease and quality-of-life impairment. Use a visual analog scale

Q Is the pain in one or more joints? Arthritis in three or more joints suggests RA

Q When does the pain occur? Rheumatoid patients have constant pain that is worse in the morning

Q How often is it painful for you to dress yourself? To get in and out of bed? To lift a cup to your lips? To walk outdoors on flat ground? To wash and dry all of your body? To bend down and pick clothing from the floor? Turn faucets? Get in and out of a car? Indicates level of impairment

Q How long do you feel stiff after you wake up? How severe is the stiffness? Indicates level of disease and quality-of-life impairment. Morning stiffness lasting over one hour is strongly indicative of RA

Q Do you feel tired, especially midafternoon? Indicates level of disease and quality-of-life impairment

Q How well are you able to carry out everyday activities? Answer will indicate functional status and quality of life

Q What medicines are you taking? The answer may affect possible treatment

Family history

Q Do any members of your family have similar symptoms or been diagnosed with RA? There is a genetic predisposition to developing RA.

Examination

- Are there any actively inflamed joints? Symmetric inflammation with swelling of the small joints in the periphery strongly suggests RA. Also indicates baseline level of disease

- Are there any mechanical joint problems, such as loss of motion, instability, malalignment, and/or deformity? Some signs are characteristic of RA. Also indicates baseline level of disease and quality of life

- Are there any rheumatoid nodules present? Presence strongly indicates RA

- Are there any extra-articular manifestations/complications? Indicates level of disease and need for additional treatment/care

- Complete history, review of systems, and a thorough general and musculoskeletal examination are essential for diagnosis and to establish level of disease

- History, joint examination, and functional assessment indicate prognosis during first 2 years of disease

A classification of global functional status has been proposed by the American College of Rheumatology:

- Class 1: completely able to perform usual daily activities
- Class 2: able to perform usual self-care and vocational activities, but limited in avocational activities
- Class 3: able to perform usual self-care, but limited in vocational and avocational activities
- Class 4: limited in usual self-care, vocational, and avocational activities

Summary of investigative tests

- ESR or C-reactive protein tests indicate level of disease activity in some patients, and elevated C-reactive protein correlates with the development of erosive disease
- Serum rheumatoid factor: tested only at baseline to establish diagnosis; may be repeated 6-12 months after disease onset if initially negative
- Complete blood count: performed at baseline before starting therapy. Also serum electrolyte and creatinine levels, hepatic and renal function tests, and stool guaiac
- Synovial fluid
- X-rays of selected involved joints (usually hands and/or feet): may have limited diagnostic value in early disease, but helps to establish a baseline from which to measure disease progression or response to therapy. Erosions are found earlier in the feet than in the hands

DIAGNOSTIC DECISION

According to the American College of Rheumatology, RA is present when four of seven criteria are present. (These criteria were developed for distinguishing established RA for inclusion into clinical studies and are not necessarily adequate for the diagnosis of early RA.)

1. Morning stiffness lasting more than one hour
2. Arthritis in three or more joints, with soft-tissue swelling or fluid
3. Arthritis of hand joints with soft-tissue swelling
4. Symmetric arthritis
5. Rheumatoid nodules
6. Serum rheumatoid factor
7. Radiographic changes consistent with RA

- Criteria 1–4 must have been present for at least 6 weeks
- Criteria 2–5 must be observed by a physician

Guidelines

The American Rheumatism Association has revised criteria for the classification of rheumatoid arthritis [1].

CLINICAL PEARLS

- Almost always involves the small joints of the hands and feet
- Virtually all patients with RA have prolonged morning stiffness
- A patient with symmetrical inflammatory arthritis of the small joints of the hands and feet very likely has RA

THE TESTS
Body fluids
ERYTHROCYTE SEDIMENTATION RATE
Description
Venous blood sample.

Advantages/Disadvantages
Advantages:
- Simple, safe sample procedure that may be combined with other tests
- Elevated levels are observed in 90% of cases
- Indicates level of disease activity

Normal
Females: 0–20mm/h; males 0–15mm/h (Westergren method).

Abnormal
- Females: >30mm/h; males >20mm/h in males (Westergren method)
- Keep in mind the possibility of a false-positive result

Cause of abnormal result
Inflammatory disease activity.

Drugs, disorders and other factors that may alter results
Many other conditions are also associated with an increase in the ESR, including:
- Many other forms of arthritis, e.g. ankylosing spondylitis and connective tissue diseases, and other inflammatory states
- Infections
- Myocardial infarction
- Neoplasms

C-REACTIVE PROTEIN
Description
- Venous blood sample
- Alternative to ESR test

Advantages/Disadvantages
Advantages:
- Simple, safe sample procedure that may be combined with other tests
- Positive test may be a positive indication in patients with no rheumatoid factor
- Indicates level of disease activity
- May correlate better with development of erosive disease than ESR

Normal
6.8–820mcg/dL.

Abnormal
- >0.7pg/mL in many cases of RA
- Keep in mind the possibility of a false-positive result

Cause of abnormal result
Inflammatory disease activity.

Drugs, disorders and other factors that may alter results
Many other conditions are also associated with increased C-reactive protein levels, including:
- Rheumatic fever
- Inflammatory bowel disease
- Bacterial infections
- Myocardial infarction
- Oral contraceptives
- Pregnancy (third trimester)
- Inflammatory and malignant diseases

RHEUMATOID FACTOR
Description
Venous blood sample.

Advantages/Disadvantages
Advantage: simple, safe sample procedure that may be combined with other tests

Disadvantages:

- Nonspecific. About 20% of patients have seronegative RA
- Rheumatoid factor is present in some people who never develop the disease (patients with systemic lupus, endocarditis, other infectious and inflammatory diseases)
- Sample needs to be sent away for analysis

Normal
Negative.

Abnormal

- Latex fixation tube dilution titer of at least 1:160 or nephelometry measurement of over 20 IU/mL
- Keep in mind the possibility of a false-positive result

Cause of abnormal result

- Rheumatoid factor test is positive in 70–80% of people with symptoms of RA
- Rheumatoid factor is present in some people who never develop the disease

Drugs, disorders and other factors that may alter results
Many other conditions may cause the presence of rheumatoid factor, including:

- Granulomatous diseases
- Chronic infections or inflammatory processes
- Liver disease
- Multiple myeloma
- Pulmonary fibrosis
- Sjögren's syndrome
- Sarcoidosis
- Subacute bacterial endocarditis
- Systemic lupus erythematosus

COMPLETE BLOOD COUNT
Description
Venous blood sample.

Advantages/Disadvantages
Advantages:

- Simple, safe sample procedure that may be combined with other tests
- Also indicates safety of certain drugs (which may affect blood cell counts) in particular patients

Normal

- WBCs: 3200–9800/mm^3 (3.2–9.8x10^9/L)
- Red blood cells: males, 4.3–5.9x10^6/mm^3 (4.3–5.9x10^{12}/L); females, 3.5–5.0x10^6/mm^3 (3.5–5.0x10^{12}/L)
- Hemoglobin: males, 13.6–17.7g/dL (136–172g/L); females, 12–15g/dL (120–150g/L)
- Hematocrit: males, 39–49% (0.39–0.49); females, 33–43% (0.33–0.43)
- Mean corpuscular hemoglobin: 27–33pg
- Mean corpuscular hemoglobin concentration: 33–37g/dL (330–370g/L)
- Platelet count: 130–400x10^3/mm^3 (130–400x10^9/L)

Abnormal

- Mild anemia (normochromic-normocytic; hemoglobin 10g/dL (100g/L)) and/or thrombocytosis often occur in RA
- Mild leukocytosis may also occur, but a drastically lowered white cell count is seen in Felty's syndrome
- Keep in mind the possibility of a false-positive result

Cause of abnormal result
May be caused by RA.

Drugs, disorders and other factors that may alter results
Thrombocytosis, mild leukocytosis, and normochromic-normocytic anemia are typical of many other chronic diseases.

SERUM ELECTROLYTE LEVELS
Description
Venous blood sample.

Advantages/Disadvantages
Advantages:
- Simple, safe sample procedure that may be combined with other tests
- Indicates presence or absence of comorbid diseases and therefore indicates safety of certain drugs in particular patients

Normal
- Sodium: 135–147mEq/L (135–147mmol/L)
- Potassium: 3.5–5mEq/L (3.5–5mmol/L)
- Calcium: 8.8–10.3mEq/L (4.4–5.15mmol/L)
- Chloride: 95–105mEq/L (95–105mmol/L)

Abnormal
- Values outside the ranges above
- Keep in mind the possibility of a false-positive result

Cause of abnormal result
Comorbid conditions or comedication.

Drugs, disorders and other factors that may alter results
Numerous conditions cause serum electrolyte imbalances. Those especially relevant to the administration of drugs for RA are the following:
- Renal insufficiency or failure
- Diuretics
- Nephrotic syndrome
- Congestive heart failure

SERUM CREATININE LEVELS
Description
Venous blood sample.

Advantages/Disadvantages
Advantages:
- Simple, safe sample procedure that may be combined with other tests
- Indicates safety of certain drugs (which may affect renal function) in particular patients

Disadvantage: sample needs to be sent away for analysis

Normal
0.6–1.2mg/dL (50–110mcmol/L).

Abnormal
- Above 1.2mg/dL (110mcmol/L)
- Keep in mind the possibility of a false-positive result

Cause of abnormal result
Raised creatinine levels are indicative of renal disease.

Drugs, disorders and other factors that may alter results
Also raised in cases of decreased renal perfusion and urinary tract infections.

Tests of function
HEPATIC FUNCTION
Description
Venous blood sample.

Advantages/Disadvantages
Advantages:
- Simple, safe sample procedure that may be combined with other tests
- Indicates safety of certain drugs (which may affect hepatic function) in particular patients

Disadvantage: sample needs to be sent away for analysis

Normal
- Bilirubin, total: 0–1.0mg/dL (2–18mcmol/L)
- Alanine aminotransferase: 0–35U/L (0.058mckat/L)
- Alkaline phosphatase: 30–120U/L (0.5–2.0mckat/L)
- Albumin: 4–6g/dL (40–60g/L)
- Prothrombin time: 10–12s

Abnormal
- Above the normal ranges for bilirubin, alanine aminotransferase, alkaline phosphatase, and prothrombin time
- Below the normal range for albumin
- Keep in mind the possibility of a falsely abnormal result

Cause of abnormal result
Hepatic disease or dysfunction.

Drugs, disorders and other factors that may alter results
Many drugs and conditions may affect hepatic function tests, including:
- Steroids
- Antibiotics
- Oral contraceptives
- Pulmonary embolism or infarction
- Congestive heart failure
- Myocardial infarction
- Narcotics
- Antihypertensive agents
- Nonsteroidal anti-inflammatory drugs (NSAIDs)
- Pregnancy
- Nephrotic syndrome
- Alcohol

RENAL FUNCTION
Description
Urinalysis.

Advantages/Disadvantages
Advantages:
- Simple, safe sample
- Indicates safety of certain drugs (which may affect renal function) in particular patients

Disadvantage: sample needs to be sent away for analysis

Normal
- Chloride: 110–250mEq/day (110–250mmol/L/day)
- Occult blood: none
- Osmolarity: 50–1200mOsm/kg
- pH: 4.6–8
- Phosphate: 0.8–2.0g/24h
- Potassium: 25–100mEq/24h
- Protein: <150mg/24h
- Sodium: 40–220mEq/day (40–220mmol/L/day)
- Specific gravity: 1.005–1.03

Abnormal
- Lowered chloride levels
- Presence of occult blood
- Decreased osmolarity
- Elevated pH
- Phosphate outside range
- Lowered potassium levels
- Raised protein levels
- Raised sodium levels
- Decreased specific gravity

Cause of abnormal result
Renal disease or dysfunction.

Drugs, disorders and other factors that may alter results
Many other forms of arthritis may cause renal disease, including systemic lupus erythematosus and vasculitis.

Other conditions and drugs that may alter results include:
- Diuretics
- NSAIDs
- Corticosteroids
- Diabetes insipidus
- Diabetes mellitus
- Aspirin
- High protein or vegetarian diet
- Antibiotics
- Antacids
- Diarrhea or vomiting
- Congestive heart failure
- Hypertension
- Hepatic failure

Imaging
X-RAYS
Description
X-rays of hand and/or foot.

Advantages/Disadvantages
Advantages:
- Allows course of disease to be monitored
- Essential in diagnosis
- Involves relatively low levels of radiation exposure

Disadvantage: may require visit to health center

Abnormal
- Early disease: soft-tissue swelling and periarticular osteopenia
- Established disease: joint-space narrowing, erosions, and deformity

Cause of abnormal result
Rheumatoid arthritis.

Special tests
SYNOVIAL FLUID ANALYSIS
Description
Synovial fluid sample.

Advantages/Disadvantages
Advantage: differentiates RA from septic arthritis, gout, or pseudogout.

Normal
- Clear appearance and sterile
- WBC count $<200/mm^3$
- Firm mucin clot formation

Abnormal
- Straw-colored, cloudy appearance, but sterile
- Poor mucin clot formation
- WBC count of $3000–50,000/mm^3$
- Decreased synovial fluid glucose
- Increased polymorphonuclear leukocyte count
- Keep in mind the possibility of a nondiagnostic abnormal result

Cause of abnormal result
Possible RA.

Drugs, disorders and other factors that may alter results
Other diseases may affect synovial fluid:
- Osteoarthritis
- Gout
- Pseudogout
- Reiter's syndrome
- Psoriatic arthritis
- Rheumatic fever
- Septic arthritis

STOOL GUAIAC
Description
Stool sample.

Advantages/Disadvantages
- Advantage: simple, safe sample
- Disadvantage: sample may need to be sent away for analysis

Normal
No occult blood.

Abnormal
- Occult blood loss indicated
- Keep in mind the possibility of a falsely abnormal result

Cause of abnormal result
Gastrointestinal bleeding.

Drugs, disorders and other factors that may alter results
NSAIDs.

CONSIDER CONSULT

- Refer to rheumatology for corticosteroid (systemic or local), 'second-line' agent, or drug combination therapy
- Refer to rheumatology to establish long-term treatment plan
- Refer to rheumatology if the treatment is effective but drug toxicity/intolerance emerges
- Refer to rheumatology if disease onset is severe and requires especially aggressive therapy
- Refer to physical/occupational therapy to establish recommendations/training and for rehabilitation following surgery
- Refer to surgery for timing and need of interventions and to co-ordinate pre- and postsurgery medication
- Refer to nursing or social welfare if the patient's independence is compromised and the patient does not have adequate support
- Referral for health education and/or clinical psychology is thought to decrease pain, increase coping ability, and decrease number of physician appointments
- Referral to podiatry may be needed if there is foot involvement

IMMEDIATE ACTION

Refer immediately to rheumatology or orthopedics if septic arthritis is suspected. Effective treatment that should be started before a firm diagnosis includes:

- Patient education
- Pain control
- Rest and exercise
- Thermotherapy
- Adjunctive drug therapy

PATIENT AND CAREGIVER ISSUES
Impact on career, dependants, family, friends

- The patient may become increasingly dependent upon others as disability progresses
- Progressive disability may also affect the ability of patients to carry out their profession

Patient or caregiver request

- **Can rheumatoid arthritis (RA) be cured?** The condition cannot be cured, but there is a good chance that it can be controlled
- **Will I be disabled?** Approx. 50% of patients will become disabled or unable to work within 10 years of diagnosis. However, keep in mind that this data is based on the treatment regimen of 10–20 years ago
- **Should I take an over-the-counter (OTC) pain killer?** The patient may be concerned about gastrointestinal side-effects
- **Do corticosteroids have bad side-effects?** Corticosteroids are associated with weight gain, fluid retention, increased blood sugar, diabetes, and bone loss. Depression or agitation may also occur

Health-seeking behavior

Has the patient been self-medicating? The patient may have been treating the pain and/or inflammation with OTC drugs, which may have hidden the symptoms for some time.

MANAGEMENT ISSUES
Goals

Early recognition and diagnosis, and timely introduction of therapy is the primary goal. Once diagnosis has been made and treatment started, goals are to:

- Control disease activity and slow rate of joint damage

- Minimize pain, stiffness, inflammation, and complications
- Improve functional status and quality of life

Management in special circumstances

RA often affects the elderly, who are more susceptible to drug side-effects and are more likely to be taking comedications.

COEXISTING DISEASE

- Peptic ulcer disease: caution is necessary with NSAIDs
- Diabetes: caution is necessary with NSAIDs
- Renal insufficiency: avoid NSAIDs

COEXISTING MEDICATION

- Insulin: be cautious using NSAIDs in patients with diabetes
- Cancer chemotherapy: may produce thrombocytopenia, in which case NSAIDs should not be used

SPECIAL PATIENT GROUPS

Pregnant patients:

- Etanercept, methotrexate, leflunomide, hydroxychloroquine, and infliximab are not recommended for pregnant patients
- Guidelines for the use of other drugs in pregnant patients may be obtained from the American College of Rheumatology [2]
- Corticosteroids may be prescribed as the principal therapy during pregnancy. Sulfasalazine may also be given during pregnancy

Elderly patients:

- Elderly patients can sometimes be managed with low-dose corticosteroids alone. Immunosuppressive therapy should be used with great caution

PATIENT SATISFACTION/LIFESTYLE PRIORITIES

- Alcohol consumption should be avoided with methotrexate
- Parenteral gold, parenteral methotrexate, local injections of corticosteroids, and infliximab administration require visits to a clinic and possible discomfort
- Etanercept is administered by subcutaneous injection
- Apheresis (Prosorba column) requires regular visits to an apheresis center
- Surgery requires recovery and rehabilitation

SUMMARY OF THERAPEUTIC OPTIONS
Choices

Treatment should always be discussed with the patient.

Adjunctive drug treatment:

- Pain control is the first consideration in therapy and should be initiated immediately, even before a diagnosis
- Acetaminophen (paracetamol) relieves pain only
- NSAIDs relieve both pain and inflammation. No one drug (including cyclo-oxygenase (COX-2) inhibitors) is categorical superior in efficacy to the others. There are substantial differences from one patient to the other with regard to the efficacy of individual agents
- Corticosteroids (usually prednisone or prednisolone) may also be given orally to treat refractory/aggressive disease, to control symptoms during special life events, and during pregnancy. Local injections (usually a long-acting compound, such as triamcinolone hexacetonide) may be given occasionally to treat persistent effusions, recover lost joint motion, or treat the most symptomatic joints early in the disease

Disease-modifying antirheumatic drugs (DMARDs) are given to control the disease process, and should be started early as irreversible damage occurs within 1–2 years of diagnosis, and early intervention (<3 months after diagnosis) improves most markers and outcome measures at 1–5 years compared with patients in whom treatment was delayed.

- Choice of agent is heavily dependent on the each patient's particular situation and each patient's preferences and concerns about risks
- Treatment must be sustained indefinitely as there is no treatment that is curative
- These compounds are slow-acting: an effect is apparent after several months
- Fertile women should use effective contraception
- Methotrexate is the most common first-choice agent. The discontinuation rate is low compared with other agents. Watch for liver and pulmonary toxicity
- Sulfasalazine is another common first-choice agent. Often used as first-choice drug to treat mild disease with no poor prognostic features. Contraindicated in sulfa-allergic patients
- Leflunomide is a newer, effective agent, which is given orally and has been shown to reduce radiographic progression. It may be combined with methotrexate
- Antimalarial drugs include hydroxychloroquine, another common first-choice agent. Often used as first-choice drug to treat mild disease with no poor prognostic features. Has low toxicity but may have relatively low efficacy and relatively ineffective in preventing radiographic damage. Requires periodic eye examinations by an ophthalmologist
- Azathioprine is a useful disease-modifying antirheumatic drug but is used less commonly than almost all other DMARDs. Complete blood count should be monitored regularly
- Parenteral gold is rarely used today
- Oral gold (auranofin) is less effective but is also less toxic than parenteral gold
- Etanercept and infliximab are new, highly effective, parenterally administered tumor necrosis factor (TNF) antagonists. They may be used to treat patients with severe disease, poor prognostic features, and refractory disease. Both are often given in combination with methotrexate. In contrast with the agents mentioned above, these TNF antagonists usually produce a rapid onset of action
- Anakinra (interleukin (IL)-1 receptor antagonist) is another biologic agent that counters the effect of IL-1, another potent proinflammatory cytokine. Although its efficacy appears to be less than that of the TNF antagonists, it may have the potential to retard radiographic progression to a greater degree than other agents
- Minocycline is sometimes used in RA. It may have a role in early, mild disease. This is an off-label indication
- Combinations of two or more agents may be beneficial
- Methotrexate has been successfully combined with leflunomide, etanercept, infliximab, and sulfasalazine/hydroxychloroquine

Other therapies:
- Physical therapy (balneotherapy, thermotherapy, dynamic exercise) and occupational therapy may be initiated before a firm diagnosis, as may lifestyle changes
- Dynamic exercise therapy is an essential part of treatment
- Splints (to immobilize acutely and severely inflamed joints until anti-inflammatory medication takes effect) and self-help devices may assist daily living
- Low-level laser therapy
- Apheresis (Prosorba column): Prosorba immunosorption has been demonstrated effective in patients with long-standing severe disease
- Complementary therapies: nutrition (eliminating food allergies, following a vegetarian diet, modifying intake of dietary antioxidants and fats/oils), supplementation with selenium and vitamin E, and curcumin (strong anti-inflammatory and antioxidant properties)

Surgical therapy can be performed to treat severe joint damage:
- Joint replacement may be considered if the patient suffers refractory pain and a marked drop in the quality of life

- Tendon reconstruction is indicated where there is tendon damage
- Synovectomy, a temporary measure, is performed as part of reconstructive surgery or may preserve joint function if drugs are ineffective
- Carpal tunnel release and resection of metatarsal heads are other highly effective procedures

Guidelines

- The American College of Rheumatology and Subcommittee on Rheumatoid arthritis guidelines. Guidelines for the management of rheumatoid arthritis 2002 update [3]
- The American College of Rheumatology. Guidelines for monitoring drug therapy in rheumatoid arthritis [2]
- American College of Rheumatology. Preliminary definition of improvement in rheumatoid arthritis [4]
- Guidelines for prescribing methotrexate have been produced by the American College of Rheumatology. American College of Rheumatology Position Statement: Methotrexate [5]
- Methotrexate for rheumatoid arthritis. Suggested guidelines for monitoring liver toxicity from the American College of Rheumatology [6]

Clinical pearls

- A DMARD should be started as soon as the diagnosis of RA is certain
- The goal of therapy should be the elimination of synovitis, not simply improving the comfort and quality of life of the patient
- Most patients with RA will require therapy with a combination of DMARDs

Never

- Never prescribe corticosteroids or 'second-line' agents without the guidance of a rheumatologist
- Do not treat acute flares of the disease without first ruling out septic arthritis

FOLLOW UP

- Regular and frequent follow up visits throughout the remaining life of the patient are essential
- Patients in remission may be seen twice a year; patients with more active disease should be seen more often
- Sessions with a rheumatologist (8–9 visits/year) have been associated with slower rates of disease progression than with sporadic specialist care
- Guidelines for monitoring drug therapy in RA been published by the American College of Rheumatology [2]

Plan for review

- Monitor the course of the disease
- Establish whether the disease is active; check for inflammatory signs and symptoms
- Periodically measure ESR and/or C-reactive protein
- Periodically take X-rays of affected joints
- Monitor for emergence of complications
- Periodically assess functional status and quality of life using questionnaires such as the Health Assessment Questionnaire
- Determine the benefits and toxicity of treatment
- Change treatment as needed

Reference

Health Assessment Questionnaire
Fries JF, SpitzP, Kraines RG, et al. Measurement of patient outcome in arthritis. Arthritis Rheum 1980;23:137–45

Information for patient or caregiver
Education is very important, and may be related to patient outcome. Information should include:
- How arthritis affects people
- How patients can be involved helping themselves
- The various treatments that physicians prescribe and how they improve outcome
- How to deal with stress (and other forms of psychologic counseling) can also be very useful

DRUGS AND OTHER THERAPIES: DETAILS
Drugs
ACETAMINOPHEN (OTC)
Very useful analgesic for symptomatic relief.

Dose
325–1000mg orally every 4h. Up to 4g/day orally may be taken without generating significant side-effects (in patients without liver disease). However, there is some recent evidence that high doses may be associated with increased gastrointestinal toxicity.

Efficacy
Effectively controls mild-to-moderate pain. However, it has no effect on inflammation.

Risks/Benefits
Risks:
- Use caution in hepatic and renal impairment
- Overdosage results in hepatic and renal damage unless treated promptly
- Overdose may lead to multiorgan failure and may be fatal
- Accidental overdosage can occur if OTC preparations containing acetaminophen are taken with prescribed drugs that contain acetaminophen

Benefit: pain is reduced quickly before the effect of 'second-line' agents is apparent

Side-effects and adverse reactions
- Acetaminophen rarely causes side-effects when used intermittently
- Gastrointestinal: nausea, vomiting
- Hematologic: blood disorders
- Metabolic: acute hepatic and renal failure
- Skin: rashes
- Other: acute pancreatitis

Interactions (other drugs)
- Alcohol ■ Anticoagulants ■ Anticonvulsants ■ Isoniazid ■ Cholestyramine ■ Colestipol ■ Domperidone ■ Metoclopromide

Contraindications
Known liver dysfunction.

Acceptability to patient
High.

Follow up plan
Monitor patient's feelings of pain.

Patient and caregiver information
- The patient/caregiver must be made aware of possible side-effects and the necessity of reporting them if they occur

- The importance of compliance with therapy must be stressed

NONSTEROIDAL ANTI-INFLAMMATORY DRUGS

- Relieve pain and inflammation, but do not modify disease progression
- No one drug has been found to be consistently superior to others; individual responses may vary
- Select according to dosing regimen, efficacy, tolerance, costs, patient's age, concomitant disease, concurrent drugs, patient's preferences
- Drugs may need to be changed occasionally to minimize side-effects and possibly increase benefits
- Combinations of NSAIDs should be avoided, because of increased risk of gastrointestinal toxicity
- One drug should be tried for 10–14 days for efficacy

Dose

- Aspirin: delayed-release, enteric-coated tablets, are indicated in patients who need the higher 15-grain (975mg) dose of aspirin in the long-term palliative treatment of mild-to-moderate pain and inflammation of arthritic and other inflammatory conditions
- Adult: one 325mg tablet 3–4 times daily
- Patients who have displayed no significant adverse effects on a long-term four times daily regimen and who receive a total daily dosage of aspirin no greater than 3.9g may be considered for a twice-daily regimen (two tablets of enteric-coated aspirin twice daily). Patients on the twice-daily enteric-coated aspirin regimen should be closely monitored for serum salicylate levels, increased incidence of central nervous system-related adverse effects, increased fecal blood loss, or any other signs or symptoms suggestive of significant blood loss
- Start slowly: for aspirin begin at 0.6–1.0mg/day

Efficacy
Effectively relieves mild-to-moderate pain.

Risks/Benefits
Risks:
- Use caution in elderly and children
- Use caution in hepatic, renal, and cardiac failure
- Use caution in bleeding disorders
- There is no evidence that final outcome is changed by NSAIDs

Side-effects and adverse reactions

- Cardiovascular system: hypertension, peripheral edema, congestive heart failure
- Central nervous system: headache, dizziness, tinnitus, fever
- Gastrointestinal: anorexia, nausea, dyspepsia, peptic ulceration, bleeding
- Genitourinary: nephrotoxicity
- Hematologic: blood cell disorders
- Hypersensitivity: rashes, bronchospasm, angioedema
- Skin: pruritus, rash

Interactions (other drugs)

- Aminoglycosides Anticoagulants Antihypertensives Baclofen Corticosteroids Cyclosporine, tacrolimus Digoxin Diuretics Lithium Methotrexate Phenylpropanolamine Warfarin

Contraindications

- Peptic ulceration Hypersensitivity to NSAIDs Coagulation defects Severe renal or hepatic disease

Evidence

- A systematic review found no significant difference between different NSAIDs for the treatment of tender joints in patients with rheumatoid arthritis [7] *Level M*
- A RCT compared celecoxib (COX-2 inhibitor) with naproxen in patients with rheumatoid arthritis. Similar efficacy was noted for the drugs, but fewer peptic ulcers were seen with celecoxib [8] *Level P*

Acceptability to patient

Medium: some patients may be unable to tolerate these drugs.

Follow up plan

- Monitor level of active synovitis
- Adverse events should be carefully monitored
- Blood levels should be monitored for aspirin
- Guidelines for monitoring drug therapy in RA been published by the American College of Rheumatology [2]

Patient and caregiver information

- The patient/caregiver must be made aware of possible side-effects and the necessity of reporting them if they occur
- The importance of compliance with therapy must be stressed

CORTICOSTEROIDS

- Prednisolone and prednisone are the systemic corticosteroids of choice (except for local injection)
- A long-acting compound, such as triamcinolone hexacetonide, is preferred for local injections
- Used as 'bridging' therapy (<3 months) when introducing DMARD, in refractory/aggressive disease (short- to moderate-term use), or during special life events
- May be used during pregnancy
- Long-term use (>3 months) is associated with toxicity; the risk/benefit ratio must be carefully considered
- Local injections may be given every 3 months or more to reduce persistent effusions (treatment of choice for Baker's cyst of the knee), recover lost joint motion, or treat the most symptomatic joints early in the disease

Dose

- Bridging therapy: approx. prednisone (or equivalent) 5–10mg/day orally
- Higher doses may be needed for patients with extra-articular complications (e.g. neuropathy, vasculitis, pleuritis, pericarditis, and scleritis)
- The dose of solutions used for local injection depends on the size of the joint. In general, 1cc for large joints such as the knee, ankle, or shoulder, 0.5cc for the wrist, and 0.25cc for small joints in the hands

Efficacy

- Highly effective in reducing joint inflammation and disease activity
- Long-term use (>3 months) may reduce radiologic progression during the first 12 months of treatment, but this does not persist
- Relief of symptoms may only be short-term (average 9 months)

Risks/Benefits

Risks:

- Slow-acting
- False-negative skin allergy tests

- Overwhelming septicemia if patient has an infection
- Loss of control of blood glucose in those with diabetes
- Use caution in elderly due to risk of diabetes and osteoporosis
- Use caution in patients with psychosis, seizure disorders, myasthenia gravis, congestive heart failure, hypertension, ulcerative colitis, peptic ulcer, esophagitis
- May mask the signs of an acute abdomen or intussusception
- Prolonged use causes adrenal suppression
- Use caution in glaucoma and renal disease
- Prednisone taken in doses higher than 7.5mg for a period of 3 weeks or longer may lead to clinically relevant suppression of the pituitary-adrenal axis

Benefit: significantly effective in reducing signs and symptoms of RA

Side-effects and adverse reactions
- Side-effects are minimized by short duration of therapy
- Cardiovascular system: hypertension, thromboembolism
- Central nervous system: insomnia, euphoria, depression, psychosis, seizures
- Endocrine: adrenal suppression, impaired glucose tolerance, growth suppression in children, Cushing's syndrome
- Eyes, ears, nose, and throat: cataract, glaucoma, blurred vision
- Gastrointestinal: dyspepsia, peptic ulceration, esophagitis, oral candidiasis, nausea, diarrhea
- Musculoskeletal: proximal myopathy, osteoporosis
- Skin: delayed healing, acne, striae

Interactions (other drugs)
- Adrenergic neurone-blockers, alpha-blockers, beta-blockers, beta-2 agonists
- Aminoglutethimide Anticonvulsants (carbemazepine, phenytoin, barbiturates)
- Antibiotics (clarithromycin, erythromycin, troleandomycin) Antidiabetics
- Antidysrhythmics (calcium channel blockers, cardiac glycosides) Antifungals (amphotericin, ketoconazole) Antihypertensives (angiotensin-converting enzyme (ACE) inhibitors, diuretics: loop and thiazide, acetazolamide; angiotensin II receptor antagonists, clonidine, diazoxide, hydralazine, methyldopa, minoxidil) Cardiac glycosides
- Cholestyramine Colestipol Cyclosporine Diuretics Isoniazid Ketoconazole
- Methotrexate NSAIDs Nitrates Nitroprusside Oral contraceptives Rifampin
- Ritonavir Saliclyates Somatropin Vaccines Warfarin

Contraindications
- Systemic infection Avoid live virus vaccines in those receiving immunosuppressive doses History of tuberculosis Cushing's syndrome Recent myocardial infarction

Evidence
- A systematic review found that short-term low-dose prednisolone (not more than 15mg/day) is more effective than placebo for the control of disease activity, and may be used intermittently in RA. Joint tenderness and pain were significantly more improved with prednisolone than NSAIDs [9] *Level M*
- A systematic review found that moderate-term prednisone treatment was more effective than placebo in the management of RA [10] *Level M*

Acceptability to patient
- High in the short-term, for oral administration, but side-effects may decrease acceptability with extended treatment
- Low for local injections: discomfort and inconvenience of meeting the practitioner decrease acceptability

Follow up plan
- Careful, regular monitoring is essential to avoid potentially dangerous toxicity
- Guidelines for monitoring drug therapy in RA been published by the American College of Rheumatology [2]
- Monitor level of synovitis and restoration of range of motion

Patient and caregiver information
- The patient/caregiver must be made aware of possible side-effects and the necessity of reporting them if they occur
- The importance of compliance with therapy must be stressed

METHOTREXATE
- The most common first choice and most widely used DMARD
- Often combined with other DMARDs: has been combined with sulfasalazine plus hydroxychloroquine, leflunomide, etanercept, infliximab, and anakinra to treat refractory disease
- Folic acid 1–2mg/day reduces oral and gastrointestinal toxicity without impairing efficacy (folinic acid 5mg once a week may also be used)

Dose
- Dosage should be individualized
- An initial test dose may be given prior to the regular dosage schedule to detect any extreme sensitivity to adverse effects
- 7.5–20mg/week orally as a single weekly oral dose, or divided into three oral dosages, given at 12-h intervals, once weekly
- Parenteral administration essential for doses >20mg/week, or in patients with gastrointestinal side-effects or refractory disease with oral methotrexate
- Gradual dose increase is recommended (2.5–5mg/week every 3–4 weeks)
- Once response has been achieved reduce to lowest possible effective dose

Efficacy
Very effective for reducing the signs and symptoms of RA as well as preventing the progression of radiographic damage.

Risks/Benefits
Risks:
- Must be administered under specialist supervision
- Serious toxic reactions are possible, which may be fatal
- Only use with severe recalcitrant, disabling disease which is not adequately responsive to other forms of therapy
- The patient should be fully informed of the risks involved
- Closely monitor for bone marrow, liver, lung, and kidney toxicity
- Use caution with infection and bone marrow depression, peptic ulceration and ulcerative colitis, and renal and hepatic impairment
- Use caution in the elderly

Benefits:
- Reduces joint inflammation and radiologic progression, and improves functional status
- Effect noticeable in 1–2 months
- Relatively low discontinuation rate
- Relatively inexpensive; monitoring for toxicity is also relatively inexpensive

Side-effects and adverse reactions
- Central nervous system: headache, seizures, dizziness, drowsiness

- Eyes, ears, nose, and throat: visual disturbances, tinnitus
- Gastrointestinal: abdominal pain, diarrhea, hepatotoxicity, nausea, vomiting, stomatitis
- Genitourinary: renal failure, urinary retention, depression of and defective spermatogenesis, hematuria
- Hematologic: blood cell disorders
- Musculoskeletal: osteoporosis, muscle pain and wasting
- Respiratory: pulmonary fibrosis
- Skin: rashes, acne, dermatitis, alopecia, hyperpigmentation, vasculitis

Interactions (other drugs)

- Alcohol
- Aminoglycosides
- Antimalarials
- Binding resins
- Co-trimoxazole
- Cyclosporine
- Etretrinate
- Live vaccines
- NSAIDs
- Omeprazole
- Penicillins
- Probenicid
- Salicylates
- Sulfinpyrazone

Contraindications

- Severe renal and hepatic impairment
- Profound bone marrow depression
- Nursing mothers, pregnancy; conception should also be avoided for 6 months after stopping
- Safety and effectiveness in pediatric patients have not been established, other than in cancer chemotherapy

Evidence

- A systematic review found that low-dose methotrexate is significantly more effective than placebo for the short-term treatment of patients with rheumatoid arthritis. Patients receiving methotrexate were more likely to withdraw due to adverse effects [11] *Level M*
- Systematic reviews have found no consistent differences between methotrexate and other DMARDs [12] *Level M*
- A systematic review found that folic acid reduces the oral and gastrointestinal side-effects of methotrexate [13] *Level M*

Acceptability to patient

- Medium: toxicity may occur, but the drug has one of the lowest discontinuation rates of the orally administered DMARDs
- Alcohol consumption should be discouraged

Follow up plan

- Monitor regularly for appearance of toxicity
- Guidelines for monitoring drug therapy in RA have been published by the American College of Rheumatology [2]
- Improvement in symptoms may be noticed as early as 1–2 months and plateaus by 3–6 months

Patient and caregiver information

- The patient/caregiver must be made aware of possible side-effects and the necessity of reporting them if they occur
- The importance of compliance with therapy must be stressed
- Alcohol should be avoided

ANTIMALARIAL DRUGS

- The patient/caregiver must be made aware of possible side-effects and the necessity of reporting them if they occur
- The importance of compliance with therapy must be stressed
- Alcohol should be avoided

Dose
- Hydroxychloroquine: 200–400mg/day orally
- Start at 400mg/day and possibly decrease to 200mg/day if definite improvement is seen
- 'Dose-loading' at a higher than normal dose for 6 weeks at the start of treatment may increase efficacy

Efficacy
Moderately efficacious.

Risks/Benefits
Risks:
- Very toxic in overdose
- Use caution in children
- Use caution in hepatic and renal disease, G6PD deficiency
- Use caution in alcoholism, patients susceptible to skin reaction, and in porphyria
- Patients should be regularly examined for retinal toxicity

Benefits:
- Reduces disease activity and joint inflammation
- Less toxic than many other DMARDs

Side-effects and adverse reactions
- Allergic reactions
- Gastrointestinal: nausea, vomiting, diarrhea, abdominal pain
- Eyes, ears, nose, and throat: irreversible retinal damage, visual disturbances, tinnitus, hearing disturbances
- Central nervous system: headache, seizures, psychosis
- Hematologic: blood cell disorders
- Musculoskeletal: myalgia, arthralgia
- Skin: pigmentation, rashes, eruptions, pruritus

Interactions (other drugs)
- Antiepileptics ▪ Cyclosporine ▪ Digoxin ▪ Mefloquine ▪ Praziquantel

Contraindications
- Avoid in psoriasis ▪ Pregnancy and breast-feeding ▪ Visual changes
- Long-term therapy in children

Evidence
- A systematic review found that hydroxychloroquine reduces disease activity and joint inflammation [4] *Level M*
- Systematic reviews have found no significant difference in efficacy between antimalarials and other DMARDs [12] *Level M*
- A RCT found that dose-loading hydroxychloroquine at a higher than normal dose for 6 weeks at the start of treatment may increase efficacy [15] *Level P*

Acceptability to patient
- High: low toxicity compared with other 'second-line' agents
- Most patients withdraw, owing to lack of efficacy

Follow up plan
- Monitor carefully for development of toxicity
- Requires periodic eye examinations

Effect should be apparent in 3–6 months

Patient and caregiver information
- The patient/caregiver must be made aware of possible side-effects and the necessity of reporting them if they occur
- The importance of compliance with therapy must be stressed

SULFASALAZINE
- Common first-choice DMARD, especially in Europe
- Enteric-coated preparations enhance tolerability

Dose
- Adult: 2–3g/day orally
- Start at 500mg/day and increase by 500mg/day at weekly intervals

Efficacy
- Moderately beneficial
- Over the first year of therapy, effectiveness is comparable with methotrexate. However, after the first year, sulfasalazine does not compare as favorably

Risks/Benefits
Risks:
- Only after critical appraisal should sulfasalazine tablets be given to patients with hepatic or renal damage or blood dyscrasias
- Concomitant relief of symptoms of coexisting gastrointestinal inflammatory disease

Benefits:
- Reduces disease activity, joint inflammation, and reduces radiologic progression
- Concomitant relief of symptoms of coexisting gastrointestinal inflammatory disease

Side-effects and adverse reactions
- Gastrointestinal: abdominal pain, diarrhea, hepatotoxicity, melena, vomiting
- Genitourinary: renal failure, urinary retention
- Hematologic: blood cell disorders
- Musculoskeletal: arthralgia, myalgia, osteoporosis
- Cardiovascular system: pericarditis, allergic myocarditis
- Central nervous system: dizziness, drowsiness, headache, seizures
- Eyes, ears, nose, and throat: blurred vision, tinnitus
- Skin: Stevens-Johnson syndrome

Interactions (other drugs)
- Digoxin Methenamine Phenytoin Tolbutamide Warfarin

Contraindications
- Contraindicated in porphyria and gastrointestinal or urinary tract obstruction Cross-hypersensitivy with salicylates Caution required in patients with renal or hepatic impairment, glucose-6-phosphate deficiency

Evidence
- A systematic review found that sulfasalazine is effective for the treatment of rheumatoid arthritis. Sulfasalazine is significantly more effective than placebo for the treatment of tender and swollen joints, and for decreasing pain and ESR [16] *Level M*

- A RCT compared sulfasalazine with placebo. Sulfasalazine significantly improved both patient and physician global assessment [17] *Level P*
- Systematic reviews found no evidence that sulfasalazine is more or less effective than other DMARDs [12] *Level M*

Acceptability to patient
Medium.

Follow up plan
- Monitor carefully for development of toxicity
- Guidelines for monitoring drug therapy in RA been published by the American College of Rheumatology [2]
- Effect should be apparent in 1–3 months

Patient and caregiver information
- The patient/caregiver must be made aware of possible side-effects and the necessity of reporting them if they occur
- The importance of compliance with therapy must be stressed

LEFLUNOMIDE
- Newer DMARD that inhibits activated T-lymphocytes
- Effectiveness in preventing radiographic progression is comparable with methotrexate

Dose
- Adult maintenance: 20mg/day, as a single dose
- If the 20mg/day dose is not well tolerated, 10mg/day may be used
- A loading dose may be used, because the half-life of the active metabolite of leflunomide is 2 weeks, so reaching a steady state would take 8 weeks. A loading dose of 100mg/day for 3 days may be used, but is associated with considerable gastrointestinal toxicity in the form of diarrhea. Giving 40mg/day for 14 days, followed by the standard dose of 20mg/day is better tolerated
- For patients already on methotrexate, patients should be started on 10mg/day, because the risk of elevated liver function tests is higher when both drugs are given concurrently. A loading dose of 100mg/day for 2 days may be given

Efficacy
Comparable with methotrexate over 2 years and with sulfasalazine at one year. However, at 2 years, sulfasalazine does not compare as favorably. There are no studies that directly compare leflunomide with etanercept or infliximab.

Risks/Benefits
Risks:
- Pregnancy must be avoided
- Use caution in patients with significant hematologic abnormalities
- Use caution in renal impairment
- May increase risk of neoplasia

Benefits:
- Reduces disease activity, joint inflammation, and radiologic progression
- Improves functional status and quality of life

Side-effects and adverse reactions
- Gastrointestinal: diarrhea
- Metabolic: elevated liver function tests (transaminases), pancytopenia

- Skin: rash, rare serious reactions, alopecia
- Other: teratogenicity

Interactions (other drugs)
- **Methotrexate (increased hepatotoxicity)** ■ **Rifampin** ■ **Vaccines (live)**

Contraindications
- **Pregnancy and breast-feeding** ■ **Known hypersensitivity to drug** ■ **Severe immunodeficiency** ■ **Bone marrow dysplasia** ■ **Severe, uncontrolled infections** ■ **Hepatic impairment, or hepatitis B or C** ■ **Not recommended for children**

Evidence
- RCTs in a systematic review consistently showed that leflunomide is more effective than placebo in improving quality of life, number of swollen joints, and radiologic progression of disease in patients with rheumatoid arthritis [18] *Level M*
- Two RCTs found no significant difference between leflunomide, sulfasalazine, and methotrexate in the control of disease progression or radiologic progression [17,19] *Level P*
- Another RCT found that methotrexate was significantly more effective than leflunomide. After 12 months, methotrexate-treated patients had a reduced number of tender and swollen joints, reduced radiologic disease progression, and lower ESR. Patient and physician global assessments were improved with methotrexate. After 2 years, there was no significant difference in the number of tender joints or patient assessment, but radiologic progression was significantly less with methotrexate [20] *Level P*

Acceptability to patient
Possibly high: low toxicity and significant activity may ensure high compliance.

Follow up plan
- Monitor carefully for development of toxicity
- Liver function needs to be checked regularly

Patient and caregiver information
- The patient/caregiver must be made aware of possible side-effects and the necessity of reporting them if they occur
- The importance of compliance with therapy must be stressed

ETANERCEPT
- Newer 'biologic' agent. Etanercept is a fully human fusion protein, consisting of two TNF receptor molecules linked by an immunoglobulin G (IgG) Fc fragment to prolong the half-life
- Clearly effective in patients unresponsive to methotrexate. In early RA, effectiveness is at least as good as (and possibly superior to) methotrexate
- Administered alone or with methotrexate

Dose
Adult: 25mg subcutaneously twice weekly.

Efficacy
- Equivalent, or superior to, methotrexate in early RA
- Efficacious in patients refractory to methotrexate

Risks/Benefits
Risks:
- Monitor patients who develop infections

- Use caution in the elderly (higher infection risk)
- Use caution with multiple sclerosis or demyelinating disease, patients with a history of recurring infections or predisposing conditions such as diabetes
- Use caution in pregnancy
- Risk of autoantibodies

Benefits:
- Reduces disease activity and joint inflammation
- Retards radiographic progression
- Symptomatic improvement occurs rapidly

Side-effects and adverse reactions
- Serious allergic reactions
- Cardiovascular: chest pain, vasodilation
- Central nervous system: demyelinating disorders, transverse myelitis, optic neuritis, paresthesia, seizures, stroke
- Gastrointestinal: altered sense of taste, anorexia, diarrhea, dry mouth
- Hematologic: blood cell disorders
- Injection site reactions
- Musculoskeletal: joint pain
- Ocular: dry eyes, ocular inflammation
- Respiratory: spontaneous reports of pulmonary diseases
- Serious infections (including tuberculosis)
- Skin: cutaneous vasculitis, pruritus, subcutaneous nodules, urticaria
- Systemic: angioedema, fatigue, fever, influenza syndrome, generalized pain, weight gain

Interactions (other drugs)
None listed.

Contraindications
- Active infection, including chronic or localized ■ Breast-feeding ■ Hypersensitivity to the drug ■ Live vaccines ■ Sepsis

Evidence
- A RCT compared etanercept with placebo for the management of active rheumatoid arthritis in patients who had not responded to other DMARDs. Patients receiving etanercept were significantly more improved compared with placebo at 3 and 6 months. A 25mg dose was more effective than 10mg. Functional status and quality of life were also improved with etanercept [21] *Level P*
- Etanercept (25mg) and placebo were compared in another RCT of patients with an inadequate response to methotrexate. Patients were allowed to continue methotrexate. Improvement was achieved in significantly more patients receiving etanercept than placebo [22] *Level P*

Acceptability to patient
Medium: the agent is quickly effective, but has to be administered subcutaneously. It is also expensive.

Follow up plan
- Monitor carefully for development of toxicity
- Serious, fatal infections have occurred, especially in patients with active pre-existing infections at the time of etanercept initiation

Patient and caregiver information

- The patient/caregiver must be made aware of possible side-effects and the necessity of reporting them if they occur
- The importance of compliance with therapy must be stressed

INFLIXIMAB

- Newer 'biologic' agent; a monoclonal antibody to TNF
- Exact role in the treatment of rheumatoid patients is yet to be decided but may be used to treat patients with severe disease, poor prognostic features, and refractory disease
- Usually coadministered with methotrexate (US Food and Drug Administration (FDA)-approved), as results with this combination are superior to those with infliximab alone. The role of substituting other DMARDs (such as sulfasalazine, leflunomide, or azathioprine) for methotrexate in combination with infliximab is not clear
- Risk of infusion reaction during administration. The risk for this can be reduced by infusing the medication slowly over 2–3h. Premedication with diphenhydramine and/or corticosteroids may be useful in preventing subsequent infusion reactions
- Risk of reactivation of tuberculosis. Infliximab should not be given to patients with a history of tuberculosis. A purified protein derivative (PPD) skin test should be administered subcutaneously prior to beginning treatment with infliximab. If the PPD is positive, the patient should be treated appropriately, and the decision to administer infliximab reassessed

Dose

- Initial regimen is 3mg/kg intravenous infusion at 0, 2, and 6 weeks, and then every 8 weeks
- Increasing the dose (above 10mg/kg has not been studied) of each infusion, or decreasing the interval between infusions from 8 to 4 weeks, are options for patients who do not improve on the standard regimen

Efficacy

Infliximab has been demonstrated to be effective in patients with long-standing RA who have not responded to methotrexate. Its role in patients with early RA has not been established.

Risks/Benefits

Risks:

- Use caution with chronic infection or history of recurrent infection
- Use caution in patients who have resided in an area where histoplasmosis is endemic
- Evaluate patients for latent tuberculosis prior to infliximab therapy
- Monitor patients for infection
- Use caution in the elderly (increased risk of infections), and in pregnancy
- Use caution with demyelinating disorders
- Medications for the treatment of hypersensitivity reactions (e.g. acetaminophen, antihistamines, corticosteroids, and/or epinephrine) should be available for immediate use in the event of a reaction
- Possible increased risk of lymphoma
- Safety and effectiveness of infliximab in patients with juvenile RA and in pediatric patients with Crohn's disease have not been established

Benefits:

- Reduces disease activity and slows radiologic progression
- Quickly and highly effective

Side-effects and adverse reactions

- Cardiovascular system: arrhythmia, atrioventricular block, bradycardia, cardiac arrest, palpitation, tachycardia, brain infarction, peripheral ischemia, pulmonary embolism, deep

thrombophlebitis, angina pectoris, cardiac failure, myocardial ischemia
- Central nervous system: exacerbation of demyelinating disorders, encephalopathy, spinal stenosis, upper motor neuron lesion, dizziness, headache, anxiety, confusion, delirium, depression, somnolence, suicide attempt
- Eyes, ears, nose, and throat: ceruminosis, endophthalmitis
- Gastrointestinal: appendicitis, Crohn's disease, diarrhea, gastric ulcer, gastrointestinal hemorrhage, intestinal obstruction, intestinal perforation, intestinal stenosis, nausea, pancreatitis, peritonitis, proctalgia, vomiting
- Genitourinary: azotemia, dysuria, endometriosis, hydronephrosis, kidney infarction, pyelonephritis, renal calculus, renal failure, ureteral obstruction
- Hematologic: thrombocytopenia, anemia, leukopenia
- Hypersensitivity: including severe reactions, infusion reactions, reactions following readministration, urticaria
- Metabolic: dehydration, pancreatic insufficiency, weight decrease, changes in liver enzymes, biliary pain, cholecystitis, cholelithiasis, cholestatic hepatitis
- Respiratory: adult respiratory distress syndrome, bronchitis, coughing, dyspnea, pleural effusion, pleurisy, pneumonia, pneumothorax, pulmonary edema, pulmonary infiltration, respiratory insufficiency, upper respiratory tract infection
- Other: lupus-like syndrome, Guillain-Barrè syndrome, optic neuritis, polyneuropathy, worsening rheumatoid arthritis, rheumatoid nodules, neoplasia, histoplasmosis, listeriosis, pneumocystosis, tuberculosis, invasive fungal infections, opportunistic infections, sepsis, lymphadenopathy, lymphangitis

Interactions (other drugs)
None listed.

Contraindications
- Active infection (clinically important) - Breast-feeding - Hypersensitivity to any murine proteins or other components - Live vaccines

Evidence
- Two RCTs found that infliximab was more effective than placebo for the treatment of rheumatoid arthritis [23,24] *Level P*
- Another RCT compared infliximab with placebo in patients with active disease not responsive to methotrexate. Patients continued with methotrexate treatment during the trial. The combination of infliximab with methotrexate was significantly more effective than placebo and methotrexate [25] *Level P*
- Short-term toxicity is low; long-term safety is unknown. The optimal dose and duration of treatment are not known [12]

Acceptability to patient
Possibly medium: the agent is highly effective but has to be administered intravenously. It is also expensive.

Follow up plan
Patients must be followed closely for infection and treatment interrupted if infection develops.

Patient and caregiver information
- The patient/caregiver must be made aware of possible side-effects and the necessity of reporting them if they occur
- The importance of compliance with therapy must be stressed

ANAKINRA

A new self-injected biologic agent, a naturally occurring inhibitor of the proinflammatory cytokine AL-1.

Dose
100mg/day subcutaneously.

Efficacy
Treatment with anakinra produces relief of signs and symptoms that is superior to placebo. Studies are underway to assess its efficacy in preventing radiographic damage from RA.

Risks/Benefits
Risk: associated with increased incidence of serious infections

Benefits:
- Reduces disease activity
- Generally well tolerated

Side-effects and adverse reactions
- Central nervous system: headache, dizziness
- Gastrointestinal: nausea, abdominal pain
- Hematologic: neutropenia
- Skin: injection site reactions
- Other: malignancies, sinusitis, influenza-like symptoms

Interactions (other drugs)
The current FDA labeling discourages the simultaneous administration of anakinra and TNF-inhibitors, because of concern that the risk of infection might be increased. Studies are currently underway to assess this risk.

Contraindications
■ Known hypersensitivity to *Escherichia coli*-derived proteins, anakinra, or any components of the product ■ Pregnancy category B ■ Breast-feeding ■ The safety and efficacy of anakinra in patients with juvenile RA have not been established

Acceptability to patient
Moderate: patients may be reluctant to give themselves daily injection.

Follow up plan
- Monitor carefully for the development of infection
- Effect should be apparent in 2–3 months

Patient and caregiver information
- The patient/caregiver must be made aware of possible side-effects and the necessity of reporting them if they occur
- The importance of compliance with therapy must be stressed

AZATHIOPRINE

A DMARD that is seldom used currently.

Dose
- Adult: initial dose should be approx. 1mg/kg (50–100mg) given as a single dose or on a twice-daily schedule. The dose may be increased, beginning at 6–8 weeks and thereafter by steps at

4-week intervals if there are no serious toxicities and if initial response is unsatisfactory. Dose increments should be 0.5mg/kg daily, up to a maximum dose of 2.5mg/kg/day. Therapeutic response occurs after several weeks of treatment, usually 6–8; an adequate trial should be a minimum of 12 weeks. Patients not improved after 12 weeks can be considered refractory. Azathioprine may be continued long-term in patients with clinical response, but patients should be monitored carefully, and gradual dosage reduction should be attempted to reduce risk of toxicities

■ Maintenance therapy should be at the lowest effective dose, and the dose given can be lowered decrementally with changes of 0.5mg/kg or approx. 25mg daily every 4 weeks while other therapy is kept constant. The optimum duration of maintenance azathioprine has not been determined

Efficacy
■ Significantly beneficial
■ No evidence regarding its prevention of radiographic progression

Risks/Benefits
Risks:
■ Use caution with bone marrow depression and infection
■ Use caution in renal or hepatic impairment
■ Severe blood cell disorders may occur
■ May increase risk of neoplasia

Benefits:
■ Reduces disease activity
■ Generally well tolerated

Side-effects and adverse reactions
■ Gastrointestinal: nausea, vomiting, diarrhea, abdominal pain, hepatic failure, jaundice
■ Genitourinary: depression of spermatogenesis
■ Hematologic: anemia, leukopenia, pancytopenia, thrombocytopenia
■ Musculoskeletal: arthralgia, myalgia, malaise
■ Skin: rash, alopecia
■ Other: fungal, bacterial, protozoal, and viral infections, may increase risk of neoplasm (skin cancer, reticulocyte or lymphomatous tumors), teratogenicity

Interactions (other drugs)
■ ACE inhibitors ■ Allopurinol ■ Anticoagulants ■ Carbamazepine ■ Clozapine ■ Co-trimoxazole (TMP-SMX) ■ Cyclosporine ■ Methotrexate ■ Nondepolarizing muscle blockers ■ Vaccines ■ Warfarin

Contraindications
■ Hypersenstitivity to the drug ■ Intramuscular injections ■ Pregnancy or breast-feeding ■ Vaccines

Evidence
A systematic review found that azathioprine appears to be significantly more effective than placebo for the reduction of disease activity. This evidence is based on a small number of patients, included in older trials. Toxicity is higher and more serious with azathioprine than with other DMARDs. There is no evidence to recommend azathioprine over other DMARDs [26] *Level M*

Acceptability to patient
Moderate: patients are often worried about the potential for the development of malignancy (although, in fact, the risk is quite low).

Follow up plan
- Monitor carefully for development of toxicity with periodic complete blood counts
- Guidelines for monitoring drug therapy in RA been published by the American College of Rheumatology [2]
- Effect should be apparent in 2–3 months

Patient and caregiver information
- The patient/caregiver must be made aware of possible side-effects and the necessity of reporting them if they occur
- The importance of compliance with therapy must be stressed

MINOCYCLINE
This is an off-label indication.

Dose
50–100mg twice daily.

Efficacy
Minocycline has mild potency, perhaps comparable with hydroxychloroquine, but probably less potent than methotrexate.

Risks/Benefits
Risks:
- Use of this drug may result in overgrowth of nonsusceptible organisms, including fungi. If superinfection occurs, the antibiotic should be discontinued
- Use caution with renal impairment
- Risk of pseudotumor cerebri (benign intracranial hypertension) in adults
- Risk of bulging fontanels in infants
- Photosensitivity manifested by an exaggerated sunburn reaction has been observed
- Central nervous system effects may make driving or operation of machinery hazardous
- Possible risk of neoplasia

Side-effects and adverse reactions
- Cardiovascular system: pericarditis
- Central nervous system: bulging fontanels in infants and benign intracranial hypertension (pseudotumor cerebri) in adults, headache, lightheadedness, dizziness, vertigo
- Gastrointestinal: anorexia, nausea, vomiting, diarrhea, glossitis, dysphagia, enterocolitis, esophagitis and esophageal ulcerations
- Metabolic: pancreatitis, inflammatory lesions (with monilial overgrowth) in the anogenital region, increases in liver enzymes, hepatitis, and liver failure
- Musculoskeletal: polyarthralgia
- Hypersensitivity and skin reactions: anaphylaxis, maculopapular erythematous rashes, exfoliative dermatitis, erythema multiforme, Stevens-Johnson syndrome, photosensitivity, pigmentation of the skin and mucous membranes, urticaria, angioneurotic edema, anaphylactoid purpura, exacerbation of systemic lupus erythematosus, pulmonary infiltrates with eosinophilia, transient lupus-like syndrome has also been reported with the capsules
- Hematologic: hemolytic anemia, thrombocytopenia, neutropenia, and eosinophilia have been reported
- Renal toxicity: dose-relelated elevations in blood urea nitrogen (BUN) have been reported
- Other: with prolonged treatment, brown-black microscopic discoloration of the thyroid glands, tooth discoloration and enamel hypoplasia during tooth development

Interactions (other drugs)
- Methoxyflurane (has been reported to result in fatal renal toxicity) ■ Anticoagulants (may depress plasma prothrombin activity) ■ Penicillin (bactericidal action may be reduced) ■ Oral contraceptives (may reduce effectiveness of contraceptives) ■ Antacids containing aluminum, calcium, or magnesium, and iron-containing preparations (may impair absorption of minocycline)

Contraindications
- Children under 8 years of age ■ Pregnancy and breast-feeding ■ Hypersensitivity to any of the tetracyclines

Evidence
RCTs have found that minocycline is more effective than placebo for disease activity control in patients with rheumatoid arthritis [12] *Level P*

Physical therapy
Plays an essential role in the therapy of RA.

BALNEOTHERAPY (HYDROTHERAPY OR SPA THERAPY)
- One of the oldest treatments for RA
- Used as an adjunct to other treatment
- Aims to soothe pain

Efficacy
- Difficult to assess because most studies have been flawed
- Possibly relieves pain

Risks/Benefits
Benefit: possibly soothing.

Evidence
A systematic review found no clear evidence for the efficacy of balneotherapy, due to methodologic flaws in RCTs. Most trials reported positive findings, but these results should be noted with caution [27] *Level M*

Acceptability to patient
High.

Follow up plan
Monitor patient response to this therapy.

Patient and caregiver information
- This therapy must be used in conjunction with other treatments
- Hot water should be treated with caution

THERMOTHERAPY
- Local application of heat and/or cold
- Aims to soothe symptoms
- Used as an adjunct to other treatment

Efficacy
Patients prefer thermotherapy to no therapy.

Risks/Benefits
Benefit: possibly provides relief of symptoms.

Acceptability to patient
High.

Follow up plan
Monitor patient response to this therapy.

Patient and caregiver information
This therapy must be used in conjunction with other treatments.

DYNAMIC EXERCISE THERAPY

- Aims to improve joint mobility, muscle strength, aerobic capacity, and functional status
- A weight-loss program should be developed for obese patients
- A daily, simple regimen drawn up by a physical therapist is recommended, even during acute flares
- May range from passive exercises to high-intensity strength training

Efficacy
Improves aerobic capacity and muscle strength.

Risks/Benefits
Benefit: improves physical capacity of patients.

Evidence
A systematic review found that dynamic exercise therapy improves aerobic capacity and muscle strength. Effects on functional status and radiologic progression are unclear [28] *Level M*

Acceptability to patient
Low: compliance with exercise regimens is notoriously low.

Follow up plan
Regular follow up meetings and supervised sessions are needed to maintain compliance and to ensure that the exercises are done correctly.

Patient and caregiver information
The importance of compliance must be stressed.

Occupational therapy
One or more sessions with an occupational therapist is recommended.

HOME THERAPY

- It is important for the patient to learn how to preserve joint function and alignment when carrying out daily activities
- Zipper pullers, long shoe horns, and devices to help patients get in and out of chairs, toilet seats, and beds, can be extremely useful

Efficacy
Often highly effective.

Risks/Benefits
Benefits:

- Helps to educate patients as to the best way of carrying out routine activities

- Helps to preserve joint function
- Occupational therapist may be able to advise about home modifications that would help the patient

Acceptability to patient
High.

Follow up plan
Further appointments with an occupational therapist may need to be made if the patient's disease progresses.

Surgical therapy
- Used to treat severe joint damage
- Can reduce pain, improve joint function and appearance, and raise functional status and quality of life
- Needs careful discussion between patient and physician before making a decision

JOINT REPLACEMENT
- Replacement of the hip and knee are indicated if mechanical structural damage from RA has become severe, and if the patient has significant functional loss
- Replacement of damaged metacarpophalangeal joints in the hands with silastic implants, usually combined with tendon transfer, is appropriate in patients for whom hand deformity seriously compromises function

Efficacy
- High, especially for hip and knee prostheses
- Ankle, elbow, and shoulder replacements are also improving

Risks/Benefits
Benefits:
- The patient is likely to regain some functional status
- Quality of life will improve

Acceptability to patient
Low.

Follow up plan
Physical and occupational therapy will be needed.

TENDON RECONSTRUCTION
To repair tendons damaged or ruptured by the disease, most frequently on the hands.

Efficacy
Early treatment has a higher success rate.

Risks/Benefits
Benefits:
- The patient is likely to regain some functional status
- Quality of life will improve

Acceptability to patient
Low.

Follow up plan
Physical and occupational therapy will be needed.

SYNOVECTOMY

- Removal of the inflamed synovial tissue at the dorsal wrist may reduce the risk of tendon rupture
- Performed prior to, or as part of, reconstructive surgery

Risks/Benefits
Benefits:
- The patient is likely to regain some functional status
- Quality of life will improve

Acceptability to patient
Low.

Follow up plan
Physical and occupational therapy will be needed.

CARPAL TUNNEL RELEASE
Efficacy
Can preserve median nerve function and relieve pain.

Risks/Benefits
Benefits:
- Relatively simple, same-day surgery
- The patient is likely to obtain relief from paresthesias
- Quality of life will improve

Acceptability to patient
High.

Follow up plan
Physical and occupational therapy will be needed.

RESECTION OF METATARSAL HEADS
Resection of metatarsal heads is indicated when forefoot pain resulting from mechanical damage cannot be controlled with orthotics, special shoes, and medications.

Efficacy
This treatment is likely to enable the patient to ambulate with considerably less pain.

Risks/Benefits
Benefits:
- The patient is likely to regain some functional status
- Quality of life will improve

Acceptability to patient
Low.

Follow up plan
Physical and occupational therapy will be needed.

Complementary therapy
NUTRITION
Elimination of food allergies, following of a vegetarian diet, and modifying intake of dietary antioxidants and fats/oils.

Efficacy
- Food allergens can definitely exacerbate RA. Commonest food allergies are wheat, corn, milk/dairy, beef, nightshade vegetables (tomato, potato, peppers, eggplant), and food additives
- Dietary fats have important influences on inflammation in the body, as precursors to inflammatory prostaglandins, thromboxanes, and leukotrienes. Altering the balance of fatty acid types can influence the propensity toward or away from inflammatory substance production. More GLA (gamma linoleic acid) and EPA (eicosapentaenoic acid) produce anti-inflammatory prostaglandins; more arachidonic acid promotes inflammatory prostaglandins. Therefore, a diet high in cold water marine fish (mackerel, herring, salmon, sardines) and possibly supplementation with omega-3-fatty acids may be beneficial to RA patients
- Dietary antioxidants are also of value – generally in the form of whole fresh fruits and vegetables. Flavonoids in these foods serve as anti-inflammatory substances and support of collagen structures

Risks/Benefits
Risk: little risk to a balanced vegetarian diet. Must watch for potential vitamin B12 deficiency.

Evidence
A single-blind RCT compared dietary manipulation vs regular diet in patients with RA. Patients in the treatment group received a gluten-free vegan diet for 3.5 months after an initial 7- to 10-day fast. The food was gradually changed to a lactovegetarian diet for the remainder of the one-year study. After 4 weeks of treatment, there was a significant improvement in symptomatic and objective measures of inflammation in the patients on the lactovegetarian diet. The benefits noted in the treatment group were still present after one year [29] *Level P*

Acceptability to patient
Major dietary changes are very difficult for many people. Following a modified vegetarian diet with the addition of marine fish may not be acceptable to some patients in terms of their personal tastes or family eating habits. If patients notice substantial improvement in symptoms, they may be motivated to make these dietary changes.

Follow up plan
Usual medical and rheumatologic care.

Patient and caregiver information
Recommend a modified vegetarian diet with added cold water fish, restrict omega-6 fatty acids (most vegetable oils) and supplement with one tablespoon of flaxseed oil daily (source of omega-3 fatty acid).

SELENIUM AND VITAMIN E
Selenium levels are reported to be low in patients with RA. Selenium is a cofactor in the activity of glutathione peroxidase, an enzyme which reduces the production of inflammatory prostaglandins and leukotrienes. These inflammatory substances are responsible for causing much of the tissue damage seen in RA.

Risks/Benefits
- Risk: high doses of vitamin E (>1000 IU/day) have been associated with increased bleeding
- Benefit: selenium has no reported toxicity

Acceptability to patient
As these supplements are readily available, nontoxic, and inexpensive, this approach is quite acceptable to patients.

Follow up plan
Regular care.

Patient and caregiver information
Good food sources of selenium are Brazil nuts, fish, and grains. However, the amount of selenium in plant foods is directly related to the selenium content of the soil it is grown in. Doses recommended for RA are selenium 200mcg/day and vitamin E 400 IU/day.

CURCUMIN (CURCUMA LONGA)
Efficacy
Curcumin has strong anti-inflammatory and antioxidant properties. It appears to have a direct anti-inflammatory effect on inhibiting leukotriene and other inflammatory mediator production, and also may potentiate the body's own cortisone-enhancing effects.

Risks/Benefits
Benefit: animals fed very high curcumin doses (3g/kg) have not evidenced any adverse effects. Curcumin is well tolerated in humans with no adverse effects reported at recommended dosages.

Acceptability to patient
Well tolerated and accepted by patients.

Follow up plan
Regular medical care.

Patient and caregiver information
Recommended dosage of curcumin is 400–600mg three times daily on an empty stomach 20min before meals. It is sometimes combined with bromelain to enhance absorption, or provided in a lipid base (e.g. lecithin, fish oil) to enhance absorption.

Other therapies
LOW-LEVEL LASER THERAPY
Divided into classes I, II, and III.

Efficacy
- Has been controversial
- Beneficial if given for at least 4 weeks

Risks/Benefits
Benefit: reduces pain and morning stiffness.

Evidence
A meta-analysis found that low-level laser therapy may be beneficial for the short-term relief of pain and morning stiffness. There was no effect on functional outcomes, range of motion, or local swelling [30] *Level M*

Acceptability to patient
High.

Follow up plan
Monitor patient response carefully.

Patient and caregiver information
The importance of compliance must be stressed.

SPLINTS
Inflamed joints, or mechanically damaged joints, may benefit from splinting, which limit joint motion. This is particularly true in the wrist and hand.

Efficacy
Splinting clearly provides comfort. Whether splinting can prevent deformity such as ulnar drift of the metacarpophalangeal joints is less clear.

Acceptability to patient
May be inconvenient.

Follow up plan
Assess inflammation.

Patient and caregiver information
Splints should be used in the manner specified by the therapist.

APHERESIS (PROSORBA COLUMN)
- Combination of plasmapheresis and exposure of plasma to staphylococcal protein A presented on the surface of a silica matrix
- Performed weekly (over 2–3h) at an outpatient facility for 12 weeks
- Labor- and time-intensive
- Requires insertion of two large-bore intravenous catheters

Efficacy
Prosorba immunosorption has been demonstrated effective in patients with longstanding severe disease.

Risks/Benefits
Benefit: reduces disease activity.

Evidence
A RCT compared Prosorba with sham apheresis in patients with RA who failed to respond to methotrexate or at least two other second-line medications. Apheresis with the Prosorba column reduced disease activity compared with sham treatment [31] *Level P*

Acceptability to patient
Low: the inconvenience and flu-like symptoms may lower acceptability.

Follow up plan
Monitor need for other therapy.

Patient and caregiver information
Stress need for compliance.

LIFESTYLE

- Midafternoon fatigue is generally relieved by a period of bed rest
- The patient should exercise daily, especially when the disease is less active
- Patients should get down to or maintain optimum bodyweight

RISKS/BENEFITS

Benefits:

- Decreases symptoms
- Places less stress on joints
- Maintains/improves joint function

ACCEPTABILITY TO PATIENT

Medium: rest should not be too difficult to encourage, but exercise has notoriously low compliance rates.

FOLLOW UP PLAN

- Patients prone to 'pushing' themselves too hard may have to be reminded to rest regularly
- Follow-up visits may be needed to maintain compliance with an exercise program

PATIENT AND CAREGIVER INFORMATION

Rest and exercise are an essential part of treatment.

EFFICACY OF THERAPIES

- The various treatments have been shown to reduce pain, inflammation, disease activity, and radiographic progression in randomized clinical trials
- The effect in any one patient is very difficult to judge because of the variability of the disease

Evidence

- There is no significant difference between different NSAIDs for the treatment of tender joints in patients with RA [7] *Level M*
- Short-term, low-dose prednisolone is more effective than placebo for the control of disease activity, and may be used intermittently in rheumatoid arthritis. Joint tenderness and pain are significantly more improved with prednisolone than NSAIDs [9] *Level M*
- Moderate-term prednisone treatment is more effective than placebo in the management of RA [10] *Level M*
- Early intervention with DMARDs has been shown to improve outcomes [12]
- Systematic reviews have found no evidence of a difference in efficacy between DMARDs for the treatment of RA [12] *Level M*
- Combinations of certain DMARDs may be more effective than using individual drugs alone. However, the evidence is conflicting, and the balance of benefits and harms varies for different combinations [12] *Level M*
- There is evidence that most DMARDs are more effective than placebo for treating joint inflammation and reducing disease activity. The effect of prolonged treatment with DMARDs has not been adequately evaluated [12] *Level M*
- Tumor necrosis factor antagonists (entanercept and infliximab) are more effective than placebo for the reduction of disease activity and joint inflammation [12] *Level P*
- A systematic review found that dynamic exercise therapy improves aerobic capacity and muscle strength. Effects on functional status and radiologic progression are unclear [28] *Level M*
- Low-level laser therapy may be beneficial for the short-term relief of pain and morning stiffness. There is no effect on functional outcomes, range of motion, and local swelling [30] *Level M*
- Dietary manipulation has been shown to improve symptomatic and objective measures of inflammation [29] *Level P*

Review period

Monitor course of disease at regular intervals.

PROGNOSIS

- Course of disease is variable and unpredictable
- Some patients experience flares and remissions; for others it is a progressive disease
- Structural damage occurs in approx. 30% of patients, leading to articular deformities and functional impairment
- Approx. 50% of patients will be disabled or unable to work within 10 years of diagnosis
- History, joint examination, and functional assessment indicate prognosis during first 2 years of disease
- Patients at highest risk of a poor outcome may have high levels of rheumatoid factor, HLA-DRB1 alleles, earlier age of onset, synovial fluid acidosis, or white blood cell (WBC) count of >50,000/mm^3, rheumatoid nodules, elevated ESR, swelling of >20 joints, and extra-articular manifestations/complications
- Life expectancy is shortened (average 3–7 years) through infections, systemic manifestations, pulmonary disease, renal disease, and gastrointestinal bleeding or perforation
- RA cannot be cured with current treatment modalities

Criteria for complete remission have been proposed by the American College of Rheumatology [32].

At least five of the following criteria must be fulfilled for at least two consecutive months:
1. Morning stiffness lasting 15min or less
2. No fatigue
3. No joint pain (by history)
4. No joint tenderness or pain on movement
5. No soft-tissue swelling in joints or tendon sheaths
6. An ESR of <30mm/h for females and 20mm/h for males

Clinical pearls
▓ Patients with RA should be started on a DMARDs as soon as the diagnosis has been established. In most cases, methotrexate is the DMARD of first choice
▓ If joint swelling (synovitis) persists, consideration should be given to additional or different DMARDs, even if the patient's symptoms have improved
▓ Combinations of DMARDs are necessary for adequate disease control in most patients

Therapeutic failure
▓ Choices of DMARDs in refractory disease include, etanercept, infliximab, and anakinra
▓ Combinations that may also be used in severe disease: methotrexate, sulfasalazine plus hydroxychloroquine or methotrexate with either leflunomide, etanercept, infliximab, or anakinra
▓ Referral to rheumatology is always indicated in refractory disease

Recurrence
▓ Choices of DMARD agents in re-emergent disease following remission include parenteral gold, oral gold (auranofin), cyclosporin (cyclosporine), azathioprine, leflunomide, etanercept, infliximab, and minocycline
▓ Combinations of either cyclophosphamide, azathioprine plus hydroxychloroquine or methotrexate, sulfasalazine plus hydroxychloroquine may also be used in severe disease
▓ Referral to rheumatology is indicated in refractory disease

Deterioration
▓ Rising, but low, level of disability should trigger a change in 'second-line' treatment
▓ Joint replacement or other surgical measures if the patient experiences unbearable pain and a marked drop in quality of life
▓ Referral to rheumatology is indicated in refractory disease
▓ Treatment of disease refractory to 'second-line' agents includes systemic corticosteroids and/or NSAIDs

COMPLICATIONS
Joint destruction and cervical instability (life-threatening) may result from articular damage. In addition, potentially serious extra-articular complications may arise:
▓ Gastrointestinal bleeding
▓ Heart failure
▓ Pericarditis
▓ Pleuritis or lung disease
▓ Anemia
▓ Low or high platelet count
▓ Eye inflammation
▓ Neuropathy
▓ Vasculitis

- Felty's syndrome is a complication of long-standing disease in 1% of sufferers. Characterized by presence of RA with splenomegaly and an abnormally low WBC count. Specific treatment not always required
- Interstitial lung disease

CONSIDER CONSULT

- Refer to rheumatology if there is pain, stiffness, or swelling that is unresponsive to NSAID therapy within 3–4 months after onset
- Refer to rheumatology if previously stable disease becomes active
- Refer to rheumatology if erosions appear/progress on X-ray at any stage of the disease
- Refer to rheumatology if there is functional deterioration affecting the quality of life
- Refer to rheumatology if there is rapid disease progression
- Refer to rheumatology if there are extra-articular manifestations/complications

PREVENTION

There is no current method of providing effective screening for rheumatoid arthritis.

PREVENT RECURRENCE
Treatment must be unbroken.

ASSOCIATIONS

American College of Rheumatology
1800 Century Place, Suite 250
Atlanta, GA 30345
Tel: (404) 633 3777
Fax: (404) 633 1870
E-mail: acr@rheumatology.org
www.rheumatology.org

National Arthritis and Musculoskeletal and Skin Diseases Information Clearing House
NIAMS/National Institutes of Health
1 AMS Circle
Bethsedsa, MD 20892-3675
Tel: (301) 495 4484
Fax: (301) 718 6366
www.nih.gov/niams/

Arthritis Foundation
1330 West Peachtree Street
Atlanta, GA 30309
Tel: (800) 283 7800 or (404) 872 7100
E-mail: webmaster@arthritis.org
www.arthritis.org

KEY REFERENCES

- Suarez-Almazar M, Foster W. Rheumatoid arthritis: Musculoskeletal disorders. In: Clinical Evidence 2001;6:927–44. London: BMJ Publishing Group
- Firestein GS. Etiology and pathogenesis of rheumatoid arthritis. In: Ruddy S, Harris ED, Sledge CB, Eds. Kelley's Textbook of Rheumatology, 6th edn. Philadelphia (PA): WB Saunders, 2001, p921–58
- Fries JF, Williams CA, Morfeld D, et al. Reduction in long-term disability in patients with rheumatoid arthritis by disease-modifying antirheumatic drug-based treatment strategies. Arthritis Rheum 1996;39:616–22. Medline
- Kremer JM, Alarcon GS, Lightfoot RW Jr, et al. Methotrexate for rheumatoid arthritis. Suggested guidelines for monitoring liver toxicity. American College of Rheumatology. Arthritis Rheum 1994;37:316–28
- Lipsky PE, van der Heijde DMF, St Clair EW, et al. Infliximab and methotrexate in the treatment of rheumatoid arthritis. N Engl J Med 2000;343:1594–602
- Kremer JM. Rational use of new and existing disease modifying agents in rheumatoid arthritis. Ann Intern Med 2001;134:695–706
- Bathon JM, Martin RW, Fleischmann RM, et al. A comparison of etanercept and methotrexate in patients with early rheumatoid arthritis. N Engl J Med 2000;343:1586–93

Evidence references and guidelines

1 Arnett FC, Edworthy SM, Bloch DA, et al. The American Rheumatism Association 1987 revised criteria for the classification of rheumatoid arthritis. Arthritis Rheum 1988;31:315–24. Available at the The American College of Rheumatology website
2 The American College of Rheumatology. Guidelines for monitoring drug therapy in rheumatoid arthritis. Arthritis Rheum 1996;39:723–31
3 The American College of Rheumatology. Guidelines for the management of rheumatoid arthritis 2002 update. Arthritis Rheum 2002;46:328–46
4 Felson DT, Anderson JJ, Boers M, et al. American College of Rheumatology: Preliminary definition of improvement in rheumatoid arthritis. Arthritis Rheum 1995;38:727–35
5 American College of Rheumatology. Position Statement: methotrexate.
6 Kremer JM, Alarcon GS, Lightfoot RW, et al. Methotrexate for rheumatoid arthritis. Suggested guidelines for mintoring liver toxicity. Arthritis Rheum 1994;37:316–28

7   Gotzsche PC. Meta-analysis of NSAIDs: contribution of drugs, doses, trial designs, and meta-analytic techniques. Scand J Rheumatol 1993;22:255–60. Reviewed in: Clinical Evidence 2001;6:894–901

8   Simon LS, Weaver AL, Graham DY, et al. Anti-inflammatory and upper gastrointestinal efects of celecoxib in rheumatoid arthritis. JAMA 1999;282:1921–8. Reviewed in: Clinical Evidence 2001;6:894–901

9   Gotzsche PC, Johansen HK. Short-term low-dose corticosteroids vs placebo and nonsteroidal antiinflammatory drugs in rheumatoid arthritis (Cochrane Review). In: The Cochrane Library, 1, 2002. Oxford: Update Software

10 Criswell LA, Saag KG, Sems KM, et al. Moderate-term, low-dose corticosteroids for rheumatoid arthritis (Cochrane Review). In: The Cochrane Library, 1, 2002. Oxford: Update Software

11 Suarez-Almazor ME, Belseck E, Shea B, et al. Methotrexate for treating rheumatoid arthritis (Cochrane Review). In: The Cochrane Library, 1, 2002. Oxford: Update Software

12 Suarez-Almazor M, Foster W. Rheumatoid arthritis: Musculoskeletal disorders. In: Clinical Evidence 2001;6:927–44. London: BMJ Publishing Group

13 Ortiz Z, Shea B, Suarez-Almazor ME, et al. Folic acid and folinic acid for reducing side effects in patients receiving methotrexate for rheumatoid arthritis (Cochrane Review). In: The Cochrane Library, 1, 2002. Oxford: Update Software

14 Suarez-Almazor ME, Belseck E, Shea B, et al. Antimalarials for treating rheumatoid arthritis (Cochrane Review). In: The Cochrane Library, 1, 2002. Oxford: Update Software

15 Furst DE, Lindsley H, Baethge B, et al. Dose-loading with hydroxychloroquine impreoves the rate of response in early, active rheumatoid arthritis: A randomized, double-blind six-week trial with eighteen-week extension. Arthritis Rheum 1999;42:357–365. Reviewed in: Clinical Evidence 2001;6:927–44

16 Suarez-Almazor ME, Belseck E, Shea B, et al. Sulfasalazine for treating rheumatoid arthritis (Cochrane Revew). In: The Cochrane Library, 1, 2002. Oxford: Update Software

17 Smolen JS, Kalden JR, Scott DL, et al. Efficacy and safelt of leflunomide compared with placebo and sulfasalazine in active rheumatoid arthritis: A double-blind, randomized, multicenter trial. Lancet 1999;353:259–66. Reviewed in: Clinical Evidence 2001;6:927–44

18 Hewitson PJ, BeBroe S, McBride A, Milne R. Leflunomide and rheumatoid arthritis: a systematic review of effectiveness, safety and cost implications. J Clin Pharm Ther 2000;25:295–302. Reviewed in: Clinical Evidence 2001;6:927–44

19 Strand V, Cohen S, Schiff M, et al. Treatment of active rheumatoid arthritis wt leflunomide compared with placebo or methotrexate. Arch Intern Med 1999;159:2542–50. Reviewed in: Clinical Evidence 2001;6:927–44

20 Emery P, Breedveld FC, Lemmel EM, et al. A comparison of the efficacy and safety of leflunomide and methotrexate for the treatment of rheumatoid arthritis. Rheumatology 2000;39:655–335. Reviewed in: Clinical Evidence 2001;6:927–44

21 Moreland W, Schiff MH, Baumgartner SW, et al. Etanercept therapy in rheumatoid arthritis. A randomized, controlled trial. Ann Intern Med 1999;130:478–86. Reviewed in: Clinical Evidence 2001;6:927–44

22 Weinblatt ME, Kremer JM, Bankhurst AD, et al. A trial of etanercept, a recombinant tumor necrosis factor receptor: Fc fusion protein, in patients with rheumatoid arthritis receiving methotrexate. N Engl J Med 1999;340:253–9. Reviewed in: Clinical Evidence 2001;6:927–44

23 Elliot MJ, Maini RN, Feldman M, et al. Randomised double-blind comparison of chimeric monoclonal antibody to tumor necrosis factor alpha (cA2) versus placebo in rheumatoid arthritis. Lancet 1994;344:1105–10. Reviewed in: Clinical Evidence 2001;6:927–44

24 Maini RN, Breedveld FC, Kalden JR, et al. Therapeutic efficacy of multiple intravenous infusions of anti-tumor necrosis factor alpha monoclonal antibody combined with low-dose weekly methotrexate in rheumatoid arthritis. Arthritis Rheum 1998;41:1552–63. Reviewed in: Clinical Evidence 2001;6:927–44

25 Maini RN, St Clair EW, Breedweld F, et al. Infliximab ((chimeric anti-tumor necrosis factor alpha monoclonal antibody) versus placebo in rheumatoid arthritis patients receiving concomitiant methotrexate: a randomized phase III trial. ATTRACT study group. Lancet 1999;354:1932–9. Reviewed in: Clinical Evidence 2001;6:927–44

26 Suarez-Almazor ME, Spooner C, Belseck E. Azathioprine for treating rheumatoid arthritis (Cochrane Review). In: The Cochrane Library, 1, 2002. Oxford: Update Software

27 Verhagen AP, de Vet HCW, de Bie RA, et al. Balneotherapy for rheumatoid arthritis and osteoarthritis (Cochrane Review). In: The Cochrane Library, 1, 2002. Oxford: Update Software

28 Van Den Ende CH, Vliet Vlieland TP, Munneke M, Hazes JM. Dynamic exercise therapy for treating rheumatoid arthritis (Cochrane Review). In: The Cochrane Library, 1, 2002. Oxford: Update Software

29 Kjeldsen-Kraugh J, Hangen M, Borchgrevnick CF, et al. Controlled trial of fasting and one-year vegetarian diet in rheumatoid arthritis. Lancet 1991;338:899–902. Medline

30 Brosseau L, Welch V, Wells G, et al. Low level laser therapy (classes I, II and III) in the treatment of rheumatoid arthritis (Cochrane Review). In: The Cochrane Library, 1, 2002. Oxford: Update Software

31 Felson DT, LaValley MP, Baldassare AR, et al. The Prosorba column for treatment of refractory rheumatoid arthritis: a randomized, double-blind, sham-controlled trial. Arthritis Rheum 1999;42:2153–9. Medline

32 American College of Rheumatology. Clinical Guidelines Committee: Guidelines for RA management. Arthritis Rheum 1996;39:713–22

FAQS
Question 1
When should disease-modifying antirheumatic drug (DMARD) therapy be administered to patients with rheumatoid arthritis (RA)?

ANSWER 1
DMARDs (such as methotrexate, sulfasalazine) should be started in every patient with RA as soon as the diagnosis can be established.

Question 2
When should prednisone or prednisolone be used in the treatment of RA?

ANSWER 2
Whenever possible, the administration of corticosteroids is avoided because of their serious long-term toxicity. However, their rapid and predictable onset of action makes them a useful 'bridge' therapy while awaiting the improvement from a DMARD.

Question 3
What is the role of the tumor necrosis factor (TNF) antagonists (etanercept and infliximab) in treating RA?

ANSWER 3
These agents are clearly appropriate in patients who have failed to respond to DMARDs such as methotrexate and sulfasalazine, and they are efficacious even in patients with long-standing disease. Whether TNF antagonists should be administered very early in disease (as 'first-line' DMARDs) is a subject of current debate.

Question 4
Should the American College of Rheumatology criteria be applied by clinicians in practice in the diagnosis of RA?

ANSWER 4
Not necessarily. These criteria are most useful for establishing the diagnosis for patients to be included in a clinical trial of an investigational therapeutic agent. However, these criteria are more accurate in making the diagnosis of established RA, rather than early RA (when aggressive treatment intervention is important). Practically speaking, a patients with symmetrical inflammatory arthritis involving the small joints of the hands (except the distal interphalangeal joints), morning stiffness, and a positive rheumatoid factor, most likely has RA.

Question 5
Is a positive rheumatoid factor essential for making the diagnosis of RA?

ANSWER 5
No. As many as 20% of patients with RA are seronegative for the rheumatoid factor. However, disease tends to be more severe in patients whose rheumatoid factor is positive.

CONTRIBUTORS
Joseph E Scherger, MD, MPH
Jane L Murray, MD
Richard Brasington Jr, MD, FACP
Deborah L Shapiro, MD

ROTATOR CUFF SYNDROME

DESCRIPTION

■ A spectrum of conditions affecting the tendons of the rotator cuff of the shoulder: supraspinatus, infraspinatus, teres minor
■ Characterized by shoulder pain, especially on abduction through a painful arc
■ Commonly caused by repetitive overhead activities such as basketball, javelin, freestyle swimming, tennis, skiing, and also occupational overuse such as painting and decorating. Certain other occupations seem to be particularly problematic for rotator cuff such as tree pruning, fruit picking, nursing, grocery clerking, long shoring, warehousing, and carpentry
■ Can usually be successfully treated in primary care with advice on rest and avoidance of high-risk exercises involving the shoulder, nonsteroidal anti-inflammatory drugs, physical therapy, or subacromial corticosteroid injection

URGENT ACTION

Septic arthritis is among the differential diagnoses of acute shoulder pain. This may need urgent consultation or referral with specialist for drainage, culturing of organisms, and recommendation for intravenous antibiotic therapy.

KEY! DON'T MISS!

Septic arthritis is among the differential diagnoses of acute shoulder pain. This requires urgent referral for specialist treatment. NEVER inject corticosteroids into a joint that may be septic.

ICD9 CODE
726.10 Rotator cuff syndrome
727.61 Rotator cuff rupture

SYNONYMS
- Shoulder impingement syndrome
- Painful arc syndrome
- Internal derangement of the subacromial joint
- Supraspinatus syndrome
- Swimmer's shoulder
- Tennis shoulder

CARDINAL FEATURES
There are no cardinal features that distinguish rotator cuff syndrome from other causes of shoulder pain. Calcific tendinitis and subacromial bursitis give very similar clinical pictures. The most common features of rotator cuff syndrome are:
- Anterolateral shoulder pain
- Painful arc between 70 and 120 degrees of abduction
- Weakness in abduction and forward flexion
- Relief of pain (usually) on the subacromial injection of lidocaine

CAUSES
Common causes
- Repetitive overuse: stressing the shoulder joint with the arm overhead is most common cause in young people. Activities such as freestyle swimming, basketball, tennis, and throwing sports often to blame. Other overuses include unaccustomed decorating, carpentry, and weight training
- Trauma: a fall on the shoulder or outstretched arm, especially in the elderly, can tear the rotator cuff tendons with symptoms identical to rotator cuff syndrome
- Abnormally shaped acromion: some patients have pronounced dip at the tip of the acromion into the subacromial space, making impingement of rotator cuff tendons more likely on lesser degrees of use
- Shoulder instability: recurrent dislocation of the shoulder can cause repeated impingement of the rotator cuff tendons

Rare causes
Secondary rotator cuff symptoms can be due to:
- Malignancy in the humeral head, glenoid fossa, acromion, or clavicle
- Subacromial bursitis
- Acromioclavicular arthritis
- Acute traumatic anterior subluxation of the humeral head
- Glenoid dysplasia
- Ehler-Danlos syndrome

Serious causes
Trauma: tears of the rotator cuff. Most occur in men over 40 involved in strenuous overhead activity with the dominant arm. A tear is suspected if shoulder pain is worse at night and wakes the patient, if active abduction of the shoulder is impossible to initiate, if the patient is unable to hold the arm actively abducted at 90 degrees, or if there is supraspinatus or infraspinatus muscle wasting on inspection of the scapula area. Referral for consideration for surgical repair is important.

Contributory or predisposing factors
- Overhead activity
- Repetitive overuse

EPIDEMIOLOGY
Incidence and prevalence
FREQUENCY
5–10% of the population will suffer from rotator cuff syndrome at some time in their lives.

Demographics
AGE
Uncommon under 20 years of age.

GENDER
More common in men than women.

DIFFERENTIAL DIAGNOSIS
Adhesive capsulitis (frozen shoulder)
FEATURES
- Anterior and posterior shoulder pain
- Active and passive movement of the glenohumeral joint greatly restricted

Biceps tendinitis
FEATURES
- Pain reproduced by resisted elbow flexion and supination
- Tenderness of the long head of biceps in the bicipital groove over the proximal anterior margin of the humerus

Glenohumeral instability
FEATURES
- Usually follows post-traumatic capsular tear
- Shoulder feels as if it 'gives out'
- Shoulder pain, discomfort, or weakness common

Glenohumeral joint arthritis
FEATURES
- Rest pain and stiffness
- Crepitus on movement
- Decreased range of passive movement

Acromioclavicular degeneration
FEATURES
- Pain and tenderness localized to the acromioclavicular joint
- Pain does not radiate usually
- Exacerbated by activity with the arm above the head or in front of the body

Septic arthritis
FEATURES
- Swelling and redness of the shoulder joint
- Fever
- NEVER inject the septic joint with corticosteroids

Referred pain
Causes of referred pain that may be confused with rotator cuff syndrome include:
- Cervical radiculopathy
- Suprascapular nerve entrapment
- Apical lung pathology
- Myocardial infarction
- Stroke
- Gallbladder disease
- Angina
- Diaphragmatic hernia
- Gastritis

SIGNS & SYMPTOMS
Signs
- Rotator cuff tenderness
- Weakness in abduction
- Weakness in forward flexion
- Wasting of the scapular muscles in chronic cases

Symptoms
- Shoulder pain
- Pain referred down deltoid
- Pain on abducting shoulder between 70 and 120 degrees (painful arc)
- Weakness
- Pain exacerbated by overhead activities, e.g. combing hair

KEY! DON'T MISS!
Septic arthritis is among the differential diagnoses of acute shoulder pain. This requires urgent referral for specialist treatment. NEVER inject corticosteroids into a joint that may be septic.

CONSIDER CONSULT
- When medical/conservative treatment fails
- Professional athlete who has to return to rigorous training activities as quickly and as healed possible

INVESTIGATION OF THE PATIENT
Direct questions to patient
Q **Where is your pain?** The pain is in the shoulder, usually the anterior or lateral areas and may radiate down the deltoid area

Q **When do you get the pain?** On trying to lift the arm above the head or away from the body to the side or in front

Q **Does the pain interfere with activities of daily living?** There may be difficulty dressing, combing hair, wiping after toilet

Q **Are you otherwise well?** There should be no suspicion of causes of referred pain to the shoulder from myocardial ischemia, gallbladder disease, or the neck

Q **Do you have any history of stomach ulcer or asthma?** Can the patient be prescribed nonsteroidal anti-inflammatory drugs (NSAIDs)?

Contributory or predisposing factors
Q **What is your occupation?** Jobs involving overhead work such as painting and decorating carry a greater risk of rotator cuff injury. Carpenters, gardeners, builders, and other manual occupations will need time away from work in order to heal the rotator cuff before resuming shoulder stresses

Q **What sports do you do?** Throwing sports such as javelin, racquet sports such as tennis, and other overhead games such as basketball all carry a high risk of rotator cuff injury. The professional sportsperson is likely to be involved in rigorous training and want to resume activities as quickly and as fully healed as possible. Referral to a specialist in sports medicine and orthopedics is indicated

Q **Have you been overusing the arm recently?** Unaccustomed overuse can cause rotator cuff syndrome and is seen in the amateur sportsperson and home maintenance fan

Examination
- **Examine both shoulders and the back.** Look for swelling and redness to exclude septic arthritis, scars of previous surgery or arthroscopy, and wasting of supraspinatus or infraspinatus muscle suggesting rotator cuff tear or suprascapular nerve palsy

- **Palpate the shoulder.** The rotator cuff is usually tender on palpation. Exclude tenderness of the acromioclavicular joint and of the long head of biceps in the bicipital groove. The joint should be neither hot nor swollen
- **Can you move the arm away from the body sideways until it is above your head?** Full abduction should be possible with a painful arc between 70 and 120 degrees. Severe restriction of movement both actively and passively is seen in adhesive capsulitis. Poor active abduction with full passive abduction suggests a tear of the rotator cuff
- **Can you point your elbow forward towards me and resist as I try to push down on your elbow?** This stress test of the supraspinatus tendon is very specific for rotator cuff syndrome. The test is positive if it reproduces the patient's pain accurately. If the patient is unable to resist (positive drop-arm test), this is highly suggestive of a tear of the rotator cuff
- **Perform a general physical exam.** Exclude septic arthritis, gallbladder tenderness and acute abdomen, cardiac decompensation of myocardial infarction, chest signs of pleural effusion, restrictive or painful neck movements of cervical spondylosis with radiculopathy

Summary of investigative tests

- Plain X-ray of the shoulder: if glenohumeral arthritis or calcific bicipital tendinitis are suspected, this will help narrow down the differential diagnosis as they both have characteristic X-ray appearances. In rotator cuff syndrome the X-ray should be normal
- Magnetic resonance imaging of the shoulder. is usually performed by a specialist and is considered if a tear of the rotator cuff is suspected. If patients fail to improve after 6 months of nonoperative therapy they should be referred to a specialist for a decision on whether to order a magnetic resonance scan. Also high-powered overhead athletes should be referred early for scanning due to the higher risk of both significancy rotator cuff tears and tears of the glenoid labrum
- Ultrasound of the shoulder is used in some centers as specialist investigation instead of MRI

DIAGNOSTIC DECISION

The diagnosis of rotator cuff syndrome is based on:
- History of unilateral shoulder pain on abduction or forward flexion especially following repetitive overhead stresses
- Examination showing reduced power on abduction or forward flexion, a painful arc between 70 and 120 degrees abduction, but with a full range of active and passive movement.

Diagnostic tests are expected to be normal in rotator cuff syndrome and are not part of routine first-line management in straightforward cases. Guidelines on examination and evaluation are available at National Guidelines Clearinghouse [1].
- Eliminate rheumatological emergencies by excluding: a history of significant trauma, a hot swollen joint, constitutional upset, marked focal or diffuse weakness, neurogenic pain and claudication pain
- Symptoms to expect include: brief morning stiffness, peak period of discomfort with use, unilaterality
- Signs to expect include: focal tenderness, stable shoulder joint, absence of multisystem disease
- Tests for rheumatoid disease are unnecessary
- Imaging is unnecessary unless: the diagnosis is in doubt, there is significant loss of joint function, pain continues despite adequate conservative management, suspicion of fracture, bone infection, or malignancy

CLINICAL PEARLS

- In middle-aged individuals, impingement of the rotator cuff and adjacent structures is likely to be the explanation for shoulder pain.
- Although rotator cuff tendinoplasty is quite common, surgery is required in a minority of cases.
- Patients with a history of repetitive overhead arm motion are at high risk for rotator cuff problems

THE TESTS
Imaging
PLAIN X-RAY OF THE SHOULDER
Advantages/Disadvantages
Advantage: plain anteroposterior view of the shoulder will demonstrate calcific bicipital tendinitis, osteoarthritis, dislocation, acromioclavicular disorder or spur and narrowing of the acromio-humeral distance in chronic rotator cuff tears. The advantage is in excluding alternative diagnoses if there is clinical uncertainty after the history and examination, or if there has been no improvement in clinical condition after 6 months of nonoperative management.

Normal
In simple rotator cuff syndrome, X-ray appearances are normal. It is therefore unnecessary to order an X-ray initially if diagnosis is not in doubt after history and examination.

Abnormal
- Chronic rotator cuff syndrome can cause the X-ray changes of subacromial sclerosis and osteophyte formation, sclerosis and cystic changes involving the greater tuberosity, and a reduction in the acromiohumeral distance
- Massive rotator cuff tears can cause the X-ray changes of superior migration of the humeral head and deformity of the greater tuberosity

Cause of abnormal result
- In chronic rotator cuff syndrome, changes are those of chronic inflammation and irritation of the rotator cuff tendon insertions on the humeral head
- In massive rotator cuff tears, the changes represent shoulder joint instability and misalignment

Drugs, disorders and other factors that may alter results
Some elderly patients with rotator cuff syndrome may have X-ray changes of coexisting osteoarthritis of the glenohumeral joint, which may confuse the diagnosis.

ULTRASOUND OF THE SHOULDER
Advantages/Disadvantages
Advantages:
- Noninvasive
- Quick
- Helps to confirm suspected rotator cuff tear

Disadvantages:
- Operator-dependent
- Normal appearances in rotator cuff sprain

Normal
Normal echogenic pattern with continuity of the rotator cuff and no effusion.

Abnormal
Rotator cuff tears give the ultrasound appearances:
- Nonvisualization of the rotator cuff
- Localized absence or focal nonvisualization
- Discontinuity
- Focal abnormal echogenicity

Cause of abnormal result
Interruption to the continuity of the rotator cuff tendons.

Drugs, disorders and other factors that may alter results
- Operator-dependent
- Patient obesity
- Subdeltoid bursal effusion

MAGNETIC RESONANCE IMAGING
Advantages/Disadvantages
Advantages:
- MRI has replaced arthrography in the investigation of shoulder pathology due to noninvasiveness, multiplanar capability, and excellent soft-tissue contrast.
- It is not a first-line investigation in simple acute cases of rotator cuff syndrome but should be considered in suspected cases of rotator cuff tear, especially massive tears.

Abnormal
MRI changes in tendinopathy are also seen in asymptomatic volunteers and must be placed in context of the clinical picture. They include increased signal less than fat, fluid within the subacromial bursa, obliteration of the peribursal fat stripe, and glenohumeral effusion.

Cause of abnormal result
Chronic irritation of the subacromial structures and the tendons themselves.

Drugs, disorders and other factors that may alter results
- Mild to moderate increases in tendon signal may be a normal variant.
- Signal changes are seen with increasing frequency in older age groups, suggesting senescent change.
- An artefact known as the 'magic angle' occurs if the tendon is angled at 55 degrees to the main magnetic field

TREATMENT

CONSIDER CONSULT

- Refer to physical therapist for exercise therapy after adequate management of pain with analgesics or NSAIDs
- Subacromial corticosteroid injection is common therapy. If the primary care physician is untrained in this technique, refer to orthopedic surgeon or rheumatologist for treatment
- Failure of nonoperative therapy after 6 months of adequate and appropriate treatment

PATIENT AND CAREGIVER ISSUES
Patient or caregiver request

- **Steroid anxiety.** Many patients are reluctant to accept the offer of a corticosteroid injection on the basis of anxiety about steroids and fear of the pain of injection
- **Medication aversion.** Some patients dislike taking oral medication generally, preferring rest, alteration of shoulder use, or physical therapy
- **Desire for specialist treatment.** Most patients with simple rotator cuff syndrome can be successfully managed entirely by the primary care physician and a physical therapist

Health-seeking behavior

- **How long have you had the problem?** Persistent symptoms for 6 months or more, despite adequate treatment, should prompt specialist referral
- **How many corticosteroid injections have been given already and over what time span?** There is a suggested limit of three to four injections over one year into the subacromial space. Any more than this carries the risk of rotator cuff thinning, bicipital tendon thinning, and capsular weakening
- **Have exercises been supervised by a physiotherapist?** Some patients do not perform exercises correctly for rotator cuff syndrome

MANAGEMENT ISSUES
Goals

- To eliminate pain
- To restore range of motion
- To resume occupational and sporting activities
- To prevent future episodes

Management in special circumstances
COEXISTING DISEASE

- Osteoarthritis of the glenohumeral joint. Apart from making the diagnosis more difficult, coexisting osteoarthritis may make exercise therapy more painful. The patient may already be taking NSAIDs. The goal of achieving full use of the shoulder may be compromised in patients who have premorbid restriction of activity due to osteoarthritis
- Patients with peptic ulcer disease, asthma, renal impairment, or allergy may be unable to tolerate NSAIDs
- A previous adverse reaction to a corticosteroid injection may preclude further use

COEXISTING MEDICATION
Many patients will already have tried an over-the-counter (OTC) NSAID. This may have been taken at a subtherapeutic dose, so advice on correct dosing may be appropriate. Changing to a therapeutic nonsteroidal dose may be indicated.

SPECIAL PATIENT GROUPS

- Athletes: particularly high-powered overhead athletes such as basketball players, javelin throwers, tennis players. Early referral indicated for management due to the risk of a rotator cuff tear

- Disabled: rotator cuff syndrome relatively common in wheelchair patients. Physical therapy adapted according to disability
- Occupation: patients using shoulder movements at work such as painters and decorators, carpenters, plasterers, etc. need early, effective treatment. Consider giving a subacromial corticosteroid injection earlier in the course of treatment to speed recovery

PATIENT SATISFACTION/LIFESTYLE PRIORITIES

- Occupation: the priority for most patients with manual occupations is to effect a speedy recovery and return to work
- Old age: patients may not wish to retain full overhead activities, especially if this means having physical therapy, injections, or more tablets. Nursing home patients may prefer to rest the shoulder and restrict use and see how things go. Watch out for adhesive capsulitis. Passive mobilization may help prevent this
- Disabled: wheelchair patients are heavily reliant on normal shoulder function for mobility and transfers. Active intervention is usually wanted

SUMMARY OF THERAPEUTIC OPTIONS
Choices

- The first choice of treatment for rotator cuff syndrome consists of rest, NSAIDs (e.g. ibuprofen, ketoprofen, naproxen, diclofenac) and modification of activities that produce pain
- If this is unsuccessful then the next line of treatment is to maintain flexibility and range of motion through physical therapy
- The place of subacromial corticosteroid injection is debatable, but for most patients this would be the next choice
- Surgical treatment is reserved for refractory shoulder cuff pain or tears

Clinical pearls

- Treatment is focused on pain reduction and improvement in range of motion
- Physical therapy, in general, is more important than NSAIDs
- Surgery is reserved for pain unresponsive to more conservative treatment

Never

Never inject corticosteroids into a shoulder that may have septic arthritis.

FOLLOW UP
Plan for review

After the initial treatment ask the patient to return if symptoms do not improve, especially if there is any residual loss of function. Follow patients through physical therapy to assess response. Ask patients to report symptoms of indigestion with nonsteroidal anti-inflammatories. Following subacromial corticosteroid injection ask the patient to report any symptoms of heat, redness, or swelling of the shoulder.

Information for patient or caregiver

- With rest, nonsteroidals, or physical therapy the patient should patiently await gradual diminution of symptoms
- Inform the patient to expect an increase in pain following subacromial corticosteroid injection for up to 48 h

DRUGS AND OTHER THERAPIES: DETAILS
Drugs
IBUPROFEN
OTC or prescription.

Dose
400–600mg three times a day.

Efficacy
Nonsteroidal anti-inflammatory. May be all that is required to relieve pain in rotator cuff syndrome.

Risks/Benefits
Risks:
- Risk of inducing gastritis, gastric hemorrhage, and renal failure especially in the elderly
- Use caution in hepatic, renal, and cardiac failure
- Use caution in bleeding disorders

Benefit: inexpensive

Side-effects and adverse reactions
- Gastrointestinal: anorexia, nausea, dyspepsia, peptic ulceration, bleeding
- Central nervous system: headache, dizziness, tinnitus
- Hypersensitivity: rashes, bronchospasm, angioedema
- Cardiovascular system: hypertension, peripheral edema
- Genitourinary: nephrotoxicity
- Hematological: blood cell disorders

Interactions (other drugs)
- Aminoglycosides ▪ Anticoagulants ▪ Antihypertensives ▪ Baclofen ▪ Corticosteroids ▪ Cyclosporine, tacrolimus ▪ Digoxin ▪ Diuretics ▪ Lithium ▪ Methotrexate ▪ Phenylpropanolamine ▪ Warfarin

Contraindications
- History of serious GI complication of NSAID ▪ Peptic ulceration ▪ Hypersensitivity to NSAIDs ▪ Coagulation defects ▪ Severe renal or hepatic disease

Acceptability to patient
Usually well tolerated by most patients.

Follow up plan
Ask patients to report any side-effects, especially GI symptoms. Monitor renal function in patients at high risk for NSAID-induced renal dysfunction.

Patient and caregiver information
NSAIDs are used as part of a combination of treatments, including rest and modification of shoulder use to reduce pain. Compliance with these other aspects of treatment is as important as the drugs themselves in effecting a cure.

KETOPROFEN
OTC and prescription.

Dose
- 50–100mg three times a day, prescription only. Do not exceed 300mg a day
- 12.5mg three to four times a day OTC

Efficacy
Mild anti-inflammatory. May be all that is required to relieve pain in rotator cuff syndrome.

Risks/Benefits
Risks:

- Use caution in elderly
- Use caution in hepatic, renal, and cardiac failure
- Use caution in bleeding disorders

Benefits:

- Risk of gastrointestinal toxicity is low
- Inexpensive

Side-effects and adverse reactions

- Gastrointestinal: anorexia, nausea, dyspepsia, peptic ulceration, bleeding
- Central nervous system: headache, dizziness, tinnitus
- Hypersensitivity: rashes, bronchospasm, angioedema
- Cardiovascular system: hypertension, peripheral edema
- Genitourinary: nephrotoxicity
- Hematological: blood cell disorders

Interactions (other drugs)

- Aminoglycosides ▪ Anticoagulants ▪ Antihypertensives ▪ Baclofen ▪ Corticosteroids ▪ Cyclosporine, tacrolimus ▪ Digoxin ▪ Diuretics ▪ Lithium ▪ Methotrexate ▪ Phenylpropanolamine ▪ Warfarin

Contraindications

- History of serious GI complication of NSAID. ▪ Peptic ulceration ▪ Hypersensitivity to NSAIDs ▪ Coagulation defects ▪ Severe renal or hepatic disease

Acceptability to patient
Usually well tolerated by most patients.

Follow up plan
Ask patients to report any Side-effects, especially gastrointestinal symptoms. Monitor renal function in patients at high risk for NSAID-induced renal dysfunction.

Patient and caregiver information
NSAIDs are used as part of a combination of treatments, including rest and modification of shoulder use to reduce pain. Compliance with these other aspects of treatment is as important as the drugs themselves in effecting a cure.

NAPROXEN
OTC and prescription.

Dose
250–500mg twice a day.

Efficacy
Nonsteroidal anti-inflammatory.

Risks/Benefits
Risks:

- Use caution in hepatic, renal, and cardiac disorders
- Use caution in elderly
- Use caution in bleeding disorders
- Use caution in porphyria

Benefits:
- Propionic acids are effective and better tolerated than most other NSAIDs
- Risk of gastrointestinal toxicity is low

Side-effects and adverse reactions
- Gastrointestinal: diarrhea, vomiting, nausea, dyspepsia, peptic ulceration
- Central nervous system: headache, dizziness, drowsiness
- Hypersensitivity: rashes, bronchospasm, angioedema
- Thrombocytopenia
- Cardiovascular system: congestive heart failure, dysrhythmias, edema, palpitations
- Genitourinary: acute renal failure

Interactions (other drugs)
- Aminoglycosides Anticoagulants Antihypertensives Corticosteroids
- Cyclosporine Digoxin Diuretics Lithium Methotrexate Phenylpropanolamine
- Probenecid Triamterene

Contraindications
- Peptic ulceration Hypersensitivity to NSAIDs Coagulation defects Do not use naproxen and naproxen sodium concomitantly

Acceptability to patient
Usually well tolerated by most patients.

Follow up plan
Ask patients to report any side-effects, especially GI symptoms. Monitor renal function in patients at high risk for NSAID-induced renal dysfunction.

Patient and caregiver information
NSAIDs are used as part of a combination of treatments, including rest and modification of shoulder use to reduce pain.

DICLOFENAC
Dose
25–50mg three times a day.

Efficacy
NSAID; good at relieving pain and stiffness.

Risks/Benefits
Risks:
- Use caution in hepatic, renal, and cardiac failure, porphyria
- Use caution in bleeding and GI disorders

Side-effects and adverse reactions
- Gastrointestinal: anorexia, nausea, dyspepsia, peptic ulceration, vomiting
- Central Nervous system: headache, dizziness, tinnitus
- Hypersensitivity: rashes, bronchospasm, angioedema
- Cardiovascular system: CHF, dysrhythmias, hypertension, and hypotension
- Eyes, ears, nose and throat: blurred vision

Interactions (other drugs)
- Aminoglycosides Anticoagulants Antihypertensives Corticosteroids Cyclosporine
- Digoxin Lithium Methotrexate Phenylpropanolamine Triamterene

Contraindications
▪ Hypersensitivity to nonsteroidal anti-inflammatories ▪ Peptic ulceration ▪ Coagulation defects

Acceptability to patient
Usually well tolerated by most patients.

Follow up plan
Ask patients to report any side-effects, especially GI symptoms. Monitor renal function in patients at high risk for NSAID-induced renal dysfunction.

Patient and caregiver information
NSAIDs are used as part of a combination of treatments, including rest and modification of shoulder use to reduce pain.

CORTICOSTEROID INJECTION
Injection into the subacromial space of corticosteroid preparations.

Dose
▪ Methylprednisolone acetate 20–80mg, single dose
▪ Triamcinolone acetonide 10–20mg, single dose
▪ May be repeated three to four times in a year in any one joint

Efficacy
Range of abduction improved by an average of 35 degrees compared with placebo, according to Cochrane Review.

Risks/Benefits
Risks:
▪ Potential risks with subacromial corticosteroid injection
▪ Iatrogenic septic arthritis
▪ Articular cartilage atrophy
▪ Tendon rupture
▪ Never inject a suspected septic shoulder with corticosteroids
▪ Overwhelming septicemia if patient has an infection
▪ Loss of control of blood glucose in those with diabetes
▪ Use caution in elderly due to risk of diabetes and osteoporosis
▪ Use caution in patients with psychosis, seizure disorders, or myasthenia gravis
▪ Use caution in congestive heart failure, hypertension
▪ Use caution in ulcerative colitis, peptic ulcer, or esophagitis
▪ Prolonged use causes adrenal suppression

Benefit: the only method of treatment for shoulder pain to satisfy the Cochrane Reviewers of scientific benefit

Side-effects and adverse reactions
Systemic complications are rare after local injection therapy. Systemic side-effects include:
▪ Gastrointestinal: dyspepsia, peptic ulceration, esophagitis, oral candidiasis, nausea, vomiting
▪ Cardiovascular system: hypertension, thromboembolism
▪ Central nervous system: insomnia, euphoria, depression, psychosis, seizures
▪ Endocrine: adrenal suppression, impaired glucose tolerance, growth suppression in children
▪ Musculoskeletal: proximal myopathy, osteoporosis
▪ Skin: delayed healing, acne, striae
▪ Eyes, ears, nose and throat: cataract, glaucoma, blurred vision

Interactions (other drugs)
Aminoglutethamide Antidiabetics Barbiturates Cholestyramine Clarithromycin, erythromycin Colestipol Cyclosporine Isoniazid Ketoconazole NSAIDs Oral contraceptives Rifampin Salicylates Troleandomycin

Contraindications
Septic arthritis Previous adverse reaction to similar preparation Systemic infection

Evidence
The Cochrane Reviewers found evidence to support the use of corticosteroid injection as a treatment for shoulder pain [2].

Acceptability to patient
The treatment is quick and effective. Some patients are averse to the idea of being injected.

Follow up plan
Advise the patient to report any heat, redness, or swelling of the shoulder. Repeat injection may be given after 2 weeks if there has been incomplete improvement.

Patient and caregiver information
Advise the patient to expect a temporary worsening of shoulder pain for 24–36 h after the injection. Improvement should follow and continue over the next 7 days. Improvement should be sustained for several months or even be permanent.

Physical therapy
PHYSICAL THERAPY
There are a number of specific exercises and physical therapy techniques that help to both reduce pain and rehabilitate the shoulder.
- Oblique rotator cuff muscle strengthening: with the arm by the side and the elbow flexed to 90 degrees the humerus is actively externally rotated against resistance. Repeating this exercise strengthens those muscles which depress the humeral head, enlarging the subacromial space and lessening impingement
- Scapular muscle strengthening: upright rowing, pull-downs and push-ups all help the scapular musculature to develop. A well-balanced scapula allows for more normal activation of the rotator cuff muscles
- Humeral positioning: a gradual increase in resisted movements of glenohumeral flexion and extension, abduction, and adduction, and internal and external rotation. These exercises are begun once the other exercises have produced humeral head depression and scapular strengthening. These movements reproduce sports and overhead work activities so need to be graded to avoid further exacerbation of subacromial impingement

Efficacy
Up to 70% chance of resolution of symptoms using these methods.

Risks/Benefits
Risk: incorrect exercises can exacerbate subacromial impingement, e.g. deltoid strengthening and pectoral muscle building. This should not occur with a well-supervised program.

Evidence
Several articles [2–4] support the role of physiotherapy in the conservative management of rotator cuff syndrome. There are no randomized controlled trials. The Cochrane Review for interventions in shoulder pain found no evidence to support or refute the efficacy of physiotherapy for shoulder pain.

Acceptability to patient
Physical therapy is time-consuming and requires some commitment from the patient to continue the exercises while unsupervised.

Follow up plan
- Re-examination to exclude rotator cuff tear if symptoms worsen
- Advice on prevention

Patient and caregiver information
To be successful, physical therapy requires commitment from the patient to continue the exercises demonstrated by the physical therapist.

Surgical therapy
SUBACROMIAL DECOMPRESSION
Either open surgery or arthroscopic decompression of the subacromial space.

Efficacy
Best results are likely in:
- A well-motivated patient over 40
- Absence of posterior capsular stiffness
- Absence of tendon signs and other shoulder pathology
- Symptoms associated with work-related injury

Risks/Benefits
Risks:
- Those of surgery in general: sepsis, bleeding, anesthetic risks, postoperative complications
- Those of shoulder surgery: brachial plexus injuries, arm swelling and weakness

Benefits: often the only option available to very refractory cases that have failed to respond to adequate physical therapy and repeated subacromial corticosteroid injections

Acceptability to patient
Patients with chronic or severe symptoms may be willing to consider surgery. Time off work of up to 10 weeks can be required after surgery.

Follow up plan
Look for signs of sepsis and bleeding in the immediate postoperative period. Surgical review at 6 weeks. Physical therapy and rehabilitation are very important aspects of recovery from this type of surgery.

Patient and caregiver information
Motivation and compliance with exercise regimens are important for postoperative recovery and rehabilitation.

LIFESTYLE
- Modification of shoulder activities helps to reduce pain
- Avoiding those movements that reproduce the pain is most useful, especially repetitive overhead arm motion

RISKS/BENEFITS
- Risk: no-risk strategy
- Benefit: seen immediately in a reduction in pain

ACCEPTABILITY TO PATIENT

Many tasks possible with unaffected arm.

FOLLOW UP PLAN

If rest is advised it is best combined with supervised exercise and rehabilitation to prevent loss of motion and strength.

PATIENT AND CAREGIVER INFORMATION

- For acute rotator cuff sprains a short period of rest is often all that is needed to effect a cure
- If symptoms persist then further treatment is available

EFFICACY OF THERAPIES

The use of analgesics, anti-inflammatories, and physical therapy is highly effective for the majority of patients. Occasionally surgery is required (for which efficacy is uncertain).

Evidence

- The only systematic review of evidence for the different treatments for shoulder pain concluded that subacromial corticosteroid injection provides a 35-degree improvement in range of abduction [2]
- In their paper on the conservative management of shoulder injuries, Morrison et al claim a 70% chance of resolution of symptoms with physiotherapy [3]
- There is insufficient evidence to support or refute all the other modalities of treatment

Review period

Monthly review during physical therapy to monitor improvement (can be undertaken by physical therapist).

PROGNOSIS

- The vast majority of patients seen in primary care with acute rotator cuff syndrome will make a full recovery within 2 weeks to 6 months
- Chronic rotator cuff syndrome (greater than 6 months of continuous symptoms) carries a worse prognosis and may result in significant impairment

Clinical pearls

- Most important factor determining successful treatment is the patient's compliance with physical therapy
- Corticosteroid injection may bring symptomatic relief when severe structural derangement of the rotator cuff is not present

Therapeutic failure

Patients suffering chronic rotator cuff symptoms despite adequate conservative management. Referral to a specialist with an interest in the surgical treatment of shoulder problems is appropriate.

Recurrence

For patients in whom rotator cuff syndrome is due to occupational use or sporting activities, recurrence is common. The therapeutic modalities are the same for each recurrence. Preventive exercises should be encouraged more in these patients.

Deterioration

Worsening of symptoms despite adequate conservative management suggests the possibility of a rotator cuff tear. Referral for ultrasound or magnetic resonance scanning is appropriate.

COMPLICATIONS

- Iatrogenic complications: gastrointestinal bleeding from nonsteroidal anti-inflammatories, septic arthritis from subacromial corticosteroid injection
- Tear of the rotator cuff due to progressive strain or massive initial disruption

CONSIDER CONSULT

Worsening symptoms despite adequate conservative treatment suggests possible rotator cuff tear. Referral for diagnostic ultrasound or MRI is appropriate.

PREVENTION

RISK FACTORS

Repetitive abduction and elevation of the shoulder is a common risk factor for rotator cuff syndrome. Three scenarios are most prevalent:

- High-powered overhead use in sportsmen, e.g. javelin, tennis, basketball, freestyle swimming
- Repeated occupational stress, e.g. carpenter, painter and decorator, plasterer
- Unaccustomed overuse, e.g. house or car maintenance

PREVENT RECURRENCE

Athletes who place their shoulders under excessive stress should be trained to warm up and stretch their rotator cuff muscles and tendons adequately before each training session or competition.

ASSOCIATIONS
American Academy of Orthopedic Surgeons
6300 North River Road
Rosemont, IL 60018-4262
Tel: (800) 824-BONES (2663)
www.aaos.org

Jefferson Health System, Thomas Jefferson University Hospital
111 South 11th Street
Philadelphia, PA 19107
Tel: (215) 955 6000

KEY REFERENCES
- American College of Rheumatology. Guidelines for the initial evaluation of the adult patient with acute musculoskeletal symptoms. Arthritis Rheum 1996;39(1):1–8
- Green S, Buchbinder R, Glazier R, Forbes A. Interventions for shoulder pain (Cochrane Review). In: The Cochrane Library, 2000, 3. Oxford: Update Software
- Morrison D, Greenbaum B, Einhorn A. Conservative management of shoulder injuries. Orthopaed Clin N Am 2000;31(2)
- Subacromial syndromes and impingement. In: Rosen. Emergency Medicine: Concepts and Clinical Practice, 4th edn. St Louis: Mosby Year Book, Inc, 1998, p732–8
- Warner J. Atlas of rotator cuff arthroscopy: rotator cuff disease. Orthoped Clin N Am 1997;28(2):251–65
- Miniaci A, Salonen D. Rotator cuff evaluation: imaging and diagnosis. Orthoped Clin N Am 1997;28(1):43–58

Evidence references and guidelines
1 American College of Rheumatology. Guidelines for the initial evaluation of the adult patient with acute musculoskeletal symptoms. Arthritis Rheum 1996;39(1):1–8. Available from the National Guidelines Clearinghouse
2 Green S, Buchbinder R, Glazier R, Forbes A. Interventions for shoulder pain (Cochrane Review). In: The Cochrane Library, 2000, 3. Oxford: Update Software
3 Morrison D, Greenbaum B, Einhorn A. Conservative management of shoulder injuries. Orthopaed Clin N Am 2000;31(2)
4 Morrison D, Frogameni A, Woodworth P. Conservative management for subacromial impingement syndrome. J Bone Joint Surg Am 1997;79:732–7

FAQS
Question 1
What causes rotator cuff syndrome?

ANSWER 1
The usual cause is impingement of the rotator cuff tendons (supraspinatus, infraspinatus, teres minor) in the subacromial space. This often follows overuse.

Question 2
Is supraspinatus tendonitis the same thing?

ANSWER 2
Supraspinatus tendonitis is the commonest pathological process involved in rotator cuff syndrome. Other synonyms are: impingement syndrome, painful arc, tennis shoulder, swimmer's shoulder.

Question 3

Is it necessary to inject the shoulder with corticosteroids?

ANSWER 3

Not always. Many cases settle with rest, physical therapy, and avoidance of the precipitating activities. If this fails then injection is usually tried next. In athletes and occupational users, an earlier injection can mean less interruption to training or work.

Question 4

When should referral to a specialist be considered?

ANSWER 4

- If the diagnosis is in doubt
- If examination suggests a rotator cuff tear
- If conservative treatment (including injection) fails after six months
- Professional athletes
- At the patient's insistence

Question 5

What exercises help?

ANSWER 5

Strengthening of the humeral head depressor muscles (latissimus dorsi) and the scapular muscles. Avoid exercises that build the deltoid as this reduces the subacromial space by elevating the humeral head.

CONTRIBUTORS

Martin L Kabongo, MD, PhD
Richard Brasington Jr, MD, FACP
Thiruvalam P Indira, MD

SARCOIDOSIS

DESCRIPTION

- A multisystem granulomatous disorder of unclear etiology characterized pathologically by the presence of noncaseating granulomas
- Wide spectrum of clinical presentation – can mimic several other diseases
- Acute or insidious onset; the latter being more serious due to progressive damage, through fibrosis, to one or more organs
- No specific therapy available. Corticosteroids are used but modify rather than prevent damage
- Granulomas can be widely distributed throughout the body without causing significant problems
- Spontaneous recovery occurs in 66% of patients

KEY! DON'T MISS!

- Uveitis needs urgent treatment to prevent blindness
- Cardiac arrhythmias need urgent referral for further investigation

BACKGROUND

ICD9 CODE
135.0 Sarcoidosis.

SYNONYMS
Löfgren's syndrome describes an acute subgroup of sarcoidosis.

CARDINAL FEATURES
Commonest presenting features are:
- Bilateral hilar lymphadenopathy
- Pulmonary infiltration
- Skin or eye lesions
- Acute onset with erythema nodosum and bilateral hilar lymphadenopathy tends to be benign and self-limiting
- Insidious onset heralds progressive fibrotic organ damage
- Organ-specific symptoms and signs can lead to confusion with other conditions
- Diagnosis is clinical with supporting evidence from investigations
- Noncaseating epithelioid cell granulomas on histology
- Elevated serum angiotensin-converting enzyme (ACE) levels

CAUSES
Common causes
Cause remains unclear although mounting evidence suggests a combination of an environmental trigger with genetic predisposition. Cases cluster within some employment groups and the disease is more common in siblings than in spouses. An infective trigger seems likely with some form of mycobacterium being the prime suspect.

EPIDEMIOLOGY
Incidence and prevalence
Sarcoidosis has a worldwide distribution; more is known about prevalence than incidence.

INCIDENCE
In Sweden from the 1960s to the 1980s, the incidence was 0.19 new cases per 1000 population/year.

PREVALENCE
In the US 0.3 per 1000.

FREQUENCY
- Swedish study suggests lifetime risk of 0.9% for men and 1.3% for women
- About 3% of African-American women develop the disease at some stage during adult life

Demographics
AGE
- May occur at any age
- 68% are under 40 at time of diagnosis
- Uncommon under 15 years or over 65

GENDER
Women affected slightly more often than men.

RACE

- In the US, African-Americans are more likely than Caucasians to suffer sarcoidosis
- The expression of the disease is also affected by race with more florid presentations in blacks and more cardiac sarcoidosis in Japanese populations

GENETICS

Precise genetic risk is not known; however, if one family member has sarcoidosis, other family members have a 16% chance of developing it.

GEOGRAPHY

Worldwide distribution but more common in Northern Europe and the US.

SOCIOECONOMIC STATUS

Sarcoidosis is more common in healthcare workers, particularly nurses, and in rural areas. This may suggest a shared environmental trigger.

DIFFERENTIAL DIAGNOSIS

Differential diagnosis depends on organ(s) damaged. This most commonly arises with progressive lung damage, hepatic granulomas and, in the acute onset cases, with other causes of erythema nodosum.

Other causes of erythema nodosum

These need to be considered when sarcoidosis presents acutely as it may be the only sign on clinical examination.

Infections:

- Bacteria (streptococci, tuberculosis, brucellosis, leprosy)
- Viruses
- *Mycoplasma*
- *Rickettsia*
- *Chlamydia*
- Fungi

Drugs:

- Sulfonamides
- Oral contraceptives

Systemic disease:

- Ulcerative colitis
- Crohn's disease
- Behçet's syndrome

Other causes of granulomatous reactions

Infection:

- Mycobacteria
- Fungi
- Spirochaetes
- Bacteria: brucellosis
- Parasites

Neoplasms:

- Lymphoma
- Carcinoma

Extrinsic allergic alveolitis:

- Animal protein (bird fancier's lung)
- Fungi (farmer's lung)

Chemicals:

- Silica
- Beryllium

Immunological disorders:

- Crohn's disease
- Primary biliary cirrhosis
- Vasculitis – Wegener's granulomatosis

SIGNS & SYMPTOMS
Signs
PHYSICAL EXAMINATION

Skin:

- Rashes – erythema nodosum, lupus pernio
- Granulomatous skin lesions – plaques, papules, subcutaneous nodules and infiltration of old surgical or traumatic scars

Lymph nodes:

- Small mobile nontender lymph nodes are found in up to 30% of cases.
- Common sites are anterior triangle of neck, supraclavicular fossae, axillae, and inguinal regions

Lower respiratory tract:

Few signs of this without testing respiratory function, but pleural involvement may give rise to a pleural effusion.

Cardiac:

- Arrhythmias
- Congestive cardiac failure

Abdominal organs:

- Spleen may be just palpable in mild cases but a large spleen may be a sign of longstanding sarcoidosis
- It is usually accompanied by hepatic enlargement, which may lead to thrombocytopenic purpura and signs of hepatic failure

Upper respiratory tract:

- Mucosal thickening in the nose is usually associated with longstanding sarcoidosis
- A discharge may be blood stained or purulent

Musculoskeletal system:

- Acute cases present with arthralgia and stiffness of large joints
- Chronic cases can show swelling of soft tissues around small joints with accompanying stiffness
- Can have acute arthritis in form of Löfgren's syndrome – triad of acute polyarthritis, hilar adenopathy and erythema nodosum
- Chronic arthritis may be seen with nondeforming arthritis

Ocular:

- Uveitis
- Conjunctival follicles

Neurological:

Bell's palsy from facial nerve damage is the commonest manifestation if the nervous system is involved.

Symptoms
Depend on organ involved, especially in rare presentations when only one organ or system is affected, e.g. cardiac involvement or small joint involvement. Half of all patients present with chronic respiratory symptoms only. The more common presenting symptoms are:

- Cough
- Breathlessness on exertion
- Chest pain

- Fatigue
- Fever
- Anorexia
- Weight loss
- Erythema nodosum or other skin rashes
- Swelling and stiffness of joints
- Nasal discharge or stuffiness
- Gritty or dry eyes with misty vision
- Dry mouth
- Löfgren's syndrome is a form of sarcoidosis presenting acutely with erythema nodosum, malaise, fever, arthralgia affecting large joints, and uveitis

KEY! DON'T MISS!
- Uveitis needs urgent treatment to prevent blindness
- Cardiac arrhythmias need urgent referral for further investigation

CONSIDER CONSULT
- Referral to a specialist is necessary in almost all cases to firmly establish the diagnosis
- Histological confirmation of the diagnosis is best done from a transbronchial biopsy as the presence of noncaseating granulomas in a single organ such as the skin is generally insufficient to confirm diagnosis. An acute onset Löfgren's syndrome can be managed without biopsy proof if the patient recovers rapidly without specific treatment

INVESTIGATION OF THE PATIENT
Direct questions to patient
Q Has the cough developed suddenly or gradually? Consider other causes of cough and try and eliminate simple respiratory infection

Q What do you mean by breathlessness? Look for gradual onset with initial dyspnea on exertion. Patient should complain of a restrictive quality

Q Have you had any respiratory problems? Asthma could mimic some of the respiratory symptoms

Q Do you have any chest pain? Patients may complain of a retrosternal feeling of tightness that can mimic cardiac pain

Q Have any of your work colleagues, friends or family had chest problems? Think about tuberculosis as an alternative cause

Q How quickly did the rash develop? Erythema nodosum typically presents acutely

Q Do you have any joint pains? Arthralgia and arthropathy presenting acutely with erythema nodosum and accompanied by fever and malaise suggests Löfgren's syndrome

Q Has this happened before? Check for a history of similar attacks that may not have been investigated and diagnosed

Q Any problems with your eyes or eyesight? Discomfort, watering, photophobia or blurring of vision might suggest uveitis, which needs prompt treatment

Q Do you have any other skin problems? A history of thickened nontender areas of skin could be granulomatous infiltration

Q Have you felt your heart beating irregularly or had any palpitations? Sarcoidosis can selectively affect the heart and arrhythmias can be life-threatening

Q What is your job? Exposure to silica or beryllium can cause similar lung problems. Farmers can suffer lung damage from fungi

Q Do you keep birds? Psittacosis can result in pulmonary symptoms

Q Have you taken any over-the-counter medicines for your symptoms? Patients may self-medicate in acute stages with nonsteroidal anti-inflammatory agents and this may mask the presentation

Contributory or predisposing factors

Q What is your occupation? Have any colleagues had similar symptoms? Environmental exposure to chemicals could suggest an alternative diagnosis

Family history

Q Have any members of your family suffered similar symptoms? A positive family history may favor sarcoidosis as a possible diagnosis

Examination

Because sarcoidosis is a multisystem disorder, examination should be generalized but with emphasis on presenting symptoms.

Q Is there evidence of erythema nodosum and painful joints? Large joints are affected in acute cases and small joints in chronic disease. Erythema nodosum presents as red, raised, tender bumps on the extensor surfaces of the legs

Q Are other rashes present? Lupus pernio describes indurated plaques with discoloration. It is most commonly seen around the nose, cheeks, lips, and ears

Q What is the patient's breathing like? Listen to the chest; decreased breath sounds suggest a pleural effusion. Wheezing is unusual and may indicate asthma, or infectious process. Basal crepitations or rales occur with heart failure secondary to cardiac infiltration

Q Is the heart functioning normally? Examine the heart to check for arrhythmias, pericardial effusion or enlargement of the heart

Q Is there evidence of liver/spleen enlargement? Palpate the abdomen for evidence of enlargement of the liver and/or spleen

Q What is the appearance of old scar tissue? Check old scars for granulomatous infiltration

Q Are the eyes functioning normally? Examine the eyes, looking for watering and redness, which would suggest uveitis. Use a slitlamp if available

Q Are the lymph nodes enlarged? Small nontender, discrete and mobile nodes are typical. Greater degrees of enlargement might suggest tuberculosis or lymphoma

Q Is there evidence of cranial nerve damage? Look especially for a unilateral facial nerve palsy

Summary of investigative tests

Sarcoidosis often needs referral for specialist care. Investigations can be generally carried out in the outpatient setting:

- Chest X-ray in all cases to grade the severity of the disease and for follow up to assess improvement or progression
- Pulmonary function tests to clarify clinical dyspnea and provide a baseline
- ECG as screening for cardiac involvement
- Echocardiography if cardiac involvement is suspected
- Peripheral blood count to assess hematological activity and if splenic involvement is suspected
- Serum chemistry – liver function studies and analysis of serum ACE to help with diagnosis and to monitor response to therapy
- Urinary calcium to assess extrathoracic involvement
- Incisional biopsy to confirm histologic diagnosis
- CT or MRI scanning to clarify X-ray findings
- Bronchial lavage in selected patients to help differentiate from other causes of chronic lung disease

DIAGNOSTIC DECISION

A diagnosis of sarcoidosis is suggested if the following criteria are present:

- A consistent clinical presentation
- Histological evidence of noncaseating epithelioid cell granulomas
- Exclusion of other agents/diseases known to cause granulomatous reactions

Guidelines
A consensus statement on sarcoidosis has been produced: 'Statement on sarcoidosis. Joint Statement of the American Thoracic Society (ATS), the European Respiratory Society (ERS) and the World Association of Sarcoidosis and Other Granulomatous Disorders (WASOG) adopted by the ATS Board of Directors and by the ERS Executive Committee, February 1999 [1].

This statement has been reviewed by the American Academy of Family Physicians [2].

THE TESTS
Body fluids
PERIPHERAL BLOOD COUNT
Description
Cuffed venous sample into an EDTA bottle.

Advantages/Disadvantages
- Advantage: abnormal hematology is seen in up to 40% of patients with sarcoidosis
- Disadvantage: they are not diagnostic but can be useful to exclude infectious process

Abnormal
- Anemia with a hemoglobin of less than 11g/dL occurs in up to 20% of patients
- Leukopenia (<4 x 10⁹/L) is rarely severe
- Thrombocytopenia (150 x 10⁹/L) is rare
- Keep in mind the possibility of a false-positive result

Cause of abnormal result
- Anemia occurs as a response to a chronic disease and is nonspecific
- Leukopenia may indicate splenomegaly or bone marrow involvement but may just show because T cells are concentrated at sites of disease
- Thrombocytopenia is also linked to splenomegaly

Drugs, disorders and other factors that may alter results
Other causes of microcytic anemia such as iron deficiency must be excluded.

SERUM CHEMISTRY
Description
Venous sample.

Normal
8.8–10.3mg/dL (2.2–2.58mmol/L).

Abnormal
- Raised serum calcium (> 10.3mg/dL)
- Raised liver enzyme levels (ALT>60 IU/L; AST>40 IU/L; Alk Phos>120 IU/L)
- Raised creatinine and urea (>1.2mg/dL and >18mg/dL)
- Raised serum ACE levels (refer to laboratory for normal values)
- Keep in mind the possibility of a false-positive result

Cause of abnormal result
- Hypercalcemia affects up to 2–10% of patients and reflects abnormalities in calcitriol production
- Liver enzymes abnormalities are caused by granulomatous infiltration of the liver
- Abnormal renal function may result from undetected hypercalcemia causing renal stones or renal failure
- Serum ACE may reflects disease activity

Drugs, disorders and other factors that may alter results
Check for evidence of excessive alcohol intake causing liver abnormalities.

URINARY CALCIUM

Description
Assessment of daily urinary output of calcium.

Advantages/Disadvantages
Disadvantage: requires 24-h collection of all urine output so can be inconvenient for the patient.

Abnormal
- Greater than 7.5mmol/day
- Keep in mind the possibility of a false-positive result

Cause of abnormal result
Impaired regulation of calcitriol production by activated macrophages and granulomas.

Tests of function
PULMONARY FUNCTION TESTS
Description
Pulmonary function tests are designed to measure the various lung volumes and diffusion capacity of the lungs.

Advantages/Disadvantages
Advantages:
- Useful to classify the disease into restrictive or obstructive pathology and help in finding the severity of disease
- Serial measurements may help gauge the response to treatment

Normal
Normal lung volumes and diffusion capacity.

Abnormal
- Reduced total lung capacity and restricted ventilatory capacity
- Impaired gas transfer
- Low compliance
- Keep in mind the possibility of a falsely positive result

Cause of abnormal result
Pulmonary infiltration.

Drugs, disorders and other factors that may alter results
Other respiratory disease such as asthma/chronic obstructive pulmonary disease.

Biopsy
INCISIONAL BIOPSY
Description
A specialist often carries out biopsy for histologic proof, but a primary care physician with appropriate expertise may take a specimen from easily accessible tissues such as lupus pernio or infiltration of scars.

Advantages/Disadvantages

Disadvantage: histology from a single skin lesion is often not considered proof and patients have to undergo further sampling by a specialist.

Abnormal
- Noncaseating epithelioid cell granuloma
- Keep in mind the possibility of a false-positive result

Cause of abnormal result
Sarcoidosis.

Imaging
CHEST X-RAY
Advantages/Disadvantages
Advantage: an important test for diagnosis and follow up of disease activity.

Abnormal
- Five stages of X-ray findings are described with the first (Stage 0) being a normal result
- Keep in mind the possibility of a falsely positive result

Cause of abnormal result
- Stage 1 bilateral hilar lymphadenopathy
- Stage 2 bilateral hilar lymphadenopathy with parenchymal infiltration
- Stage 3 parenchymal infiltration without hilar lymphadenopathy
- Stage 4 advanced fibrosis with evidence of honeycombing, hilar retraction, bullae, cysts, and emphysema

ECHOCARDIOGRAPHY
Advantages/Disadvantages
Advantage: non-invasive test that can pick up early signs of cardiac involvement.

Abnormal
- Echocardiography can identify reduced left ventricular function, valve abnormalities, pericardial effusion and ventricular aneurysms
- Keep in mind the possibility of a false-positive result

Cause of abnormal result
Granuloma formation.

Other tests
ECG
Advantages/Disadvantages
Advantages:
- May be normal
- A 24-hour tracing using a Holter monitor or event monitor may be used if arrhythmias are suspected

Abnormal
- May show arrhythmias or heart block
- Keep in mind the possibility of a false-positive result

Cause of abnormal result
Sarcoid granulomas in the myocardium.

TREATMENT

IMMEDIATE ACTION

If uveitis is suspected, referral to an ophthalmologist is necessary. Use of corticosteroid eye drops may prevent permanent damage.

MANAGEMENT ISSUES
Goals

- Reduce pain and swelling related to erythema nodosum and joint involvement in acute cases
- Initiate treatment for eye involvement
- Patient referral for diagnostic studies (biopsy, pulmonary function tests etc)
- In approaching management in chronic cases, the physician should assess whether the disease is stable or likely to progress and whether therapy will be of any benefit

Management in special circumstances

Cardiology referral if cardiac involvement is suspected.

SUMMARY OF THERAPEUTIC OPTIONS
Choices

Therapy should be individualized based on clinical presentation. Although systemic corticosteroids suppress granulomas and may speed up resolution in acute cases, granulomas may resolve spontaneously and side-effects of therapy must be considered. Steroids also reduce symptoms and slow disease progression in chronic cases but there is no proof that they prevent the development of fibrosis.

- NSAIDs such as ibuprofen reduce pain from erythema nodosum or joint involvement and any associated fever – specific treatment is of little value in the acute presentation
- Selective cyclo-oxygenase-2 (COX-2) inhibitors are preferred in patients with history of gastroesophageal reflux disease (GERD), peptic ulcer, or gastritis
- Topical corticosteroid therapy such as fluticasone may be all that is required in mild cases of erythema nodosum
- Ophthalmic corticosteroids such as betamethasone eye drops can be used for treating uveitis
- The ideal dose for systemic corticosteroids like prednisolone has not been established in any clinical trials therefore dose and duration of therapy needs to be tailored for each individual patient. Corticosteroids remain the first choice when treatment is indicated but do not always produce a response. In responders the dose can be gradually tapered to find the minimum effective dose. Treatment is generally continued for at least 12 months
- Second-line therapy is needed for cases that do not respond to corticosteroids after a 3 month trial. It can also be used in addition to corticosteroid as steroid-sparing therapy if high corticosteroid doses are necessary to maintain improvement. Methotrexate and azathioprine seem to be the best choices on the basis of safety and efficacy. These drugs should only be initiated under specialist supervision
- Address lifestyle issues

Guidelines

A consensus statement on sarcoidosis has been produced: 'Statement on sarcoidosis. Joint Statement of the American Thoracic Society (ATS), the European Respiratory Society (ERS) and the World Association of Sarcoidosis and Other Granulomatous Disorders (WASOG) adopted by the ATS Board of Directors and by the ERS Executive Committee [1].

This statement has been reviewed by the American Academy of Family Physicians [2].

FOLLOW UP

- Essential whether patients are being actively treated or not
- Should be most intensive in first 2 years after diagnosis to allow assessment of prognosis and decide on the need or otherwise for therapy. Based on X-ray staging, stage 1 requires 6-monthly follow up. Stages 2 through 4 require 3-monthly reassessments or more frequently if having therapy. In these cases, follow up should continue for at least 3 years after discontinuation of treatment
- Follow up comprises general examination, chest X-ray, lung function tests, blood tests as indicated by extent of disease; more involved investigation depends on organs affected
- Patients who have undergone splenectomy should have pneumococcal vaccination (prevents life-threatening encapsulated infections)

Information for patient or caregiver

Patients need to be told about the need to be reassessed earlier than a planned follow up if they suffer any new symptoms.

DRUGS AND OTHER THERAPIES: DETAILS
Drugs
IBUPROFEN

Indicated for symptomatic relief of pain from erythema nodosum and joint involvement. Will also reduce fever.

Dose
Oral: 200–800mg three times daily after meals, usual dose 400mg four times daily.

Efficacy
Pain begins to ease within 1–2 h.

Risks/Benefits
Risk: use caution in hepatic, renal and cardiac failure

Benefits:
- Faster onset of action than colchicines
- Inexpensive

Side-effects and adverse reactions
- Gastrointestinal: anorexia, nausea, dyspepsia, peptic ulceration
- Central nervous system: headache, dizziness, tinnitus
- Hypersensitivity: rashes, bronchospasm, angioedema

Interactions (other drugs)
- Aminoglycosides ▪ Antihypertensives ▪ Corticosteroids ▪ Cyclosporin ▪ Digoxin
- Lithium ▪ Methotrexate ▪ Phenylpropanolamine ▪ Diuretics ▪ Warfarin

Contraindications
- Peptic ulceration ▪ Hypersensitivity to NSAIDs ▪ Coagulation defects

Acceptability to patient
High.

Follow up plan
Monitor response and advise patient as needed when dosing can be used.

BETAMETHASONE EYE DROPS

To treat pain and inflammation from uveitis. This can be initiated in primary care but should be followed up by a specialist.

Dose

One drop to each eye every 1–2 h until symptoms controlled then reduce frequency to twice daily.

Efficacy

Quickly reduces pain and blurring of vision.

Risks/Benefits

Risks:

- Caution needed in long-term use (10 days or more); may lead to secondary ocular infections, glaucoma, optic nerve damage, cataract
- May mask signs of pre-existing or secondary ocular infection
- Caution needed in pregnancy and lactation
- Safe use in children has not been established

Side-effects and adverse reactions

- Glaucoma
- Optic nerve damage
- Cataract formation
- Superinfection of the eye
- Corneal and scleral perforation
- Stinging or burning on application

Interactions (other drugs)

None recorded.

Acceptability to patient

- Usually well tolerated
- Some patients find it unpleasant
- Those with painful hand joints my need a carer to instill them.

Follow up plan

Follow up by specialist to assess response and determine the duration of treatment.

FLUTICASONE

Available as cream, inhaler, and nasal spray. May be used in mild disease if systemic corticosteroids are not indicated. Evidence base is not sound as some studies have shown little effect.

Dose

- Cream (0.05%) applied once daily
- Inhaler 100–250mcg twice daily
- Nasal spray 100mcg to each nostril once daily

Efficacy

Needs to be assessed for each individual patient.

Risks/Benefits

Risks:

- Not suitable for use in children (risk of growth retardation)

- Use caution after recent nasal surgery
- Use caution in pregnancy and lactation

Benefit: good for relief of moderate to severe allergic rhinitis

Side-effects and adverse reactions
- Nasal irritation, epistaxis, taste and smell disturbances
- Raised intra-ocular pressure

Interactions (other drugs)
No significant interactions recorded.

Contraindications
- Hypersensitivity to the fluticasone. ■ Active varicella infection ■ Untreated nasal infection
- Pulmonary TB

Acceptability to patient
Usually well tolerated and patients prefer to try topical preparations to avoid systemic side-effects.

Follow up plan
Review after 4 weeks to assess efficacy.

PREDNISOLONE
Dose
Initially 20–40mg/day although higher doses are used for cardiac involvement. After 1–3 months, depending on response, dose can be tapered down to 5–10mg/day.

Efficacy
- Some patients do not respond at all
- In others, symptomatic relief may be noted only after several weeks
- Effect on disease progression is not clear

Risks/Benefits
Risks:
- Overwhelming septicemia if patient has an infection
- Loss of control of blood glucose in those with diabetes
- Prolonged use causes adrenal suppression

Side-effects and adverse reactions
- Side-effects are minimized by short duration of therapy
- Gastrointestinal: dyspepsia, peptic ulceration, oesophagitis, oral candidiasis
- Cardiovascular system: hypertension, thromboembolism
- Central nervous system: insomnia, euphoria, depression, psychosis
- Endocrine: adrenal suppression, impaired glucose tolerance, growth suppression in children
- Musculoskeletal: proximal myopathy, osteoporosis
- Skin: delayed healing, acne, striae
- Eyes, ears, nose, and throat: cataract, glaucoma, blurred vision

Interactions (other drugs)
- Aminoglutethamide ■ Barbiturates ■ Cholestyramine ■ Clarithromycin, erythromycin
- Colestipol ■ Isoniazid ■ Ketoconazole ■ NSAIDs ■ Oral contraceptives ■ Rifampin
- Salicylates ■ Troleandomycin

Contraindications
- Systemic infection ▪ Avoid live virus vaccines in those receiving immunosuppressive doses

Acceptability to patient
Patients are cautious about 'steroid' use (press coverage: anabolic steroid use in athletes; severe side-effects due to over prescribing of topical steroids when first introduced) so the benefits have to be explained.

Follow up plan
Frequency of follow up is judged on an individual patient basis.

Patient and caregiver information
- Patient must be fully aware that corticosteroids occurring naturally in the body will be suppressed and that treatment must not be discontinued without medical advice
- Patient should avoid high-salt diet
- Corticosteroid treatment cards must be carried to ensure correct treatment is given in the case of an accident or other emergency
- Medalert bracelets are useful

METHOTREXATE
Usually used under specialist supervision either to reduce dose of steroids or as sole agent in cases that do not respond to steroids.

Dose
- An initial test dose of 2.5mg is given to check for hypersensitivity
- 7.5mg once a week increased according to response to a maximum of 20mg once a week

Efficacy
Acts to suppress rather than cure the disease.

Risks/Benefits
Risks:
- Use caution with infection and bone marrow depression
- Use caution with peptic ulceration and ulcerative colitis
- Use caution with renal and hepatic impairment
- Use caution with the elderly
- Use caution in pregnancy

Side-effects and adverse reactions
- Central nervous system: dizziness, drowsiness, headache, seizures
- Eyes, ears, nose, and throat: blurred vision, tinnitus
- Gastrointestinal: abdominal pain, diarrhoea, hepatotoxicity, melena, vomiting
- Genitourinary: depression of and defective spermatogenensis, hematuria, renal failure, urinary retention
- Hematologic: anemia, hemorrhage, leukopenia, pancytopenia, thrombocytopenia
- Metabolic: increased serum uric acid
- Musculoskeletal: arthralgia, myalgia, osteoporosis
- Respiratory: pneumonitis, pulmonary fibrosis
- Skin: acne, dermatitis, hyperpimentation, vaculitis

Interactions (other drugs)
- Aminoglycosides ▪ Antimalarials ▪ Binding resins ▪ Co-trimoxazole ▪ Cyclosporin
▪ Ethanol ▪ Etretrinate ▪ Live vaccines ▪ NSAIDS ▪ Omeprazole ▪ Penicillins
▪ Probenicid ▪ Salicylates ▪ Sulfinpyrazone

Contraindications
- Severe renal and hepatic impairment ▪ Profound bone marrow depression ▪ Nursing mothers

Acceptability to patient
Nausea may limit its use, as can the thought of having repeated liver biopsies.

Follow up plan
Regular monthly blood tests to monitor liver function.

Patient and caregiver information
Patients must tell all other physicians who might treat them that they are on this drug.

AZATHIOPRINE
Used only under specialist supervision either to reduce dose of steroids or as sole agent in cases that do not respond to steroids.

Dose
- Initially up to 3mg/kg daily reduced according to response
- Maintenance 1–3mg daily

Efficacy
Limited evidence for efficacy.

Risks/Benefits
Risks:
- Use caution with bone marrow depression and infection
- Use caution in pregnancy and nursing mothers

Side-effects and adverse reactions
- Gastrointestinal: esophagitis, hepatotoxicity, nausea, pancreatitis
- Genitourinary: depression of spermatogenensis
- Hematologic: anemia, leukopenia, pancytopenia, thrombocytopenia
- Musculoskeletal: arthralgia, muscle wasting
- Skin: rash
- Miscellaneous: fungal, bacterial, protozoal and viral infections, may increase risk of neoplasm (skin cancer, reticulocyte or lymphomatous tumours)

Interactions (other drugs)
- Allopurinol ▪ Warfarin

Contraindications
No significant contraindications recorded.

Acceptability to patient
Usually well tolerated, regular blood tests necessary to check for marrow suppression.

Follow up plan
Monthly blood tests and assessment of efficacy with tapering of dose.

LIFESTYLE
- Encourage patients with liver abnormalities to abstain from alcohol, depending on the degree of liver damage

- Encourage patients to cease smoking
- Advise avoidance of high-salt diet when on corticosteroid therapy
- Advise low-calcium diet for patients with hypercalcemia

RISKS/BENEFITS
Risk: to avoid malnutrition, a dietitian should supervise dietary manipulation.

ACCEPTABILITY TO PATIENT
Will need support to overcome withdrawal effects from smoking.

FOLLOW UP PLAN
Confirm nonsmoking status at each visit and inquire about diet.

PROGNOSIS

- Spontaneous recovery is the rule for about 66% of patients with 10–30% suffering chronic or progressive disease
- Of those treated with corticosteroids (up to 50%), the vast majority stabilize or improve. Relapse occurs in 16–74% after reduction or cessation of therapy
- Between 10 and 20% of patients have permanent disability from either pulmonary or extrapulmonary disease
- Deaths are reported as being between 1 and 5% of cases and occur from pulmonary, neurological or cardiac involvement

COMPLICATIONS

Complications are due to involvement of specific organs such as cardiac, neurologic, ophthalmologic, and respiratory system.

PREVENTION

Sarcoidosis is not specifically preventable in the general population.

ASSOCIATIONS
National Sarcoidosis Resource Center
PO Box 1593
Piscataway, NJ 08855-1593
Tel: (732) 699 0733
Fax: (732) 699 0882

Sarcoidosis Online Sites
A very useful site with details of many medical and lay sites dealing with sarcoidosis.

The National Sarcoidosis Foundation
268 Martin Luther King Blvd.
Newark, NJ 07102
Tel: (800) 223 6429
Fax: (201) 877 2850

Sarcoidosis - Grand Rounds at Baylor
Pictures and examples of sarcoidosis.

National Center for Immunology and Respiratory Medicine
Pictures and examples of sarcoidosis.

KEY REFERENCES
- James, DG. Descriptive definition and historic aspects of sarcoidosis. Clin Chest Med 1997; 18:663
- Gottlieb, JE, Israel, HL, Steiner, RM et al. Outcome in sarcoidosis: The relationship of relapse to corticosteroid therapy. Chest 1997; 111:623
- Mitchell, DN. Sarcoidosis. Medicine 1998; 26:43–9
- ATS Guidelines: Statement on sarcoidosis. Am J Respir Crit Care Med 1999: 160:736–55 (available at http://thoracic.org/)
- Newman, LS, Rose, CS, Maier, LA. Sarcoidosis. New Engl J of Med 1997; 336:17:1224–34

Evidence references and guidelines
1   ATS Guidelines: Statement on sarcoidosis. Am J Respir Crit Care Med 1999: 160:736–55
2   Morey SS. Practice guidelines: American Thoracic Society: issues consensus statement on sarcoidosis. Am Fam Physician 2000;61:553–4, 556

FAQS
Question 1
What happens if I get pregnant?

ANSWER 1
Sarcoidosis generally has no effect on pregnancy but it may worsen after delivery. The baby is not at risk.

Question 2
What causes sarcoidosis?

ANSWER 2
The cause is currently unknown. Many different environmental causes have been looked at which might work in combination with an in-built genetic tendency. Infections such as tuberculosis and similar diseases have been looked at closely without any proof that they are involved.

Question 3

Is there a cure for sarcoidosis?

ANSWER 3

Most cases resolve spontaneously. There is no cure. The treatments available may only help to speed up the natural healing process.

Question 4

Is there any screening available for sarcoidosis?

ANSWER 4

As it is a rare disease, it would be unnecessary and expensive to set up a screening service. In the days of mass chest X-ray for TB screening, many cases of sarcoidosis were detected. Most of these did not produce any symptoms and the X-ray findings returned to normal over a few years.

Question 5

Is it safe to play sport with sarcoidosis?

ANSWER 5

Yes, there are no general problems with any sports. If you have joint disease it would be better to swim than jog, and lung disease might limit how much you can do. Exercise is important in building your endurance and resilience to the effects of the disease.

CONTRIBUTORS

Fred F Ferri, MD, FACP
Richard Brasington Jr, MD, FACP
Dinnesh Khanna, MD

SCLERODERMA

DESCRIPTION

- Rare, multisystem, chronic disorder of unknown cause, characterized by tissue fibrosis (especially skin thickening), small blood vessel vasculopathy (especially Raynaud's phenomenon), and autoimmunity
- Diffuse and limited scleroderma are characterized by both cutaneous and visceral involvement; lower risk of early visceral involvement in limited scleroderma
- Localized scleroderma is characterized by cutaneous involvement only (itself divided into morphea and linear scleroderma)
- Systemic sclerosis sine scleroderma is characterized by visceral involvement only (rare)
- No cure exists; treatment is limited to management

URGENT ACTION

- Hospitalize immediately if renal hypertension (also referred to as renal crisis) or severe pulmonary involvement is suspected
- Large, deep ulceration in the fingers accompanied by intense pain is indicative of deep tissue infarction secondary to Raynaud's phenomenon; immediate treatment is essential

KEY! DON'T MISS!

Signs of renal or pulmonary involvement should lead to immediate hospitalization.

ICD9 CODE
710.2 (Morphea 701.0).

SYNONYMS
- Systemic sclerosis
- Progressive systemic sclerosis
- Morphea only applies to localized scleroderma affecting the skin

CARDINAL FEATURES
- Rare, multisystem, chronic disorder of unknown cause, characterized by tissue fibrosis (especially skin thickening), small blood vessel vasculopathy (especially Raynaud's phenomenon), and autoimmunity
- No cure exists; treatment is limited to management
- Condition is loosely divided into subtypes which set the course of the disease once established; it does not progress from one established subtype to another
- Diffuse scleroderma: characterized by rapid (<1-2 years) skin thickening on the extremities, face, and trunk in a symmetric pattern; greater risk of early visceral involvement
- Limited scleroderma: characterized by gradual skin thickening limited to distal extremities, and face; lesser risk of early visceral involvement; when calcinosis, Raynaud's phenomenon, esophageal dysphagia, and telangiectasis accompany the limited skin involvement; it is often referred to as CREST syndrome
- Localized scleroderma is divided into morphea and linear
- Morphea scleroderma features oval plaque(s) of hard skin, 0.5-12 inches in diameter; usually on the trunk alone; generalized morphea occurs when very hard and dark plaques are widely spread over the body
- Linear scleroderma, which may coincide with morphea, features bands of skin induration; a line running down the forehead is sometimes called en coup de sabre ('sword stroke')
- Systemic sclerosis sine scleroderma: visceral involvement without skin thickening (rare)
- May overlap with other connective tissue diseases (mixed connective tissue disease)

CAUSES
Common causes
- Causes of most cases are unknown, but all are associated with autoimmunity
- Some evidence suggests that pregnancy, or estrogen, confers a predisposition; virus infections have also been suggested

Rare causes
Scleroderma and scleroderma-like conditions have been linked to exposure to:
- Silica dust (from mines)
- Polyvinyl or vinyl chloride
- Epoxy resins
- Aromatic hydrocarbons (e.g. toluene, benzine, trichloroethylene)
- Pentazocine
- Chemotherapy (bleomycin, vinblastine)
- Contaminated rapeseed oil - caused a scleroderma-like condition in 20,000 people in Madrid in the 1980s

Other rare causes of scleroderma-like syndromes:
- Ingestion of L-tryptophan-containing foods, possibly due to a contaminant (eosinophilic myalgia syndrome)
- Morphea sometimes caused by radiotherapy

Contributory or predisposing factors
Autoimmune history in patient or close relatives.

EPIDEMIOLOGY
Incidence and prevalence
Rare condition.

INCIDENCE
0.01-0.02/1000.

PREVALENCE
0.1-0.3/1000.

Demographics
AGE
- Unusual in children and young men
- Incidence peaks at 30-40 years
- Localized scleroderma is more common in children and teenagers

GENDER
Women:men - 4:1.

RACE
- Limited and diffuse scleroderma is more frequent in African-American women
- Localized scleroderma is more common in Caucasians than African-Americans
- Relatively high prevalence (0.472/1000) in Choctaw Native Americans (Oklahoma, US)

GENETICS
- Suggested linkages with HLA-A1, -B8, -DR1, -DR3, -DR3/DR52, -DR5, and limited scleroderma and HLA-DR1; strong associations shown with C4AQ0 and DQA2
- However, disease is rarely inherited (<2% of cases); familial links may depend more on environmental factors

DIFFERENTIAL DIAGNOSIS

- Early scleroderma can be very difficult to distinguish from other connective tissue diseases
- Cause of unexplained pulmonary fibrosis, biliary cirrhosis, pulmonary or renal hypertension, or cardiomyopathy should also be investigated

Primary Raynaud's phenomenon

Primary Raynaud's phenomenon occurs in 10-15% of the population, but almost all patients do not develop scleroderma. Other secondary causes of Raynaud's phenomenon should be taken into account, including thoracic outlet syndrome, vibration disease, peripheral vascular disease, carcinoid syndrome, cold agglutinin disease, cold injury, cryoglobulinemia, and dermatomyositis.

FEATURES
- Delineated, symmetric, triphasic color change (white, blue, then red) of fingers in response to cold, stress, or vibration
- Toes, nose, and ears may also be affected
- Age at onset <30 years
- Mild-to-moderate severity (gangrene rare)
- Normal nailfold capillaries
- Negative antinuclear antibody titer

Rheumatoid arthritis

Rheumatoid arthritis may mimic scleroderma in early stages.

FEATURES
- Symmetric polyarthralgia, most often in hands and feet
- Joint effusions, tenderness, and restricted movement usually present in early stages
- Prolonged morning stiffness (over one hour)
- Chronic, inflamed joints
- Systemic symptoms often present: fatigue, possible mild anemia, or mild leukocytosis
- Positive rheumatoid factor test (but also positive in 30-50% of scleroderma patients)
- Raynaud's phenomenon may be present

Systemic lupus erythematosus

Systemic lupus erythematosus may mimic scleroderma in early stages.

FEATURES
- Malar or discoid rash
- Alopecia
- Constitutional features such as fatigue, fever
- Nasal or oropharyngeal ulcerations
- Anemia, thrombocytopenia, or leukopenia (predominantly a lymphopenia)
- Tender, swollen, or effusive joints (usually peripheral)
- Myalgia
- Serositis (pleuritis, pericarditis, serositis)
- Heart murmur
- Conjunctivitis, sicca syndrome
- Raynaud's phenomenon may be present

Polymyositis

Polymyositis may mimic scleroderma in early stages.

FEATURES

- Muscular weakness
- Dysphagia
- Fatigue
- Arthralgia
- Myalgia
- Cardiac abnormalities
- Raynaud's phenomenon may be present
- An overlap condition, sclerodermatomyositis (distinguished by tight skin and muscle weakness), is sometimes indistinguishable from true scleroderma

Chronic graft-versus-host disease

Skin thickening of chronic graft-versus-host disease may especially mimic scleroderma.

FEATURES

- Generalized skin thickening
- Skin rash
- Alopecia
- Hepatic dysfunction
- Oral lichenoid lesions
- Sicca complex
- Obliterative bronchiolitis
- Gastrointestinal (GI) motility disorders

Amyloidosis

Skin thickening on fingers and hands of amyloidosis may particularly mimic scleroderma.

FEATURES

- Skin thickening on fingers and hands
- Nephrotic syndrome
- Hepatomegaly
- Carpal tunnel syndrome
- Macroglossia
- Malabsorption
- Unexplained diarrhea or constipation
- Peripheral neuropathy
- Cardiomyopathy

Porphyria cutanea tarda

Skin thickening of porphyria cutanea tarda may especially mimic scleroderma.

FEATURES

- Cutaneous photosensitivity: fluid-filled vesicles and bullae develop on sun-exposed areas
- Calcinosis and skin thickening may also occur

Eosinophilic fasciitis

Eosinophilic fasciitis is also known as Shulman's syndrome.

FEATURES

- More common in men
- Rapid onset of pain and swelling of extremities frequently follows unusual physical exertion/trauma
- Progressive stiffening of limbs and trunk

- Inflammation and fibrosis pucker the skin and form deep venous tracks
- Skin is erythematous and shiny; 'orange peel' appearance is common over affected areas
- Carpal tunnel syndrome
- Joint contractures
- No Raynaud's phenomenon or visceral involvement

Scleredema

Scleredema is also known as scleredema adultorum of Buschke. It may closely mimic skin changes of scleroderma.

FEATURES

- Occurs mostly in children
- May be associated with Streptococcal infection
- Usually resolves in 6-12 months
- Thick, hardened skin that first appears on the trunk and then spreads distally in a painless process (spares hands)
- Puffy hands may develop
- Can be transient following infection, or more permanent associated with diabetes mellitus (50% of cases)
- No Raynaud's phenomenon or visceral involvement

Scleromyxedema

Scleromyxedema is also known as papular mucinosis or lichen myxedematosus. It may closely mimic skin changes of scleroderma.

FEATURES

- Usual age of onset is 30-70 years
- Widespread thickening and hardening of the skin
- Yellowish or pale red papules are characteristic
- Mucin deposition noted on pathology
- Paraproteinemia (usually IgG lambda)
- No Raynaud's phenomenon or visceral involvement

SIGNS & SYMPTOMS
Signs

Disease has an insidious onset and affects many organ systems.

Skin involvement:

- Initial sign in 70% of cases is Raynaud's phenomenon
- Fingertip ulcers, scars, or even gangrene may be present in severe cases
- Skin disease starts with edematous phase (lasts for several weeks) - nonpitting edema plus inflammation, advancing proximally from fingers and hands
- Fibrotic stage (lasts months or years) then ensues with skin gradually becoming firm, thickened, and bound to the underlying tissue
- Involvement of fingers is typical (sclerodactyly)
- Flexion contractures on the hands, wrists, and elbows
- Tightened skin on the face may result in a mask-like appearance, the opening of the mouth becoming smaller and vertical furrowing appearing around the mouth
- Affected skin becomes dry and coarse with secondary loss of hair, oil, and sweat glands
- Hyper- or hypopigmentation of the skin; 'salt and pepper' or tanned appearance is common
- Calcinosis (calcium deposits in the skin, possibly ulcerated) is typical later; usually found on the fingertips and over bony eminences
- Telangiectasias on hands, forearms, face, lips, and tongue are also typical but frank vasculitis is rarely seen

Joint involvement:

- Symmetrical polyarthralgia resembling rheumatoid arthritis in early disease
- Tendinitis with friction rubs over joints, especially knees, may be apparent in advanced diffuse scleroderma; indicative of poor prognosis
- Resorption of bone, particularly apparent in fingertips, may occur

Gastrointestinal involvement:

- Esophageal dysfunction is the most frequent visceral disturbance (90% of patients)
- Barrett's esophagus occurs in 30% of patients due to esophageal reflux (associated with increased risk of stricture or adenocarcinoma)
- Malabsorption due to anaerobic bacterial overgrowth may cause weight loss
- Signs of pneumatosis cystoides intestinalis or biliary cirrhosis may also be apparent
- Rectal prolapse occurs in rare cases

Pulmonary involvement:

- Pulmonary function is abnormal in >60% of patients; 10-30% of patients with diffuse or limited scleroderma develop severe lung disease, the leading cause of mortality in scleroderma
- Fine early inspiratory crackling rales may be heard
- Nonproductive cough is a late symptom

Cardiac involvement (usually silent until late in the disease):

- 15-20% of patients with limited or diffuse scleroderma develop heart problems
- Signs of congestive heart failure, ventricular gallops, sinus tachycardia, and/or occasional pericardial friction rubs
- Pericarditis (often with effusion) is apparent in 10% of patients, but present in 40-60% of cases
- Signs of pulmonary hypertension may result from involvement of pulmonary arteries

Renal involvement:

- 15-20% of patients with limited or diffuse scleroderma develop severe kidney problems
- Acute renal failure resulting from intimal hyperplasia of interlobular and arcuate arteries; usually heralded by abrupt onset of malignant hypertension (hypertensive renal crisis)
- Limited cutaneous scleroderma is sometimes known as the CREST syndrome if at least three of the following five signs are present - calcinosis, Raynaud's phenomenon, esophageal dysmotility, sclerodactyly, telangiectasias

Symptoms

Raynaud's phenomenon usually precedes discernable fibrosis:

- Color changes, pain, and/or numbness in fingers and/or toes (or even cheeks, nose, and ears) in response to cold, stress, or vibration
- Painful ulcers are a late complication

Cutaneous involvement:

- Overt disease first announced by edematous phase (lasts for several weeks) - swollen, puffy, intensely itchy skin, accompanied by general malaise, advancing proximally from fingers and hands
- Edematous phase followed by fibrotic stage (lasts months or years) - skin gradually becomes firm, thickened, and bound to the underlying tissue
- Involvement of fingers is typical (sclerodactyly)
- Skin also thickens, removing skin creases and causing a shiny appearance over bone
- Flexion contractures

- Thickened skin on the face may result in a mask-like appearance, the opening of the mouth becoming smaller, and vertical furrowing appearing around the mouth; may result in chewing difficulties (also due to dry mouth)
- Affected skin becomes dry and coarse secondary to loss of hair, oil, and sweat glands
- Dryness of eyes/mouth, or eye burning, itching, and discharge (sicca complex)
- Painful white lumps under the skin that can leak, erupting chalky fluid, and leaving painful ulcers that may become infected; typically found on the fingertips and over bony eminences (calcinosis)
- Small, red spots (telangiectasis) on hands, forearms, face, lips, and tongue
- Frank vasculitis rarely seen
- Vaginal changes may make intercourse painful

Musculoskeletal involvement:
- >50% of patients complain of joint pain, aching, and/or swelling during early stages (especially in the extremities); a symmetric polyarthralgia resembling rheumatoid arthritis
- Generalized muscle pain, stiffness, and weakness is another common initial symptom; tendinitis may also occur
- Later disuse atrophy may lead to muscular weakness
- Crepitus may be apparent over the joints, especially the knees, in advanced diffuse scleroderma; indicative of poor prognosis

Gastrointestinal involvement:
- Esophageal dysfunction is the most frequent visceral disturbance (90% of patients)
- Dysphagia
- Esophageal reflux/heartburn
- Appetite loss and feelings of bloating after meals
- Malabsorption due to anaerobic bacterial overgrowth may lead to weight loss, diarrhea, constipation, pseudo-obstruction, fatigue, and/or flatulence
- Rectal prolapse and fecal incontinence may rarely occur
- Symptoms of pneumatosis cystoides intestinalis or biliary cirrhosis may be apparent

Pulmonary involvement:
- Initially asymptomatic, gradually progressing to painless dyspnea, initially apparent on exertion
- Wheezing, tiredness, and nonproductive cough may be apparent
- Swollen feet may be an indicator of pulmonary involvement

Cardiac involvement:
- Pericarditis is symptomatic in 10% of patients, but present in 40-60% of cases
- Symptoms of pulmonary or renal hypertension (especially dangerous complications) or congestive heart failure may occur

Other:
- Renal involvement may cause symptoms of acute renal failure
- Impotence may also result from vascular involvement

ASSOCIATED DISORDERS
- Often associated with other connective tissue diseases: mixed connective tissue disease classically contains features of all the above conditions plus scleroderma; Sjögren's syndrome
- Lung carcinoma occurs at a higher rate than expected in systemic sclerosis patients

KEY! DON'T MISS!
Signs of renal or pulmonary involvement should lead to immediate hospitalization.

CONSIDER CONSULT

Refer to rheumatology if a connective tissue disease is suspected. This is important because of the difficulty in diagnosis and danger of visceral involvement.

INVESTIGATION OF THE PATIENT
Direct questions to patient

Q Do your fingers or toes change color in response to cold, vibration, or stress? Intense attacks of Raynaud's phenomenon accompanied by gangrene or ulceration with the specific color changes being pallor, cyanosis, and then erythema

Q Can you tell me about patches of unusual skin on your body? The presence and pattern of sclerodermatous skin and telangiectasis assists the diagnosis

Q Do you have any painful white lumps under the skin? Calcinosis is typical of scleroderma

Q Do you have difficulty making a fist, eating, or using any other of your joints? Provides information about extent of disease and level of impairment

Q Are your eyes and mouth affected? Sicca complex may be present

Q Do you suffer from heartburn or have problems swallowing? Esophageal complications are very common in scleroderma

Q Does your body ache? Joint involvement is common, especially in early disease

Q Does eating lead to bowel problems? Loss of appetite, bloating after meals, diarrhea, constipation, and/or flatulence may result from GI involvement

Q Have you lost weight recently? Weight loss may point to malabsorption

Q Are you often tired, out of breath, or do you have swollen feet? These symptoms may be due to pulmonary involvement

Contributory or predisposing factors

Q Have you ever been diagnosed with an autoimmune disease? A personal history of autoimmune disease can be associated with scleroderma

Family history

Q Do any of your family have an autoimmune disease? A familial history of autoimmune disease can be associated with scleroderma

Examination

- Full physical examination. Are there signs of hypertension? Weight loss may indicate malabsorption
- Perform an examination of the skin. Check for digital pitting, presence of painful ulcers, telangectasia, calcinosis, and loss of fingertip tissue consistent with severe Raynaud's phenomenon secondary to scleroderma
- Check for range of motion and swelling in joints. Indicates extent of disease and functional impairment
- Full respiratory examination. Check for fine early inspiratory crackling rales characteristic of pulmonary fibrosis; wheezing and nonproductive cough may also be heard
- Check for cardiac involvement. Signs of congestive heart failure, ventricular gallops, sinus tachycardia, and/or occasional pericardial friction rubs

Summary of investigative tests

- Nailfold capillary test: useful to detect capillary changes typical of scleroderma
- Skin biopsy: very useful in differential diagnosis by showing the presence of fibrosis
- Autoantibody profile: can aid in diagnosing scleroderma but results must be supported by other evidence; normally performed by a specialist

Joint involvement:
Joint X-rays - usually performed if osteopenia or arthritis is suspected.

Heart involvement:
- Electrocardiogram (ECG) - may detect early pulmonary hypertension or other cardiac changes
- Right-sided heart catheterization - confirms diagnosis and may also detect myocardial disease or pericarditis; normally performed by a specialist

Respiratory involvement:
- Pulmonary function tests - often show restrictive lung disease before symptoms arise
- High resolution chest computed tomography (CT) scan - may reveal underlying pulmonary fibrosis; normally performed by a specialist
- Bronchoscopy with biopsy, a gallium lung scan, and bronchoalveolar lavage - may yield further information; normally performed by a specialist

Renal involvement:
- Routine biochemistry tests - may reveal renal involvement
- Blood count - useful to detect anemia or thrombocytopenia possibly heralding renal disease; urinalysis may also reveal signs
- Renal biopsy may be required; normally performed by a specialist

Gastrointestinal involvement:
- Barium swallows and cine-esophagograms - useful tests for esophageal strictures, but direct measurement of esophageal motility by esophageal manometry may be needed if source of symptoms is not clear, e.g. to rule out Barrett's esophagus; normally performed by a specialist
- Barium meals - useful for monitoring motility of the lower GI tract; endoscopy may also be performed; normally performed by a specialist
- Malabsorption is best detected as impaired D-xylose absorption or increased quantitative fecal fat elimination; jejunal cultures and bile acid test are useful in the diagnosis of bacterial overgrowth; normally performed by a specialist

DIAGNOSTIC DECISION
There is a 97% degree of certainty if one major or two minor criteria are present:
- Major criterion - sclerodermatous involvement of the skin proximal to the metacarpophalangeal or metatarsophalangeal joints
- Minor criteria - sclerodactyly, digital pitted scars or tissue loss at fingertips, or bibasilar pulmonary fibrosis

Severe nailfold capillary abnormalities have been proposed to markedly increase the sensitivity of the criteria for systemic scleroderma.

- Presence of severe Raynaud's phenomenon and visceral involvement are further key signs. A skin biopsy is also extremely useful in differential diagnosis
- The term undifferentiated connective tissue disease is reserved for patients without diagnostic criteria for any one condition. It may develop into scleroderma, systemic lupus erythematosus, or rheumatoid arthritis, or remain undifferentiated

CLINICAL PEARLS
- Raynaud's phenomena is very common in the general population and is not usually associated with an underlying connective tissue disorder
- Raynaud's phenomena may be precipitated by emotional stress

THE TESTS
Body fluids
BLOOD BIOCHEMISTRY
Description
Blood test assessing various markers of renal function.

Advantages/Disadvantages
Advantages:
- Simple, inexpensive test
- Quick and relatively noninvasive

Disadvantages:
- Requires laboratory analysis of blood constituents
- Information is nonspecific for renal disease

Normal
- Sodium: 135-147mEq/L
- Potassium: 3.5-5mEq/L
- Urea nitrogen (BUN): 8-18mg/dL (3-6.5mmol/L)
- Creatinine: 0.6-1.2mg/dL (50-110mmol/L)

Abnormal
Outside normal reference values.

Cause of abnormal result
Renal failure may alter all parameters.

Drugs, disorders and other factors that may alter results
- Hypotension
- Dehydration
- Congestive heart failure
- Urinary tract infection
- Rhabdomyolysis
- Ketonemia
- Aminoglycosides, cephalosporins
- Hydantoin
- Diuretics
- Methyldopa

BLOOD COUNT
Description
Venous blood sample.

Advantages/Disadvantages
Advantage: simple, routine examination

Disadvantages:
- Requires laboratory analysis
- Results must be substantiated by other evidence

Normal
- Red blood cells: men 4.3-5.9x10^6/mm^3; women 3.5-5x10^6/mm^3
- Hemoglobin: men 13.6-17.7g/dL; women 12-15g/dL

- Hematocrit: men 39-49%; women 33-43%
- Platelets: 130-400x10³/mm³

Abnormal
Values below the normal ranges.

Cause of abnormal result
- Anemia may be caused by GI bleeding (secondary to engorged GI vessels or internal telangiectasis) or may herald renal failure
- Thrombocytopenia may herald renal disease

Drugs, disorders and other factors that may alter results
- There are many causes of anemia and thrombocytopenia
- Anemia caused by GI bleeding secondary to NSAID intake is especially likely in this condition

AUTOANTIBODY PROFILE
Description
Blood sample required for the following antibody profile:
- Antinuclear antibody (homogenous, speckled, or nucleolar pattern)
- Native DNA antibody
- Anti-Sm
- Anti-nRNP
- Rheumatoid factor
- Anticentromere
- Extractable nuclear antibody to SCL 70

Advantages/Disadvantages
Advantage: important for diagnosing scleroderma

Disadvantages:
- Serum sample required
- Specialist analysis must be performed by a laboratory
- Result must be supported by other evidence to confirm diagnosis

Normal
Negative to the antibodies.

Abnormal
- Antinuclear antibody (homogenous, speckled, or nucleolar pattern) - positive in scleroderma and other connective tissue diseases such as systemic lupus erythematosis
- Native DNA antibody - negative in scleroderma
- Anti-Sm - negative in scleroderma, specific for systemic lupus erythematosus
- Anti-nRNP - positive in 20% of scleroderma patients
- Rheumatoid factor - positive in 30%
- Anticentromere - positive in 10-90%
- Extractable nuclear antibody to SCL 70 - positive in 30%

Cause of abnormal result
Scleroderma has this specific autoantibody profile.

Drugs, disorders and other factors that may alter results
- Other autoimmune diseases have specific autoantibodies profiles: rheumatoid arthritis, mixed connective tissue disease, primary biliary cirrhosis, systemic lupus erythematosis

- As there is overlap between disease presentations and autoantibody profiles, interpretation is best left to a specialist

Tests of function

PULMONARY FUNCTION TEST

Description

Measurements of carbon monoxide diffusion in the lung, forced expiratory volume in one second, forced vital capacity, respiratory volume, total lung capacity, and bronchiodilator response.

Advantages/Disadvantages

Advantages:

- Can usually be performed in the primary care center
- Simple, noninvasive testing

Disadvantage: results must be substantiated with other data

Normal

Normal values for age and gender.

Abnormal

- Reduced forced vital capacity, carbon monoxide diffusion, and total lung capacity
- Normal to reduced forced expiratory volume in one second, and respiratory volume
- Negative bronchiodilator response
- Isolated low diffusing capacity and reduced lung volume are most common findings in early disease

Cause of abnormal result

In the scleroderma patient: interstitial fibrosis.

Drugs, disorders and other factors that may alter results

- Asthma
- Chronic obstructive airways disease
- Other causes of pulmonary fibrosis

URINANALYSIS

Description

Urine sample.

Advantages/Disadvantages

Advantage: simple, routine test

Disadvantages:

- Requires laboratory analysis
- Results must be substantiated by other data

Normal

Absence of protein or microscopic blood in urine.

Abnormal

Presence of protein and microscopic blood in urine.

Cause of abnormal result
Renal failure.

Drugs, disorders and other factors that may alter results
- Congestive heart failure
- Hypertension
- Cancer of prostate, renal pelvis, or bladder
- Myeloma
- Waldenstrom's macroglobulinemia
- Trauma or lesions
- Renal disease, calculi, and prostatitis
- Menstrual contamination
- Hematopoietic disorders, aspirin, and anticoagulants

Biopsy
SKIN BIOPSY
Description
Biopsy of affected skin area(s).

Advantages/Disadvantages
Advantage: very helpful in differential diagnosis

Disadvantages:
- Requires laboratory analysis
- Painful for patient
- Cannot distinguish between localized and systemic disease

Normal
Absence of fibrosis.

Abnormal
- Increase in compact collagen fibers in the reticular dermis
- Epidermal thinning
- Loss of rete pegs
- Atrophy of dermal appendages
- Large infiltrations of T lymphocytes into the dermis and subcutis, which may also be the site of severe fibrosis

Imaging
JOINT X-RAY
Description
X-rays of hands and other affected joints.

Advantages/Disadvantages
Advantages:
- Enables bony abnormalities to be observed
- May be useful in differential diagnosis

Disadvantage: exposes patient to radiation

Abnormal
Osteopenia visible as bone resorption, especially on fingertips.

Special tests
NAILFOLD CAPILLARY TEST
Description
Capillaries of the nailfolds are examined using a wide-angle microscope or an ophthalmoscope after immersion oil has been applied to skin surface.

Advantages/Disadvantages
Advantages:
- Useful to detect capillary changes and provide a positive diagnosis
- Noninvasive
- Cost-effective

Disadvantage: results are not conclusive for scleroderma

Normal
Normal reticular pattern observed.

Abnormal
Dilated, tortuous capillaries mixed with areas of capillary loss.

Cause of abnormal result
- Scleroderma
- Systemic lupus erythematosus
- Polymyositis/dermatomyositis

Other tests
ELECTROCARDIOGRAM (ECG)
Description
- Standard ECG test
- Ambulatory (Holter) ECG monitoring may yield more information

Advantages/Disadvantages
Advantages:
- May detect asymptomatic cardiac involvement
- Inexpensive and may be performed in primary care center

Abnormal
Signs of congestive heart failure, pericarditis, arrhythmias, and/or hypertension.

Cause of abnormal result
Fibrosis of heart or blood vessels.

Drugs, disorders and other factors that may alter results
There are numerous causes of ECG changes.

TREATMENT

CONSIDER CONSULT
Refer to rheumatology for treatment recommendations and administration of immunosuppressive medications.

IMMEDIATE ACTION
If visceral involvement is suspected, patient should be referred immediately to rheumatology for treatment.

PATIENT AND CAREGIVER ISSUES
Forensic and legal issues
Treatment for end-stage disease: parenteral nutrition or organ transplant.

Impact on career, dependants, family, friends
- Patient may become less independent due to flexion contractures and arthritic changes
- Mental support is often required

Patient or caregiver request
- **Is the disease curable?** No, but it can be managed very effectively
- **Are steroids dangerous?** Patient may confuse corticosteroids with anabolic steroids abused by athletes. However, corticosteroids can lead to long-term side-effects and patient needs to be counseled about these effects. Additionally, high-dose steroid use has been associated with precipitation of renal failure in this population
- **Are painkillers bad for my stomach?** Patient may be concerned about GI side-effects, especially in the light of existing problems

Health-seeking behavior
- **Have you previously been to see another physician?** The disease presents widely and over time; therefore, patient may have visited another physician about a different symptom of the same disorder
- **Have you been taking over-the-counter (OTC) painkillers?** This may affect the presentation; also, patient may not have consulted in the early stages

MANAGEMENT ISSUES
Goals
- To ensure early diagnosis of overall disease by a specialist
- To base treatment on patient's symptoms and to follow up closely
- To provide rapid and effective intervention for visceral complications

Management in special circumstances
COEXISTING DISEASE
- NSAIDs should be prescribed with care to patients with thrombocytopenia, congestive heart failure, cirrhosis (especially sulindac), or renal insufficiency
- Systemic corticosteroids should be prescribed with care to patients with hypertension, congestive heart failure, recent myocardial infarction, hypertension, hypothyroidism, renal impairment, or untreated infections
- Methotrexate should be prescribed with care to patients with significant lung, liver, or kidney impairment, or to heavy consumers of alcohol
- Cyclosporin should be prescribed with care to patients with compromised renal function, or to those taking NSAIDs
- Cyclophosphamide should be prescribed with care to patients with renal impairment

COEXISTING MEDICATION

- NSAIDs interact with methotrexate, cardiac glycosides, angiotensin-converting enzyme (ACE) inhibitors, cyclosporin, diuretics, beta-blockers, and corticosteroids
- Corticosteroids interact with NSAIDs, diuretics, cyclosporin, and cyclophosphamide
- Methotrexate interacts with NSAIDs and diuretics
- Cyclophosphamide interacts with antiarrhythmics, corticosteroids, and NSAIDs
- Cyclosporin interacts with corticosteroids, calcium channel blockers, diuretics, antidepressants, and antiarrhythmic drugs

SPECIAL PATIENT GROUPS

Pregnant women:

- Women are not advised to get pregnant during the first 3 years of the disease; following this period, in the absence of organ problems, it is generally safe to conceive
- Pregnant patients should be monitored closely by a specialist, plus an obstetrician experienced in supervising high-risk pregnancies
- Pregnant patients should use all medication with caution; the advice of a physician should be sought

Elderly and children:
Elderly patients and children are more at risk of side-effects of all drugs.

PATIENT SATISFACTION/LIFESTYLE PRIORITIES

- Metaclopramide may cause drowsiness
- Corticosteroids: the side-effects can result in poor compliance. Patient requires counseling concerning the risks and benefits of long-term corticosteroid treatment

SUMMARY OF THERAPEUTIC OPTIONS
Choices

- No therapy has been consistently shown to modify the course of the disease
- Treatment is confined to aggressive management of individual complications

General complications:

- Renal, cardiac, and pulmonary hypertension complications should be under specialist treatment
- Raynaud's phenomenon can be treated with nifedipine and iloprost
- Avoid smoking and cold exposure
- Constipation and diarrhea should be treated with usual therapies
- Patients with any chronic illness are liable to depression, which should be pre-empted with mental support. Antidepressants may be indicated
- Renal complications and crisis should be treated with ACE inhibitors, including captopril

Cutaneous involvement:

- Skin management - affected skin areas should be treated with oil-based moisturizers (especially after bathing). Applying sunscreen before going outside, employing humidifiers to moisten the air during the winter months, and avoiding very hot baths or showers with harsh soaps can protect the skin. Using gloves to handle household cleaners or other caustic chemicals and protecting the skin from mechanical injury aids in skin disease management
- Topical corticosteroids and antihistamines may relieve pruritus during early disease
- Ulcer management - traumatic and ischemic ulcers are treated with topical antibiotics, periodic cleansing with soap and water, and local dressing
- Telangiectasias may be treated with laser therapy
- Facial disfigurement can be at least partially countered with special cosmetics and/or plastic surgery (but not in areas where the disease is active)

Musculoskeletal involvement:

- NSAIDs (ibuprofen) are first choices to treat inflammation and pain. Their use is limited by concerns over the renal and GI issues encountered in this disease; low-dose corticosteroids (prednisolone) are a second choice (do not alter course of disease); methotrexate is a third choice
- Physical therapy is very important to strengthen the joints, maintain function and flexibility, and increase blood flow to affected regions
- Occupational therapy is also important so that the patient continues to be independent in daily life; affected joints should be protected to reduce physical stress

Oral involvement:

- Dental care - caries should be avoided by regular brushing and flossing, and by having regular dental check-ups
- Mouth should be kept moist by drinking lots of water, sucking ice chips, sugarless gum and hard candy, and avoiding alcohol-based mouthwashes

Gastrointestinal involvement:

- Esophageal reflux should be avoided by dietary management including measures to reduce esophageal reflux
- Proton-pump inhibitors, such as omeprazole, are used for esophageal reflux
- Esophageal strictures may need periodic dilation in refractory dysphagia
- Gastroplasty may prevent esophageal reflux if all other treatments have failed
- Laser therapy may be required to control bleeding from engorged gastric vasculature
- Parenteral nutrition may be necessary as a last resort in severe bowel disease

Pulmonary involvement:

- Influenza and pneumonia vaccination is essential protection for the patient with pulmonary impairment
- Cyclophosphamide is a first choice for treating pulmonary fibrosis with alveolitis (early disease) and it may be supplemented by low doses of corticosteroids. Its use and administration should be guided by a specialist
- Lung or kidney transplants may be considered in end-stage disease

Current early investigations include the use of recombinant human relaxin, autologous stem cell transplantation, cyclosporine, colchicine, and thalidomide.

Clinical pearls

Use of D-penicillamine, at one time (1970s-90s) the most commonly used medication for scleroderma, has been called into question following the randomized prospective trial of 1999. Many have abandoned it completely.

FOLLOW UP

- Careful and regular follow up with a specialist is essential due to the risk of visceral involvement
- New visceral involvement tends to occur in the early stages of diffuse scleroderma, and in late limited scleroderma

Plan for review

- Blood pressure should be regularly monitored by the patient, as well as by the primary care physician, so that renal hypertension may be detected early
- Blood counts
- Urinalysis
- Renal and pulmonary function

Information for patient or caregiver

- Diagnosis may take a long time
- Disease has no cure; it can only be managed
- Spontaneous remission, however, does sometimes occur
- Compliance with treatment is essential
- Scleroderma is not contagious, and is rarely inheritable
- Joining a support group can be very beneficial, and patient should stay connected with friends and family
- Try to lead as normal a life as possible, pacing yourself as necessary
- Any change in the condition should be reported

DRUGS AND OTHER THERAPIES: DETAILS
Drugs
TOPICAL CORTICOSTEROIDS
Corticosteroid available in cream form is suitable to treat pruritus.

Dose
Apply to affected area twice daily.

Efficacy
Effective at relieving pruritus.

Risks/Benefits
Risks:

- Ineffective at reducing edema and inflammation
- Does not alter course of disease
- Simple dosing regimen allows for better patient compliance, also allows for application directly to area affected
- Systemic absorption of topical corticosteroids has produced reversible hypothalamic-pituitary-adrenal (HPA) axis suppression, manifestations of Cushing's syndrome, hyperglycemia, and glucosuria in some patients
- Therefore, patients receiving a large dose of a potent topical steroid applied to a large surface area or under an occlusive dressing should be evaluated periodically for evidence of HPA axis suppression
- Pediatric patients may absorb proportionally larger amounts of topical corticosteroids and, thus, be more susceptible to systemic toxicity
- If irritation develops, topical corticosteroids should be discontinued

Benefits:

- Relieves pruritus
- Use of topical formulation reduces risk of systemic toxicity

Side-effects and adverse reactions
Skin: burning, itching, irritation, dryness, folliculitis, hypertrichosis, acneiform eruptions, hypopigmentation, perioral dermatitis, allergic contact dermatitis, maceration of the skin, secondary infection, skin atrophy, striae, miliaria.

Interactions (other drugs)
None listed.

Contraindications

- Should be used during pregnancy only if the potential benefit justifies the potential risk to the fetus ▪ Use on face, axilla, or groin

Acceptability to patient
Low incidence of side-effects coupled with effective relief of pruritus makes this therapy an acceptable treatment.

Follow up plan
Monitor relief of symptoms.

Patient and caregiver information
- Must be aware of possible side-effects and the need to report them
- Importance of compliance with therapy must be stressed

IBUPROFEN
- NSAID
- Simple dosing regimen and good tolerance
- NSAIDs should be prescribed with great care to patients with poor renal function
- Cyclo-oxygenase-2 (OX-2) inhibitors are as effective as ibuprofen but cause less GI ulceration, platelet toxicity, and ulceration complications (but dyspepsia is as frequent)

Dose
Adult oral dose: 400mg four times daily to achieve anti-inflammatory effects.

Efficacy
More effective than placebo in treating inflammation and pain.

Risks/Benefits
Risks:
- Use caution in elderly
- Use caution in hepatic, renal, and cardiac failure
- Use caution in bleeding disorders
- There is no evidence that final outcome changed by NSAIDs

Benefits:
- Relieves inflammation and pain
- Good tolerance and simple dosing regimen
- Relatively cheap, relatively safe, and effective

Side-effects and adverse reactions
- Cardiovascular system: hypertension, peripheral edema
- Central nervous system: headache, dizziness, tinnitus
- Gastrointestinal: anorexia, nausea, dyspepsia, peptic ulceration, bleeding
- Genitourinary: nephrotoxicity
- Hematologic: blood cell disorders
- Hypersensitivity: rashes, bronchospasm, angioedema

Interactions (other drugs)
- Aminoglycosides ■ Anticoagulants ■ Antihypertensives ■ Baclofen ■ Corticosteroids ■ Cyclosporine, tacrolimus ■ Digoxin ■ Diuretics ■ Lithium ■ Methotrexate ■ Phenylpropanolamine ■ Warfarin

Contraindications
- Peptic ulceration ■ Hypersensitivity to any pain reliever or antipyretic (including NSAIDs)
- Coagulation defects ■ Severe renal or hepatic disease

705

Acceptability to patient
Patients may not be able to tolerate these drugs. In this population, the risks of renal and GI side-effects may be particularly unacceptable.

Follow up plan
Carefully monitor for appearance of side-effects.

Patient and caregiver information
- Must be made aware of possible side-effects and need to report them
- Importance of compliance with therapy must be stressed

PREDNISOLONE
- Used to treat inflammation and pain
- Can also be used to treat pulmonary fibrosis

Dose
- Adult oral dose: 10mg per day
- Higher doses, which may be necessary to treat myositis, should be administered by a specialist

Efficacy
Generally more effective than placebo in reducing inflammation and pain.

Risks/Benefits
Risks:
- Overwhelming septicemia if patient has an infection
- Loss of control of blood glucose in those with diabetes
- Prolonged use causes adrenal suppression
- Use caution in elderly due to risk of diabetes and osteoporosis
- Use caution in patients with psychosis, seizure disorders, or myasthenia gravis
- Use caution in congestive heart failure, hypertension
- Use caution in ulcerative colitis, peptic ulcer, or esophagitis

Benefits:
- Reduces pain and inflammation
- Improves pulmonary fibrosis

Side-effects and adverse reactions
- Side-effects are minimized by short duration of therapy
- Cardiovascular system: hypertension, thromboembolism
- Central nervous system: insomnia, euphoria, depression, psychosis
- Endocrine: adrenal suppression, impaired glucose tolerance, growth suppression in children
- Eyes, ears, nose, and throat: cataract, glaucoma, blurred vision
- Gastrointestinal: dyspepsia, peptic ulceration, oesophagitis, oral candidiasis
- Musculoskeletal: proximal myopathy, osteoporosis
- Skin: delayed healing, acne, striae

Interactions (other drugs)
- Adrenergic neurone blockers, alpha-blockers, beta-blockers, beta-2 agonists
- Aminoglutethamide ▪ Anticonvulsants (carbamazepine, phenytoin, barbiturates)
- Antibiotics (clarithromycin, erythromycin, troleandomycin) ▪ Antidiabetics
- Antidysrhythmics (calcium channel blockers, cardiac glycosides) ▪ Antifungals (amphotericin, ketoconazole) ▪ Antihypertensives (ACE inhibitors, diuretics: loop and thiazide, acetazolamide; angiotensin II receptor antagonists, clonidine, diazoxide, hydralazine,

methyldopa, minoxidil) ▪ Cardiac glycosides ▪ Cholestyramine ▪ Colestipol ▪ Cyclosporine ▪ Diuretics ▪ Isoniazid ▪ Ketoconazole ▪ Methotrexate ▪ NSAIDs ▪ Nitrates ▪ Nitroprusside ▪ Oral contraceptives ▪ Rifampin ▪ Ritonavir ▪ Saliclyates ▪ Somatropin ▪ Vaccines ▪ Warfarin

Contraindications
▪ Systemic infection ▪ Avoid live virus vaccines in those receiving immunosuppressive doses ▪ History of tuberculosis ▪ Cushing's syndrome ▪ Recent myocardial infarction

Acceptability to patient
Acceptability is reduced by side-effect profile.

Follow up plan
Carefully monitor for appearance of side-effects.

Patient and caregiver information
▪ Must be made aware of possible side-effects and need to report them
▪ Importance of compliance with therapy must be stressed
▪ Patient must not stop taking this medication unless under close medical supervision
▪ Patient requires a steroid card stating the dose of medication and medical information that is useful stating he is unwell

METHOTREXATE
▪ Disease-modifying drug used to treat severe myositis associated with the disease. Although it may help treat the myositis associated with overlap syndromes, its use in early systemic sclerosis cannot be recommended
▪ Its institution and use should be determined by a specialist
▪ This is an off-label indication
▪ Targets inflammatory agents of the disease and fibroblasts
▪ Several weeks are required before it takes effect
▪ Folic acid 1mg/day decreases oral and GI toxicity without impairing efficacy

Dose
▪ Adult oral dose: 7.5mg once weekly to a maximum 20mg once weekly under specialist guidance
▪ Use the lowest effective dose once response is achieved

Efficacy
Thought to be more effective than other drugs in suppressing inflammation and pain.

Risks/Benefits
Risks:
▪ Must be administered under specialist supervision
▪ Serious toxic reactions are possible, which may be fatal
▪ Only use with severe recalcitrant, disabling disease which is not adequately responsive to other forms of therapy
▪ The patient should be fully informed of the risks involved
▪ Closely monitor for bone marrow, liver, lung, and kidney toxicity
▪ Use caution with infection and bone marrow depression
▪ Use caution with peptic ulceration and ulcerative colitis
▪ Use caution with renal and hepatic impairment
▪ Use caution with the elderly

Benefits:
- Reduces inflammation and pain
- Treats myositis effectively

Side-effects and adverse reactions
- Central nervous system: headache, seizures, dizziness, drowsiness
- Eyes, ears, nose, and throat: visual disturbances, tinnitus
- Gastrointestinal: abdominal pain, diarrhea, hepatotoxicity, nausea, vomiting, stomatitis
- Genitourinary: renal failure, urinary retention, depression of and defective spermatogenensis, hematuria
- Hematologic: blood cell disorders
- Musculoskeletal: osteoporosis, muscle pain and wasting
- Respiratory: pulmonary fibrosis
- Skin: rashes, acne, dermatitis, alopecia, hyperpigmentation, vasculitis

Interactions (other drugs)
- Aminoglycosides ▪ Antimalarials ▪ Binding resins ▪ Co-trimoxazole ▪ Cyclosporin ▪ Ethanol ▪ Etretrinate ▪ Live vaccines ▪ NSAIDS ▪ Omeprazole ▪ Penicillins ▪ Probenicid▪ Salicylates ▪ Sulfinpyrazone

Contraindications
- Severe renal and hepatic impairment ▪ Profound bone marrow depression
- Nursing mothers, pregnancy, and avoid conception for 6 months after stopping
- Safety and effectiveness in pediatric patients have not been established, other than in cancer chemotherapy

Acceptability to patient
Drug takes several weeks to produce a response, with high toxicity reducing the use of this disease-modifying drug.

Follow up plan
- Carefully monitor for appearance of side-effects
- Monitor liver function tests and complete blood count throughout therapy

Patient and caregiver information
- Must be made aware of possible side-effects and need to report them
- Importance of compliance with therapy must be stressed
- Alcohol consumption should be discouraged
- Blood monitoring is required
- Folic acid supplementation is required

NIFEDIPINE
- Calcium antagonist used to treat Raynaud's disease
- Effective treatment with good tolerability
- This is an off-label indication

Dose
Adult oral dose: 10mg three times daily.

Efficacy
Effective in treatment of Raynaud's disease in patients with scleroderma.

Risks/Benefits

Risks:

- Nifedipine should be used during pregnancy only if the potential benefit justifies the potential risk to the fetus
- Use caution when administering to patients with congestive heart failure, hypotension, and aortic stenosis
- Use caution when administering to patients with hepatic and renal disease
- Use caution when administering to the elderly
- Use caution with recent beta-blocker withdrawal

Benefits:

- Useful to treat Raynaud's disease
- Good tolerability and good side-effect profile
- Can be used long-term
- Inexpensive

Side-effects and adverse reactions

- Cardiovascular system: bradycardia, peripheral edema, palpatations
- Central nervous system: dizziness, headache, paresthesias
- Gastrointestinal: constipation, nausea, dry mouth, dyspepsia
- Genitourinary: nocturia, polyuria, sexual dysfunction
- Respiratory: cough, dyspnea
- Skin: alopecia, pruritus, rash

Interactions (other drugs)

- Anticoagulants
- Barbiturates
- Beta-blockers
- Cimetidine, ranitidine
- Carbamazepine
- Cardiac glycosides
- Diltiazem
- Doxasozin
- Fentanyl
- Grapefruit juice
- H_2 antagonists
- Insulin
- Lansoprazole
- Magnesium
- Phenytoin
- Quinidine
- Theophylline
- Vincristine

Contraindications

- Severe coronary artery disease
- Recent myocardial infarction
- Hypertensive emergencies
- Pregnancy category C
- Safety and efficacy in pediatric patients have not been established

Acceptability to patient

Acceptable due to their effectiveness and low risk of side-effects. May be slightly less tolerable to the scleroderma patient with GI reflux, which calcium channel blockers can make worse.

Follow up plan

Monitor patient for appearance of side-effects or new symptoms of Raynaud's phenomenon.

Patient and caregiver information

- Administer on an empty stomach
- Importance of compliance with therapy must be stressed

OMEPRAZOLE

Proton-pump inhibitor used to relieve esophageal reflux.

Dose

Adult oral dose: 10-20mg daily prior to eating.

Efficacy
Effective in treatment of esophageal reflux in patients with scleroderma.

Risks/Benefits
Risks:
- Use caution in the elderly and children
- Gastric malignancy may still be present even if symptoms lessen with treatment

Benefits:
- Useful to treat esophageal reflux
- Good tolerability and good side-effect profile
- Can be used long-term

Side-effects and adverse reactions
- Central nervous system: headache, dizziness
- Gastrointestinal: nausea, vomiting, diarrhea, constipation, flatulence, abdominal pain, hepatitis, pancreatitis
- Genitourinary: interstitial nephritis, gynecomastia, urinary problems, urinary infections
- Hematologic: agranulocytosis, thrombocytopenia, anemia, neutropenia, and other blood cell disorders
- Hypersensitivity: angioedema, rashes, anaphylactoid reactions
- Skin: purpura, Stevens-Johnson syndrome, alopecia, erythema multiforme

Interactions (other drugs)
- Calcium channel antagonists (nifedipine, nimodipine, nisoldipine, nitrendipine)
- Carbamazepine ▪ Cefpodoxime, cefuroxime ▪ Clarithromycin ▪ Diazepam ▪ Digoxin
- Enoxacin ▪ Glipizide, glyburide ▪ Itraconazole, ketoconazole ▪ Methotrexate
- Phenytoin ▪ Sucralfate ▪ Tacrolimus ▪ Tolbutamide ▪ Warfarin

Contraindications
- Pregnancy and breast-feeding ▪ Gastric carcinoma ▪ Hepatic impairment

Acceptability to patient
Acceptable due to its high effectiveness and low risk of side-effects.

Follow up plan
Carefully monitor for appearance of side-effects or esophageal reflux symptoms.

Patient and caregiver information
- Must be made aware of need to take the medication before eating
- Importance of compliance with therapy must be stressed

CAPTOPRIL
- ACE inhibitor used to treat renal disease associated with scleroderma
- Very effective agent for renal crisis in scleroderma patients
- This is an off-label indication

Dose
Adult oral dose: 6.25–12.5mg three times daily initially and titrate dose to a maximum of 50mg three times daily.

Efficacy
Effective in treatment of renal disease and complications in patients with scleroderma.

Risks/Benefits
Risks:
- Use caution in patients receiving diuretics
- First dose may cause hypotension in those on diuretics, on a low-sodium diet or dialysis, who are dehydrated or have heart failure
- Use caution in atherosclerosis where renal artery stenosis could be present
- Use caution in renal impairment
- Use caution in breast-feeding
- Use caution in angioedema

Benefits:
- Useful to treat complications of renal disease
- Good tolerability
- Can be used long-term
- Inexpensive

Side-effects and adverse reactions
- Cardiovascular system: hypotension, angioedema, vasculitis
- Central nervous system: headache, dizziness, fatigue, paresthesias, fever, malaise
- Gastrointestinal: nausea, vomiting, diarrhea, constipation, dyspepsia, hepatitis, altered liver function tests, cholestatic jaundice, pancreatitis
- Genitourinary: renal impairment
- Hematologic: blood cell dyscrasias
- Musculoskeletal: myalgia, arthralgia
- Respiratory: dry cough, upper respiratory tract infections
- Skin: rash, photosensitivity

Interactions (other drugs)
- Adrenergic neurone blockers - Alcohol - Alpha-blockers - Alprostadil - Angiotensin II receptor antagonists - Antacids - Antidiabetics (insulin, metformin, sulfonylureas) - Antihypertensives (beta-blockers, clonidine, diazoxide, hydralazine, methyldopa, minoxidil, nitrates, nitroprusside) - Anxiolytics and hypnotics - Baclofen, tizanidine - Calcium channel blockers - Cyclosporine - Corticosteroids - Diuretics - Estrogens - Heparins - Levodopa - Lithium - NSAIDs - Phenothiazines - Potassium salts

Contraindications
- Pregnancy - Aortic stenosis - Renovascular disease

Acceptability to patient
Acceptable due to its effectiveness and good tolerability.

Follow up plan
Renal function must be monitored within 2 weeks after initiating therapy.

Patient and caregiver information
- Must be made aware of need for renal function monitoring within 2 weeks of initiating therapy
- Importance of compliance with therapy must be stressed

Physical therapy
PHYSICAL THERAPY
Exercise, such as swimming, to strengthen the joints, maintain function and flexibility, and increase blood flow to the affected regions is a very important component of the long-term management of scleroderma.

Risks/Benefits
Benefit: improves prognosis and maintains patient independence.

Acceptability to patient
Compliance with exercise is notoriously low.

Follow up plan
Monitor compliance regularly.

Patient and caregiver information
Importance of compliance with therapy must be stressed.

Occupational therapy
OCCUPATIONAL THERAPY
- Patient should be helped to live independently in a way that will preserve joint function
- Use of self-help devices should also be taught

Risks/Benefits
Benefit: preserves independence and functional abilities.

Acceptability to patient
High acceptability as benefits of occupational therapy are clearly apparent to patients.

Follow up plan
Ability to carry out daily activities should be monitored, and patients require regular occupational therapy sessions.

Patient and caregiver information
Importance of compliance with therapy to maintain improvements must be stressed.

Surgical therapy
GASTROPLASTY
- Treatment for esophageal reflux refractory to medical treatment
- Provides long-term relief of esophageal reflux

Risks/Benefits
Risks:
- Invasive technique requiring surgery
- Surgical complications can occur

Benefit: reduces esophageal reflux and provides long-term relief of symptoms

Acceptability to patient
Low acceptability as the surgery will affect eating habits.

Follow up plan
Monitor esophageal function.

Patient and caregiver information
- Reasons for recommending this treatment must be fully explained
- Dietary modification will be required

Other therapies
PATIENT COUNSELING
- Stress management, psychotherapy/counseling, and education about the disease are important to allow patients to cope with this disease
- Patient counseling needs to be ongoing, especially if disease is rapidly progressing

Risks/Benefits
Benefit: reduces risk of depression and improves prognosis.

Acceptability to patient
High.

Follow up plan
Monitor for signs of depression.

Patient and caregiver information
Depressive thoughts and feelings of inability to cope should not be hidden and may be signs of an illness that can be treated.

LASER THERAPY
- Used to remove internal or external telangiectasis
- May be used to treat engorged GI blood vessels

Risks/Benefits
Benefits:
- Removes unsightly telangiectasis
- Removes sources of GI bleeding

Acceptability to patient
High.

Follow up plan
Blood counts should be performed periodically to monitor GI bleeding.

Patient and caregiver information
Symptoms of anemia should be reported immediately.

VACCINATION
Vaccination against influenza and pneumonia.

Risks/Benefits
Benefit: protects against influenza and pneumonia.

Acceptability to patient
High.

Follow up plan
Annual influenza vaccinations are required.

Patient and caregiver information
- Must report any symptoms of chest infection
- Must be informed of need for annual influenza vaccinations

EFFICACY OF THERAPIES

- Much can be done to improve the lifestyle of those with scleroderma
- Dramatic developments include the ability to reverse kidney disease by prompt use of angiotensin-converting enzyme (ACE) inhibitors and modern methods of renal transplantation

Review period

6 months.

PROGNOSIS

- 5- and 10-year survival rates are 80-85% and 60-65%, respectively
- Course is often slow, variable, and unpredictable
- Mortality and severe disability are caused by visceral involvement, particularly of the heart, lungs, and/or kidneys (<30% of all patients)
- Prognosis is worse for diffuse scleroderma (10-year survival rate of 40-60%) than for limited scleroderma (>70%), primarily due to greater risk of early visceral involvement
- Limited scleroderma is relatively benign, but visceral involvement tends to develop eventually; digital amputations may be necessary due to severe ischemic vascular disease
- Other poor prognostic indicators include later age at onset, African-American or Native American race, absence of Raynaud's phenomenon, or tendon friction rubs
- Aggressive antihypertensive therapy has improved survival rates following onset of renal crisis to >2 years
- Better prognosis is associated with a longer edematous phase
- Decreased hand function often occurs due to joint disfigurement or finger ulceration
- Skin changes in diffuse scleroderma commonly peak in 3-5 years and then stabilize; musculoskeletal symptoms and wellbeing usually improve after this initial period
- Skin changes in limited scleroderma are usually very gradual and irreversible, but may start as generalized skin patches, which then retreat to the face and hands
- Localized scleroderma generally fades away in 3-5 years, but dark skin patches and muscle weakness may persist
- After many years, the skin in diffuse scleroderma usually softens and returns to normal thickness, or thins and atrophies; hair and sweat glands always remain absent
- Complete remission in diffuse scleroderma is rare and established organ damage tends to remain, although more serious visceral damage is unlikely unless previous damage leaves the organs vulnerable to further deterioration

Clinical pearls

- Skin findings usually stabilize or even diminish after several years, even without treatment
- Lung carcinoma has been found at higher than expected rates

COMPLICATIONS

- Arrhythmias: ventricular ectopy, strongly associated with sudden death, is found in 50-70% of patients with pulmonary or cardiac involvement
- Biliary cirrhosis; usually associated with limited scleroderma
- Carpal tunnel syndrome and other entrapment neuropathies as a result of polyarthralgia
- Congestive heart failure due to pulmonary hypertension and secondary cor pulmonale, or cardiomyopathy; chronic and difficult to treat
- Dental decay occurs more frequently due to a smaller oral opening and a dry mouth; damage to oral connective tissue can loosen teeth
- Depression: typical of chronic disease, absence of consistently effective treatment, and disfigurement
- Esophagitis and Barrett's esophagus (associated with increased risk of bleeding, stricture, and adenocarcinoma)

- Ischemic ulcerations and gangrene associated with Raynaud's phenomenon
- Impotence due to vascular involvement
- Interstitial pulmonary fibrosis (with or without alveolitis) resulting in progressive acute and chronic pulmonary failure; more common in diffuse scleroderma
- Malabsorption syndrome
- Myositis and tendinitis, especially in early disease
- Osteopenia is common: resorption of digital tufts most frequently seen
- Pericarditis
- Pneumatosis cystoides intestinalis (ominous prognosis) or sacculations of the intestine may follow deterioration of the GI tract
- Polyarthralgia
- Primary hypothyroidism (25% of patients)
- Pulmonary hypertension is the most dangerous complication (mean duration of survival 2 years); prognosis is poor if coupled with severe lung fibrosis. Detection is difficult until advanced; heralded by worsening dyspnea and eventual appearance of right-sided heart failure. Typically associated with limited scleroderma after 10-20 years (10% of patients)
- Renal hypertension is progressive and dangerous, but usually reversible, especially with appropriate treatment with an ACE inhibitor. Renal failure is usually heralded by malignant hypertension, but may occur in normotensive cases. More common in diffuse scleroderma

CONSIDER CONSULT

Refer to rheumatology if patient does not respond to therapy, or if complications occur, particularly renal, cardiac, and pulmonary hypertension complications.

PREVENTION

This disease cannot be prevented.

RISK FACTORS
Family history: slight relation to risk shown.

MODIFY RISK FACTORS
Generally not applicable.

Lifestyle and wellness
DIET
- Avoid spicy or fatty foods, alcohol, and caffeine
- Moist, soft food
- Avoid tight clothing
- Eat small and frequent meals
- Chew foods thoroughly
- Keep upright for at least one hour after eating
- Do not eat 3-4h before bedtime
- Elevate head of the bed to reduce esophageal reflux

ENVIRONMENT
Avoid exposure to trigger substances.

RESOURCES

ASSOCIATIONS
American Academy of Dermatology
930 E.Woodfield Road
Schaumburg, IL 60173-4927
Mailing address:
PO Box 4014
Schaumbaurg, IL 60168-4014
Tel: (847) 330 0230
Fax: (847) 330 0050
www.aad.org

American College of Rheumatology
1800 Century Place, Suite 250
Atlanta, GA 30345
Tel: (404) 633 3777
Fax: (404) 633 1870
E-mail: acr@rheumatology.org
www.rheumatology.org

Arthritis Foundation
1330 West Peachtree Street
Atlanta, GA 30309
Tel: (404) 872 7100 or (800) 283 7800
www.arthritis.org

National Institute of Arthritis and Musculoskeletal and Skin Diseases Information Clearinghouse
NIAMS/National Institutes of Health
1 AMS Circle
Bethedsa, MD 20892-3675
Tel: (301) 495 4484 or (877) 226 4267 (free call)
Fax: (301) 718 6366
E-mail: niamsinfo@mail.nih.gov
www.niams.nih.gov

Scleroderma Foundation
12 Kent Way, Suite 101
Byfield, MA 01922
Tel: (978) 463 5843 or (800) 722 4673
Fax: (978) 463 5809
E-mail: sfinfo@scleroderma.org
www.scleroderma.org

Scleroderma Research Foundation
2320 Bath Street, Suite 315
Santa Barbara, CA 93105
Tel: (805) 563 9133 or (800) 441 CURE
Fax: (805) 563-2402
E-mail: srfcure@srfcure.org
www.srfcure.org

United Scleroderma Foundation
734 E Lake Avenue
Watsonville, CA 95076-3566

KEY REFERENCES

- American College of Rheumatology. Scleroderma Fact Sheet. Available at http://www.rheumatology.org/patients/factsheet/scler.html
- Arthritis Foundation Disease Center. Scleroderma. Available at http://arthritis.org/conditions/diseasecenter/scleroderma.asp
- Drake LA, Dinehart SM, Farmer ER, et al. Guidelines of care for scleroderma and sclerodermoid disorders. J Am Acad Dermatol 1996;35:609-14
- Lonzetti LS. Updating the American College of Rheumatology preliminary classification criteria for systemic sclerosis: addition of severe nailfold capillaroscopy abnormalities markedly increases the sensitivity for limited scleroderma. Arthritis Rheum 2001;44:735-6
- Mayo Clinic. Scleroderma. Available at http://www.mayoclinic.com/invoke.cfm?id=DS00362
- National Institute of Arthritis and Musculoskeletal and Skin Diseases. Handout on Health: Scleroderma. Available at http://www.niams.nih.gov/hi/topics/scleroderma/scleroderma.htm
- Subcommittee for scleroderma criteria of the American Rheumatism Association and Therapeutic Criteria Committee. Preliminary criteria for the classification of systemic sclerosis (scleroderma). Arthritis Rheum 1980;23:581-90
- Clements PJ, Furst DE, Wong WK, et al. High dose versus low dose D penicillamine in early diffuse systemic sclerosis. Arthritis Rheum 1999;42:1194
- Thompson AE, Shea B, Welch V, et al. Calcium channel blockers for Raynaud's phenomenon in systemic sclerosis. Arthritis Rheum 2001;44:1841-7
- Pope JE, Bellamy N, Seibold JR, et al. A randomized, controlled trial of methotrexate versus placebo in early diffuse scleroderma. Arthritis Rheum 2001;44:1351-8
- Kahl LE. Raynaud's phenomemon, it may signal systemic disease. Diagnosis 1985;7:30-8

FAQS
Question 1
What is the role of D-penicillamine in systemic sclerosis?

ANSWER 1
The use of D-penicillamine, at one time (1970s-90s) the most commonly used medication for scleroderma, has been called into question following a randomized prospective trial in 1999. However, a number of retrospective studies have found improved skin thickness and survival with its use. Many have abandoned it completely following the prospective study.

Question 2
What is the role of nailfold capillaroscopy?

ANSWER 2
By examining the nailfold capillaries, early microvascular abnormalities may be identified, which allows earlier diagnosis of scleroderma. By adding this technique to current criteria, the sensitivity for the diagnosis of scleroderma increases. Patients with scleroderma will have dilated tortuous capillaries with avascular areas.

Question 3
What is the role for methotrexate in scleroderma?

ANSWER 3
The use of methotrexate in early systemic sclerosis cannot be recommended. Preliminary reports on its effect on skin scores are conflicting and marginal at best. Its use by a specialist should be reserved for severe myositis associated with an overlap syndrome.

CONTRIBUTORS
Fred F Ferri, MD, FACP
Maria-Louise Barilla-LaBarca, MD
Keith M Hull, MD, PhD

SEPTIC ARTHRITIS

DESCRIPTION

- Infection of a joint space, usually monoarticular
- May be caused by a wide variety of organisms
- Bacterial septic arthritis is classified as nongonococcal or gonococcal
- Requires urgent diagnosis and treatment with parenteral antibiotics and aspiration or surgical drainage
- Other causes include viruses, mycobacteria, and fungi (not covered here)

URGENT ACTION

Arthrocentesis and aspirate examination essential to:

- Confirm diagnosis
- Identify causative organism
- Determine antibiotic sensitivity
- Ensure effectiveness of therapy

KEY! DON'T MISS!

- Any patient with monoarticular arthritis should be considered to have septic arthritis until proven otherwise
- Signs and symptoms may be minimal in children, immunosuppressed patients, and elderly patients. Extensive, rapid joint destruction will occur if infection is not diagnosed and treated with appropriate parenteral antibiotics and drainage of necrotic material
- In patients with conditions such as rheumatoid arthritis, osteoarthritis, and crystal arthropathy, signs and symptoms of joint infection may mistakenly be attributed to exacerbation of underlying disorder

BACKGROUND

ICD9 CODE
711.0 Pyogenic arthritis, site unspecified.

SYNONYMS
- Infectious arthritis
- Suppurative arthritis
- Pyogenic arthritis

CARDINAL FEATURES
- Presents as a painful, usually swollen joint
- Often accompanied by fever, chills, malaise
- Knee joint most frequently affected, then hip, then shoulder
- Other joints, e.g. sternoclavicular joint, may be affected in intravenous drug abusers
- Characteristics vary according to causative organism and with age and condition of patient
- Cartilage and bone destruction will ensue if untreated

In gonococcal arthritis:
- Initial bacteremic stage with fever, polyarthralgia, positive blood culture
- Septic joint stage with monoarthritis or oligoarthritis, joint pain, and effusion as above
- Papular or petechial rash and tenosynovitis in two-thirds of patients

In children:
- Neonates and younger children may have coexisting osteomyelitis due to anatomy of immature joint
- Children have monoarticular involvement; neonates are more likely to present with polyarticular disease
- Decreased/absent range of motion of affected limb may be the only sign; fever and swelling of joint may or may not occur

CAUSES
Common causes
Bacterial arthritis:
- Most likely causative organism depends on age and clinical condition of patient
- Gonococcal arthritis is caused by *Neisseria gonorrhoeae*
- Nongonococcal arthritis is usually caused by *Staphylococcus aureus* followed by group B streptococci and *Streptococcus pneumoniae*
- In immunosuppressed and intravenous drug-abusing patients, infection may be with Gram-negative organisms such as *Haemophilus influenzae*, *Salmonella* spp., or *Pseudomonas aeruginosa*
- Hematogenous spread is most common
- Direct inoculation (trauma, surgery) can occur
- Contiguous spread from adjacent osteomyelitis, cellulitis, tenosynovitis, or bursitis can occur

Nonbacterial arthritis:
- Viral arthritis may be caused by parvovirus, hepatitis B, hepatitis C, rubella virus, adenovirus, Epstein-Barr virus, coxsackieviruses

Rare causes
- Anaerobic infections (with peptococcus, peptostreptococcus, *Bacteroides fragilis*, or *Fusobacterium* spp.) may occur, usually after trauma, in prosthetic joints, in immunocompromised patients, or after gastrointestinal surgery for malignancy; infections are polymicrobial in around 50% cases

- *Borrelia burgdorferi* causes Lyme disease arthritis
- *Treponema pallidum* causes syphilitic arthritis
- *Mycobacterium tuberculosis* causes tuberculous arthritis
- Fungal arthritis is usually chronic and may be caused by *Candida* spp., *Coccidioides immitis, Histoplasma capsulatum, Cryptococcus neoformans, Blastomyces dermatitidis, Sporothrix schenckii*, or *Aspergillus fumigatus*

Contributory or predisposing factors
Gonococcal arthritis:
- Young individual with venereal exposure
- Concurrent mucosal gonococcal infection

Nongonococcal arthritis:
- The very old
- The very young
- Pre-existing arthritis, particularly rheumatoid arthritis patients taking corticosteroids (note that these patients may also have multijoint involvement)
- Prosthetic joint
- Trauma
- Diabetes mellitus
- Skin and other infections
- Joint surgery
- Immunosuppression
- Chronic debilitating disease (liver disease, malignancy, AIDS)
- Intravenous drug abuse

EPIDEMIOLOGY
Incidence and prevalence
INCIDENCE
- 0.02–0.05/1000 per year in the general population (about half due to *N. gonorrhoeae*)
- 0.3–0.4/1000 per year in patients with rheumatoid arthritis
- 0.4–0.68/1000 per year in patients with joint prosthesis

PREVALENCE
3–30/1000.

Demographics
AGE
- Nongonococcal septic arthritis more common at extremes of age
- Around two-thirds of children with joint infection are less than 2 years of age
- Gonococcal arthritis more common in young adults

GENDER
- No gender difference in nongonococcal cases
- Gonococcal arthritis occurs in 0.6% women and 0.1% men with gonorrhea

GEOGRAPHY
Incidence lower in European countries than in US; much higher in Africa, Latin America, and Asia.

DIFFERENTIAL DIAGNOSIS

- Any patient with monoarticular arthritis should be considered to have septic arthritis until proven otherwise
- Very many conditions may present as acute monoarticular arthritis
- Remember that septic arthritis may be superimposed on other arthropathies
- Additional differential diagnoses must be considered in children

Gout

Monosodium urate crystals are deposited in tissues due to primary or secondary hyperuricemia.

FEATURES

- Mainly lower extremities affected, classically MP joint of great toe
- Physical findings resemble cellulitis
- Marked soft-tissue tenderness
- Mild leukocytosis and raised erythrocyte sedimentation rate (ESR)
- Synovial aspirate cloudy, inflammatory, with urate crystals
- More information in acute gout and chronic gout

Pseudogout

Pseudogout is caused by deposition of calcium pyrophosphate dehydrate crystals in joint hyaline and fibrocartilage.

FEATURES

- Symptoms similar to those of gout
- Peak age 65–75 years
- Fever is common
- Tendon calcification (chondrocalcinosis) may be present
- May present as acute arthritis or chronic arthritis with acute exacerbations
- Crystal analysis of synovial fluid reveals rhomboid crystals of calcium pyrophosphate

Other crystal arthropathies

Both hydroxyapatite arthropathy and calcium oxalate-induced arthritis may mimic an intra-articular infectious process.

FEATURES

Diagnosis based on synovial fluid crystal identification.

Other infectious arthritides

Distinguishing features of other infectious arthritides are as follows:

FEATURES

- Nonbacterial infectious arthritis can occur as part of Lyme disease or tuberculosis
- Viral causes include parvovirus, hepatitis B, hepatitis C, rubella virus, adenovirus, Epstein-Barr virus, coxsackieviruses
- Occasionally, fungi are the infectious agents, e.g. *Candida* spp., *C. immitis, H. capsulatum, C. neoformans, B. dermatitidis, S. schenckii, A. fumigatus*
- Generally runs a more indolent course than bacterial arthritis

Trauma

Consider as differential diagnosis in children and in adults.

FEATURES

- History of fall may be reported
- Localized pain, swelling, loss of motion
- White blood cell (WBC) count may be raised but usually <50,000/mm^3 (50x109/L)
- Plain X-ray or bone scan usually reveals fracture
- Synovial fluid may contain red blood cells (RBCs) and WBCs but is not purulent

Periarticular infectious processes

Periarticular disorders such as bursitis and cellulitis may mimic some of the features of septic arthritis.

FEATURES

- Erythema, warmth, and tenderness may be present
- Palpation of joint line not specifically painful
- Stressing the joint does not produce pain

Osteoarthritis

Osteoarthritis is essentially a chronic degenerative joint disorder but occasionally presents as an acutely painful joint with effusion.

FEATURES

- Usually widely distributed
- Signs of widespread disease, e.g. Heberden's nodes
- History of previously painful joint
- Often crepitus

Monoarticular presentations of rheumatic disease

- Conditions that typically cause polyarthritis may present initially as monoarthritis; these include rheumatoid arthritis and sarcoidosis
- Seronegative spondyloarthropathies that may present with monoarthritic symptoms include Reiter's syndrome, psoriatic arthritis, ankylosing spondylitis, and arthritis of inflammatory bowel disease

Bacterial endocarditis

Subacute bacterial endocarditis may present with signs and symptoms similar to those of septic arthritis.

FEATURES

- Low-grade fever and malaise
- Cardiac murmurs
- Splenomegaly
- Petechiae on conjunctivae, palate, buccal mucosae, upper extremities
- Nonspecific findings include splinter hemorrhages, Roth's spots, Osler's nodes, Janeway lesions
- Bacteremia
- Elevated ESR; rheumatoid factor positive in around 50% of cases

Rheumatic fever

Rheumatic fever is a multisystem disease following group A streptococcal throat infection.

FEATURES

- Age 5–15 years at first attack; possible relapses later
- Acute rheumatic attack follows 1–5 weeks after streptococcal pharyngitis
- Fever
- Migratory polyarthritis, typically severe for one week
- Carditis
- Subcutaneous nodules over extensor tendons and bony prominences
- Increased antistreptococcal antibody titers
- Positive throat culture
- Elevated ESR and C-reactive protein (CRP); leukocytosis

Polymyalgia rheumatica

Polymyalgia rheumatica is a rheumatic disorder of unknown etiology.

FEATURES

- Rare in patients under 50 years of age
- Neck, shoulder, low back, and thigh pain common
- Morning stiffness lasting 2–3h
- Malaise, low-grade fever
- Synovitis may be present
- Temporal arteritis commonly coexists
- Rheumatoid factor negative
- Elevated ESR
- Rapid response to low-dose steroids

Transient synovitis of the hip in children

Most common cause of acute hip pain in children between 3 and 10 years of age.

FEATURES

- Peak incidence in children between 5 and 6 years of age
- Child limps or cannot bear weight
- Complains of pain in hip, thigh, or knee
- Onset abrupt or insidious
- Symptoms resolve spontaneously after a few days
- ESR and WBC count elevated but usually not to same levels as in septic arthritis

Juvenile rheumatoid arthritis

Juvenile rheumatoid arthritis is an arthritis beginning before 16 years of age.

FEATURES

- Articular findings may be minimal
- History of joint pain, worse in mornings
- May be accompanied by spiking fevers and rash that appears in evenings
- Increased ESR
- High peripheral WBC count

Legg-Calvè-Perthes disease

Legg-Calvè-Perthes disease is a self-limiting disease of unknown etiology.

FEATURES

- Most common in boys 4–9 years of age
- Child limps
- Complains of pain in knee

- Reduced range of motion
- Trendelenburg gait
- Pelvic plain films show bone fragmentation and joint-space widening

Slipped capital femoral epiphysis

Slipped capital femoral epiphysis is a developmental disorder.

FEATURES
- Most common in adolescents (11–16 years of age)
- Obligate external rotation of involved lower extremity when hip is flexed
- Radiographic findings may be minimal
- Laboratory results usually normal

SIGNS & SYMPTOMS
Signs

Adults with nongonococcal arthritis:
- Usually monoarticular, most commonly involving the knee or hip
- Joint swollen, erythematous, and warm
- Patient may be febrile

In gonococcal arthritis (in addition to above):
- May follow migratory or oligoarticular pattern
- Tenosynovitis and skin rash may be present

In young children:
- Restricted movement of a joint (pseudoparalysis)
- Irritability
- Low-grade or no fever

Symptoms

Acute course, depending on infectious agent:
- Severe joint pain
- Swelling
- Tenderness
- Fever

Chronic course:
- Gradual swelling
- Slight or no erythema
- Aching pain

Immunosuppressed, elderly, or debilitated patients: systemic symptoms may be minimal.

ASSOCIATED DISORDERS
- Mode of onset in patients with joint prosthesis usually much less acute
- Patients with rheumatoid arthritis often have less acute presentation, but usually more than one joint is involved

KEY! DON'T MISS!
- Any patient with monoarticular arthritis should be considered to have septic arthritis until proven otherwise
- Signs and symptoms may be minimal in children, immunosuppressed patients, and elderly patients. Extensive, rapid joint destruction will occur if infection is not diagnosed and treated

with appropriate parenteral antibiotics and drainage of necrotic material
- In patients with conditions such as rheumatoid arthritis, osteoarthritis, and crystal arthropathy, signs and symptoms of joint infection may mistakenly be attributed to exacerbation of underlying disorder

CONSIDER CONSULT
- All patients with infection of a prosthetic joint should be referred to their orthopedic surgeon for thorough investigation and possible removal of prosthesis.

INVESTIGATION OF THE PATIENT
Direct questions to patient
Q How quickly did the symptoms start? Onset usually abrupt
Q Do you have symptoms of fever? Patient usually febrile, often with chills
Q Which joint is affected? Usually monoarticular, and usually knee or hip
Q Is the pain mild/moderate or severe? Pain typically severe, especially on attempted movement
Q (In children) Any reluctance to move the joint/limb? May be the only symptom apart from fractiousness in a young child

Contributory or predisposing factors
Q Are there any venereal symptoms? Gonococcal arthritis is one of the most common forms of the condition
Q Is there any history of arthritis? Arthritis, especially rheumatoid, predisposes to septic arthritis
Q Has the patient had previous joint surgery? Sepsis occurs in 0.5–2.3% of patients who have had joint replacement surgery
Q Are there signs of recent trauma? An infected laceration or hematoma may provide a source of blood-borne infection
Q Is there any other current infectious process? Urinary, respiratory tract, or skin infections, for example, may result in embolic seeding of pathogens
Q Is there any concurrent constitutional condition? Diabetes mellitus and other debilitating disorders (e.g. cancer, AIDS) predispose to the condition
Q Is there a history of complement deficiency or other immunodeficiency? Patients with IgA deficiency, x-linked agammaglobulinemia, common variable immunodeficiency, and hyper-IgM immunoglobulin deficiency are at risk for septic arthritis (due to the normal causative agents). Patients with deficiency of terminal complement components (C5–9) leave patients at risk for recurrent *Neisseria* infections

Examination
- Is the patient well/unwell? Suspect septic arthritis in an ill patient
- Check temperature. Infection of the joint may be associated with fever
- Inspect affected joint and record skin color, tenderness, effusion, signs of tracking infection, and local lymphadenopathy
- Look for any source of sepsis, e.g. pressure sores, varicose ulcers in the elderly, otitis, tonsillitis, impetigo in the child, venereal infection in the young adult. Localized infection elsewhere in the body can disseminate to joints
- Look for evidence of generalized joint disease. Patients with other arthropathies have increased risk for septic arthritis
- Look for stigmata of crystal arthropathies: gouty tophi, chondrocalcinosis; gout is a major differential diagnosis

Summary of investigative tests
- Hematologic investigations: complete blood count may reveal contributory debilitating disorders, and raised WBC count will help confirm infective process; ESR and CRP level are usually raised

- Arthrocentesis with laboratory examination of synovial fluid is essential
- Synovial tissue biopsy may be taken at arthroscopy for microscopic examination and culture and may reveal causative organism when synovial fluid culture is negative
- Blood culture may reveal causative organism and help confirm results of synovial fluid culture
- Any other site of possible sepsis should be sampled for bacteriologic examination: urethral swab may reveal gonococcal infection; throat and nasal swabs may help identify a causative organism arising in these sites
- Plain X-ray has limited value in diagnosis of septic arthritis but may aid in detection of underlying disease
- Ultrasound may be used to detect effusion of the hip in infants with suspected septic arthritis
- Computed tomography (CT) scanning may be used for early diagnosis of suspected infections of spine, hips, and sternoclavicular and sacroiliac joints (usually performed by a specialist)
- Technetium and gallium scintigraphy may be useful if deep-seated joint involved but cannot distinguish inflammation from infection (usually performed by a specialist)

DIAGNOSTIC DECISION

- Diagnosis rests on urgent laboratory investigation of aspirated joint fluid allied with signs and symptoms of joint infection
- Imaging procedures and other investigations are appropriate only in obscure or difficult cases
- Retain high index of suspicion in patients who are elderly, young, immunocompromised, or who have rheumatoid arthritis or osteoarthritis, all of whom may have nonspecific signs and symptoms

Be alert for four features in a child who presents with hip pain of 1–3 days' duration and/or a limp:

- History of fever
- Difficulty bearing weight
- Peripheral WBC count >12,000 cells/mm^3
- ESR >40mm/h

Probability of septic arthritis is:

- 99.6% for children with all four of above factors
- 93.1% for those with any three of above factors

Guidelines

The American Academy of Family Physicians have produced a guideline, which includes information on septic arthritis [1].

CLINICAL PEARLS

- Children have a higher incidence of hip involvement with septic arthritis
- Children often have an adjacent osteomyelitis
- Intravenous drug users with septic arthritis often have involvement at atypical sites, such as sternocostal articulations and symphysis pubis

THE TESTS
Body fluids
HEMATOLOGIC INVESTIGATIONS
Description
Venous blood sample analyzed for:

- WBC count
- ESR
- CRP level

Advantages/Disadvantages
Advantages:
- Useful indicators of infection
- Quick, inexpensive tests

Disadvantage: nonspecific

Normal
WBC count:
- Adults: 3200–9800/mm^3 (3.2–9.8x10^9/L)
- Neonates: 5000–21,000/mm^3 (5–21x10^9/L)
- Children: 5000–13,500/mm^3 (5–13 5x10^9/L)

ESR:
- Men: 0–15mm/h
- Women: 0–20mm/h

CRP level: 6.8–820mcg/dL (68–8200mcg/L)

Abnormal
- WBC elevation occurs in about 50% of cases, usually >50,000/mm^3
- WBC elevation less likely in gonococcal cases and in debilitated patients with rheumatoid arthritis
- ESR usually raised but normal in 20% cases
- CRP usually elevated
- Keep in mind the possibility of a false-positive result

Cause of abnormal result
Inflammatory processes in infected joint.

Drugs, disorders and other factors that may alter results
- WBC count elevated in any infection or inflammatory process
- ESR raised in most infections and inflammatory states
- CRP level raised in rheumatoid arthritis, rheumatic fever, inflammatory bowel disease, bacterial infections, inflammatory diseases
- Laboratory technique may affect results

EXAMINATION OF SYNOVIAL FLUID
Description
Arthrocentesis and synovial fluid examination is mandatory in cases of joint effusion where an infectious process is being considered.

All fluid aspirated should be sent for:
- Aerobic and anaerobic bacterial cultures
- Gram stain
- Cell count with differential leukocyte count
- Glucose level (compared with serum glucose level)
- Note: first three points are in order of priority if only a small amount of fluid obtained

Inoculate blood culture bottles immediately after joint aspiration to try to secure survival of fastidious organisms. If gonococcal arthritis is suspected, synovial fluid cultures should be done on chocolate agar.

Advantages/Disadvantages

Disadvantages:

- Aspiration of joint may be technically difficult but is essential
- Aspiration of the hip may have to be performed under fluoroscopic or ultrasonographic control
- Culture negative in 20–25% of clinically suspected cases and up to 50% of gonococcal cases
- Synovial fluid glucose levels not specific for septic arthritis and may be also very low in other inflammatory, but not infectious, arthritides

Normal

Normal synovial fluid:

- Pale yellow color
- Clear
- Normally viscous
- Cell count 200–1000/mm^3
- Predominant cells mononuclear
- Synovial fluid: serum glucose ratio 0.8–1.0
- Gram stain reveals no organisms
- Culture negative

Abnormal

Inflammatory fluid – noninfectious:

- Yellow color
- Turbid
- Viscosity reduced
- Cell count 3000 to >10,000/mm^3
- Predominant cells polymorphonuclear leukocytes
- Gram stain reveals no organisms
- Culture negative

Inflammatory fluid – infectious:

- Yellow color
- Turbid, purulent
- Viscosity reduced
- Cell count 10,000 to >100,000/mm^3
- Predominant cells polymorphonuclear leukocytes
- Synovial fluid: serum glucose ratio <0.5
- Gram stain may reveal organisms
- Culture may be positive

Keep in mind the possibility of a falsely abnormal result.

Cause of abnormal result

Infection of joint space by micro-organisms.

Drugs, disorders and other factors that may alter results

- Prior treatment with antibiotics or glucocorticoids may modify the inflammatory process
- Septic arthritis may result in increased precipitation and release of crystals: search for an infectious agent should not be abandoned if crystals found
- For synovial fluid: serum glucose ratio patient must not have eaten for 6h, and no intravenous solutions should be infusing because these factors alter result

BLOOD CULTURE
Description
Blood should be cultured routinely. In gonococcal arthritis, it should be cultured on chocolate agar.

Advantages/Disadvantages
Advantage: blood culture may reveal causative organism.

Normal
No growth.

Abnormal
- Growth of organism
- Keep in mind the possibility of a false-positive result

Cause of abnormal result
Positive in up to 50% of *S. aureus* infections but less frequently with other organisms.

Drugs, disorders and other factors that may alter results
- Prior treatment with antibiotics will reduce the chance of successful culture
- Sampling and laboratory technique can affect results

OTHER BACTERIOLOGIC INVESTIGATIONS
Description
Cultures from possible *foci* of infection, e.g. nose, throat, ureter, urine, skin lesions. Use Thayer Martin media for urethral and pharyngeal cultures in cases of suspected gonococcal infection.

Advantages/Disadvantages
Disadvantage: bacterial growth from these sites will not necessarily be diagnostic of the causative organism.

Normal
No growth, or growth of commensals.

Abnormal
- Growth of organism other than commensal
- Keep in mind the possibility of a false-positive result

Cause of abnormal result
Hematogenous spread to joint.

Drugs, disorders and other factors that may alter results
- Prior treatment with antibiotics will reduce the chance of successful culture
- Sampling and laboratory technique can affect results

Biopsy
SYNOVIAL BIOPSY
Description
Synovial tissue obtained at arthroscopy for microscopic analysis and culture.

Advantages/Disadvantages
Advantage: cultures of tissue may be positive despite negative synovial fluid cultures.

Normal
Normal microscopic appearance, negative culture.

Abnormal
- Causative organism may be grown
- Large numbers of neutrophils more common in septic arthritis than in other inflammatory arthropathies
- Keep in mind the possibility of a false-positive result

Cause of abnormal result
Inflammation, infection.

Drugs, disorders and other factors that may alter results
- Prior use of antibiotics may reduce the chances of successful culture
- Sampling and laboratory technique may affect result

Imaging
PLAIN X-RAY
Advantages/Disadvantages
- Advantage: plain X-rays are of limited use in diagnosing septic arthritis but can help distinguish underlying disease
- Disadvantage: safety depends on area being imaged; low back X-ray is equivalent to >12 months background radiation and should only be taken when essential

Normal
No bone changes; no displacement of soft-tissues.

Abnormal
- Medial displacement of obturator tendon suggests effusion in hip joint
- Widening of joint space may be evident at first
- Erosion of bone may appear at margins of joints early in septic arthritis
- Disuse of a limb will cause early osteopenia
- Narrowing of joint space will eventually occur

Cause of abnormal result
Articular inflammatory processes.

Drugs, disorders and other factors that may alter results
Pre-existing joint disease – rheumatoid arthritis, osteomyelitis, osteoarthritis – may coexist and may mask radiologic appearance of septic arthritis.

ULTRASONOGRAPHY
Advantages/Disadvantages
Advantages:
- Greater sensitivity than plain radiographs
- Most useful in diagnosis of effusion in the infant hip

Disadvantage: nonspecific for septic arthritis

Normal
No abnormality.

Abnormal
- Demonstration of joint effusion, displacement of tissues
- Keep in mind the possibility of a false-positive result

Cause of abnormal result
Inflammatory processes in joint space.

Drugs, disorders and other factors that may alter results
Transient synovitis, septic arthritis, juvenile rheumatoid arthritis, and Legg-Calvè-Perthes disease all cause joint effusion in children.

TREATMENT

CONSIDER CONSULT

- In general, all cases of septic arthritis should be referred for immediate hospital admission. Rarely, an extremely compliant patient with a very sensitive organism might be treated as an outpatient
- All cases of septic arthritis with suspected or confirmed underlying rheumatic disease should be referred to a specialist for management

IMMEDIATE ACTION

Joint aspiration may be undertaken prior to hospital admission, but any undue delay in inoculation and incubation of culture medium may compromise identification of causative organism.

PATIENT AND CAREGIVER ISSUES
Patient or caregiver request

Patients (or parents) may question the necessity for referral or hospital admission.

Health-seeking behavior

Prior medication with antibiotics, e.g. for upper respiratory infection in a child, may make identification of causative organism impossible.

MANAGEMENT ISSUES
Goals

Achieving the following management goals will help minimize joint damage and ensure optimal restoration of function:

- Early diagnosis
- Early institution of empiric antibiotic therapy after arthrocentesis
- Early drainage of joint

Management in special circumstances

COEXISTING DISEASE

Glycemic control will require careful monitoring in patients with diabetes mellitus.

COEXISTING MEDICATION

Oral glucocorticoid treatment for rheumatoid arthritis must be optimized.

SPECIAL PATIENT GROUPS

Neonates:

Early diagnosis and treatment are particularly important to avert destruction of the cartilaginous femoral head.

Patients with joint prosthesis:

- Implantation of joint prosthesis is followed by infection in 1–5% cases
- Infection most likely in first 3 months
- Most common agents are *S. epidermidis* (40%), *S. aureus* (20%), and streptococcal species (20%)
- Treatment will most likely require removal of prosthesis

PATIENT SATISFACTION/LIFESTYLE PRIORITIES

Most patients will expect return to full range of motion and function.

SUMMARY OF THERAPEUTIC OPTIONS
Choices

- All cases require parenteral antibiotics – inpatient treatment is recommended
- Empiric antibiotic therapy (drug choice based on Gram stain) is employed until results of

bacteriologic studies available

- For gonococcal arthritis, first-choice therapy is ceftriaxone or spectinomycin in penicillin-allergic patients
- For nongonococcal arthritis, Gram-positive cases should be treated with nafcillin and Gram-negative cases with a third-generation cephalosporin and an aminoglycoside. Most patients will benefit from specialist guidance
- All nongonococcal cases will also require repeated needle aspiration or surgical drainage of the joint, either by arthroscopy or arthrotomy; these procedures are usually performed by a specialist
- Postpone nonsteroidal anti-inflammatory drugs (NSAIDs) for 24h to allow cultures to grow and permit repeat arthrocentesis if first is nondiagnostic
- Most patients require physical therapy with immobilization/remobilization regimen, usually performed by a specialist

Clinical pearls

- Patients with gonococcal arthritis should also be treated for silent chlamydia infection (e.g. doxycycline 100mg orally twice daily for 7 days; if pregnant, use erythromycin)
- Septic arthritis involving the hips and shoulders requires surgical drainage

Never

Never embark upon conjectural antibiotic therapy without:

- Arthrocentesis and urgent submission of aspirate for laboratory examination
- Bacteriologic sampling of likely sources of infection, including blood culture

FOLLOW UP
Plan for review

As the condition settles with appropriate antibiotic therapy, joint drainage, and management of any comorbid conditions, outpatient follow up and review can be considered; continuing oral antibiotics and rehabilitation of the joint will be necessary.

Information for patient or caregiver

- Long-term oral antibiotics may be required to prevent recurrence
- Weight control (if a weight-bearing joint) may be needed

DRUGS AND OTHER THERAPIES: DETAILS
Drugs
CEFTRIAXONE
For gonococcal arthritis.

Dose

- 1g intravenously every 24h
- Generally followed by oral preparations after improvement

Efficacy
Effective in most cases of gonococcal arthritis.

Risks/Benefits
Risks:

- Single-dose regimen allows directly observed therapy and ensures compliance
- Provides sustained, high bactericidal levels in blood
- Use caution with hypersensitivity to penicillins
- Use caution with renal disease and anaphylaxis

Side-effects and adverse reactions
- Central nervous system: headache, sleep disturbance, confusion, dizziness
- Gastrointestinal: anorexia, nausea, diarrhea, abdominal pain
- Genitourinary: nephrotoxicity
- Hematologic: bone marrow suppression
- Skin: rash

Interactions (other drugs)
- **Warfarin** **Aminoglycosides** **Loop diuretics** **Vancomycin** **Polymyxin B**

Contraindications
Infant less than one month of age.

Acceptability to patient
Side-effects may cause compliance problems with oral therapy.

Follow up plan
- Oral therapy as outpatient after inpatient parenteral therapy
- Specialist guidance is usual

Patient and caregiver information
- Patients should be warned of common side-effects
- Patients must be informed of importance of completing oral course of antibiotics

SPECTINOMYCIN
- For gonococcal arthritis
- For patients with penicillin allergy

Dose
2g intramuscularly every 12h.

Risks/Benefits
Risks:
- Expensive
- Use parenterally only
- Definitive treatment with single dose

Benefit: for patients with penicillin allergy

Side-effects and adverse reactions
- Central nervous system: dizziness, headache, pain at injection site
- Gastrointestinal: nausea, vomiting
- Hematologic: anemia
- Skin: rashes

Interactions (other drugs)
None listed.

Contraindications
Allergy to aminoglycosides.

Follow up plan
- Oral therapy as outpatient after inpatient parenteral therapy
- Specialist guidance is usual

Patient and caregiver information
- Patients should be warned of common side-effects
- Patients should be informed of importance of completing full course of oral antibiotics

NAFCILLIN
Usually the agent of choice for Gram-positive organisms.

Dose
- Adult: 1g every 4h, intravenously over 1h to avoid vein irritation
- Infants and children <40kg: 25mg/kg intramuscularly given twice daily
- Neonates: 10mg/kg intramuscularly given twice daily

Efficacy
Nafcillin is generally effective against *S. aureus* and a range of streptococci, including *S. pyogenes* and *S. pneumoniae*.

Risks/Benefits
Risks:
- Use caution in imipenem and cephalosporin hypersensitivity, hepatic disease, and history of gastrointestinal disease
- Use caution in breast-feeding

Benefit: usually effective where penicillinase is produced

Side-effects and adverse reactions
- Central nervous system: seizures
- Gastrointestinal: nausea, vomiting, diarrhea, elevated hepatic enzymes, pseudomembranous colitis
- Genitourinary: interstitial nephritis, renal tubular necrosis, nephrotic syndrome
- Hematologic: neutropenia, thrombocytopenia, leukopenia
- Skin: rash, maculopapular rash, urticaria, Stevens-Johnson syndrome, purpura, vasculitis, toxic epidermal necrosis, exfoliative dermatitis, injection site reaction, phlebitis

Interactions (other drugs)
- Aminoglycosides
- Probenecid
- Rifampin
- Warfarin

Contraindications
Penicillin hypersensitivity.

Acceptability to patient
Side-effects may be difficult to tolerate.

Follow up plan
Complete blood count and urinalysis during therapy to ensure early detection of serious adverse effects.

Patient and caregiver information
Patients should be warned of common side-effects.

Physical therapy
IMMOBILIZATION/REMOBILIZATION REGIMEN
- Usually joint is immobilized in the position of function for the first 2–3 days
- Thereafter, gentle, gradually increasing passive movement is applied

Efficacy
Early mobilization helps return to normal function.

Risks/Benefits
- Risk: no risks in physical therapy applied to these patients
- Benefit: preserves muscle bulk and bone density, and prevents adhesions

Acceptability to patient
Pain control may be required.

Follow up plan
Ongoing physical therapy may be required after resolution of infection.

Patient and caregiver information
Patient should be advised to perform recommended exercises at home.

Surgical therapy
- Gonococcal arthritis can usually be treated effectively with antibiotics alone
- Joint aspiration should be performed in all other varieties of infectious arthritis
- Choice lies between repeated aspiration through a wide-bore needle and surgical drainage, either by arthroscopy or arthrotomy

NEEDLE ASPIRATION OF JOINT
Joint is aspirated through wide-bore needle.

Efficacy
Effectively removes damaging accumulations of debris and pus.

Risks/Benefits
Risk: may need to be performed under fluoroscopic control in difficult joints, e.g. the hip

Benefits:
- Needle aspiration is usually relatively simple in expert hands
- General anesthesia not required, and morbidity rate is low

Follow up plan
Should be repeated at least once a day with strict attention to leukocyte count. If it is not going down after a couple of days, patients will likely require surgical drainage.

Patient and caregiver information
Patient should be aware that procedure is repeated daily during the initial course of the disease.

SURGICAL DRAINAGE
Surgical drainage is performed if response to aspiration is unfavorable and repeat aspiration reveals no decrease in synovial leukocyte count over 24–48h. The choice lies between arthroscopy and arthrotomy.

Efficacy
Surgical drainage is effective. It is usually considered mandatory in:
- Septic arthritis of the hip in infants, in whom joint damage begins early and proceeds rapidly
- Infected joint prostheses

Risks/Benefits
Risks:
- General anesthetic required
- May lead to scarring and restriction of joint movement

Benefits:
- Joint can be fully cleared of pus and debris
- Loculations can be broken
- Irrigation and drainage tubes can keep joint free of destructive cells and enzymes

Acceptability to patient
Some patients may have concerns about postoperative scarring.

Follow up plan
Physical therapy with immobilization/remobilization regimen.

Patient and caregiver information
Removal of damaging infected material from the joint is of equal importance to antibiotic treatment.

OUTCOMES

EFFICACY OF THERAPIES

For patients with prosthetic joint infections, cure rates without removal is poor. Therefore treatment of most prosthetic joint infections will require removal of the prosthesis along with surgical debridement and antibiotics.

In the uncomplicated case, rapid clinical improvement is usually attained by:

- Early diagnosis
- Swift commencement of effective antibiotic treatment
- Drainage of the joint

The one factor most responsible for poor outcome is delay in diagnosis and treatment.

Evidence

PDxMD are unable to cite evidence that meets our criteria for evidence.

PROGNOSIS

Overall, 60–65% cases of septic arthritis recover completely, i.e. full range of movement and no pain. In about one-third of cases there is:

- Reduced mobility
- Ankylosis
- Pain on movement
- Chronic infection, or overwhelming infection and death

Clinical pearls

Patients with polyarticular presentations tend to have poorer outcomes.

Therapeutic failure

- The great majority of these cases will have been referred early for orthopedic diagnosis and management
- Otherwise, if patient fails to improve in 1–2 days after aspiration, empiric antibiotic therapy, and immobilization, orthopedic referral should be urgently considered

Recurrence

Recurrence rate is about 7% in patients with rheumatoid arthritis.

COMPLICATIONS

In children, epiphyseal damage may cause:

- Impaired growth
- Length discrepancy

In all cases, complications include:

- Infection of periarticular structures
- Sinus formation
- Avascular necrosis of femoral head
- Ankylosis
- Long-term degenerative arthritis of affected joint

In elderly and immunocompromised patients especially, complications include: systemic sepsis

CONSIDER CONSULT

- Most cases of therapeutic failure will have been referred early for orthopedic diagnosis and management
- Otherwise, if patient fails to improve in 1–2 days after aspiration, empiric antibiotic therapy, and immobilization, orthopedic referral should be urgently considered

PREVENTION

RISK FACTORS

Adult patients most at risk are those with:

- Rheumatoid arthritis on glucocorticoids: septic arthritis with overlying rheumatoid arthritis is common, particularly when patient is immunosuppressed
- Prosthetic joint or recent joint surgery: any surgery on a joint carries a risk for infection
- Immunosuppression or chronic debilitating disease, e.g. diabetes mellitus: immunosuppression increases risk for infection
- History of intravenous drug abuse: increases risk for hematogenous spread of microorganisms

MODIFY RISK FACTORS

- Physician should have high index of suspicion in all at-risk patient groups
- For patients with prosthetic joints, early identification and treatment of oropharyngeal infections

Lifestyle and wellness

ALCOHOL AND DRUGS

Discourage intravenous drug abuse.

DIET

Good glycemic control should be emphasized in patients with diabetes mellitus.

SEXUAL BEHAVIOR

Safer sex practices should be encouraged.

PREVENT RECURRENCE

Reassess coexisting disease

Maintain high degree of patient awareness in vulnerable groups, e.g. HIV-positive, immunocompromised, diabetic, and those with rheumatoid arthritis or other debilitating conditions.

INTERACTION ALERT

- Optimize dosage of glucocorticoids in rheumatoid arthritis patients
- Ensure optimal glycemic control in patients with diabetes mellitus

ASSOCIATIONS
National Office of the Arthritis Foundation
1330 West Peachtree Street
Atlanta, GA 30309
Tel: (404)8727100
Arthritis Answers: (800) 2837800
www.arthritis.org

KEY REFERENCES

- Anon. Clinical aspects of septic arthritis. In Rosen F, ed. Emergency medicine: concepts and clinical practice, 4th edn. St Louis (MO): Mosby-Year Book, 1998
- Brower AC. Septic arthritis. Radiol Clin North Am 1996;34:293–309
- Carreno Perez L. Septic arthritis. Best Pract Res Clin Rheumatol 1999;13:37–58
- Cimmino MA. Recognition and management of bacterial arthritis. Drugs 1997;54:50–60
- Cucurull E, Espinoza LR. Gonococcal arthritis. Rheumatol Dis Clin North Am 1998;24:305–22
- Dubost JJ, Soubrier M, Sauvezie B. Pyogenic arthritis in adults. Joint Bone Spine: Rev Rheum 2000;67:11–21
- Graif M, Schweitzer ME, Deely D, Matteucci T. The septic versus nonseptic inflamed joint: MRI characteristics. Skeletal Radiol 1999;28:616–20
- Hart JJ. Transient synovitis of the hip in children. Am Fam Physician 1996;54:1587–91,1595–6
- Kocher MS, Zurakowski D, Kasser JR. Differentiating between septic arthritis and transient synovitis of the hip in children: an evidence-based clinical prediction algorithm. J Bone Joint Surg 1999;81:1662–70
- Kortekangas P. Bacterial arthritis in the elderly, an overview. Drugs Aging 1999;14:165–71
- Lyon RM, Evanich TD. Culture-negative septic arthritis in children. J Pediatr Orthoped 1999;19:655–9
- Perry CR. Septic arthritis. Am J Orthoped 1999;28:168–78
- Pioro MH, Mandell BF. Septic arthritis. Rheumatol Dis Clin North Am 1996;23:239–58
- Sack K. Monarthritis: differential diagnosis. Am J Med 1997;10291a0;30S–34S
- Salzbach R. Pediatric septic arthritis. AORN J 1999;70:998, 991–1002
- Schumacher HR. Arthrocentesis of the knee. Hosp Med 1997;33:60–4
- Shiv VK, Jain AK, Taneja K, Bhargava SK. Sonography of the hip joint in infective arthritis. Can Assoc Radiol J 1990;41:76–8
- Stimmler MM. Infectious arthritis. Postgrad Med 1996;99:127–31,135–9
- Till SH, Snaith ML. Assessment, investigation and management of acute monoarthritis. J Acc Emerg Med 1999;16:355–61
- Wener MH. Synovial fluid analysis http://www.rheumatology.org (Accessed 23 October 2000)
- Weston VC, Jones AC, Bradbury N, et al. Clinical features and outcome of septic arthritis. Ann Rheum Dis 1999;58:214–9
- Williams KD. Infectious arthritis. In: Canale, ed. Campbell's operative orthopedics. St Louis (MO): Mosby-Year Book; 1998
- Youssef PP, York JR. Septic arthritis. Aust NZ J Med 1994;24:307–11

Guidelines
1 Leet A, Skaggs DL. Evaluation of the acutely limping child. Am Fam Physician 2000;61:1011–8

FAQS
Question 1
When does a joint need surgical drainage?

ANSWER 1
Hips, shoulders, and joints from which it is difficult to aspirate fluid should be immediately referred for surgical drainage. Additionally, any joint in which it is difficult to aspirate fluid (e.g. because of loculations) and any infected joint that does not show a decrease in WBC count after 1–2 days should be surgically drained. Finally, prosthetic joints and associated osteomyelitis are complicating factors requiring surgical consultation.

Question 2

What is the role of plain radiographs in the diagnosis of septic arthritis?

ANSWER 2

The only information gained from a plain radiograph is to document underlying or associated disease (rheumatoid arthritis, osteomyelitis). Changes from septic arthritis will take weeks to be seen on plain films.

Question 3

How do you culture for *Neisseria gonorrhoeae*?

ANSWER 3

Thayer Martin media (urethral and pharyngeal cultures) or chocolate agar (blood and synovial fluid cultures).

CONTRIBUTORS

Joseph E Scherger, MD, MPH
Maria-Louise Barilla-LaBarca, MD

SJÖGREN'S SYNDROME

SUMMARY INFORMATION

DESCRIPTION

- Chronic, slowly progressive, inflammatory autoimmune disease characterized by lymphocytic (CD4+) infiltration of exocrine glands, especially the salivary and lacrimal glands, and sometimes the pancreas
- May develop independently of a connective tissue disease (primary Sjögren's syndrome), or associated with other disorders (secondary Sjögren's syndrome)
- Characteristic autoantibodies to the ribonucleoprotein complexes Ro(SS-A) and La(SS-B) are present in most patients

URGENT ACTION

If nonHodgkin's lymphoma is suspected, refer immediately to oncology.

KEY! DON'T MISS!

- Unilateral salivary gland enlargement, or an especially hard or nodular gland, may be a sign of salivary gland tumor, even if Sjögren's syndrome is diagnosed
- Pseudolymphoma or frank lymphoma should also be suspected in cases of persistent salivary gland enlargement, progressive lymphadenopathy, or lung nodules
- Glomerulonephritis may be a sign of overlapping, systemic lupus erythematosus, or cryoglobulinemia
- In cases of myalgia and fatigue, Hashimoto's thyroiditis should be suspected

BACKGROUND

ICD9 CODE
710.2 Sjögren's syndrome.

SYNONYMS
- Sjögren syndrome
- Sicca syndrome

CARDINAL FEATURES
- Chronic inflammatory autoimmune disease characterized by lymphocytic infiltration and sometimes destruction of exocrine glands, especially the salivary and lacrimal glands, and sometimes the pancreas
- May range from involvement of lacrimal and salivary glands only, through involvement of other exocrine glands, to full systemic disease
- May develop independently of a connective tissue disease (primary Sjögren's syndrome), or associated disorders (secondary Sjögren's syndrome)
- Characteristic autoantibodies to the ribonucleoprotein complexes Ro(SS-A) and La(SS-B) are present in most patients

CAUSES
Common causes
No cause has been convincingly demonstrated for the primary disease.

Contributory or predisposing factors
- Genetic predisposition – associated with certain haplotypes
- Female gender – 90% of cases in women
- Middle to old age – most common in women in 30s and 40s

EPIDEMIOLOGY
Incidence and prevalence
There are only few data available.

INCIDENCE
Unknown.

PREVALENCE
- Primary disease: 0.5–3.0/1000
- Secondary disease: approximately as for primary disease
- Nonspecific keratoconjunctivitis sicca and xerostomia are more common: up to 40/1000

FREQUENCY
Affects up to one-third of autoimmune disease patients, including:
- 20–30% of patients with systemic lupus erythematous
- 20–25% of patients with rheumatoid arthritis
- 20% of patients with scleroderma

Demographics
AGE
- Incidence peaks in the fifth through the eighth decades, but may be seen in patients of all ages, including children (rare)
- Prevalence in persons aged 60 years or older: 20–50/1000

GENDER
Female:male 9:1.

RACE
Tends to affect Caucasians, although all races are affected.

GENETICS
- Heritable predisposition shown by higher than normal incidence in families
- Immunogenetic studies have revealed many alleles that may affect susceptibility, disease severity, and production of autoantibodies, in different ethnic groups

GEOGRAPHY
Uniform distribution.

SOCIOECONOMIC STATUS
Unknown.

DIFFERENTIAL DIAGNOSIS

Differential diagnosis is difficult because the signs and symptoms of Sjögren's syndrome may have many causes. Diuretics, tricyclic antidepressants, antihistamines, antipsychotics, and others may all cause dry mouth. The following disorders are those most commonly confused with Sjögren's syndrome.

Viral infections
FEATURES

- Keratoconjunctivitis sicca may occur in asymptomatic carriers of human T-lymphotropic virus 1
- Bilateral parotid gland enlargement may occur in viral infections including mumps, influenza, Epstein-Barr virus, coxsackievirus, and cytomegalovirus

Chronic conjunctivitis
FEATURES

- Injection and edema of the conjunctivae with conjunctival injection, edema, and discharge
- Xerophthalmia may occur
- Clear cornea
- Vision typically normal
- Dry eyes, even with keratoconjunctivitis sicca, may occur in the absence of the diagnosis of Sjögren's syndrome

Chronic blepharitis
Blepharitis due to meibomian gland dysfunction or plugging with excessive ocular lubricants may present a similar ocular picture to Sjögren's syndrome.

FEATURES

- Diffusely erythematous eyelids with exudate at the eyelash bases
- Thickened eyelid margins, with loss and misdirected growth of eyelashes, and overflow or dryness of meibomian glands
- Frequent associated conjunctivitis but without discharge
- Chalazia are possible
- Superficial punctate erosions of the inferior corneal epithelium are frequent
- Xerophthalmia may occur

Diabetes mellitus
FEATURES

- Xerostomia
- Polyuria, polydipsia
- Diabetic retinopathy
- Neuropathic arthropathy (bone or joint deformity from repeated trauma secondary to peripheral neuropathy)
- Cataracts and glaucoma are common
- Peripheral neuropathy
- Autonomic neuropathy
- Nephropathy
- Foot ulcers
- Necrobiosis lipoidica diabeticorum
- Bilateral parotid gland enlargement may occur

Anxiety
FEATURES

- Xerostomia
- Anxious disposition
- Excessive worry
- Sleep disturbances
- Muscle tension
- Fatigue
- Tension headaches
- Difficulty in concentration
- Irritable bowel syndrome
- Associated psychiatric illness or substance abuse is common

Fibromyalgia
FEATURES

- Tender nodules at any of 18 defined sites on the body, including the low cervical area
- Musculoskeletal pain and stiffness
- Paresthesias
- Nonrefreshing sleep
- Easy fatigability
- Symptoms of oral dryness (especially in patients taking medications with anticholinergic side-effects, such as amitriptyline)

Hepatitis C infection
FEATURES

- Hepatomegaly
- More than 75% of patients may have mild symptoms without jaundice. Others may have jaundice and dark urine
- Rare splenomegaly, cryoglobulinemia, or immune complex disease (including vasculitis, glomerulonephritis, and Hashimoto's thyroiditis)
- Xerophthalmia and xerostomia may also occur

Hyperlipidemia
Types II, IV, and V, in particular, may induce bilateral parotid gland enlargement.

FEATURES

Depending on the type involved, features may include the following:
- Xanthomas
- Xanthelasmas
- Hepatomegaly
- Splenomegaly
- Lipemia retinalis
- Arcus cornea
- Obesity
- Bilateral parotid gland enlargement
- Pancreatitis can occur

Hepatic cirrhosis
FEATURES

Depending on the cause, the features may include the following:

Dermatological signs:
Jaundice, palmar erythema, spider angiomata, ecchymosis, dilated superficial periumbilical veins, increased pigmentation, xanthomas, and needle tracks.

Ocular signs:
- Kayser-Fleischer rings (characteristic of Wilson's disease), scleral icterus
- Fetor hepaticus
- Gynecomastia in males

Abdominal signs:
Tender hepatomegaly; small, nodular liver; palpable, nontender gall bladder; palpable spleen; ascites; venous hum auscultated over periumbilical veins

Rectal signs:
- Hemorrhoids, guaiac-positive stools
- Testicular atrophy in males
- Pedal edema
- Arthropathy
- Flapping tremor
- Choreoathetosis
- Dysarthria
- Bilateral parotid gland enlargement may occur

Chronic pancreatitis
FEATURES
- Persistent/recurrent, radiating epigastric pain
- Peripancreatic pain with muscle guarding
- Marked weight loss
- Bulky, greasy, foul-smelling stools
- Epigastric mass and/or jaundice may also be present
- Bilateral parotid gland enlargement may occur

Chronic sialadenitis
May mimic salivary gland involvement of Sjögren's syndrome, and the nonspecific changes that are seen on biopsy may be confused with the focal lymphocytic infiltrates typical of Sjögren's syndrome.

FEATURES
- Painful and swollen salivary gland
- Increased pain on eating
- Erythema and tenderness at duct opening, with purulent discharge (may be absent with obstruction)
- Induration and pitting of skin

Sarcoidosis
Sarcoidosis may present a very similar clinical picture to Sjögren's syndrome.

FEATURES
- Bilateral parotid gland enlargement
- Noncaseating granuloma in minor salivary gland biopsies
- Pulmonary features (dry cough, dyspnea, chest discomfort)
- General malaise, fatigue, with weight loss and anorexia
- Ocular features (blurred vision, discomfort, keratoconjunctivitis sicca, conjunctivitis, iritis, uveitis)
- Dermatologic features (erythema nodosum, macules, papules, subcutaneous nodules, hyperpigmentation)
- Cardiac features (arrhythmias, cardiomyopathy)
- Splenomegaly and hepatomegaly

- Arthropathy
- Cranial nerve palsies
- Diabetes insipidus

Acromegaly
FEATURES
- Coarse features, and coarse, greasy skin
- Spadelike, fleshy, and moist hands and feet
- Prognathism (with possible underbite)
- Carpal tunnel syndrome
- Excessive sweating
- Arthralgias and osteoarthritis
- Hypertension
- Skin tags
- History of large shoe, glove, or hat size
- Weakness and decreased exercise capacity
- Headaches
- Diabetes mellitus
- Visual field defects
- Bilateral parotid gland enlargement may occur

HIV infection
A syndrome sometimes associated with HIV infection, diffuse infiltrative lymphocytosis syndrome, presents a clinical picture indistinguishable from Sjögren's syndrome.

FEATURES
- Predominant in young males
- Acute infection: typically fever, sore throat, lymphadenopathy, headache, rash
- Chronic asymptomatic phase: typically lymphadenopathy, weight loss, diarrhea, skin disorders
- Advanced disease: various infections and malignancies
- Diffuse infiltrative lymphocytosis syndrome may cause keratocytosis sicca, and enlargement and infiltration of the salivary glands (CD8+ lymphocytes) with xerostomia

Neurologic conditions
May lead to impaired lacrimal gland or eyelid function.

FEATURES
Xerophthalmia.

Amyloidosis
FEATURES
- Bilateral parotid gland enlargement
- Symmetric polyarthritis
- Peripheral neuropathy
- Carpal tunnel syndrome
- Nephrotic syndrome
- Pulmonary involvement (dyspnea, fatigue)
- Gastrointestinal involvement (diarrhea, macroglossia, malabsorption, hepatomegaly, weight loss)
- Cardiac involvement (congestive heart failure, peripheral edema, hepatomegaly)
- Vascular involvement (easy bleeding, periorbital purpura)

Hypovitaminosis A
FEATURES
- Xerophthalmia
- Xeroderma
- Follicular hyperkeratosis
- Lowered resistance to infection
- Nyctalopia
- Anorexia
- Sterility

SIGNS & SYMPTOMS
Signs
Sjögren's syndrome has a very broad clinical presentation:
- Xerophthalmia and xerostomia: commonest clinical presentations in adults
- Bilateral parotid gland swelling: commonest sign at onset in children

Ocular involvement (keratoconjunctivitis sicca, inflammation of the corneal epithelium associated with dryness):
- Xerophthalmia, with dullness of the corneal light reflex in severe cases
- Redness of the eye
- Conjunctival or pericorneal injection
- Mucinous discharge
- Irregularity of corneal light reflex
- Enlargement of the lacrimal glands (rare)
- Ocular complications include corneal ulceration, vascularization, opacification, and perforation (rare)

Oral involvement:
- Fissures on tongue and lips (cheilosis)
- Absent or cloudy saliva in sublingual vestibule
- Dry, erythematous, 'parchment-like' tongue, and oral mucosa
- Sticky oral mucosa (tongue depressor may adhere to surfaces)
- Atrophy of filiform papillae on lingual dorsum
- Increased dental caries
- Possible candidiasis (may also be present in the vagina)
- Bilateral, parotid gland enlargement (25–66% of primary disease patients; rare in secondary disease), sometimes accompanied by erythema, or superimposed infection

Other exocrine gland involvement (less frequent):
- Decreased mucous secretions in the respiratory tree may lead to dry cough, hoarseness, chronic/recurrent bronchitis, and pneumonitis
- Decreased exocrine secretions in the gastrointestinal (GI) tract may lead to signs of atrophic gastritis, or subclinical pancreatitis (acute or chronic pancreatitis is rare)
- Dry skin (xerosis)
- Extraglandular involvement is found in one-third of patients and is more common with primary disease (it is especially rare in secondary patients with rheumatoid arthritis) – generally mild or subclinical
- Low-grade fever is frequent

Skin involvement (38% of primary disease sufferers):
- Annular lesions – common
- Photosensitivity – common

- Allergic drug eruptions – common
- Vasculitis as nonthrombocytopenic purpura
- Recurrent urticaria
- Maculopapular erythematous lesions
- Skin ulcerations
- Subcutaneous nodules (renal, pulmonary, and GI involvement are also possible)
- Raynaud's phenomenon
- Lymphadenopathy (14–20% of primary disease patients) – pseudolymphoma and non-Hodgkin's lymphoma may also develop

Pulmonary involvement (14–20% of primary disease patients; usually mild):
- Dyspnea
- Lymphocytic alveolitis
- Lymphocytic interstitial pneumonitis and fibrosis
- Chronic obstructive lung disease
- Bronchiolitis obliterans organizing pneumonia
- Pleurisy, serositis – rare
- Pulmonary vasculitis – rare

Renal involvement (9–12% of primary disease sufferers; usually mild) may lead to overt disease:
- Hyposthenuria
- Renal tubular dysfunction with or without tubular acidosis (which may rarely manifest as recurrent renal colic, hypokalemic muscular weakness, osteomalacia rickets, nephrocalcinosis, renal calculi, and compromised renal function)
- Fanconi's syndrome
- Glomerulonephritis (also rare, may be a sign of coexistent systemic lupus erythematosus or cryoglobulinemia)
- Splenomegaly (3–14% of primary disease patients)

Hepatic involvement (5–6% of primary disease sufferers; usually subclinical), liver biopsy may reveal signs of:
- Primary biliary cirrhosis (diagnosis by biopsy)
- Hepatomegaly or hepatitis C infection may also occur

Peripheral neuropathy and mononeuritis multiplex (2–20% of primary disease patients; usually of moderate severity): manifestations include:
- Hearing loss
- Carpal tunnel syndrome
- More rarely, central nervous system disorders occur
- Hashimoto's thyroiditis and other autoimmune endocrinopathies sometimes occur

Laboratory abnormalities:
- Mild, normochromic and normocytic anemia is common
- Elevated erythrocyte sedimentation rate (ESR)
- Polyclonal hypergammaglobulinemia (70–80% of sufferers)
- Autoantibodies against the ribonucleoprotein complexes Ro(SS-A) and La(SS-B) are present in most patients (and positive in about 10–15% of normals)
- Rheumatoid factor positive (50–75% of patients)
- Abnormal renal acidification due to renal involvement (30% of primary disease sufferers)
- Leukopenia (22% of primary disease sufferers)
- In secondary disease, signs of associated disorders will be present

Symptoms

Sjögren's syndrome has a very broad clinical presentation:

- Xerophthalmia and xerostomia are the commonest clinical presentations in adults
- Bilateral parotid gland swelling is the commonest symptom at onset in children

Ocular involvement (keratoconjunctivitis sicca):

- Sensation of dry eye – very common
- Sandy/gritty, itching, or burning sensation (typically worse at the end of the day) – very common
- Redness of the eye
- Blurred vision and ocular fatigue (reading or watching television may be difficult)
- Mucinous discharge, particularly noticeable on awakening
- Photophobia, and/or inability to tolerate smoke or air drafts
- 'Filmy' sensation that interferes with vision

Oral involvement:

- Dry mouth (xerostomia) and lips – very common
- Need to drink frequently
- Difficulty in chewing and swallowing dry food (the so-called 'cracker test')
- Inability to speak continuously
- Sore or burning sensation
- Reddening of tongue and other mucosal surfaces
- Increased dental caries
- Problems in wearing complete dentures
- Changes in taste and smelling
- Bilateral parotid gland enlargement (25–66% of primary disease cases; rare in secondary disease), sometimes accompanied by fever, tenderness, erythema, or superimposed infection
- Symptoms of oral candidiasis (may also be present in the vagina)
- Noncardiac chest pain due to gastroesophageal reflux (perhaps also due to altered esophageal motility)

Other exocrine gland involvement (less frequent):

- Respiratory tract involvement (frequent, but usually mild): dry nose, throat, or trachea (leading to dry cough or hoarseness) – chronic/recurrent bronchitis, or pneumonitis, may also result
- Decreased exocrine secretion in the GI tract may lead to symptoms of atrophic gastritis, or subclinical pancreatitis (acute or chronic pancreatitis is rare)
- Dry skin (xerosis)
- Dyspareunia due to dryness of vaginal mucosa

Extraglandular involvement (30% of patients; generally mild or subclinical) more common in primary disease:

- Fatigue and low-grade fever are frequent
- At least one episode of distal, nonerosive, lupus-like arthropathy (60% of primary disease sufferers) sometimes followed by Jaccoud's arthropathy (polymyositis is rare)

Skin involvement (38% of primary disease sufferers):

- Annular lesions – common
- Photosensitivity – common
- Allergic drug eruptions – common
- Vasculitis as nonthrombocytopenic purpura
- Recurrent urticaria
- Maculopapular erythematous lesions

- Skin ulcerations
- Raynaud's phenomenon (37% of primary disease patients; without telangiectasia or digital ulcerations) usually from very early in the disease
- Lymphadenopathy (14–20% of primary disease patients): pseudolymphoma and nonHodgkin's lymphoma may also develop
- Pulmonary involvement (14–20% of primary disease patients; usually mild): dyspnea, cough, exacerbation of chronic obstructive lung disease, and bronchiolitis obliterans organizing pneumonia (pleurisy, serositis, and pulmonary vasculitis are rare)
- Renal involvement (9–12% of primary disease sufferers; usually mild) may rarely manifest as recurrent renal colic, hypokalemic muscular weakness, osteomalacia rickets, renal calculi, or signs of glomerulonephritis
- Hepatic involvement (5–6% of primary disease sufferers) may rarely manifest as fatigue, anorexia, weight loss, abdominal pain
- Acute abdominal pain may be due to microangiitis involving the small intestine
- Peripheral neuropathy and mononeuritis multiplex (2–20% of primary disease patients; usually of moderate severity): manifestations include hearing loss and carpal tunnel syndrome
- More rarely, central nervous system disorders occur
- Hashimoto's thyroiditis and other autoimmune endocrinopathies sometimes occur
- In secondary disease, symptoms of associated disorders will occur

ASSOCIATED DISORDERS

Secondary Sjögren's syndrome is associated with several autoimmune disorders including the following:

- Rheumatoid arthritis
- Mixed connective disease
- Primary biliary cirrhosis
- Systemic lupus erythematosus
- Scleroderma
- Polymyositis

KEY! DON'T MISS!

- Unilateral salivary gland enlargement, or an especially hard or nodular gland, may be a sign of salivary gland tumor, even if Sjögren's syndrome is diagnosed
- Pseudolymphoma or frank lymphoma should also be suspected in cases of persistent salivary gland enlargement, progressive lymphadenopathy, or lung nodules
- Glomerulonephritis may be a sign of overlapping, systemic lupus erythematosus, or cryoglobulinemia
- In cases of myalgia and fatigue, Hashimoto's thyroiditis should be suspected

CONSIDER CONSULT

- Refer for biopsy of minor salivary gland and serum autoantibody test to confirm diagnosis
- Refer to oncology if nonHodgkin's lymphoma is suspected

INVESTIGATION OF THE PATIENT
Direct questions to patient

Q Do you have any eye problems? Patient may recite characteristic symptoms of keratoconjunctivitis sicca

Q Do your eyes feel sandy or gritty, as if something might be in them?

Q Do you have any problems with your mouth and throat? Are they dry? Would you be able to eat a saltine cracker without it sticking to the inside of your mouth? Patient may recite symptoms of xerostomia and xerotrachea

Q Have you been having dental problems? Increased dental caries is a sign of Sjögren's syndrome that the patient may only think to mention to a dentist

◻ **Have any of your glands swollen recently, especially at the side of your neck?** Glandular swelling is a sign of lymphadenopathy, and recurrent parotid glandular swelling may not be evident at the time of consultation

◻ **Are you taking any medication?** Exclude medications (e.g. antihistaminergic, antidepressive, antipsychotic, and antihypertensive agents) as a cause of symptoms

◻ **Have you had radiation therapy or any other exposure to radiation?** Exclude radiation injury as a cause of symptoms

◻ **Are you suffering from an infection?** Several bacterial and viral infections may cause similar symptoms to Sjögren's syndrome

◻ **What is your age?** Elderly patients may suffer from age-related exocrine gland dysfunction

◻ **Do you spend a long time in front of the computer?** Long periods working in front of a computer, particularly in a place of low humidity, can cause ocular dryness

◻ **Are you feverish or feeling tired?** Fever and fatigue are very common features of Sjögren's syndrome

◻ **Do you ever have problems with your joints?** Episodes of arthropathy are common in the disorder, and carpal tunnel syndrome may also occur

◻ **Do you suffer from dry skin? Do you have any problems with your skin?** Skin features are common in the disorder

◻ **Do you have difficulty breathing? How do your lungs feel?** Mild pulmonary involvement is common

◻ **Have you ever been diagnosed with Raynaud's phenomenon? Are your fingers very sensitive to the cold?** Raynaud's phenomenon often occurs in Sjögren's syndrome

◻ **Do you have any abdominal pain?** Gastrointestinal involvement may occur

◻ **What effect do your symptoms have on your daily life?** Sjögren's syndrome may have a profound impact on the quality of life

Contributory or predisposing factors

◻ **Are there signs or symptoms of associated disorders?** Their presence suggests secondary Sjögren's syndrome

◻ **Is the patient a middle-aged or elderly female?** The syndrome is commonest in this demographic group

Family history

◻ **Have the disease or symptoms been identified in the patient's immediate family?** A heritable predisposition to the disorder has been shown

Examination

▫ **Check for ocular and oral involvement.** Signs consistent with Sjögren's syndrome are usually clear

▫ **Check for glandular swelling.** Parotid glandular swelling is a common sign of the disorder, especially in children, in whom it is the commonest sign at onset. Lymphadenopathy and nonHodgkin's lymphoma may also occur

▫ **Check for signs of other exocrine involvement,** for example, cough, hoarseness, signs of bronchitis, dyspnea

▫ **Check body temperature.** Low-grade fever is common in this disorder

▫ **Examine joints** for sign of joint tenderness or swelling

▫ **Examine skin for dryness and lesions.** Skin involvement is common and obvious

▫ **Is breathing labored?** Mild pulmonary involvement is common

▫ **Are the spleen or liver palpable?** Splenomegaly or hepatomegaly may occur

▫ **Check for blink abnormality.** Blink abnormality may cause dryness of the eye

▫ **Is the patient breathing through the mouth for any reason?** Mouth breathing may cause xerostomia and xerotrachea

Summary of investigative tests

- Schirmer's test. Use to confirm xerophthalmia. Can be performed by primary care physician
- Rose bengal score. More sensitive than the Schirmer's test, performed by an ophthalmologist
- Unstimulated whole saliva collection. Use to confirm xerostomia
- Serum autoantibody assay.
- ANA and Anti-Ro(SSA). Positive in most patients
- Minor salivary gland biopsy (lower lip). The definitive pathologic proof of the diagnosis. The parotid gland itself is rarely biopsied

DIAGNOSTIC DECISION

Differential diagnosis can be difficult because many disorders share signs and symptoms with Sjögren's syndrome. Xerophthalmia and xerostomia alone DO NOT positively diagnose this disorder.

Diagnostic criteria: these are in evolution; at least two sets of criteria exist.

The modified European Community Study Group criteria require either:
- Positive minor salivary gland biopsy or
- Positive serum autoantibody assay for Ro(SS-A) and La(SS-B) autoantibodies for the positive diagnosis of Sjögren's syndrome.

The biopsy must be interpreted by a pathologist experienced in diagnosing Sjögren's syndrome. Biopsies from non-specific sialadenitis patients are sometimes difficult to distinguish from those taken from Sjögren's syndrome patients

Criteria are described in a 1999 paper [1].

CLINICAL PEARLS

- A positive 'cracker test' is very suggestive of this diagnosis. Ask the patient if he or she would be able to chew and swallow a dry cracker
- A foreign-body sensation in the eye often indicates dryness

THE TESTS
Body fluids
SERUM AUTOANTIBODY ASSAY
Description
Blood is taken for assay of autoantibodies directed against Ro(SS-A) and La(SS-B) antigens, as well as antinuclear antibody (ANA).

Advantages/Disadvantages
Advantage: noninvasive test

Disadvantages:
- Poor sensitivity: anti Ro(SS-A) sensitivity 50–80%; anti La(SS-B) sensitivity 30–60%; ANA sensitivity over 50%
- False-positive results may occur, especially with the ANA
- False-positives for anti-Ro(SS-A) may occur with lupus syndromes

Normal
- Absence of specific autoantibodies
- Keep in mind the possibility of a false-negative result

Abnormal
- Presence of specific autoantibodies
- Keep in mind the possibility of a false-positive result

Cause of abnormal result
- Sjögren's syndrome
- Systemic lupus erythematosus

Drugs, disorders and other factors that may alter results
Numerous medications are associated with a positive ANA.

Biopsy
MINOR SALIVARY GLAND BIOPSY
Description
A biopsy is taken of one or more minor salivary glands in the inner lower lip. The parotid gland itself is rarely biopsied.

Advantages/Disadvantages
Disadvantage: must be interpreted by a pathologist familiar with Sjögren's syndrome.

Normal
Score of one or less foci (clusters of at least 50 round cells) per $4mm^2$ tissue.

Abnormal
- Score of more than one focus (at least 50 round cells) per $4mm^2$ tissue
- Keep in mind the possibility of a false-positive result

Cause of abnormal result
- Lymphocytic infiltration of minor salivary glands
- Nonspecific sialadenitis
- Sjögren's syndrome

Drugs, disorders and other factors that may alter results
Diffuse infiltrative lymphocytosis syndrome (DILS), sometimes associated with HIV infection, may cause a false-positive result.

Special tests
SCHIRMER'S TEST
Description
- A strip of Whatman No. 41 filter paper is folded and placed in the lower conjunctival sac
- Length of moistened portion is measured after 5 min

Advantages/Disadvantages
Advantage: easily performed by the primary care physician

Disadvantages:
- Positive result does not positively diagnose Sjögren's syndrome
- Correct performance of this test is actually quite difficult
- Reflex corneal tearing can lead to a false-negative result

Normal
The moistened portion measures at least 15mm.

Abnormal
- The moistened portion measures less than 8mm
- Keep in mind the possibility of a false-positive result

Cause of abnormal result
Xerophthalmia.

Drugs, disorders and other factors that may alter results
Many conditions may cause xerophthalmia. Those that are most likely to be confused with Sjögren's syndrome are the following:
- Chronic conjunctivitis
- Chronic blepharitis
- Fibromyalgia
- Hepatitis C or human T-lymphotropic virus 1 infection
- Diffuse infiltrative lymphocytosis syndrome (sometimes associated with HIV infection)
- Neurologic conditions causing lacrimal gland or eyelid dysfunction
- Hypovitaminosis A

Numerous drugs may cause xerophthalmia. They include the following common classes:
- Antihistaminergic agents
- Antihypertensive agents
- Antidepressant agents
- Antipsychotic agents

ROSE BENGAL SCORE
Description
- Uptake of Rose bengal indicates devitalized corneal epithelium
- Rose Bengal solution (25ml) is placed in the inferior fornix of the eye, and the patient is asked to blink twice
- Number of red spots counted and scored (1+: sparsely scattered; 2+: densely scattered; 3+: confluent) in three areas (lateral conjunctiva, nasal conjunctiva, and cornea)

Advantages/Disadvantages
Advantage: accurate in diagnosing keratoconjunctivitis sicca, the consequence of xerophthalmia

Disadvantages:
- This test should be performed by an ophthalmologist, and generally only by a cornea specialist
- Positive result does not positively diagnose Sjögren's syndrome

Normal
Sum of scores four or less in each eye.

Abnormal
- Sum of scores at least four in at least one eye
- Keep in mind the possibility of a false-positive result

Cause of abnormal result
Keratoconjunctivitis sicca.

Drugs, disorders and other factors that may alter results
Many conditions may cause xerophthalmia. Those that are most likely to be confused with Sjögren's syndrome are the following:
- Chronic conjunctivitis

- Chronic blepharitis
- Fibromyalgia
- Hepatitis C or human T-lymphotropic virus 1 infection
- Diffuse infiltrative lymphocytosis syndrome (sometimes associated with HIV infection)
- Neurologic conditions causing lacrimal gland or eyelid dysfunction
- Hypovitaminosis A

Numerous drugs may cause xerophthalmia. They include the following common classes (usually medicines with anticholinergic properties):
- Antihistaminergic agents
- Antihypertensive agents
- Antidepressant agents
- Antipsychotic agents

UNSTIMULATED WHOLE SALIVA COLLECTION
Description
- Patient is instructed to fast overnight and refrain from brushing teeth, rinsing mouth, or smoking tobacco for at least one hour beforehand
- Saliva is collected in calibrated conical tubes for 15 min

Advantages/Disadvantages
- Advantage: accurate in diagnosing xerostomia

Disadvantages:
- Positive result does not positively diagnose Sjögren's syndrome
- Questionable results when performed infrequently

Normal
At least 1.5ml of saliva.

Abnormal
Less than 1.5ml of saliva.

Cause of abnormal result
Xerostomia.

Drugs, disorders and other factors that may alter results
Many conditions may cause xerostomia. Those that are most likely to be confused with Sjögren's syndrome include the following:
- Diabetes mellitus
- Anxiety
- Fibromyalgia
- Hepatitis C infection
- Diffuse infiltrative lymphocytosis syndrome (associated with HIV infection)

Numerous drugs may cause xerostomia. They include the following common classes:
- Antihistaminergic agents
- Antihypertensive agents
- Antidepressant agents
- Antipsychotic agents

TREATMENT

CONSIDER CONSULT
- Refer to a rheumatologist, and to an ophthalmologist (ocular complaints) or a dentist (frequent caries)
- Suspected or confirmed nonHodgkin's lymphoma in the setting of rapid progression of lymphadenopathy
- Functional deterioration
- Chronic musculoskeletal pain that is poorly responsive to treatment therapy
- Treatment of children
- Pregnancy

IMMEDIATE ACTION
If nonHodgkin's lymphoma is suspected, refer immediately to oncology.

PATIENT AND CAREGIVER ISSUES
Patient or caregiver request
- **Can the condition be cured?** No: the symptoms can only be managed
- **Will non-steroidal anti-inflammatory drugs (NSAIDs) induce side-effects?** Possibly: any side-effects must be reported immediately if they occur
- **Is steroid treatment dangerous?** These are not anabolic steroids, abused by athletes, but they do have side-effects, which must be reported immediately if they occur
- **Is cyclophosphamide treatment dangerous?** It can have serious side-effects, but the patient should be strictly managed to control them as much as possible

Health-seeking behavior
- **How long has the patient waited before consulting a physician?** A long period may have elapsed because of the slow onset of the disorder
- **Has the patient had any complementary therapy?** Some complementary therapies may be effective in managing the symptoms
- **Have you visited any other physicians for this disorder?** The condition may already be diagnosed, previous treatments may affect future choices, and information about compliance may be available

MANAGEMENT ISSUES
Goals
- To reduce symptoms
- To prevent complications
- To monitor and treat systemic involvement
- To refer cases of nonHodgkin's lymphoma if and when it arises
- To treat the associated disorder in cases of secondary Sjögren's syndrome

Management in special circumstances
COEXISTING DISEASE
- Pilocarpine (Salagen) may increase saliva production and reduce symptoms of dry mouth. It should be given with caution to patients with renal calculi, renal impairment, or biliary tract disorders. Dosages should also be reduced for those with hepatic impairment
- Cemiviline (Evoxac) is a new agent which also increases saliva production
- Hydroxychloroquine is often prescribed, as it may have some utility as a 'disease-modifying agent'

SPECIAL PATIENT GROUPS
Children and pregnant women should be referred for treatment.

PATIENT SATISFACTION/LIFESTYLE PRIORITIES

Patients taking hydroxychloroquine need to have a baseline ophthalmologic exam, which must be repeated every 6–12 months.

SUMMARY OF THERAPEUTIC OPTIONS
Choices
Xerophthalmia:
- Lifestyle changes should be instituted immediately
- First choice of treatment is use of eye lubricants, especially those preparations that are free of preservatives (as preservatives may irritate the eye).
- Second line of treatment is oral pilocarpine
- Third line of treatment is punctal occlusion by an ophthalmologist

Xerostomia:
- Lifestyle changes should be instituted immediately
- First line of treatment is frequent use of sialogogues such as sugarless lemon drops to stimulate saliva production
- Second line would be use of oral medications such as pilocarpine or cemivilene
- Dental prophylaxis must also be instituted

Other manifestations:
- Propionic acid gel may be used to treat vaginal dryness
- First choice to treat musculoskeletal symptoms or painful parotid gland swelling are NSAIDs
- Hydroxychloroquine is second choice to treat musculoskeletal symptoms and may be beneficial for some other systemic manifestations
- Systemic corticosteroids and/or cyclophosphamide can be used to treat severe systemic manifestations such as vasculitis, always by or in consultation with a rheumatologist
- Amoxicillin and clavulanic acid may be used when infection is superimposed on swelling of the parotid gland
- All complications should be treated as needed
- In the case of secondary disease, the primary autoimmune disease should be treated

Clinical pearls
- Symptoms of dry eyes should be treated with frequent administration of artificial tears; preparations free of preservatives are often better tolerated
- Two oral preparations are available to treat symptoms of dry mouth: Salagen (pilocarpine) and Evoxac (cemiviline)
- Hydroxychloroquine is sometimes helpful for systemic problems and is associated with very little toxicity

Never
- Never prescribe systemic corticosteroids or cyclophosphamide unless all previous options have been exhausted and a specialist has been consulted
- Never administer corticosteroid eye drops without the supervision of an ophthalmologist

FOLLOW UP
Frequency based on severity of disease, associated conditions, and medicines.

Plan for review
The patient should have regular consultations with an ophthalmologist, a rheumatologist, and a dentist, as well as the primary care physician: to monitor disease progress, the appearance of complications, drug side-effects, and coexisting disease.

Information for patient or caregiver

- Treatment is symptomatic or preventive, and the disorder will never be cured
- The correct use of drugs, preventive dental care, and other lifestyle measures should be communicated
- Deterioration or the appearance of side-effects should be reported immediately

DRUGS AND OTHER THERAPIES: DETAILS
Drugs
PILOCARPINE

To be prescribed if initial nonpharmacologic measures are ineffective, or in the case of moderate disease.

Dose
5mg four times daily.

Efficacy
Improves symptoms of xerophthalmia, xerostomia, and other xeroses.

Risks/Benefits
Benefit: pilocarpine is relatively safe, and its benefits outweigh any risks.

Side-effects and adverse reactions
- Ears, eyes, nose and throat: visual disturbances, stinging, twitching, induced myopia, conjunctival irritation
- Gastrointestinal: nausea, vomiting, diarrhea, salivation
- Central nervous system: headache
- Respiratory: bronchospasm

Interactions (other drugs)
Topical NSAIDs.

Contraindications
- Acute iritis Some secondary forms of glaucoma Uveitis

Evidence
Its efficacy in treating xerophthalmia and xerostomia has been well documented. It is sometimes useful in treating xerophthalmia as well, [2].

Acceptability to patient
- Subjective improvement takes several weeks to occur
- Causes sweating

Follow up plan
Patient should be monitored for signs of improvement and emergence of side-effects.

Patient and caregiver information
- Patient should be warned that subjective improvement may lag behind objective improvement
- Pilocarpine impairs dark adaptation, and therefore caution should be taken if driving at night
- The patient should be made aware of the side-effects and the need to report their occurrence immediately

CORTICOSTEROID EYEDROPS
Used for short-term, pulse treatment of severe ocular symptoms, only under the supervision of an ophthalmologist.

Dose
This should be determined by the ophthalmologist.

Efficacy
Relieves symptoms and reduces objective measures.

Risks/Benefits
Risk: steroid cataract, red eye, and steroid glaucoma may follow prolonged use.

Side-effects and adverse reactions
- Eyes, ears, nose and throat: cataract, glaucoma, blurred vision, thinning of the cornea and sclera
- Skin: delayed healing, acne, striae
- Gastrointestinal: dyspepsia, peptic ulceration, esophagitis, oral candidiasis, nausea, diarrhea
- Cardiovascular system: hypertension, thromboembolism
- Central nervous system: insomnia, euphoria, depression, psychosis
- Endocrine: adrenal suppression, impaired glucose tolerance, growth suppression in children, Cushing's syndrome
- Musculoskeletal: proximal myopathy, osteoporosis

Interactions (other drugs)
- Adrenergic neurone blockers, alpha-blockers, beta-blockers, beta-2 agonists
- Aminoglutethamide Anticonvulsants (carbamazepine, phenytoin, barbiturates)
- Antidiabetics Antidysrhythmics (calcium channel blockers, cardiac glycosides)
- Antifungals (amphotericin, ketoconazole) Antihypertensives (ACE inhibitors, diuretics: loop and thiazide, acetazolamide; angiotensin II receptor antagonists, clonidine, diazoxide, hydralazine, methyldopa, minoxidil) Cyclosporine Erythromycin Methotrexate NSAIDs Nitrates Nitroprusside Oral contraceptives Rifampin Ritonavir Somatropin Vaccines

Contraindications
Systemic infection.

Acceptability to patient
'Steroids' have a negative connotation for some patients.

Follow up plan
Patient will need careful monitoring for cataracts and increased intraocular pressure if treatment is required for more than 2 weeks.

Patient and caregiver information
The patient should be made aware of the side-effects and the need to report their occurrence immediately.

NONSTEROIDAL ANTI-INFLAMMATORY DRUGS
Dose
- Ibuprofen: 400–600mg orally every 6 h
- Indomethacin: 25–50mg orally every 8 h
- Celecoxib: 100–200mg orally twice a day

Efficacy
- These drugs are normally effective in controlling mild-to-moderate pain
- May need to be combined with hydroxychloroquine to control painful parotid gland swelling

Risks/Benefits
Risks:
- All currently available NSAIDs have unwanted effects especially in the elderly
- Substantial individual variation in clinical response to NSAIDs
- Have a range of actions: anti-inflammatory, analgesic, anti-pyretic
- Use caution in renal, cardiac, and hepatic impairment

Side-effects and adverse reactions
- Gastrointestinal: diarrhea, dyspepsia, nausea, vomiting, gastric bleeding and perforation
- Skin: rashes, urticaria, photosensitivity
- Genitourinary: reversible renal insufficiency, renal disease (high doses over long periods)
- Respiratory: worsening of asthma
- Ears, eyes, nose, and throat: tinnitus, decreased hearing
- Central nervous system: headache, dizziness

Interactions (other drugs)
Antihypertensives (ACE inhibitors, adrenergic neurone blockers, alpha-blockers, angiotensin-II receptor antagonists, beta-blockers, clonidine, diazoxide, diuretics, hydralazine, methyldopa, minoxidil, nitroprusside) Antidysrhythmics (calcium channel blockers, cardiac glycosides) Antiplatelet agents (clopidogrel, ticlopidine) Aspirin Baclofen Cyclosporine Corticosteroids Heparins Ketorolac Lithium Methotrexate Moclobemide NSAIDs Nitrates Pentoxifylline (oxpentifylline) Phenindione Phenytoin Quinolones Ritonavir Sulphonylureas Tacrolimus Zidovudine

Contraindications
Pregnancy and breast-feeding Coagulation defects

Acceptability to patient
Some patients may be unable to tolerate these drugs.

Follow up plan
Regular follow up consultations are vital to detect the emergence of any side-effects.

Patient and caregiver information
The patient should be made aware of the side-effects and the need to report their occurrence immediately.

HYDROXYCHLOROQUINE
Used to treat musculoskeletal (if NSAIDs fail) and dermatological symptoms, and other systemic manifestations.

Dose
200–400mg/day.

Efficacy
- May reduce lymphoproliferation, arthropathy, dermatological features, and recurrent swelling of parotid/lymph glands
- Long-term efficacy has not been studied systematically
- Does not improve ocular or oral symptoms

Risks/Benefits
Risks:
- Prescribe with caution – the benefits have not been conclusively demonstrated and the side-effects may be severe

- Very toxic in overdose
- Use caution in children
- Use caution in hepatic and renal disease
- Use caution in G6PD deficiency
- Use caution in alcoholism
- Use caution in patients susceptible to skin reactions
- Use caution in porphyria

Side-effects and adverse reactions
- Ears, eyes, nose, and throat: irreversible retinal damage, visual disturbances, tinnitus, hearing disturbances
- Gastrointestinal: nausea, vomiting, diarrhea, abdominal pain
- Central nervous system: headache, seizures, psychosis
- Hematological: blood cell disorders
- Musculoskeletal: myalgia, arthralgia
- Skin: pigmentation, rashes, eruptions, pruritus

Interactions (other drugs)
- **Antiepileptics** ■ **Cyclosporine** ■ **Digoxin** ■ **Mefloquine** ■ **Praziquantel**

Contraindications
- **Pregnancy and breast-feeding** ■ **Visual changes** ■ **Long-term therapy in children**

Evidence
Benefit has been demonstrated in one trial, [3].

Acceptability to patient
The possible side-effects may reduce compliance.

Follow up plan
Follow closely with regular ophthalmologic examinations to monitor for retinal toxicity.

Patient and caregiver information
The patient should be made aware of the side-effects and the need to report their occurrence immediately.

SYSTEMIC CORTICOSTEROIDS
Used to treat serious systemic complications, severe interstitial pulmonary disease, glomerulonephritis, or vasculitis.

Dose
High doses tapered down to lowest effective dose, e.g. prednisolone 0.5–1.0mg/kg/day.

Efficacy
- Effective in controlling systemic manifestations
- Does not improve lacrimal or salivary gland function

Risks/Benefits
Risks:
- Prescribe only with extreme caution after previous measures have failed – side-effects can be serious
- Slow-acting
- False-negative skin allergy tests. Overwhelming septicemia if patient has an infection.

- Loss of control of blood glucose in those with diabetes
- Use caution in elderly due to risk of diabetes and osteoporosis
- Use caution in patients with psychosis, seizure disorders, or myasthenia gravis
- Use caution in congestive heart failure, hypertension
- Use caution in ulcerative colitis, peptic ulcer, or esophagitis

Side-effects and adverse reactions
- Side-effects are minimized by short duration of therapy
- Gastrointestinal: dyspepsia, peptic ulceration, esophagitis, oral candidiasis, nausea, diarrhea
- Cardiovascular system: hypertension, thromboembolism
- Central nervous system: insomnia, euphoria, depression, psychosis
- Endocrine: adrenal suppression, impaired glucose tolerance, growth suppression in children, Cushing's syndrome
- Musculoskeletal: proximal myopathy, osteoporosis
- Skin: delayed healing, acne, striae
- Eyes, ears, nose and throat: cataract, glaucoma, blurred vision

Interactions (other drugs)
- Adrenergic neurone blockers, alpha-blockers, beta-blockers, beta-2 agonists
- Aminoglutethamide Anticonvulsants (carbamazepine, phenytoin, barbiturates)
- Antidiabetics Antidysrhythmics (calcium channel blockers, cardiac glycosides)
- Antifungals (amphotericin, ketoconazole) Antihypertensives (ACE inhibitors, diuretics: loop and thiazide, acetazolamide; angiotensin II receptor antagonists, clonidine, diazoxide, hydralazine, methyldopa, minoxidil) Cyclosporine Erythromycin Methotrexate
- NSAIDs Nitrates Nitroprusside Oral contraceptives Rifampin Ritonavir
- Somatropin Vaccines

Contraindications
- Systemic infection Avoid live virus vaccines in those receiving immunosuppressive doses

Evidence
Shown to be effective in a controlled clinical trial, [4].

Acceptability to patient
- 'Steroids' have a negative connotation for some patients
- The risk or occurrence of severe side-effects may reduce compliance

Follow up plan
Monitor closely for the emergence of side-effects.

Patient and caregiver information
The patient should be made aware of the side-effects and the need to report their occurrence immediately.

AMOXICILLIN AND CLAVULANIC ACID
- Used when infection is superimposed on parotid gland swelling
- Combine with NSAIDs and local moist heat

Dose
Amoxicillin 500mg and clavulanic acid 125mg orally every 8 h for 7 days.

Efficacy
The combination is effective in treating most commonly occurring infections of the parotid gland.

Risks/Benefits
Risks:
- Use caution if history of hypersensitivity to cephalosporins
- Use caution in renal failure
- Avoid use in mononucleosis

Benefit: the combination is effective in treating many infections, and side-effects are usually mild

Side-effects and adverse reactions
- Gastrointestinal: diarrhea, abdominal pain, psuedomembranous colitis
- Eyes, ears, nose, and throat: black tongue, oral thrush
- Central nervous system: headache, nausea
- Hematologic: bone marrow suppression
- Respiratory: anaphylaxis
- Skin: allergic rashes, erythema multiforme

Interactions (other drugs)
- Atenolol ■ Chloramphenicol ■ Macrolide antibiotics ■ Methotrexate
- Oral contraceptives ■ Tetracyclines

Contraindications
No known contraindications.

Acceptability to patient
Diarrhea may limit tolerability.

Follow up plan
Monitoring is essential, in particular to detect the emergence of hepatic side-effects.

Patient and caregiver information
- The patient should be made aware of the side-effects and the need to report their occurrence immediately
- The full course of treatment must be taken

Surgical therapy
Used only if pharmacologic methods fail.

PUNCTAL OCCLUSION
- A means of preserving what tears the patient produces
- Used only in severe cases of xerophthalmia

Efficacy
May reduce ocular symptoms.

Risks/Benefits
- Risk: the operation has few risks
- Benefit: the success of surgery may be predicted through the prior use of punctal plugs, which are removable

Acceptability to patient
This minor operation should have few acceptability problems.

Follow up plan
Review success of treatment.

Other therapies

EYE LUBRICANTS

- First choice treatment for mild xerophthalmia
- Commercially available eye drops (e.g. 0.5% methylcellulose) may be used as needed (generally every 1–3 h) during the day
- Ointments may provide longer protection at night

Efficacy
Generally effective in providing relief.

Risks/Benefits
- Risk: irritation may occur due to the presence of certain preservatives, which may mimic original symptoms. This can be avoided with preservative-free tears
- Benefit: provides symptomatic relief and prevents corneal ulceration and conjunctivitis

Acceptability to patient
More viscous preparations may blur vision and leave residue on lashes. These are most useful at bedtime.

Follow up plan
Monitor need for pharmacologic treatment.

Patient and caregiver information
- Patient may have to test many preparations to determine the optimum personal choice
- The need to report worsening symptoms should be stressed

PROPIONIC ACID GEL
Used to treat vaginal dryness.

Efficacy
Usually effective.

Risks/Benefits
Risk: there are no risks associated with this treatment.

Acceptability to patient
There are no acceptability problems associated with this treatment.

Follow up plan
Monitor the need for further treatment.

Patient and caregiver information
- Patient may have to test many preparations to determine the optimum personal choice
- The need to report worsening symptoms should be stressed

DENTAL PROPHYLAXIS
- Meticulous oral hygiene and prophylactic measures taken in co-operation with a dentist are essential
- Topical fluoride-containing varnishes are effective

Efficacy
In the general population of patients with Sjögren's syndrome, these measures prevent dental caries.

Risks/Benefits
Risk: there are no known risks associated with these treatments.

Evidence
Fluoride-containing varnishes have been shown to be more effective in preventing dental demineralization than placebo, [5].

Acceptability to patient
Some patients avoid dental consultations.

Follow up plan
Regular consultations with a dentist are essential for prevention of caries.

Patient and caregiver information
Preventive measures are essential to prevent rampant caries in this patient population.

LIFESTYLE
- Stop smoking (associated with increased xerostomia symptoms)
- Avoid dry or windy environments, or those with dust, smoke, or low levels of humidity
- Improve oral hygiene
- Avoid sugar-containing food
- Stop mouth breathing
- Limit drying medications

RISKS/BENEFITS
There are no risks associated with these changes and the benefits may be great.

ACCEPTABILITY TO PATIENT
Cessation of smoking: poor.

FOLLOW UP PLAN
Regular follow up visits may be needed to improve patient motivation.

PATIENT AND CAREGIVER INFORMATION
The importance of these measures should be stressed.

OUTCOMES

PROGNOSIS

- The primary syndrome is benign in most patients, who may have difficulty in determining when the disease began, and not necessarily progressive
- The disease can take 8–10 years to progress from the appearance of nonspecific symptoms to specific, clinical presentation
- Secondary disease in adults may occur late in the course of the primary disease; in children, Sjögren's syndrome may precede the associated disorders by years
- Ophthalmologic and oral manifestations usually remain constant
- Women of childbearing age should be counseled about the increased risk of delivering a child with neonatal systemic lupus erythematosus and congenital complete heart block

Clinical pearls

Primary Sjögren's syndrome should be considered in a patient with a positive ANA and clinical features suggestive of a connective tissue disease but in whom systemic lupus erythematosis cannot be diagnosed.

COMPLICATIONS

- Increased risk (relative risk >40) of lymphoproliferative disorders, including lymphadenopathy, and nonHodgkin's lymphoma (prevalence: 2.5–6%). May occur even after years of apparently benign disease, and is observed mostly in patients with systemic disease with rapidly progressive lymphadenopathy enlargement
- Oral or vaginal candidiasis
- GI complications include atrophic atrophic gastritis, and pancreatitis
- Musculoskeletal complications include lupus-like arthropathy, Raynaud's phenomenon, polymyositis, splenomegaly, primary biliary cirrhosis, hepatomegaly, and hepatitis C infection
- Ocular complications include corneal ulceration, vascularization, opacification, and perforation (rare)
- Pulmonary complications include lymphocytic interstitial pneumonitis and fibrosis, chronic obstructive lung disease, Bronchiolitis obliterans organizing pneumonia – pleurisy, serositis, and pulmonary vasculitis
- Renal complications include renal colic, hypokalemic muscular weakness, osteomalacia rickets, nephrocalcinosis, renal calculi, compromised renal function, Fanconi's syndrome, and glomerulonephritis
- Neurological complications include peripheral neuropathy (hearing loss and carpal tunnel syndrome may occur), mononeuritis multiplex, and central nervous system disorders
- Hashimoto's thyroiditis and other autoimmune endocrinopathies sometimes occur

PREVENTION

The disorder cannot be prevented.

SCREENING
Screening is not appropriate for this disease due to the difficulty of differential diagnosis.

RESOURCES

ASSOCIATIONS

American College of Rheumatology
1800 Century Place
Atlanta, GA 30345
Tel: (404) 633 3777
Fax: (404) 633 1870
www.rheumatology.org

The Arthritis Foundation
1330 West Peachtree Street
Atlanta, GA 30309
Tel: (404) 872 7100
www.arthritis.org
See website for local telephone and fax numbers

Sjogren's Syndrome Foundation
366 North Broadway
Jericho, NY 11753
Tel: (800) 475-6473
Fax: (516) 933-6368

KEY REFERENCES

- Talal N. Sjögren's syndrome and connective tissue diseases associated with other immunological disorders. In: McCarty and Koopman, eds. Arthritis and Allied Conditions, 12th edn. Philadelphia: Lea and Febiger, 1993
- Fox RI. Sjögren's syndrome. In: Textbook of Rheumatology, 5th edn. Philadelphia: WB Saunders, 2001
- Anaya J-M, Talal N. Sjögren's syndrome and connective tissue diseases associated with other immunologic disorders. In: Koopman WJ, ed. Arthritis and Allied Conditions: A Textbook of Rheumatology, 13th ed. Baltimore: Williams & Wilkins; 1997, p1561–80
- Bell M. Sjögren's syndrome: a critical review of clinical management. J Rheumatol 1999;26:2051–61
- Table of Vitamins. In: Dorland's Illustrated Medical Dictionary. 28th edn. Philadelpia: WB Saunders: 1994, p1834
- El-Mallakh RS. Anxiety (generalized anxiety disorder). In: Ferri FF, editor. Ferri's Clinical Advisor. Instant Diagnosis and Treatment. St Louis, Mosby, 2000, p51
- Ferri FF. Sjögren's syndrome. In: Ferri FF, editor. Ferri's Clinical Advisor. Instant Diagnosis and Treatment. St Louis, Mosby, 2000, p538
- Fox RI, Saito I. Criteria for diagnosis of Sjögren's syndrome. Rheum Dis Clin North Am 1984;20:391–407
- Fox RI. Treatment of primary Sjögren's syndrome with hydroxychloroquine. Am J Med 1988;85:62–7
- Fox RI. Antimalarial Drugs. In: Koopman WJ, editor. Arthritis and Allied Conditions: A Textbook of Rheumatology, 13th edn. Baltimore: Williams & Wilkins; 1997, p671–8
- Fox RI. Current issues in the diagnosis and treatment of Sjögren's syndrome. Curr Opin Rheumatol 1999;11:364–71
- Fox RI, Stern M, Michelson P. Update in Sjögren's syndrome. Curr Opin Rheumatol 2000;12:391–8
- Hochberg MC. Sjögren's Syndrome. In: Goldman L, Bennett JC, editors. Cecil Textbook of Medicine, 21st edn. Philadelphia: WB Saunders; 2000
- Koby M. Conjunctivitis. In: Ferri FF, editor. Ferri's Clinical Advisor. Instant Diagnosis and Treatment. St Louis, Mosby, 2000, p153
- Masci JR. Human immunodeficiency virus. In: Ferri FF, editor. Ferri's Clinical Advisor. Instant Diagnosis and Treatment. St Louis, Mosby, 2000, p287
- Mercier LR. Fibromyalgia. In: Ferri FF, editor. Ferri's Clinical Advisor. Instant Diagnosis and Treatment. St Louis, Mosby, 2000, p225
- Moutsopoulos HM. Sjögren's syndrome. In: Fauci AS, Braunwald E, Isselbacher KJ, Wilson JD, Martin JB, Kaspar DL, et al, editors. Harrison's Principles of Internal Medicine, 14th edn. International Edition. New York: McGraw-Hill; 1998, p1901–4
- Antibacterials. In: Parfitt K, ed. Martindale: The Complete Drug Reference, 32nd edn. London: The Pharmaceutical Press; 1999, p112–270

▦ Antimalarials. In: Parfitt K, ed. Martindale: The Complete Drug Reference, 32nd edn. London: The Pharmaceutical Press; 1999, p422–42

▦ Antineoplastics and immunosuppressants. In: Parfitt K, editor. Martindale: The Complete Drug Reference, 32nd edn. London: The Pharmaceutical Press; 1999, p470–572

▦ Corticosteroids. In: Parfitt K, ed. Martindale: The Complete Drug Reference, 32nd edn. London: The Pharmaceutical Press; 1999, p1010–51

▦ Parasympathomimetics. In: Parfitt K, ed. Martindale: The Complete Drug Reference, 32nd edn. London: The Pharmaceutical Press; 1999, p1386–1400

▦ Stabilising and suspending agents. In: Parfitt K, ed. Martindale: The Complete Drug Reference, 32nd edn. London: The Pharmaceutical Press; 1999, p1470–5

▦ Pedersen A. LongoVital in the treatment of Sjögren's syndrome. Clin Exp Rheumatol 1999;17:533–8

▦ Vitali C. The European Community Study Group on diagnostic criteria for Sjögren's syndrome. Sensitivity and specificity of tests for ocular and oral involvement in Sjögren's syndrome. Ann Rheum Dis 1994;563:637–47

▦ Vivino FB. Pilocarpine tablets for the treatment of dry mouth and dry eye symptoms in patients with Sjögren syndrome: a randomized, placebo-controlled, fixed-dose, multicenter trial. P92–01 Study Group. Arch Intern Med 1999;159:174–81

▦ Wutz BJ. Acromegaly. In: Ferri FF, ed. Ferri's Clinical Advisor. Instant Diagnosis and Treatment. St Louis, Mosby, 2000, p18

▦ Wutz BJ. Hyperlipoproteinemia, primary. In: Ferri FF, ed. Ferri's Clinical Advisor. Instant Diagnosis and Treatment. St Louis, Mosby, 2000, p297

▦ Zaura-Arite E. Effects of fluoride- and chlorhexidine-containing varnishes on plaque composition and on demineralization of dentinal grooves in situ. Eur J Oral Sci 2000;108:154–61

Evidence references and guidelines

1 Fox RI. Current issues in the diagnosis and treatment of Sjögren's syndrome. Curr Opin Rheumatol 1999;11:364–7

2 Vivino FB. Pilocarpine tablets for the treatment of dry mouth and dry eye symptoms in patients with Sjögren syndrome: a randomized, placebo-controlled, fixed-dose, multicenter trial. P92–01 Study Group. Arch Intern Med 1999;159:174–81

3 Fox RI. Treatment of primary Sjögren's syndrome with hydroxychloroquine. Am J Med 1988;85:62–7

4 Fox RI, Datiles M, et al. Prednisone and piroxicam for the treatment of primary Sjögren's syndrome. Clin Exp Rheumatol 1993;11:149–56

5 Zaura-Arite E. Effects of fluoride- and chlorhexidine-containing varnishes on plaque composition and on demineralization of dentinal grooves in situ. Eur J Oral Sci 2000;108:154–61

FAQS
Question 1
If a patient has dry eyes and mouth and positive serologies, can I diagnose Sjögren's syndrome?

ANSWER 1
Symptoms of dry eyes and dry mouth are present in most patients with Sjögren's syndrome, but are not sufficient to make the diagnosis.

Question 2
Aside from symptomatic treatment of dry eyes and dry mouth, is any other systemic treatment appropriate for Sjögren's syndrome?

ANSWER 2
Hydroxychloroquine is often prescribed, and may be of benefit for a number of systemic manifestations.

Question 3
When should corticosteroids or cyclophosphamide be used in Sjögren's syndrome?

ANSWER 3
These agents are appropriate only for severe manifestations such as vasculitis, and should be prescribed only by a rheumatologist.

Question 4

When should I suspect underlying lymphoma in a patient with Sjögren's syndrome?

ANSWER 4

The development of lymphoma is suggested by sudden change in peripheral lymphadenopathy, or reduction in immunoglobulin levels or the titer of rheumatoid factor.

CONTRIBUTORS

Russell C Jones, MD, MPH
Richard Brasington Jr, MD, FACP
Brigid Freyne, MD

SYSTEMIC LUPUS ERYTHEMATOSUS

SUMMARY INFORMATION

DESCRIPTION

- Systemic lupus erythematosus (SLE) is a chronic multisystemic disease of autoimmune origin
- Characteristically affects skin and joints, although any system can be involved
- Commonly affects women aged 20–45 years but may affect all age groups and males too
- The American College of Rheumatology (formerly the American Rheumatism Association) criteria for diagnosis of SLE must include four or more of the following: malar rash, discoid rash, photosensitivity, oral ulcers, arthritis, serositis, renal disorder, neurologic disorder, hematologic disorder, immunologic disorder, antinuclear antibody (ANA)

URGENT ACTION

Urgent referral is mandatory if there is impaired function of the cardiac, respiratory, renal, or neurologic systems, or if there is life-threatening infection.

KEY! DON'T MISS!

- Coexisting infection must not be missed
- Renal involvement must always be screened for
- Patients with SLE are likely to suffer from premature atherosclerosis, so primary care physicians should actively control blood pressure, hyperlipidemia, insulin resistance, and other modifiable risk factors for atherosclerosis
- Premenopausal women with SLE may have myocardial infarctions

BACKGROUND

ICD9 CODE
710.0 Systemic lupus erythematosus.

SYNONYMS
- SLE
- Lupus

CARDINAL FEATURES
Cardinal features are difficult to define, as patterns of presentation are individual to the patient. SLE is a disease that is characterized by flare-ups and remissions, and virtually any body system can be involved.

There is a wide variation in severity of the disease.

Cardinal features are best summed up from the American College of Rheumatology 1982 disease criteria. At least four of the first 11 below must be present. These were not designed to be used as diagnostic criteria but are useful for comparing homogeneous populations:
- Malar rash: fixed erythema, flat or raised, over the malar eminences, tending to spare the nasolabial folds
- Discoid rash: erythematous, raised patches with adherent keratotic scaling and follicular plugging; atrophic scarring may occur in older lesions
- Photosensitivity: skin rash as a result of unusual reaction to sunlight, by patient history or physician observation
- Oral ulcers: oral or nasopharyngeal ulceration, usually painless, observed by physician
- Arthritis: nonerosive arthritis involving two or more peripheral joints, characterized by tenderness, swelling, or effusion
- Serositis: (a) pleuritis – convincing history of pleuritic pain or rubbing heard by a physician or evidence of pleural effusion; or (b) pericarditis – documented by electrocardiogram or rub or evidence of pericardial effusion
- Renal disorders: (a) persistent proteinuria greater than 0.5g/day or greater than 3+ (dipstick) if quantitation not performed; or (b) cellular casts – may be red cell, hemoglobin, granular, tubular, or mixed
- Neurologic disorder: (a) seizures in the absence of offending drugs or known metabolic derangements, e.g. uremia, ketoacidosis, or electrolyte imbalance; or (b) psychosis in the absence of offending drugs or known metabolic derangements, e.g. uremia, ketoacidosis, or electrolyte imbalance
- Hematologic disorder: (a) hemolytic anemia with reticulocytosis; or (b) leukopenia $<4000/mm^3$ total on two or more occasions; or (c) lymphopenia $<1500/mm^3$ on two or more occasions; or (d) thrombocytopenia $<100,000/mm^3$ in the absence of offending drugs
- Immunologic disorder: (a) positive LE cell preparation; or (b) anti-DNA: antibody to native DNA in abnormal titer; or (c) anti-Sm: presence of antibody to Sm nuclear antigen; or (d) false-positive serologic test for syphilis known to be positive for at least 6 months and confirmed by *Treponema pallidum* immobilization or fluorescent treponemal antibody absorption test
- Antinuclear antibody (ANA): an abnormal titer of ANA by immunofluorescence or an equivalent assay at any point in time and in the absence of drugs known to be associated with 'drug-induced lupus' syndrome. Presence of positive ANA is a cardinal feature but is not specific for SLE

In addition:
- Constitutional symptoms: fatigue, fever, malaise, weight loss
- Other skin rashes: including calcified nodules, vasculitis, leg ulceration, and ulcers in the hair with or without alopecia

- Sicca syndrome: dry eyes/mouth and Raynaud's phenomenon are common
- Cardiac involvement: pericardial rub in pericarditis and heart murmurs if there is endocarditis or valvular thickening/dysfunction
- Hypertension: systemic and pulmonary
- Other features: including lymphadenopathy, splenomegaly, venous and arterial thrombosis

CAUSES
Common causes
The cause is unknown. Research involves:

- The role of viruses
- Hormonal factors (the female predominance and peak incidence in women of childbearing age is circumstantial evidence for hormonal factors in the pathogenesis of SLE)
- Genetic abnormalities (they may create a tendency for autoimmune responses which are then triggered by additional factors, such as viruses or sunlight)
- Environmental (virus, sunlight)
- Immune complex formation – many of the clinical manifestations are due to the effects of circulating immune complexes on various tissues or to the direct effects of antibodies to cell surface components

Serious causes
SLE may be potentially life-threatening. Death most frequently occurs from nephritis or infection.

Contributory or predisposing factors
Research suggests that many factors contribute to the immune dysfunction shown in lupus. These factors include:

- Genetic factors: evidence for genetic predisposition is shown by a concordance rate in monozygotic twins of around 30–50%
- Hormonal factors: evidence for hormonal influence can be adduced from the recognized fluctuations with flare-ups in the postovulatory phase of the menstrual cycle. Pregnancy often exacerbates the disease (especially in those with nephritis or hypertension)
- Environmental factors (e.g. ultraviolet light and sunlight): evidence for photosensitivity comes from the fact that sunlight precipitates SLE, particularly skin disease
- Infectious agents are thought to possibly induce autoimmune responses by molecular mimicry
- Drug-induced lupus syndrome: a syndrome with an SLE-like picture may be produced by several drugs, including procainamide, hydralazine, isoniazid, chlorpromazine, and methyldopa. Most patients improve on withdrawal of the offending drug

EPIDEMIOLOGY
Incidence and prevalence
The incidence and prevalence of SLE varies across the world by race and ethnicity as well as geography.

INCIDENCE
- Varies from 0.018 to 0.076/1000 per year in the US
- In northern Europe it has been reported to be 0.04/1000

PREVALENCE
- Worldwide ranges from 0.029 to 4/1000
- Variable reporting results in a range from 0.146 to 0.508 cases per 1000, with an average of 0.2/1000 in the US

Demographics

AGE
- Childbearing years (20–45) see the highest frequency (80% of cases)
- Can occur in all age groups, although uncommon before 8 years of age
- Under age 15, the reported incidence is 0.005/1000 in the US

GENDER
Reported female to male ratios vary from 3:1 to 9:1 in adults, and are as low as 2:1 in prepubertal children.

RACE
- More common in African-Americans than Caucasians: US prevalence rates of up to 2.5/1000 have been measured in Native Americans, Hispanics, Asians, and African-American patients
- Certain communities have a higher prevalence rate - the Western Cape of South Africa has a high rate amongst those of mixed ancestry, but it is rare amongst the rural African population of South Africa

GENETICS
- No proven genetic transmission: genetic makeup may predispose to SLE
- Definite family relationships have been noted and some genetic profiles described

GEOGRAPHY
More common in countries where there is an indigenous African population.

SOCIOECONOMIC STATUS
None identified.

DIAGNOSIS

DIFFERENTIAL DIAGNOSIS
The differential is massive, and will depend upon which system(s) is (are) involved at presentation. It is important to distinguish SLE from other multisystemic conditions, particularly rheumatoid arthritis and fibromyalgia. These are the only differentials cited in detail here.

- Arthralgia/arthropathy: rheumatoid arthritis, mixed connective tissue disorder, psychogenic rheumatism, other arthropathies
- Fever and malaise: fever of unknown origin, endocarditis, malignancy, chronic fatigue syndrome, subacute bacterial infections, viral infections, poisoning
- Chest symptoms: myocardial infarction, pulmonary embolism, adult respiratory distress syndrome (ARDS), chest infections including tuberculosis
- Neurologic: stroke (either hemorrhagic or ischemic), epilepsy, and other neurologic complaints
- Skin lesions: scleroderma, discoid lupus (can occur in absence of systemic disease)
- Renal symptoms: glomerulonephritis and other renal conditions
- Abdominal pain: lymphoproliferative disorder, abdominal blunt trauma, constipation
- Hematologic: hemolytic anemia, immune or thrombotic thrombocytopenia, lymphoma
- Vasculitis: other vasculitides

These lists are not exhaustive.

Rheumatoid arthitis
Rheumatoid arthritis is a chronic multisystem inflammatory disease of unknown etiology.

FEATURES
- Characteristic features are persistent inflammatory synovitis, usually involving peripheral joints in a symmetrical distribution
- Early in the disease, painful joint effusions restricting movement are common, as is prolonged morning stiffness. In late disease, characteristic deformities can occur (subluxation, dislocation, joint contractures)
- Systemic involvement may be marked, with fevers, anorexia, splenomegaly, pericarditis, vasculitis, and uveitis
- A raised rheumatoid factor occurs in 80% of cases after 2 years, (can be only 50% at onset), often with raised erythrocyte sedimentation rate (ESR) and C-reactive protein (CRP) level
- Radiographs usually reveal soft-tissue swelling and osteopenia in early disease, while they later show joint-space narrowing, erosion, and deformity as the articular surface is destroyed

Fibromyalgia
Fibromyalgia is a poorly defined pain disorder of unknown etiology.

FEATURES
- Characteristic tender points
- Referred pain, arthralgias, and myalgias
- Associated sleep disturbance (nonrestorative sleep) which can be seen on sleep study testing
- Mainly found in women aged 30–50 years (9:1 female:male ratio)
- Symptoms come and go for years
- Not life-threatening and no associated organ damage

SIGNS & SYMPTOMS
Signs
- Fever: low-grade fever (active disease) or high fever (possible infection). Constitutional symptoms occur in 70–85% of patients

- Skin rashes (55–90% of patients): malar rash – fixed erythema sparing the nasolabial fold; 'butterfly rash' – characterized by erythema, edema, and photosensitivity; tends to exacerbate with flares; discoid rash – erythematous patches with keratotic scaling. In subacute cutaneous lupus erythematosus: erythematous papules or plaques with slight scaling that may mimic psoriasis; plaques may merge to form polycyclic or annular lesions; associated with antibody to Ro(SS-A)
- Mucocutaneous ulcers (20–50% of patients): in nose and mouth
- Joints (60–90% of patients): the polyarthritis is usually mild, symmetrical, nonerosive, and nondeforming. Tenderness, edema, and effusions occur. Often there is swelling over the proximal phalanges. Tendinitis and myositis can occur. Joint deformity is uncommon: when present in hands, ulnar deviation is the typical deformity
- Cardiac: hypertension (including pulmonary), murmurs (systolic reported in 70% cases), rubs, pericardial effusion (20–30% of patients), cardiac failure (myocarditis or infarction)
- Vasculitic (10–35% of patients): vasculitis with digital infarcts and splinter hemorrhages
- Raynaud's phenomenon (20–60% of patients): may be complicated by digital ulcers
- Pulmonary: pleural rub and chest signs secondary to pleuritis (20–45% of patients), infiltrates, or hemorrhage
- Abdominal (20–50% of patients): tenderness, enlarged liver and spleen
- Lymphadenopathy (25–60% of patients)
- Central nervous system (25–50% of patients): sensory or sensorimotor neuropathies may occur. Signs of a stroke may be apparent. Mood disorders, psychosis, and seizures can occur. Many less common neurologic signs can also be present

Symptoms
- Fever: low-grade fever (active disease) or high fever (possible infection)
- Malaise and chronic fatigue
- Skin rashes: malar rash – fixed erythema sparing the nasolabial fold; discoid rash – erythematous patches with keratotic scaling
- Scalp lesions and alopecia
- Photosensitivity to sunlight and ultraviolet light
- Mucocutaneous: ulcers in nose and mouth
- Pain and swelling of the joints: the polyarthritis is usually symmetrical, nonerosive, and nondeforming. Tenderness, edema, and effusions occur. Often there is swelling over the proximal phalanges
- Arthralgia: pain may be severe in the joints with nothing to find clinically other than tenderness. Morning stiffness is common
- Chest complaints: hemoptysis, dyspnea, orthopnea, chest pain
- Vasculitic rashes and splinters in the nail: vasculitis with digital infarcts and splinter hemorrhages
- Peripheral extremity changes induced by cold: Raynaud's phenomenon may be complicated by digital ulcers
- Abdominal pain and tenderness: enlarged liver and spleen. Constipation (may be drug induced). Chronic abdominal pain may be due to recurrent vascular insults, peritoneal serositis, and/or chronic pancreatitis
- Sensory or sensorimotor neuropathies: symptoms of a stroke may be apparent. Spinal cord disease may mimic multiple sclerosis
- Cerebral symptoms: mood disturbance, cognitive dysfunction, agoraphobia, headache (occasionally migrainous), fits, movement disorders (St Vitus' dance), memory loss, and many others
- Dry eyes and mouth
- Symptoms of thrombosis: more common in patients with SLE (lupus anticoagulant)

There may be other symptoms depending on which organ the autoantibodies are attacking. Symptoms of infection may also be present. Patients with SLE are likely to suffer from premature atherosclerosis and are more susceptible to osteonecrosis and to infection, as are those treated with steroids.

ASSOCIATED DISORDERS

- Raynaud's phenomenon
- Sicca syndrome

KEY! DON'T MISS!

- Coexisting infection must not be missed
- Renal involvement must always be screened for
- Patients with SLE are likely to suffer from premature atherosclerosis, so primary care physicians should actively control blood pressure, hyperlipidemia, insulin resistance, and other modifiable risk factors for atherosclerosis
- Premenopausal women with SLE may have myocardial infarctions

CONSIDER CONSULT

Confirmation of the diagnosis by a rheumatologist is advisable.

INVESTIGATION OF THE PATIENT
Direct questions to patient

Specific questioning:

- Q Do you suffer with fevers or fatigue? How much does this interfere with your daily life? Fatigue is the most common and debilitating symptom
- Q Do you suffer with joint pains? How long do these generally last? What is their severity/associated handicap? Arthralgia is one of the commonest initial complaints (53%). Between 53 and 95% of SLE sufferers have arthralgia. SLE is a fluctuating disease
- Q Do you suffer with rashes? Are they ever related to sunshine or ultraviolet (UV) light? Where do they occur? Skin rashes occur in up to 90% of patients. A detailed description and occasionally photos shown by the patient will help to identify the rash. The typical rash is the 'butterfly rash'
- Q Do you suffer with ulcers? Inquire specifically about oral ulcers
- Q Have you had any hair loss? A significant amount of hair on the pillow after sleeping is a useful benchmark
- Q Do you have any mood disturbance or seizures? There is a broad spectrum of neurologic and psychiatric complaints that can occur in SLE
- Q What medication are you taking? Certain drugs cause SLE-like syndromes and fixed drug reactions that can look like lupus rashes
- Q Does anyone in the family suffer with a rheumatologic complaint or other illness? Inquire specifically about lupus, rheumatoid arthritis, and thyroid conditions
- Q For women: have you had any miscarriages? Women with SLE tend to have an increased rate of miscarriage
- Q Do your fingers and toes suffer in the cold, and in what way? Be sure to ask specifically about Raynaud's phenomenon

Systems enquiry:
As SLE can affect any body system, it is worth running through the systems with the standard medical history questions to pick up any specific problems. In particular, be alert for cardiac, respiratory, and renal involvement.

Contributory or predisposing factors

Q **Is there a family history of SLE?** There is a genetic predisposition to SLE, shown by a concordance rate in monozygotic twins of around 30–50%

Q **Have there been any associated hormonal changes, in particular pregnancy?** It is recognized that fluctuations with flare-ups correlate with the postovulatory phase of the menstrual cycle in some patients. Pregnancy often exacerbates the disease, especially in those with nephritis or hypertension

Q **Does sunlight act as a trigger?** Sunlight particularly precipitates skin disease

Q **Does stress exacerbate the condition?** Stress is not the cause; however, both stress and fatigue are known to precipitate flare-ups

Q **Are any drugs being taken?** A syndrome of an SLE-like picture may be produced by several drugs (drug-induced lupus)

Family history

Q **Does any one in the family suffer with a rheumatologic complaint or other illness?** Inquire specifically about lupus, rheumatoid arthritis, and thyroid conditions. There is a concordance rate in monozygotic twins of around 30–50%.

Examination

General examination:

Q **Does the patient look generally well?** Look for signs of anemia or lymphadenopathy

Q **Is the patient febrile?** If the temperature is greater than 102°F (39°C), a source of infection should be sought

Q **Are there any splinter hemorrhages or vasculitic lesions?** There may also be signs of Raynaud's phenomenon

Q **Are there any rashes present?** Malar rash or discoid

Q **Are there any mucocutaneous ulcers?** These are a common occurrence in SLE

Q **Is there a cushingoid appearance?** This results from long-term corticosteroid use

A detailed survey of the musculoskeletal system is often necessary:

Q **Are there any joint or muscle abnormalities?** Swelling, tenderness, and edema may be present. Patients already treated may be on steroids with resultant muscular weakness and/or osteonecrosis. Myositis can occur in SLE and it may not just be due to corticosteroid treatment

Screen all systems for abnormalities:

Q **Is the cardiac function normal?** Listen for murmurs and rubs as well as checking for hypertension

Q **Is the respiratory function normal?** Listen for chest abnormalities

Q **Is the abdominal system normal?** Look for organomegaly

Q **Is the renal system normal?** Check for edema, proteinuria, and hypertension

Q **Is there any abnormality in the neurologic system?** Look for signs of neuropathy or stroke

Summary of investigative tests

Although the diagnosis may be made on grounds of history and examination, laboratory tests are essential for confirmation. They may also be useful in evaluating a flare-up:

▪ Complete blood count: leukopenia is a good index of disease activity; also lymphopenia, anemia of chronic disease, evidence of hemolytic disease. Thrombocytopenia occurs in 30–50% of cases and may be severe (as a result of antiplatelet autoantibodies, antiphospholipid antibodies, or marrow suppression due to drugs or disease)

▪ Acute phase reactants – ESR and CRP: may be elevated in disease activity. The ESR is usually elevated in active disease or inflammation and infection

▪ Complete chemistry panel: to evaluate electrolytes, liver, and kidney function

- Autoantibody screen: presence of antinuclear antibody (ANA) is the cardinal feature. Although ANA-negative SLE can rarely occur, a negative ANA will call the diagnosis into question. Measurement of ANA subtypes may also be performed
- Antibodies to double-stranded DNA (dsDNA): antibody to dsDNA is more specific for lupus and often correlates with disease activity and nephritis
- Extractable nuclear antibodies: anti-Ro(SS-A) associated with Sjögren's syndrome, subacute cutaneous lupus erythematosus, and increased photosensitivity in SLE; anti-La(SS-B) associated with Sjögren's syndrome; anti-Sm (highly specific but not sensitive – seen in 30%)
- Antihistone antibodies: if drug-induced lupus is suspected
- Measurement of other autoantibodies should be guided by clinical manifestations such as petechiae, anemia, cerebritis, thyroid abnormalities, and coagulopathy. Antiphospholipid antibody (anticardiolipin antibody and lupus anticoagulant) is present in 30% of SLE patients and is associated with recurrent thromboembolism and miscarriage
- In SLE patients, rheumatoid factor is positive in 40% of cases
- A complement screen should also be performed (C3, C4). C3 and C4 decrease in disease activity, with which they often correlate better than the ESR and CRP. Serum immunoglobulins may also be measured
- Urinalysis: pyuria, hematuria, proteinuria, granular casts occur with the onset of renal involvement
- Partial thromboplastin time: may be elevated (lupus anticoagulant or antiphospholipid antibody)
- Appropriate radiographs: for joint involvement
- Electrocardiogram: for cardiac involvement, if appropriate
- Chest X-ray: for pulmonary symptoms
- Additional tests: for specific symptoms, e.g. neuropathic changes can be investigated with an electromyogram with nerve conduction velocities

Further studies may be indicated, including echocardiogram or renal biopsy, if appropriate.

DIAGNOSTIC DECISION

- Diagnosis is based on clinical findings aided by results of laboratory tests
- The typical course of the disease shows exacerbations and remissions
- The mean length of time between onset of symptoms and diagnosis is 5 years

Diagnosis is made when four or more of the following criteria are present. Note, however, that this list was not designed as diagnostic criteria, but it is useful in comparing homogeneous patient groups:

- Malar rash
- Discoid rash
- Photosensitivity
- Oral ulcers
- Arthritis
- Serositis
- Renal disorders
- Neurologic disorder
- Hematologic disorder
- Immunologic disorder
- Antinuclear antibody

CLINICAL PEARLS

- Drug-induced lupus typically spares the kidneys
- Antihistone antibodies are found in both SLE and drug-induced lupus. The lack of antihistone antibodies virtually excludes the possibility of drug-induced lupus

THE TESTS
Body fluids
AUTOANTIBODY TESTS

Description
Venous blood sample. A number of specialized tests (including DNA binding/fluorescence) are performed to establish whether the antibody is present.

Advantages/Disadvantages
Advantages:
- Blood test relatively easy to perform
- Quick
- Acceptable to most patients

Disadvantages:
- May be false-positives
- Each antibody is not disease-specific

Normal
The normal range for ANA titer varies between laboratories, but it is usually less than 1:40 or 1:80. Note that 5% of normal people may have a titer between 1:160 and 1:320.

Abnormal
ANA — a titer of greater than 1:40 or 1:80 (note: 5% of normal people may have a positive ANA).

Cause of abnormal result
Abnormal results for ANA occur in:
- SLE
- Chronic active hepatitis
- Rheumatoid arthritis
- Scleroderma
- Mixed connective tissue disease
- Necrotizing vasculitis
- Sjögren's syndrome
- Tuberculosis
- Pulmonary interstitial fibrosis

Abnormal results for antihistone occur in:
- SLE
- Drug-induced SLE (95%)
- Rheumatoid arthritis

Abnormal results for dsDNA occur in:
- SLE
- Rarely seen in other diseases

Abnormal results for other antibodies also occur in other diseases. Consultation with a rheumatologist may be required for interpretation.

Drugs, disorders and other factors that may alter results
Factors that can give a positive titer of ANA:
- Drugs: (phenytoin, ethosuximide, primidone, methyldopa, hydralazine, carbamazepine, penicillin, procainamide, chlorpromazine, griseofulvin, thiazides)
- Age over 60

TREATMENT

CONSIDER CONSULT

- Treatment for SLE should be carried out in conjunction with a specialist when feasible, and depending on the involvement of specific organs, the patient may need co-management with other specialists, particularly a nephrologist
- In women of childbearing years, especially those considering a pregnancy, specialist obstetric consultation is advisable

IMMEDIATE ACTION

Cardiac, pulmonary, hematologic, and neurologic symptoms may be life- and/or organ-threatening. They should therefore be evaluated urgently by specialists as appropriate.

PATIENT AND CAREGIVER ISSUES
Forensic and legal issues

SLE presenting with psychiatric manifestations may require emergency management following the appropriate guidelines.

Impact on career, dependants, family, friends

- As with any chronic disease, the impact of SLE on the patient's family is likely to be considerable. The unpredictable nature of the disease contributes to this
- Avoidance of sunshine can strain family relationships, e.g. on holiday
- Psychiatric manifestations can have marked effects on the family
- Dialysis (renal involvement) may be difficult for the family to accommodate to
- Conception and miscarriage issues may strain relationships
- Unpredictable levels of fatigue can be frustrating and poorly understood
- Patients with SLE should avoid smoking, which can worsen the consequences of vasculopathy (such as that seen in Raynaud's phenomenon) and atherosclerosis

Patient or caregiver request

Is it safe to be on steroids for SLE? Many patients will be aware of the steroid debate and the myriad side-effects of long-term use, but in many situations corticosteroids are life-saving. They may also significantly improve the quality of life for SLE patients. The patient and clinician will need to weigh the risks and benefits in each case, and possibly in each flare-up. Long-term use of higher-dose corticosteroids should be avoided, if possible, by controlling disease activity with steroid-sparing immunosuppressive medications.

Health-seeking behavior

Many patients seek alternative therapies as an adjunct to conventional therapy. In general, none is of proven benefit.

MANAGEMENT ISSUES
Goals

- To control the disease process (keeping disease flare-ups to a minimum)
- To limit complications
- To encourage the patient to manage his or her disease and live as full a life as possible (this includes recognizing a flare-up and presenting immediately so that it can be quickly damped down, and maintaining joints in maximal condition)

Management in special circumstances

- Pregnancy may enhance the risk of flare-ups in SLE, especially if disease activity is not quiescent before conception

- Osteoporosis is a major problem for SLE patients. Adequate intake of calcium and vitamin D is essential, and patients on long-term corticosteroid therapy should be given preventive therapy (mainly bisphosphonates in preventive doses)

COEXISTING DISEASE
- Any coexisting disease or organ impairment may adversely affect the condition of the lupus patient
- Infections pose a highly significant risk, as lupus patients are immunocompromised, both by the disease and by some of the drugs used to treat it

COEXISTING MEDICATION
- A number of drugs have a negative impact on renal function and will complicate the care of SLE patients with renal involvement
- It may be difficult to distinguish between drug-induced renal impairment and SLE-related disease

SPECIAL PATIENT GROUPS
Pregnancy:
- The frequency of flare-ups in pregnant SLE patients is slightly higher than in nonpregnant patients. These flare-ups occur in the second and third trimester and, most commonly, shortly after the delivery. Most flare-ups are mild, involving joint and skin symptoms, but 10–20% have severe flare-ups with major organ involvement
- In those with pre-existing stable lupus nephritis, pregnancy does not adversely affect renal function in the long term
- Flare-ups may be difficult to diagnose in pregnancy because many symptoms (such as hair loss, edema, facial erythema, fatigue, anemia, raised ESR, and musculoskeletal pain) are common to both

Management of lupus in pregnancy:
- Involves shared care between the obstetrician and other physicians involved in the management. Regular monitoring of lupus disease activity and fetal growth parameters are essential. Uterine artery Doppler blood flow examination at 20–24 weeks is usually performed, and umbilical artery blood flow is checked from 24 weeks
- Active lupus is associated with an increased risk of preterm delivery and small-for-gestational-age babies
- Lupus renal disease may predispose to pre-eclampsia and intrauterine growth retardation and, if active, leads to more frequent fetal losses
- Note that it can be difficult to differentiate between renal flare-ups and pre-eclampsia
- These maternal and fetal factors support the need for treatment of flare-ups
- SLE patients with antibodies to Ro(SS-A) have an increased risk of delivering a baby with neonatal lupus syndrome (skin rash and heart block mainly) and thus the proper monitoring and precautions should be undertaken
- Patients should avoid caffeine as it has been shown to increase risk of miscarriage, of which SLE patients are already at greater risk
- Patients with SLE should also avoid smoking, which can worsen the consequences of vasculopathy such as that seen in Raynaud's phenomenon

Drug treatment in lupus pregnancy:
- Lupus flare-ups may be treated with corticosteroids during pregnancy
- For women with anticardiolipin antibodies or lupus anticoagulant, self-injected low-dose heparin is sometimes used

PATIENT SATISFACTION/LIFESTYLE PRIORITIES

- Patient response to drugs used in the management of SLE is idiosyncratic, with the possible exception of corticosteroids
- The effect of treatment on the overwhelming fatigue often experienced by lupus patients is limited and unpredictable

SUMMARY OF THERAPEUTIC OPTIONS
Choices

General:

- Careful and frequent clinical and laboratory evaluation is needed to tailor the medical regimen and to provide prompt recognition and treatment of a flare-up
- Lupus is a lifelong illness and patients should be monitored indefinitely
- It is important to actively control blood pressure, hyperlipidemia, insulin resistance, and hyperglycemia, as well as other modifiable risk factors for atherosclerosis. Primary care physicians should realize that premenopausal women with SLE could have myocardial infarctions

Choice of therapy is based on the type and severity of the disease:

- Conservative symptomatic therapy (when manifestations are mild) and lifestyle modifications: general supportive measurements such as avoidance of fatigue, getting adequate sleep, use of sun block, and avoidance of sunshine (e.g. by wearing a hat, long sleeves). Nonsteroidal anti-inflammatory drugs (NSAIDs) are used to control arthralgia, arthritis, serositis, and fever; they should not be used in patients with active nephritis, and patients with SLE tend to have an increased sensitivity to the toxic effect of these drugs on the kidney and liver. Hydroxychloroquine is used in the control of skin lesions, arthralgia, arthritis, alopecia, and malaise
- Topical glucocorticoids: may help isolated skin lesions (ideally, should be started on the advice of a dermatologist)
- Systemic glucocorticotherapy: use is reserved for life-threatening manifestations such as glomerulonephritis, central nervous system involvement, thrombocytopenia, hemolytic anemias. It may also be used when the disease is debilitating and not responding to conservative therapy. Corticosteroid regimens vary and ideally should be under specialist advisement. Too rapid withdrawal of corticosteroids may result in a flare-up or in an addisonian crisis
- Immunosuppressive therapy: the indications for this are life-threatening manifestations of SLE (e.g. glomerulonephritis, central nervous system involvement, thrombocytopenia, and hemolytic anemias), inability to reduce corticosteroid dose without resulting flare-up, and severe corticosteroid side-effects. The choice of an immunosuppressive (cyclophosphamide, azathioprine) is individualized to the clinical situation and would usually be made by a specialist
- Transplantation: in specialist hands, kidney transplantation and chronic hemodialysis have been used successfully to treat patients with renal lupus
- Anticoagulation: may be necessary in thrombotic conditions (antiphospholipid syndrome). In warfarin treatment, the target international normalized ratio (INR) is 3.0–3.5
- Anti-infectives will be necessary to treat ordinary and opportunistic infections. The antibiotic or antiviral used should reflect the site of infection and the suspected causal agent
- Psychiatric therapy may be appropriate in some patients
- Physical therapy and occupational therapy may be appropriate if joint (especially hand) function is limited. These therapies may form an important part of individualized care plan for some SLE patients
- Other treatments for complications arising from SLE that may require specialist intervention include (but are not limited to) pericardial tamponade and pulmonary hemorrhage; professional counseling may be of value to many SLE patients

Clinical pearls

■ Complement deficiencies may be associated with SLE-like disease
■ The arthritis of SLE does not result in erosions
■ The swan neck deformities of SLE can be distinguished from those seen in rheumatoid arthritis in that SLE the deformities can be reduced whereas in rheumatoid arthritis they cannot

Never

Never stop corticosteroid therapy suddenly in SLE.

FOLLOW UP

Frequent follow up is essential in patients with SLE. The interval will vary with the severity of the disease, the type of treatment, and the presence of a flare-up.

Plan for review

■ Tailored to each patient
■ The importance of urgent contact with physician at onset of flare-up must be stressed

Information for patient or caregiver

■ Treatment should be followed as per the instruction of the physician, especially when steroid therapy is used (do not stop suddenly)
■ Report any side-effects or indicators of a flare-up immediately
■ The treatment does not constitute a cure but is aimed at relieving symptoms and bringing about remission

DRUGS AND OTHER THERAPIES: DETAILS
Drugs
NONSTEROIDAL ANTI-INFLAMMATORY DRUGS

■ Many NSAIDs can be used for the treatment of pain in mild to moderate SLE
■ Ibuprofen is usually the initial choice. Since the effects of NSAIDs tend to be patient-specific, other options include fenoprofen, flurbiprofen, mefenamic acid, ketoprofen, indomethacin, and piroxicam

Dose
Ibuprofen: orally (before food), titrating dose to pain response:

■ 400mg every 4–6h
■ 600mg every 6h
■ 800mg every 8h
■ Not to exceed 3.2g/day
■ Note that the lower doses are sufficient for analgesia but that the higher doses are necessary for reducing inflammation

Efficacy
Response is variable and patient-specific. If response is suboptimal, change to alternative NSAID.

Risks/Benefits
Risks:

■ Use caution in elderly
■ Use caution in hepatic, renal, and cardiac failure, and bleeding disorders
■ There is no evidence that final outcome of SLE is changed by NSAIDs

Benefits:

■ Good pain control in some patients
■ May also help reduce swelling associated with arthralgia and arthritis
■ May help in serositis and fever

Side-effects and adverse reactions
- Cardiovascular system: hypertension, peripheral edema, congestive heart failure
- Central nervous system: headache, dizziness, tinnitus, fever
- Gastrointestinal: anorexia, nausea, dyspepsia, peptic ulceration, bleeding
- Genitourinary: nephrotoxicity
- Hematologic: blood cell disorders
- Hypersensitivity: rashes, bronchospasm, angioedema
- Skin: pruritus, rash

Interactions (other drugs)
- Aminoglycosides · Anticoagulants · Antihypertensives · Baclofen · Corticosteroids
- Cyclosporine, tacrolimus · Digoxin · Diuretics · Lithium · Methotrexate
- Phenylpropanolamine · Warfarin

Contraindications
- Peptic ulceration · Hypersensitivity to any pain reliever or antipyretic (including NSAIDs)
- Coagulation defects · Severe renal or hepatic disease

Acceptability to patient
Usually acceptable to patients. Side-effects, especially gastric irritation, may limit use.

Follow up plan
follow up plan should be individualized to:
- Check symptom control
- Check side-effects
- Discuss patient concerns

Patient and caregiver information
- Regular medication helps in pain control
- Report any side-effects promptly
- Check with physician before taking any other medicines, including those bought over the counter

HYDROXYCHLOROQUINE
Hydroxychloroquine, and occasionally other antimalarials, may be used as conservative therapy in SLE.

Dose
- 400mg in one or two doses depending on the response (takes several weeks)
- Maintenance: 200–400mg/day

Efficacy
Can help in the control of skin symptoms, arthralgia associated with SLE.

Risks/Benefits
Risks:
- Very toxic in overdose
- Use caution in children and in patients susceptible to skin reactions
- Use caution in hepatic and renal disease, glucose-6-phosphate dehydrogenase deficiency, alcoholism, and porphyria

Benefits:
- Useful in the control of skin lesions, arthralgia, arthritis, alopecia, and malaise
- Well tolerated

Side-effects and adverse reactions
- Gastrointestinal: nausea, vomiting, diarrhea, abdominal pain
- Eyes, ears, nose, and throat: irreversible retinal damage, visual disturbances, tinnitus, hearing disturbances
- Central nervous system: headache, seizures, psychosis
- Hematologic: blood cell disorders
- Musculoskeletal: myalgia, arthralgia
- Skin: pigmentation, rashes, eruptions, pruritus

Interactions (other drugs)
- **Antiepileptics** ▪ **Cyclosporine** ▪ **Digoxin** ▪ **Mefloquine** ▪ **Praziquantel**

Contraindications
- **Pregnancy and breast-feeding** ▪ **Visual changes** ▪ **Long-term therapy in children**

Acceptability to patient
Usually acceptable to patients. Side-effects may limit use.

Follow up plan
follow up plan should be individualized to:
- Check symptom control
- Check side-effects
- Discuss patient concerns
- Include ophthalmologic examination every 6 months

Patient and caregiver information
- Regular medication helps in the control of symptoms
- Report any side-effects promptly, especially muscle weakness, visual disturbance, hearing difficulty, or ringing in the ears
- Check with physician before taking any other medicines, including those bought over the counter
- Advise patient to avoid intense sunlight and to continue with sun block and protective clothing even if skin condition improves

LIFESTYLE
- Sun block: waterproof sun block should be applied liberally every 2h during sun exposure. Patients with SLE should not only wear sun block but should also avoid intense sun exposure and wear protective clothing
- Smoking: patients with Raynaud's phenomenon should avoid smoking and keep hands warm at all times, e.g. by wearing gloves in cold weather
- Avoidance of stress and fatigue: these can result in disease flares
- Encouragement of exercise within the limits of the patient's fatigue levels (important for maintenance of bone density)

RISKS/BENEFITS
Benefits:
- Reduction of provoking factors may help reduce flare-ups
- Maintenance of bone density by exercise (and diet) avoids osteoporosis (a common complication in later life)

ACCEPTABILITY TO PATIENT
Patients often adapt to their limited and fluctuating energy levels by pacing themselves, thereby improving their quality of life. Initially, especially in a young person, this can be very frustrating. With time, the benefits of pacing become apparent.

FOLLOW UP PLAN

Patients with SLE need frequent follow up with attention to the agreed individual treatment and lifestyle program.

PATIENT AND CAREGIVER INFORMATION

The importance of pacing to conserve energy and of avoiding stress, fatigue, and sunlight must be emphasized.

EFFICACY OF THERAPIES

SLE has a wide clinical spectrum. The efficacy of the various therapies is therefore difficult to state because of varying clinical pattern and severity.

Review period

This can be variable and is highly dependent on the manifestation(s) being treated.

PROGNOSIS

- Prognosis is variable depending upon the systems involved
- Those with mild disease affecting only the joints and the skin tend to have a good outlook
- More severe disease with major organ involvement has a worse prognosis.
- Mortality in the first 5 years tends to be from active SLE or infection. After the first 5 years, mortality tends to be the result of coronary heart disease, end-stage renal failure, or severe infection without active SLE

Clinical pearls

SLE patients treated with corticosteroids are at higher risk of avascular necrosis of the femoral head.

Therapeutic failure

Initiation of second-line therapy in SLE may benefit from specialist consultation or evaluation and will depend on individual pattern of organ involvement and severity of illness.

Recurrence

Because SLE is a chronic lifelong disease of flare-ups and remissions, it is not appropriate to refer to recurrence.

Deterioration

Deterioration of the patient will be either because of infection or progressive organ damage.

Terminal illness

SLE patients may become terminally ill because of end-stage organ damage, e.g. heart failure, renal failure. This will require management by a multidisciplinary team specialized in management of the terminally ill patient.

COMPLICATIONS

Complications arise from infection and involvement of other organs. Treatment is aimed at the appropriate area.

CONSIDER CONSULT

- Refer all suspected flare-ups, life-threatening infections, or complications
- Patients with osteonecrosis of the hip should be referred to an orthopedic surgeon for possible total hip replacement

PREVENTION

Prevention of SLE is not possible
Compliance with medication and avoidance of aggravating factors (sun, stress, and fatigue) may help reduce flare-up rate

ASSOCIATIONS

Lupus Foundation of America
1300 Piccard Drive, Suite 200
Rockville, MD 20850-4303
Tel: (301) 670 9292
Toll-free: (800) 558 0121
Fax: (301) 670 9486
www.lupus.org

KEY REFERENCES

- Mills JA. Systemic lupus erythematosus. N Engl J Med 1994;330:1871–18
- Boumpas DT, Austin HA, Fessler BJ, et al. Systemic lupus erythematosus: emerging concepts. Part 1. Renal, neuropsychiatric, cardiovascular, pulmonary and hematologic Disease. Ann Intern Med 1995;122:940–50
- Boumpas DT, Austin HA, Fessler BJ, et al. Systemic lupus erythematosus: emerging concepts. Part 2. Dermatologic and joint disease, the antiphospholipid antibody syndrome, pregnancy and hormonal therapy, morbidity and mortality and pathogenesis. Ann Intern Med 1995;123:42–53
- Waltuk J, Buyon JP. Autoantibody-associated congenital heart block: outcome in mothers and children. Ann Intern Med 1994;120:544–51
- Petri M, Lakatta C, Magder L, Goldman D. Effect of prednisone and hydroxychloroquine on coronary risk factors in SLE: a longitudinal data analysis. Am J Med 1994;96:254
- Tan EM. The LE cell and its legacy. Clin Exp Rheumatol 1998;16:652–8
- Hargraves MM, Morton RH. Presentation of two bone marrow elements: the 'tart' cell and the LE cell. Proc Mayo Clin 1948;23:25–8

FAQS
Question 1
What complement abnormalities are associated with the development of lupus or a lupus-like syndrome?

ANSWER 1
Deficiency of the early complement components (C1q, C2, C4) has been associated with the development of lupus in both animal models and humans.

Question 2
How can the hand deformities of rheumatoid arthritis be differentiated from those of lupus?

ANSWER 2
Rheumatoid arthritis is an erosive disease with fixed deformities. SLE, on the other hand, does not show erosive changes on X-rays, and the deformities can be reduced painlessly.

Question 3
What are the official criteria for the diagnosis and classification of lupus?

ANSWER 3
Cardinal features are best summed up from the American College of Rheumatology 1982 disease criteria. At least four of the criteria below must be present. Note that these criteria were not designed as diagnostic criteria; however, they are useful in comparing a homogeneous population of patients.
- Malar rash: fixed erythema, flat or raised, over the malar eminences, tending to spare the nasolabial folds
- Discoid rash: erythematous, raised patches with adherent keratotic scaling and follicular plugging; atrophic scarring may occur in older lesions

- Photosensitivity: skin rash as a result of unusual reaction to sunlight, by patient history or physician observation
- Oral ulcers: oral or nasopharyngeal ulceration, usually painless, observed by physician
- Arthritis: nonerosive arthritis involving two or more peripheral joints, characterized by tenderness, swelling, or effusion
- Serositis: (a) pleuritis – convincing history of pleuritic pain or rubbing heard by a physician or evidence of pleural effusion; or (b) pericarditis – documented by electrocardiogram or rub or evidence of pericardial effusion
- Renal disorders: (a) persistent proteinuria greater than 0.5g/day or greater than 3+ (dipstick) if quantitation not performed; or (b) cellular casts – may be red cell, hemoglobin, granular, tubular, or mixed
- Neurologic disorder: (a) seizures in the absence of offending drugs or known metabolic derangements, e.g. uremia, ketoacidosis, or electrolyte imbalance; or (b) psychosis in the absence of offending drugs or known metabolic derangements, e.g. uremia, ketoacidosis, or electrolyte imbalance
- Hematologic disorder: (a) hemolytic anemia with reticulocytosis; or (b) leukopenia <4000/mm^3 total on two or more occasions; or (c) lymphopenia <1500/mm^3 on two or more occasions or (d) thrombocytopenia <100,000/mm^3 in the absence of offending drugs
- Immunologic disorder: (a) positive LE cell preparation; or (b) anti-DNA: antibody to native DNA in abnormal titer; or (c) anti-Sm: presence of antibody to Sm nuclear antigen; or (d) false-positive serologic test for syphilis known to be positive for at least 6 months and confirmed by *Treponema pallidum* immobilization or fluorescent treponemal antibody absorption test
- Antinuclear antibody (ANA): an abnormal titer of antinuclear antibody by immunofluorescence or an equivalent assay at any point in time and in the absence of drugs known to be associated with 'drug-induced lupus' syndrome. Presence of positive ANA is a cardinal feature but is not specific for SLE

Question 4
What is the LE cell?

ANSWER 4
It is a neutrophil that has engulfed nuclear material.

CONTRIBUTORS
Mary Jo Groves, MD
Maria-Louise Barilla-LaBarca, MD
Elizabeth C Hsia, MD

TENDINITIS

DESCRIPTION

- Painful inflammation of a tendon usually occurring near its point of insertion into the bone or at its point of muscular origin
- Inflammation often extends into the surrounding bursal tissues
- Commonly affects frequently used tendons of upper limb and shoulder
- The most frequent are supraspinatus tendinitis, De Quervain's tenosynovitis (inflammation of the abductor pollicis longus and extensor pollicis brevis tendons – the tendons on the radial side of the lower forearm), patellar tendinitis (jumpers' knee), and Achilles tendinitis
- Usually an acute condition, but may become chronic or recurrent

URGENT ACTION

Septic arthritis is an important differential diagnosis. Consider immediate referral to a rheumatologist for joint aspiration and culture where deep tissue infection is suspected.

BACKGROUND

ICD9 CODE
726.90 Tendinitis.

SYNONYMS
- Rotator cuff tendinitis also known as supraspinatus syndrome
- Patellar tendinitis may be termed jumpers' knee
- Osgood-Schlatter's disease is strictly an apophysitis rather than a tendinitis
- Tendinitis may also be referred to as tenosynovitis where synovial sheaths are also involved – hence De Quervain's tenosynovitis in the case of tendinitis of the abductor pollicis longus and extensor pollicis brevis tendons

CARDINAL FEATURES
- Painful inflammation of a tendon usually occurring at the point of insertion into bone or at the point of muscle origin
- Inflammation may extend to surrounding bursal tissues
- Often associated with overuse injury, workplace trauma or sporting activity
- Commonly affects tendons of the upper limb and shoulder but the Achilles tendon is also commonly affected
- Usually self-limiting, but may become recurrent or chronic
- May restrict mobility of the affected limb significantly – but not usually associated deformity

CAUSES
Common causes
- Repetitive activity or trauma
- Sporting injury

Rare causes
- Thyroid disease
- Diabetes mellitus
- Renal transplantation
- *Neisseria gonorrhoeae infection*: many patients with disseminated gonococcal infection have tenosynovitis involving the tendon sheath of the hands or the Achilles tendon

Contributory or predisposing factors
- Repetitive occupational overuse
- Sports injuries

EPIDEMIOLOGY
Incidence and prevalence
PREVALENCE

Prevalence of calcific tendinitis is high, affecting 2.7–8.0% of the general population.

Demographics
AGE
- Tendinosis (degenerative change in tendons) increases with age so most tendinitis increases with advancing years
- Tendinitis may be provoked by work practices so often seen in those approaching retirement in susceptible occupations
- Highest incidence of calcific tendinitis tends to occur in the fifth decade

GENDER

- Degenerative tendinitis occurs slightly more frequently in males
- Calcific tendinitis occurs equally in both sexes

SOCIOECONOMIC STATUS

Manual laborers are prone to tendinitis due to repetitive overuse injury in the work environment.

DIFFERENTIAL DIAGNOSIS
Tendinitis may affect a number of anatomical sites. The differential diagnosis includes inflammation of other articular or periarticular organs.

Bursitis
FEATURES
- Swelling, especially if the affected bursa is superficial
- Local exquisite tenderness with pain on pressure
- Pain with joint movement
- Occasionally referred pain
- Occasional palpable fibrocartilaginous bodies
- Often difficult to differentiate between tendinitis and bursitis, because the two conditions often co-exist

Infectious tenosynovitis
FEATURES
- Occurs mainly in the hand
- Tenderness and swelling are tracking along synovial lines proximally, instead of the insertion
- Marked pain, swelling and reddening of the overlying skin
- Elevated erythrocyte sedimentation rate (ESR) and white blood cell count

Osteoarthritis
FEATURES
- Very common slow onset disease characterized by articular cartilage loss and growth of bony spurs (osteophytes) at the joint margins
- Deep aching pain in affected joints made worse with activity
- Most commonly affected joints are knee, hip, distal interphalangeal joints of the hand, cervical and lumbosacral joints of the spine
- Short lived (15 min) stiffness on awakening and after prolonged periods of inactivity
- Pain with range of motion
- Bony joint enlargement
- Crepitus – creaking sound as joint is moved
- Presence of nodular swellings in the distal (Heberden's nodes) or proximal (Bouchard's nodes) interphalangeal joints

Septic arthritis
FEATURES
- Rapid onset
- Swollen, painful, hot and red joints
- Severely limited range of motion of the joint
- Febrile at presentation
- Most commonly affected joints are knees and hip
- Single joint affected in 80–90% of cases

Avulsion of the tendon
FEATURES
- Loss of function of affected muscle
- X-rays may indicate a portion of bone avulsed with tendon

Rheumatoid arthritis
FEATURES
- Multiple symmetrical small joint involvement, most often in the hands and feet
- Joint effusions, tenderness and restricted movement usually present in the early stages
- Prolonged morning stiffness
- Persistent inflammation (more than 6 weeks)
- Systemic symptoms often present
- Elevated ESR and C-reactive protein

SIGNS & SYMPTOMS
Signs
- Inflammation over the affected tendon
- Tenderness over the affected tendon
- Erythema and local heat over the affected area

Symptoms
- Pain over the area of inflammation; may be present at rest, but is worsened by activity
- Brief, focal morning stiffness
- Occasionally restricted movement of the muscles attached to the tendon

ASSOCIATED DISORDERS
- Bursitis
- Rheumatoid arthritis
- Gout
- Psoriatic arthritis
- Osgood-Schlatter disease: a prevalent form of patellar tendinitis associated with inflammation of the tibial apophysis in pediatric patients

CONSIDER CONSULT
Aspiration is advisable if there is concern about underlying infection or to obtain fluid for crystal analysis, including calcium pyrophosphate dihydrate crystals

INVESTIGATION OF THE PATIENT
Direct questions to patient
Q Has there been trauma to the affected area? Tendinitis often caused by repetitive overuse injury or a sporting injury
Q Is there pain at rest? Peak periods of pain and discomfort occur with use
Q Do symptoms worsen after sustained activity? If symptoms are associated with particular activity (e.g. work practice or sporting activity), would expect reduction in symptoms during holiday/weekend or off season
Q Do you suffer from morning stiffness? Morning stiffness is brief and focal with tendinitis
Is there tenderness over the affected area? Tenderness is focal
Q Do you have any systemic signs or symptoms, such as fever or rash? Tendinitis is not associated with any systemic symptoms

Contributory or predisposing factors
Q Is there a history of repetitive overuse with regard to occupation or sporting activity? Overuse may cause inflammation in specific tendons
Q Is there a history of previous trauma? This may predispose to tendinitis
Q Is there a history of thyroid disease or diabetes mellitus? Both disorders may predispose to calcific tendinitis
Q Have any joints been swollen? There is an association of tendinitis with seronegative arthritis

Examination

Q **Is the patient well/unwell?** If systemically unwell, suspect infectious tenosynovitis or septic arthritis

Q **Check temperature.** Pyrexia suggests infection

Q **How many regions are affected?** Tendinitis generally involves one joint region

Q **Is there inflammation at the joint?** Tenderness and pain at the joint proper indicative of arthritis rather than tendinitis, which is localized to the side of the joint where tendon insertion occurs

Q **Is there tenderness to palpation?** Tendinitis may be suggested by tenderness to palpation along the course of the tendon, or when the tendon is stretched over its range of motion against resistance

Q **Check range of motion at affected tendon/joint.** Reduced active range of motion and preserved passive range suggests tendinitis

Summary of investigative tests

- Plain radiography may be supportive of clinical evidence of osteoarthritis at a target joint
- Sonography scanning is a sensitive, safe, and inexpensive technique to demonstrate tendinitis. The procedure is highly dependent on the skill of the operator
- Magnetic resonance imaging (MRI) may be used to identify muscular tears, tendinitis, and joint inflammation. This investigation is relatively expensive

DIAGNOSTIC DECISION

- Physical examination will help to distinguish between inflammatory and noninflammatory conditions
- Little morning stiffness, only one or two symptomatic areas, no pain at rest, worsened symptoms after sustained activity and no signs or symptoms of systemic disease suggests local mechanical problems such as tendinitis
- Point tenderness, reduced active range of motion, and preserved passive range of motion suggests soft-tissue disorders, including tendinitis
- Tendinitis generally involves only one joint region
- Physical examination is usually diagnostic in tendinitis
- Specialized imaging such as MRI may be useful and can reveal tears and inflammation but sonography should be considered in the first instance where clinical examination is insufficient to confirm the diagnosis

The American College of Rheumatology has published diagnostic guidelines, [1].

CLINICAL PEARLS

- Tendinitis should be considered when the symptoms are periarticular, rather than joint-centered
- Tendinitis is often self-limiting - attention should be paid to predisposing factors (such as muscle imbalance, poor posture or work practice) in an attempt to reduce the risk of recurrence

THE TESTS
Imaging
MAGNETIC RESONANCE IMAGING
Advantages/Disadvantages
Advantages:

- Excellent resolution of soft-tissues
- May reveal the presence of muscular tears, inflammation and joint effusions

Disadvantages:

- Expensive

- Some patients find MRI scanners claustrophobic
- Cannot be used where patient has magnetic prosthesis or implant

Abnormal
Altered signal from soft-tissues on various scanning protocols (e.g. T2 weighting).

Cause of abnormal result
Inflammation or degenerative changes in the structure of tendon and surrounding connective tissue.

Drugs, disorders and other factors that may alter results
Artifacts and false-positive results if technique is not accurately carried out: a blurred tendon margin frequently seen if there is incorrect alignment between the transducer and tendon

PLAIN RADIOGRAPHY
Advantages/Disadvantages
Advantages:

- May be supportive of clinical evidence of osteoarthritis at target joint
- Superior subluxation of the humerus at the acromioclavicular joint is circumstantial evidence of supraspinatus rupture

Disadvantages: in general, tendinitis is difficult to visualize on plain films.

Abnormal

- Calcific deposits may be visualized in calcific tendinitis
- Superior humeral migration indicates supraspinatus tear
- Thickening of the Achilles tendon may be demonstrated on plain films

Cause of abnormal result
Radiopaque calcific deposits, loss of the supraspinatus muscle or thickening of the Achilles tendon.

SONOGRAPHY
Advantages/Disadvantages
Advantages:

- Sensitive, noninvasive, safe and widely available
- Accuracy close to MRI scans for supraspinatus tendinitis
- Dynamics of the tendon during contraction may be assessed, thus providing both functional and anatomical information
- Tendons easily distinguishable from surrounding tissues because of high collagen content
- Inexpensive

Disadvantages:

- The utility of this diagnostic technique is very operator-dependent
- Deep tendons are less amenable to investigation with sonography

Normal
Sonographic features of normal tendons characterized by a relatively homogeneous pattern.

Abnormal

- Loss of fibrillar echo texture
- Focal or diffuse tendon thickening
- Focal hypoechoic areas

- Irregular and ill-defined borders
- Microruptures and peritendinous edema

Cause of abnormal result
- Focal or diffuse thickening reflect inflammation-induced edematous swelling of the tendon
- Focal or diffuse hypoechoic areas inside the tendon reflect tendon degeneration and/or intratendinous tear
- Focal or confluent hypoechoic areas may contain synovial fluid, blood, fat or proteinaceous material
- Loss of defined margin may reflect chronic tendinitis

Drugs, disorders and other factors that may alter results
Artifacts and false-positive results if technique is not accurately carried out: a blurred tendon margin frequently seen if there is incorrect alignment between the transducer and tendon.

TREATMENT

CONSIDER CONSULT
- Refer to occupational or physical therapists for implementation of exercise and activity programs and help with assistive devices as necessary
- Surgical consultation only considered if patient fails to respond to conservative treatment methods and there is a surgically remediable lesion

IMMEDIATE ACTION
Consider the possibility of septic arthritis and refer urgently to a rheumatologist for joint aspiration and culture if infection of the joint is suspected.

PATIENT AND CAREGIVER ISSUES
Patient or caregiver request
- Many sports personalities are often out of action as a result of tendinitis, and so patients may have gleaned ideas about causes or treatments from news reports
- Patients may consider taking over-the-counter (OTC) nonsteroidal anti-inflammatory drugs (NSAIDs) but may be concerned with gastrointestinal health risks

Health-seeking behavior
- **Has the patient stopped the inciting activity?** Carrying on with inciting activity may exacerbate problem, resulting in tendon tears or complete rupture – (relative) rest of the affected part for a short time may well be curative
- **Has the patient been self-medicating?** Self-medication with OTC NSAIDs may alleviate pain, so patients often do not present in the early stages
- **Has the patient altered his or her workstation or sporting activity?** A change in occupational ergonomics or sporting technique may relieve pain and tension at affected areas
- **Has the patient undergone a long period of rest/inactivity?** Rest alleviates pain initially, but prolonged periods of rest may be detrimental

MANAGEMENT ISSUES
Goals
- To relieve pain
- To reduce inflammation
- To rest the local joint

Management in special circumstances
COEXISTING DISEASE
Tendinitis does not exclude coexisting arthropathies: check whether the patient is receiving medication for these.

COEXISTING MEDICATION
Is the patient already self-medicating with OTC NSAIDs? If so, these should be withdrawn if other medications prescribed by physician.

PATIENT SATISFACTION/LIFESTYLE PRIORITIES
- Pain during activity may prevent patient from carrying out normal activities of daily living and from working
- Patients must address physical activities and working conditions (ergonomics) that result in repetitive tendon injury
- Disability prevents patients from working, affects quality of life and may cause other problems such as depression, low self-esteem, financial difficulties

SUMMARY OF THERAPEUTIC OPTIONS
Choices

- Rest and/or immobilization is initial treatment, except for tendinitis of the shoulder, where immobilization may result in development of frozen shoulder
- Ice packs during initial few days reduce pain and swelling
- Assistive devices and supports for patients with functional impairments may be needed: slings and splints for the upper extremity and braces, cranes and/or crutches for the lower limbs
- Patient education helps to explain the problem and improves outcome
- Exercise therapy: including range of motion exercises, but should only be started once patient is free of pain. Later, physiotherapists will attempt to restrengthen and balance muscle groups to reduce incidence of recurrence
- Therapeutic ultrasound (using a different frequency of sonography from the frequency that is used for diagnosis) or 'shock wave therapy' may be helpful in relieving pain
- Hydrotherapy is helpful to many patients
- Simple analgesics and NSAIDs such as aspirin, ibuprofen, piroxicam, indomethacin, naproxen, tenoxicam and fenoprofen, are usually adequate
- Local injectable corticosteroids such as methylprednisolone (in combination with lidocaine), prednisolone or triamcinolone often result in dramatic relief
- Surgery may be considered if all conservative measures have failed. Surgery may be especially helpful in patients with recurrent rotator cuff tendinitis who have sharp bony spurs on the underside of the acromioclavicular joint
- Lifestyle changes to improve fitness carry the potential benefits of improved flexibility, increased physical activity, and wellbeing and cardiovascular fitness

Clinical pearls

- Judicious use of NSAIDs is beneficial for most patients with tendinitis but older patients appear to prefer topical presentations such as rubs and sprays
- Physical and occupational therapy may be especially helpful to educate the patient to prevent recurrence

Never

Never inject corticosteroids directly into a tendon, as this may precipitate tendon rupture.

FOLLOW UP
Plan for review

- Follow range of motion studies and functional status at regular intervals
- Calcific tendinitis usually responds to 2–3 days of rest
- Monitor symptoms: usually subside within a few days to weeks with simple treatment
- If symptoms fail to improve with simple analgesics and NSAIDs within 4–6 weeks, glucocorticoid injections should be considered
- Patients with recurring symptoms must be instructed to avoid inciting activities that strain susceptible anatomic structures by overuse
- Surgical procedures seldom necessary; however, with structural rupture or failure to respond to conventional treatment, surgical excision or repair may be considered. Local guidelines for referral to surgery will vary

Information for patient or caregiver

- Patient education leaflet available
- Patient must be made aware that recovery from tendinitis requires active participation in the treatment program
- Repeated pain and limitation of function may ensue if an exercise program is not taken seriously

DRUGS AND OTHER THERAPIES: DETAILS
Drugs
ASPIRIN
Dose
Enteric-coated; 650mg every 6 h, or 975mg every 8 h, orally.

Efficacy
Equal efficacy to fenoprofen in acute tendinitis.

Risks/Benefits
Risks:
- Use caution in anemia, Hodgkin's disease, bleeding disorders
- Use caution with gout, hepatic, and renal disease
- Use caution with asthma, nasal polyps, nasal allergies
- Use caution with children and teenagers (Reye's syndrome)

Benefit: simple dosing regimen allows for better patient compliance

Side-effects and adverse reactions
- Central nervous system: dizziness, headache
- Eyes, ears, nose, and throat: hearing loss and tinnitus
- Gastrointestinal: abdominal pain, nausea, dyspepsia, hepatotoxicity
- Hematologial: bleeding disorders, thrombocytopenia
- Respiratory: hyperpnea, asthma
- Skin: angioedema, bruising, rash, urticaria

Interactions (other drugs)
- ACE inhibitors Acetazolamide Antacids Corticosteroids Diltiazem Ethanol
- Griseofulvin Methotrexate Oral anticoagulants Probenecid Sulfinpyrazone
- Sulfonylureas Warfarin

Contraindications
- Hypersensitivity to salicylates, NSAIDS or tartrazine Gastrointestinal bleeding
- Hemophilia Hemorrhagic states

Acceptability to patient
High.

Follow up plan
Monitor for gastrointestinal side-effects

IBUPROFEN (OTC)
Dose
600–800mg up to 3 or 4 times a day for conventional tablet; 1200mg twice daily for sustained-release formulation.

Efficacy
Significantly effective compared with placebo.

Risks/Benefits
Risk: use caution in hepatic, renal and cardiac failure

Benefits:
- Faster onset of action than colchicines
- Inexpensive

Side-effects and adverse reactions
- Gastrointestinal: anorexia, nausea, dyspepsia, peptic ulceration
- Central nervous system: headache, dizziness, tinnitus
- Hypersensitivity: rashes, bronchospasm, angioedema

Interactions (other drugs)
- Aminoglycosides ■ Antihypertensives ■ Corticosteroids ■ Cyclosporin ■ Digoxin
- Lithium ■ Methotrexate ■ Phenylpropanolamine ■ Diuretics ■ Warfarin

Contraindications
- Peptic ulceration ■ Hypersensitivity to NSAIDs ■ Coagulation defects

Acceptability to patient
High.

Follow up plan
Monitor patient for gastrointestinal side-effects.

PIROXICAM
Dose
10–20mg daily, orally. 0.5% gel, topically applied.

Efficacy
Significant improvement in pain scores and joint motion and reduced tenderness compared with placebo.

Risks/Benefits
- Risk: use caution in hepatic, renal and cardiac failure
- Benefit: faster onset of action than colchicines

Side-effects and adverse reactions
- Gastrointestinal: anorexia, nausea, dyspepsia, peptic ulceration
- Central nervous system: headache, dizziness, tinnitus
- Hypersensitivity: rashes, bronchospasm, angioedema
- Thrombocytopenia

Interactions (other drugs)
- Aminoglycosides ■ Antihypertensives ■ Corticosteroids ■ Cyclosporin ■ Digoxin
- Lithium ■ Methotrexate ■ Phenylpropanolamine ■ Diuretics ■ Warfarin

Contraindications
- Peptic ulceration ■ Hypersensitivity to NSAIDs ■ Coagulation defects ■ Porphyria

Acceptability to patient
High.

Follow up plan
Monitor patient for signs of gastrointestinal side-effects.

INDOMETHACIN

Dose

25–50mg 3 times daily, orally; topical 4% spray 3–5 times daily for 14 days.

Efficacy

- Topical spray showed clear efficacy compared with placebo in objective and subjective symptoms
- Sustained-release formulation as effective as conventional indomethacin, but may promote patient compliance since it need only be given once or twice daily
- Evidence for the use of NSAIDs is reviewed by BMJ Clinical Evidence [2]

Risks/Benefits

- Risk: use caution in hepatic and cardiac failure, epilepsy, psychiatric disorders and parkinsonism
- Benefit: faster onset of action than colchicines

Side-effects and adverse reactions

- Gastrointestinal: anorexia, nausea, dyspepsia, peptic ulceration
- Central nervous system: headache, dizziness, tinnitus
- Hypersensitivity: rashes, bronchospasm, angioedema
- Thrombocytopenia

Interactions (other drugs)

- Aminoglycosides ■ Antihypertensives ■ Corticosteroids ■ Cyclosporin ■ Digoxin
- Lithium ■ Methotrexate ■ Phenylpropanolamine ■ Diuretics ■ Warfarin

Contraindications

- Renal failure ■ Hypertension ■ Peptic ulceration ■ Hypersensitivity to NSAIDs
- Coagulation defects

Acceptability to patient

High.

Follow up plan

Monitor patient for signs of gastrointestinal side-effects.

NAPROXEN

Dose

10% topical gel; 250–500mg twice daily, orally, followed by 500mg twice daily thereafter

Efficacy

Generally good; the gel has been shown to have superior efficacy ratings in subjective complaints.

Risks/Benefits

- Risk: use caution in hepatic, renal and cardiac failure
- Benefit: faster onset of action than colchicines

Side-effects and adverse reactions

- Gastrointestinal: anorexia, nausea, dyspepsia, peptic ulceration
- Central nervous system: headache, dizziness, tinnitus
- Hypersensitivity: rashes, bronchospasm, angioedema
- Thrombocytopenia

Interactions (other drugs)
- Aminoglycosides
- Antihypertensives
- Corticosteroids
- Cyclosporin
- Digoxin
- Lithium
- Methotrexate
- Phenylpropanolamine
- Diuretics
- Warfarin

Contraindications
- Peptic ulceration
- Hypersensitivity to NSAIDs
- Coagulation defects

Acceptability to patient
High.

Follow up plan
Monitor for signs of gastrointestinal side-effects.

TENOXICAM
Dose
20mg, periarticular injection, once weekly.

Efficacy
Alleviates pain and improves shoulder mobility in rotator cuff tendinitis.

Risks/Benefits
Risk: use caution in hepatic, renal and cardiac failure, porphyria

Side-effects and adverse reactions
- Gastrointestinal: anorexia, nausea, dyspepsia, peptic ulceration
- Central nervous system: headache, dizziness, tinnitus
- Hypersensitivity: rashes, bronchospasm, angioedema

Interactions (other drugs)
- Aminoglycosides
- Antihypertensives
- Corticosteroids
- Cyclosporin
- Digoxin
- Lithium
- Methotrexate
- Phenylpropanolamine
- Diuretics
- Warfarin

Contraindications
- Peptic ulceration
- Hypersensitivity to NSAIDs
- Coagulation defects

Acceptability to patient
Medium.

FENOPROFEN
Dose
300–600mg 3–4 times/day, up to 3.2g/day, orally.

Efficacy
As effective as aspirin but better tolerated.

Acceptability to patient
High.

Follow up plan
Monitor patient for signs of gastrointestinal side-effects.

TRIAMCINOLONE

Dose

20mg/cc suspension in 1cc ampules, subacromially in supraspinal tendinitis.

Efficacy
- Similar in efficacy to oral indomethacin
- Longer duration of activity than methylprednisolone

Risks/Benefits

Risks:
- Full aseptic precautions are essential
- Second-line therapy
- Does not provide quick response; may take several hours for relief
- Risk of infection with intra-articular injection
- Risk of joint destruction and sepsis if septic arthritis is misdiagnosed as gout

Side-effects and adverse reactions
- Pain at injection site
- Flushing

Interactions (other drugs)
- Antidiabetics Isoniazid Rifampicin Salicylates

Contraindications

Local or systemic infection.

Acceptability to patient

Medium: usually, lidocaine or bupivacaine needs to be administered first to alleviate injection pain.

Follow up plan

Monitor joint mobility; once mobility has been regained, strengthening exercises must be started.

Patient and caregiver information

Steroid injection may worsen symptoms after the anesthetic effects subside; improvement likely to follow within 48 h.

METHYLPREDNISOLONE

Dose

40mg/cc suspension in 1cc ampules, subacromial injection.

Efficacy

Similar onset of action to triamcinolone, but shorter duration of action.

Risks/Benefits

Risks:
- Overwhelming septicemia if patient has an infection. Loss of control of blood glucose in those with diabetes
- Prolonged use causes adrenal suppression

Side-effects and adverse reactions
- Side-effects are minimized by short duration of therapy
- Gastrointestinal: dyspepsia, peptic ulceration, oesophagitis, oral candidiasis
- Cardiovascular system: hypertension, thromboembolism

- Central nervous system: insomnia, euphoria, depression, psychosis
- Endocrine: adrenal suppression, impaired glucose tolerance, growth suppression in children
- Musculoskeletal: proximal myopathy, osteoporosis
- Skin: delayed healing, acne, striae
- Eyes, ears, nose, and throat: cataract, glaucoma, blurred vision

Interactions (other drugs)
- Aminoglutethamide ▪ Barbiturates ▪ Cholestyramine ▪ Clarithromycin, erythromycin
- Colestipol ▪ Isoniazid ▪ Ketoconazole ▪ NSAIDs ▪ Oral contraceptives ▪ Rifampin
- Salicylates ▪ Troleandomycin

Contraindications
- Systemic infection ▪ Avoid live virus vaccines in those receiving immunosuppressive doses

Acceptability to patient
Medium: usually lidocaine or bupivacaine administered first to alleviate injection pain.

Follow up plan
Monitor joint mobility; once mobility has been regained, strengthening exercises must be started.

Patient and caregiver information
Steroid injection may worsen symptoms after the anesthetic effects subside; improvement likely to follow within 48 h.

PREDNISOLONE
Dose
2–5mg injection into tendon sheath.

Efficacy
Medium potency.

Risks/Benefits
Benefit: useful at superficial injection sites.

Acceptability to patient
Medium.

Physical therapy
Physical therapy is the mainstay of treatment for tendinitis, especially around the shoulder, elbow, and knee.

EXERCISE
Exercise programs aim at restoration of range of motion and thereafter at strengthening and 'balancing the flexor and extensor local muscle groups to reduce the chance of recurrent injury.

Efficacy
Considered good but evidence is lacking because of the difficulties associated with designing suitable trials.

Risks/Benefits
Risks:
- Loss of compliance with exercise program over extended period is high
- No significant clinical risks associated with standard well supervised physical therapy

Acceptability to patient
High.

Follow up plan
- Monitor range of motion
- Encourage patient to continue with exercise program

Patient and caregiver information
It is important to warm up and stretch before starting an exercise program.

ICE PACKS
May be useful adjunctive therapy.

Efficacy
Excellent for reducing pain and swelling in early, acute phase.

Risks/Benefits
- Risk: ice burn may occur if ice applied directly to skin or left in contact longer than advised

- Benefit: ice pack applied for 15–20 minutes reduces swelling and pain

Acceptability to patient
High.

Follow up plan
- Monitor pain and swelling
- Ice packs should only be used for a few days
- If pain persists, consider drug therapy

Patient and caregiver information
- Ice packs reduce pain and swelling in early stages
- Heat should only be used during chronic phases and does not reduce swelling

THERAPEUTIC ULTRASOUND
Ultrasound may be used at different power and frequency from that used diagnostically to reduce pain and inflammation.

Efficacy
- There is controversy over the efficacy of therapeutic ultrasonography, and effects appear to be operator-dependent
- There may also be a large placebo effect
- In one study, calcium deposits resolved in 19% of treated shoulders and decreased in 50% of treated shoulders after 6 weeks of therapy
- There are as yet few large studies to confirm the place of ultrasonography in soft-tissue therapeutics

Risks/Benefits
Benefit: possible reduction in pain and improved quality of life compared with sham (no) treatment.

Acceptability to patient
High.

SHOCK WAVE THERAPY
Recently developed high-power focal ultrasound equipment may act as a 'lithotripter', shatter calcific deposits and possibly have beneficial effects on noncalcific tendinitis.

Efficacy
Few studies but the trial below reports relief of pain from 5–58% after one or two treatments. These results need to be confirmed.

Risks/Benefits
Risk: high energy ultrasound may be uncomfortable but radiation risk is minimal.

Acceptability to patient
High.

Follow up plan
Monitor patient's functional improvement.

HYDROTHERAPY
Efficacy
Generally good at providing relief and increasing mobility.

Risks/Benefits
Risk: few risks if therapy is properly supervised by a qualified therapist.

Acceptability to patient
Usually high.

Occupational therapy
SUPPORT FOR PATIENTS WITH FUNCTIONAL IMPAIRMENT
Efficacy
Difficult to evaluate because treatment is highly individually tailored.

Risks/Benefits
Benefits:
- Evaluating patient's ability to perform activities of daily living providing appropriate assistive devices and most importantly advice.
- May help in supporting exercise programs as needed to improve joint function and reduce disability

Acceptability to patient
High.

Patient and caregiver information
Patient should understand that recovery from tendinitis requires self-help.

ASSISTIVE DEVICES AND AIDS FOR DAILY LIVING
Efficacy
High.

Risks/Benefits
Risk: using a sling for any more than 3 or 4 days in patients with supraspinatus tendinitis may predispose to an adhesive capsulitis (frozen shoulder) and restricted mobility

Benefits:

- The use of heel pads may alleviate symptoms of Achilles tendinitis but should be used in conjunction with a physical therapy program
- Splints may be useful for immobilization of forearm extension in De Quervain's tenosynovitis or around the knee for patellar tendinitis

Acceptability to patient
Usually good.

Follow up plan
Monitor for improving mobility after 24–48 h.

Surgical therapy
ACROMIOPLASTY

- In cases of recurrent supraspinatus tendinitis, some patients benefit from a 'decompression' procedure. This may be achieved by open surgery or a 'keyhole' operation
- Spurring of the underside of the acromion may be trimmed and pain levels substantially reduced by making more space for the rotator cuff

Efficacy
In one study, pain ratings decreased substantially after surgery involving removal of calcium deposits and acromioplasty.

Risks/Benefits
Risk: scarring, muscle atrophy and loss of function, continuing pain, infection

Acceptability to patient
Low except in selected patients.

Follow up plan
Surgical follow up is required.

LIFESTYLE
Lifestyle changes to increase fitness carry potential benefits in almost all patients.

RISKS/BENEFITS
Benefits of exercise: improved flexibility, physical activity and wellbeing, and cardiovascular fitness.

ACCEPTABILITY TO PATIENT
Medium: adherence to exercise programs often low.

FOLLOW UP PLAN

- After first symptoms of tendinitis, develop an exercise plan starting with simple and interesting program aimed at keeping compliance high
- Monitor adherence to exercise program
- Full, range-of-motion exercises encouraged once mobility has improved

PATIENT AND CAREGIVER INFORMATION
Educate the patient that prevention of recurrence may relate directly to his ability to complete the exercise treatment plan – ideally this should be ongoing.

EFFICACY OF THERAPIES

A combination of an initial period of rest and/or ice packs, followed by a supervised exercise program with NSAID therapy is usually effective in the treatment of tendinitis.

Review period

Follow range-of-motion studies and pain/swelling at regular intervals: symptoms will usually subside after a few days to a few weeks.

PROGNOSIS

- The great majority of tendinitis cases subside without complications
- Orthopedic referral is necessary if symptoms persist despite all therapeutic approaches.

Clinical pearls

Patients whose occupations aggravate their symptoms and have poor workplace support are often refractory to therapy.

Therapeutic failure

- Consider local injection of corticosteroids if the patient is unresponsive to NSAIDs or simple analgesics
- Surgery is indicated in very few patients

PREVENTION

RISK FACTORS

Age: the structure of tendons changes with age; the elasticity of tendons falls significantly after middle age

Repetitive strain: manual laborers and clerical workers are prone to tendinitis, owing to repetitive actions in the work environment

MODIFY RISK FACTORS
Lifestyle and wellness
PHYSICAL ACTIVITY

Warming up and stretching becomes increasingly important with advancing age and with progressively higher activity levels

Correct warm up is considered to substantially reduce soft-tissue (tendon) injuries in the sports arena

ENVIRONMENT
Avoid repetitious tasks in the workplace.

SCREENING
General screening for tendinitis is not necessary.

PREVENT RECURRENCE

Advise a short period of rest and/or immobilization if flare-up occurs

Application of ice packs for 15–20 minutes for the first few days reduce pain and swelling

If necessary, use an assistive device such as a sling or brace for a few days only

Initiate a supervised exercise program after the inflammation has subsided

Consider NSAIDs therapy if pain persists

Consider local instillation of corticosteroids only if NSAIDs or simple analgesia is unsuccessful

Refer for surgical consultation if all conservative methods are unsuccessful

ASSOCIATIONS
American College of Rheumatology
1800 Century Place, Suite 250
Atlanta, GA 30345
Tel: (404) 633 3777
Fax: (404) 633 1870
www.rheumatology.org

Arthritis Foundation
1330 West Peachtree Street
Atlanta GA 30309
Tel: (404) 872 7100
www.arthritis.org

KEY REFERENCES

- Adebajo AO, Nash P, Hazleman BL. A prospective double blind dummy placebo controlled study comparing triamcinolone hexacetonide injection with oral diclofenac 50 mg tds in patients with rotator cuff tendinitis. J Rheumatol 1990;17:1207–10.
- American College of Rheumatology. Guidelines for the Initial evaluation of the adult patient with acute musculoskeletal symptoms. Arth Rheum 1996;39:1–8
- Ebenbichler GR, Erdogmus CB, Resch KL, et al. Ultrasound therapy for calcific tendinitis of the shoulder. N Engl J Med 1999;340:1533–8
- Friis J, Jarner D, Toft B, et al. Comparison of two ibuprofen formulations in the treatment of shoulder tendonitis. Clin Rheumatol 1992;11:105–8
- Goroll, Primary Care Medicine, 3rd Ed
- Heere LP. Piroxicam in acute musculoskeletal disorders and sports injuries. Am J Med 1988;84:50–5
- Itzkowitch D. Peri-articular injection of tenoxicam for painful shoulders: a double-blind, placebo-controlled trial. Clin Rheumatol 1996;15:604–9
- Jerosch J, Strauss JM, Schmiel S. Arthroscopic Treatment of calcific tendinitis of the shoulder. J Shoulder Elbow Surg 1998;7:30–7
- Loew M, Daecke W, Kusnierczak D, et al. Shock wave therapy is effective for chronic calcifying tendinitis of the shoulder. J Bone Joint Surg Br 1999;81:863–7
- McIlwain HH. Fenoprofen calcium versus aspirin in the treatment of acute inflammatory soft-tissue injuries. J Med 1985;16:429–38
- Moore RA. Quantitative Systemic review of topically applied non-steroidal anti-inflammatory drugs. BMJ 1998;316:333–8
- Rochwerger A , et al. Surgical management of calcific tendinitis of the shoulder. An analysis of 26 cases. Clin Rheumatol 1999;18:313–6
- Stanley KL; Weaver JE. Pharmacologic management of pain and inflammation in athletes. Clinics in Sports Med 1998;1
- Torstensen TA, Meen HD, Stiris M. The effect of medical exercise therapy on a patient with chronic supraspinatus tendinitis. diagnostic-ultrasound tissue regeneration: a case study. J Orthop Sports Phys Ther 1994;20:319–27
- Valtonen EJ. Subacromial triamcinolone mexacetonide and methylprednisolone injections in treatment of supra spinal tendinitis. A comparative trial. Scand J Rheumatol Suppl 1976;16:1–13
- White RH, Paull DM, Fleming KW. Rotator cuff tendinitis: comparison of subacromial injection of a long-acting corticosteroid versus oral indomethacin therapy. J Rheumatol 1986;13:608–13

Evidence references and guidelines
1 American College of Rheumatology. Guidelines for the Initial evaluation of the adult patient with acute musculoskeletal symptoms. Arth Rheum 1996;39:1–8
2 Golzche PC. Nonsteroidal anti-inflammatory drugs. In: Clinical Evidence, 2000, 3. London: BMJ Publishing Group

CONTRIBUTORS

Richard Brasington Jr, MD, FACP
Shane Clarke, MD
Daniel J Derksen, MD

Index

Index